Central Service
Technical Manual

Eighth Edition

Disclaimer

This publication is designed to provide accurate and authoritative information in regard to the subject matter covered. It is sold with the understanding that the publisher is not engaged in rendering legal, accounting or other professional service. If legal advice or other expert assistance is required, the services of a competent professional person should be sought.

From the Declaration of Principles jointly adopted by the American Bar Association and a Committee of Publishers and Associations.

The authors are solely responsible for the contents of this publication. All views expressed herein are solely those of the authors and do not necessarily reflect the views of the International Association of Healthcare Central Service Materiel Management (IAHCSMM).

Nothing contained in this publication shall constitute a standard, an endorsement or recommendation of IAHCSMM. IAHCSMM also disclaims any liability with respect to the use of any information, procedure or product, or reliance thereon by any member of the healthcare industry.

Foreword

The Central Service Technical Manual was first published in 1969 by the International Association of Healthcare Central Service Materiel Management. This eighth edition carries on the legacy of all previous editions, evolving and advancing to keep pace with changes impacting the profession. Current and relevant content is essential for professionals working in today's fast-paced departments who must stay educated and well informed if they are to successfully prepare and distribute medical devices for healthcare facilities and third party reprocessors.

This latest edition follows a similar layout and design to the seventh edition, which CS professionals found to be user friendly and invaluable. Some of these design elements include:

- Learning objectives that introduce the chapter and briefly outline the learning expectations in each chapter.

- Extensive use of the "green box" key terms that define new and important terms throughout the text.

- A glossary that not only contains all the terms introduced in the manual, but also many other terms important in today's dynamic CS environment.

Additionally, this fully revised Central Service Technical Manual, Eighth Edition, provides the latest information on all critical aspects of the discipline, including:

- Updates on standards and regulations.

- Expanded content on endoscopes and sterilization.

- Two new chapters: Monitoring and Recordkeeping, and Personal and Professional Development.

As with past versions, this eighth edition continues with its goal of helping CS professionals learn the science behind the discipline, as well as the why's and the how's behind CS-related processes and practices to help those working in the discipline succeed on the job and keep quality and patient safety at the forefront. As with all previous editions, this latest version was written with the following constituencies at the forefront:

- CS technicians studying to enhance their skills.

- Certified CS technicians looking for solutions for daily operational problems, and answers to questions on how to improve the products and services being delivered.

- Today's students (members of tomorrow's healthcare team) who are studying in preparation of assuming a position within the CS profession.

This new edition will help students become recognized for their knowledge of and dedication to the continually evolving roles of CS technicians. In keeping with tradition, this edition will also serve to influence the careers of certified professionals, many of whom have worked to distinguish themselves in their chosen field. Further, it will serve as a valuable study guide today and as a vital, enduring educational resource for CS professionals of all titles and tenures.

Acknowledgments

Developing any technical book relies heavily on the latest standards, regulations and guidelines that drive the industry. For the Central Service Technical Manual, Eighth Edition, these include:

- The Association for the Advancement of Medical Instrumentation (AAMI), including standards ST79, ST58, ST41 and ST91.

- Surveying agencies, including the Centers for Medicare and Medicaid Services (CMS) and The Joint Commission (TJC).

- Federal agencies, including the Centers for Disease Control and Prevention (CDC), the U.S. Food and Drug Administration (FDA) and the Occupational Safety and Health Administration (OSHA).

- Professional organizations, including the Association of periOperative Registered Nurses (AORN) Inc., the Association for Professionals in Infection Control and Epidemiology Inc. (APIC) and the Society for Gastroenterology Nurses and Associates (SGNA) Inc.

In addition, no successfully developed textbook would come to fruition without the assistance of its many dedicated, knowledgeable and talented contributors. Numerous association members, medical product and device representatives and other professionals devoted their knowledge, time and expertise to help ensure that this eighth edition would become the very best Central Service Technical Manual to date.

Following in the footsteps of the seventh edition, this eighth edition was written and revised "by the industry, for the industry." The development process began approximately 24 months before this edition was published. Volunteer members of IAHCSMM's Professional Development Resource Council (PDRC) assisted the process in the following ways:

- Reviewing the content of the previous seventh edition textbook.

- Compiling data from several sources (member, instructor and student surveys, and changes in standards and technologies).

- Determining additional subject matter that was needed.

- Suggesting the organizational structure and layout for the manual and its chapters.

The following authors, researchers and photographers generously donated their time and expertise to the development of the Central Service Technical Manual, Eighth Edition:

Gregory Agoston	Kay Huston
James Akers	Susan Klacik
Pamela Alexander	Stephen Kovach
Julie Armistead	Bill Kras
Paula Barrett	Angela Lewellyn
Nola Bayes	Julia Lynch
Michelle Bellefeuille	Ivy Magruder
Bruce Bird	Farrah Marsh
Lindsay Brown	Colleen McIntier
Mattie Castro	Curtis McNeil
Anna Clarkson	Andrew Mikos
David Craig	Thomas Overbey
Sandra Cullen	Timothy Parsons
Kimberly Davis	Sandra Ponce
Scott Davis	Gene Ricupito
Gail Doyle	Cheron Rojo
Mark Duro	Jean Sargent
Debra Ebert	Rudy Serrato
Sheryl Eder	Kristin Sims
Elizabeth Franz	Alfred Spath, Jr.
Ryan Furtado	Charles Stewart
Maliwan Gritiyutanont	Larry Talapa
Amanda Hayes	Ray Taurasi
Susan Heyward	Anthony Thurmond
David Hilliker	Lisa Venegas
Genan Holder	Don Williams
Lisa Huber	Linda Williams
Tracy Humpheys	Julie Williamson

No publication can be finalized until it is reviewed by subject matter experts to help ensure the content is accurate and current. The following individuals were instrumental in reviewing the eighth edition:

Cheri Ackert-Burr

Steve Adams

Susan Adams

James Akers

Pam Alexander

Connie Anderko

Laura Bardowski

Dewey Barker

Nola Bayes

Darla Bernard

Bruce Bird

Linda Breadmont

Joyce Burris

Etta Bushong

Gwendolyn Byrd

Mattie Castro

Josephine Colacci

Davina Cowlard

Danny Davis

Scott Davis

Debra Ebert

Sheryl Eder

Lori Ferrer

Elizabeth Franz

Rudy Gonzales

Ellen Gray

Sharon Greene-Golden

Jacqueline Harles

Amanda Hayes

Cathy Hayton

Susan Heyward

Helen Holiday

Lisa Huber

Tracy Humphreys

Kay Huston

Barbara Jackson

David Jagrosse

Lorrie Johnson

Wilhelmina Jones

Roxanne Kasper

Susan Klacik

Genti Koci

Marcy Konja

Patti Koncur

Valerie Kozik

Bruce Krolinkowski

Diane Larson

Angela Lewellyn

Tanya Lewis

Natalie Lind

Steve Maley

Elaine Mather

Curtis McNeil

Erica Meeks

Karen Nauss

Jill Nelson

Jack Ninemeier

Warren Nist

Patricia Nothum

Delores O'Connell

Mary Olivera

Malinda Osborn

Donna Perez

Carol Petro

Lana Phillips

Christina Poston

Jan Prudent

Dawn Rooney

Jean Sargent

Nicholas Schmitz

Linda Schultz

Donna Serra

Rudy Serrato

Kristin Sims

Alfred Spath, Jr.

Charles Stewart

Larry Talapa

Patricia Vanni

Lisa Venegas

Jane Wagers

Jeff Warren

Don Williams

Linda Williams

Julie Williamson

The development of this textbook required significant time and input from the following healthcare companies (listed in alphabetical order) who provided authors, reviewers, researchers and photographers, including (listed in alphabetical order):

3M Health Care

Advanced Sterilization Products (ASP), a division of Ethicon Inc.

Aesculap Inc.

Case Medical Inc.

Censis Technologies Inc.

Crosstex/SPSmedical Supply Corp.

Envision Inc.

Getinge USA Inc.

Halyard Health Inc. (formerly Kimberly-Clark Health Care)

Healthmark Industries Company Inc.

Integrated Medical Systems International (IMS), a subsidiary of STERIS Corp.

KARL STORZ Endoscopy-America Inc.

Key Surgical

Medline Industries Inc.

Mobile Instrument Service and Repair Inc.

OneSOURCE Document Site

Ruhof Corp.

Spectrum Surgical Instrument Repair, a subsidiary of STERIS Corp.

STERIS Corp.

STRYKER Corp.

TSO3 Inc.

Ultra Clean Systems Inc.

IAHCSMM would like to thank all who contributed to the development of the Central Service Technical Manual, Eighth Edition, including CS departments and healthcare facilities that allowed us to take photographs for inclusion in this manual. These facilities were instrumental in enhancing the visual content of this manual.

It is because of each and every contributor that the Central Service Technical Manual, Eighth Edition, is sure to become a valuable and trusted educational resource for professional development and knowledge advancement.

Contents

Chapter 2
Medical Terminology for Central Service Technicians

Chapter 3
Anatomy for Central Service Technicians

Chapter 4
Microbiology for Central Service Technicians

Chapter 5
Regulations and Standards

Chapter 6
Infection Prevention 101

Chapter 10
Surgical Instrumentation

Table of Contents

Chapter 13
Point-of-Use Processing

Chapter 14
High-Temperature Sterilization 301

Chapter 17
Monitoring and Recordkeeping for Central Service

Chapter 18
Quality Assurance

Table of Contents

Chapter 19
Managing Inventory within the Central Service Department 391

Chapter 22
Safety and Risk Management for Central Service

Chapter 23
Success through Communication 451

Chapter 24
Personal and Professional Development for Central Service 467

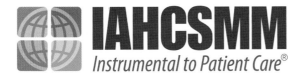

IAHCSMM
Instrumental to Patient Care®

The International Association of Healthcare Central Service Materiel Management

The International Association of Healthcare Central Service Materiel Management (IAHCSMM) is the premier organization for professionals working in the Central Service (CS) discipline. IAHCSMM was established in 1958, as a nonprofit corporation headquartered in Chicago, Ill. IAHCSMM represents more than 23,000 CS professionals in the U.S. and abroad. These individuals work throughout the healthcare industry—in hospitals, ambulatory surgery centers, clinics and dental offices, and as CS consultants, representatives for device manufacturer and third party reprocessors. IAHCSMM is committed to promoting patient safety by providing educational and professional development opportunities to the CS profession.

A BRIEF HISTORY

One of IAHCSMM's primary roles is to provide education to CS professionals. Prior to the mid-1940s, sterilization services for hospital departments were performed by surgical nurses in the surgery department. The American College of Surgeons began a movement to standardize and centralize the preparation, sterilization, handling and storage of all surgical instruments and supplies into one unit. As a result, CS departments were created.

The CS profession continues to evolve at a rapid pace, with new surgical items being introduced regularly. The processing of robotic, endoscopic, complex orthopedic, spinal and other related instruments and equipment requires special skills and knowledge of decontamination and sterilization processes.

By necessity, CS training has also changed from an on-the-job, hands-on model to a more formal course of study. This *Central Service Technical Manual, Eighth Edition*, is designed to provide CS technicians with information needed to understand the basic concepts of decontamination, sterilization, sterility maintenance and related processes, so they are better equipped to handle the increasingly specialized requirements of medical device reprocessing.

IAHCSMM MISSION STATEMENT

IAHCSMM's mission is to promote patient safety worldwide by raising the level of expertise and recognition for those in the Central Service profession. IAHCSMM accomplishes this:

- By providing educational, professional development, certification, communication and representation opportunities for Central Service professionals.

- Through collaboration efforts with allied partners, members and associates.

- Through advocacy initiatives for public policy changes.

IAHCSMM EDUCATIONAL OPPORTUNITIES

The Association's mission statement emphasizes that the provision of educational opportunities for its membership is a high priority. Held in the spring each year, IAHCSMM's Annual Conference and Expo combines the annual membership meeting with five days of educational offerings for technicians, managers and others affiliated with the field of CS.

IAHCSMM chapters also provide educational seminars to reach as many CS technicians as possible. Together, these educational offerings help technicians and managers keep up to date on the latest trends, standards, regulations and recommended practices, and provide an opportunity for these individuals to network with other CS professionals in their region.

At both the national and local level, vendors play a significant role in making educational

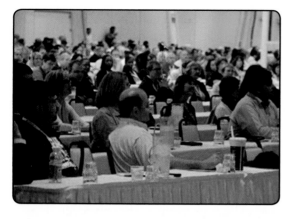

offerings possible for CS professionals. Along with sponsoring exhibits where they bring the latest information on products and services available to CS, they also provide financial support for many of IAHCSMM's educational offerings, such as continuing education lessons, educational videos and online education.

The vast majority of IAHCSMM's educational offerings are developed for CS professionals by CS professionals. The result is practical and useful information that has a direct application to the field of CS.

IAHCSMM PUBLICATIONS

IAHCSMM publishes several comprehensive and informative textbooks for the CS profession. These publications are developed as needs are identified by the membership, and as new processes and technologies enter the workplace.

Central Service Technical Manual, Eighth Edition, is designed to provide information on

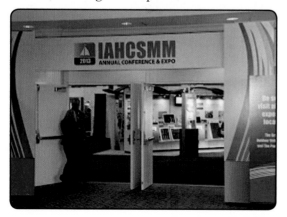

decontamination and sterilization theories and basic CS practices.

Central Service Leaderhip Manual provides valuable information for CS leaders at all levels of leadership.

Instrument Specialist Manual provides detailed information about the proper inspection, care and handling of commonly-used instruments, as well as specialty instruments.

The CS Dictionary is a useful pocket reference for all CS professionals.

The texts are used in the U.S. and several other countries. The *Central Service Technical Manual, Seventh Edition*, is available in Chinese, Japanese and Spanish translations. The *Central Service Leadership Manual* is available in Chinese.

IAHCSMM INFORMATION EXCHANGE

CS professionals require the most current information to remain effective on the job. This information is vital for keeping CS professionals informed about new products and changes in recommended practices. IAHCSMM provides the following methods for the sharing of information and ideas.

Communiqué is the Association's bi-monthly publication. With features such as "President's Message," "Technician's Exchange," "Self-Study Lesson Plans," "Hot Topics," information about upcoming meetings, and news from IAHCSMM chapters—not to mention, articles on a wide variety of CS-related subjects—*Communiqué* is a valuable tool for every CS professional.

Central Source is the Association's bi-monthly electronic publication that provides news and information that enhances CS professionals' knowledge and keeps them abreast of changes that impact the field. Popular features include: "Ask the Expert," "Certification Corner," "Educator Update," "Orthopedic Council Query" and "Breaking News."

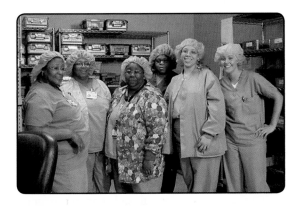

IAHCSMM's website, www.iahcsmm.org, is an immediate source of a wide variety of helpful professional information. The website allows members and certificants to renew certifications, complete online lesson plans, purchase publications and access references and resources, and stay abreast of late-breaking news, upcoming events, advocacy initiatives and much more.

One of the most popular features of the website is the Discussion Forum. This real-time feature allows users to post questions about many issues CS professionals encounter each day. Responses are provided by other forum users, many of whom face the same challenges.

IAHCSMM CERTIFICATION AND PROFESSIONAL DEVELOPMENT

Attaining certification is a positive first step in one's personal professional development efforts. Those pursuing a career in CS continually strive for recognition as professionals. IAHCSMM supports certification and recognizes it as an important component to patient safety. Professionals work in an occupation that requires extensive knowledge and skills, and a profession involves membership limited to individuals with formal education in a specialized body of knowledge. A profession is typically controlled by licensing, registration, and/ or certification. Individuals working in the CS profession certainly meet those requirements.

IAHCSMM maintains high educational and certification standards. As the professional and technical requirements of the CS profession have become more demanding, IAHCSMM has developed certification programs to address these evolving demands.

For many CS technicians, the right combination of education and experience has led to certification. Certification is the formal recognition of specialized knowledge, skills and experience in CS. It is demonstrated by clinical experience in CS and by successful completion of a multiple choice exam, which tests knowledge needed to perform everyday tasks in the CS profession. Certification assures the public that minimum competency standards were met, and recognizes those who have attained those standards.

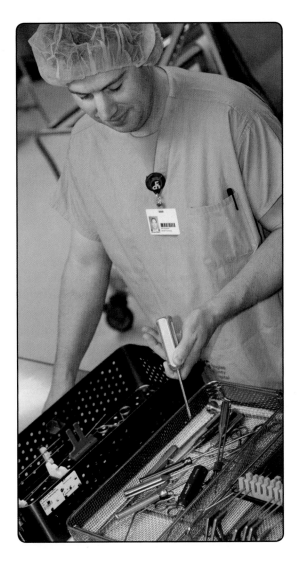

IAHCSMM offers several certifications including:

- **Certified Registered Central Service Technician (CRCST)**—Emphasis is on reprocessing concepts and current standards and practices. Attaining CRCST status also requires a minimum of 400 clinical hours of hands-on experience and successful completion of the CRCST certification exam.

- **Certified Instrument Specialist (CIS)**—Emphasis is on identifying, handling and processing surgical instrumentation. One must first have the CRCST credential before attaining this certification.

- **Certification in Healthcare Leadership (CHL)**—Emphasis is on supervisory responsibilities, including recruitment, selection, orientation and training, communication, leadership, motivation and other related concepts. One must first have the CRCST credential before attaining this certification.

Maintaining each of these certifications requires proof of continuing education that must be earned and then submitted at the time of annual certification renewal.

Fellowship in Central Service (FCS)—an honorable distinction also available to CS professionals. By demonstrating professional accomplishments and writing a research paper, and successfully completing an oral interview, applicants may achieve the FCS, which is the highest designation for CS professionals.

To learn more about IAHCSMM certifications and Fellowship, visit: www.iahcsmm.org.

In addition to certification, IAHCSMM provides several additional opportunities for professional development. Opportunities for involvement include local IAHCSMM chapters, and serving on national committees, projects, events or the IAHCSMM Executive Board. These opportunities provide an ability to learn, grow professionally and network with professional colleagues.

IAHCSMM ORGANIZATIONAL STRUCTURE

Active membership in IAHCSMM is open to anyone employed in healthcare CS or Materiel Management departments. Associate membership is open to anyone who, by virtue of their occupation, has an allied relationship with CS Materiel Management departments.

Although it is not required for membership, many IAHCSMM members form local chapters that offer independent meetings and provide educational offerings.

Information about local chapters or about forming a chapter can be found at www.iahcsmm.org.

The elected local chapter Presidents, or their designees, serve as chapter representatives and comprise the IAHCSMM Board of Directors. This Board convenes during the Annual Conference, and elects representatives to the Executive Board from among its members.

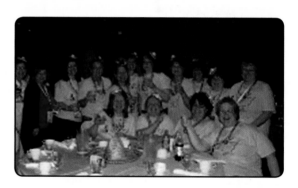

The Executive Board is comprised of the Association's President, President-Elect, Secretary-Treasurer and Executive Director, as well as the elected representatives from the Board of Directors. Responsibilities of the Executive Board include transacting administrative and financial business of the Association, planning the Annual Conference, updating educational materials, maintaining working relationships with allied associations, and interacting with committees, chapters and members.

IAHCSMM's Education Department is responsible for developing and monitoring all IAHCSMM educational programs to ensure that all materials are timely, consistent, and accurate. The Executive Board, the Education Department and Subject Matter Experts (SMEs) work together to:

- Provide various types of education, as identified by member needs.

- Develop the educational program for the association's Annual Conference.

- Develop and update all of the Association's educational resources.

Another important facet of education is the Corporate Advisory Committee (CAC). The Association's elected officers and Executive Director meet with the CAC to plan annual vendor exhibits and education, and consider other issues relating to corporate sponsors.

IAHCSMM AND ALLIED HEALTHCARE ASSOCIATIONS

IAHCSMM represents the CS profession and fosters relationships with several allied associations, such as The Association for the Advancement of Medical Instrumentation (AAMI), the Association of periOperative Registered Nurses (AORN), Association of Surgical Technologists (AST), the Association of Professionals in Infection Control and Epidemiology (APIC) and the Society of Gastroenterology Nurses and Associates (SGNA).

These allied healthcare associations focus on patient safety and infection prevention goals. Improving patient outcomes requires that all healthcare professionals within each specialty work together to achieve these goals.

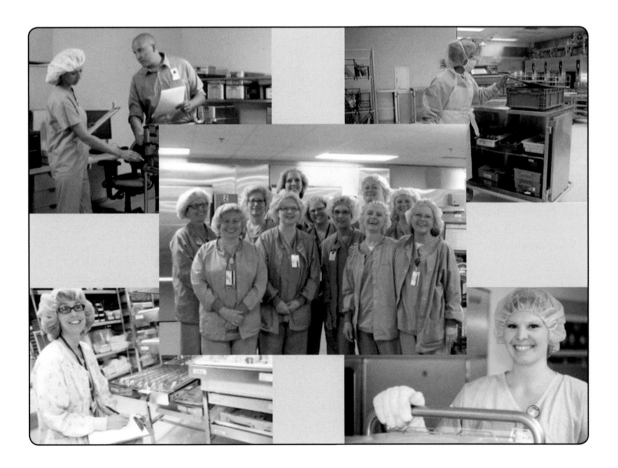

IAHCSMM AND THE FUTURE

IAHCSMM leadership strives to improve the professional status of individuals working in the CS profession. They are continually looking for ways to enhance the CS profession. Current issues include:

- Advocating certification for CS technicians in all 50 states.

- Continually updating and improving educational resources.

- Advocating standards and best practices that protect the patient.

- Providing opportunities for career growth and professional development.

The CS environment is dynamic and fast paced, and the work is challenging and highly technical. Inefficiencies in productivity, errors and poor quality outputs are costly to hospitals and can be life-threatening to patients. The performance of every person in every CS department has a direct impact on patient and employee safety. The profession is truly an evolving occupational discipline. CS professionals should take great satisfaction in knowing that their efforts, service, special skills and commitment to doing what's right are a part of every surgical procedure, patient recovery, birth and patient discharge. IAHCSMM's motto, **"Instrumental to Patient Care®,"** accurately reflects CS professionals' valuable contributions and commitment.

Chapter 1

Introduction to Central Service

Learning Objectives

As a result of successfully completing this chapter, readers will be able to:

1. Explain the importance of the Central Service department, with an emphasis on the service provided and the role of CS in quality patient care

2. Review the work flow process in an effectively organized Central Service department

3. Identify basic knowledge and skills required for effective Central Service technicians

4. Define job responsibilities of Central Service technicians

5. Discuss the role of education and training in the field of Central Service

INTRODUCTION

The majority of medical procedures require the use of supplies, instruments and/or equipment. Some items are used once and then discarded, while others are reused multiple times. Reusable items must be thoroughly cleaned, inspected, disinfected, and/or sterilized before they can be used to treat other patients. The Central Service (CS) department in a healthcare facility performs these important reprocessing activities.

Advancing Technologies

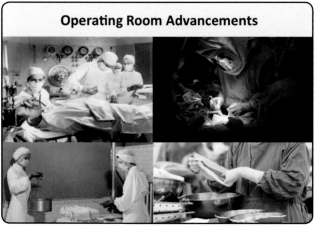

Figure 1.1

Medical technology is rapidly advancing. The medical devices used in the Operating Room (OR) and throughout the healthcare facility have changed dramatically over the years. (See **Figure 1.1**) As these devices become more complex, the same can be said of the methods required to reprocess them. (See **Figure 1.2**)

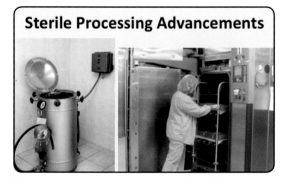

Figure 1.2

Like the entire medical field, the CS profession has evolved significantly throughout the years. The advances experienced in patient treatment and care have come with advances in the medical devices used to provide those services. Today's increasingly sophisticated medical devices require more complex handling and processing, which has resulted in many changes for CS technicians. These changes have not happened overnight, but have been introduced steadily throughout the past years. For example, one need only to look back a short time to identify changes that have enabled **minimally invasive procedures**. (See **Figure 1.3**) These procedures provide many benefits to patients, including shortened stays, smaller incisions, reduced trauma and shorter recovery times. These procedures require complex instrumentation and that instrumentation requires complex processing protocols.

Medical technologies will continue to advance, devices will become more complex and CS technicians will be required to keep up with advances. This chapter will provide an introduction to the field of CS, and an overview of the knowledge and skills required to meet the demand for timely, safe and functional medical devices.

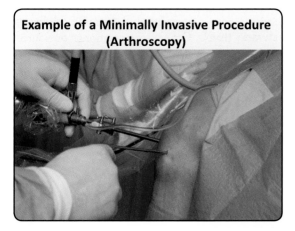

Figure 1.3

> **Minimally invasive procedure** A surgical procedure done in a manner that causes little or no trauma or injury to the patient; it is often performed through a cannula using lasers, endoscopes or laparoscopes. Compared with other procedures, minimally invasive procedures involve smaller incisions, less bleeding, smaller amounts of anesthesia, less pain and minimal scarring.

The "Central" in Central Service

The term "central" suggests that services are centralized. Processing soiled goods and sterilizing devices so they are ready for the next procedure is typically conducted in one centralized location. Many healthcare facilities find an increased demand for processing services, partially as a result of a growing trend: the use of more reusable and more complex medical devices. In addition, many facilities have expanded to clinics, ambulatory surgery centers, professional offices, and other service venues that may be remote from the facility's main location.

In response to this growing demand for processing services, satellite processing units with centralized management have been established. Others have consolidated (centralized) services into an entire **integrated delivery network (IDN).** Other organizations outsource required services to specialized businesses. Regardless of where processing activities are conducted, quality practices must be standardized in compliance with CS policies and procedures to enable standards of practice to be consistent and uniform.

> **Integrated delivery network (IDN)** A system of healthcare providers and organizations that provides (or arranges to provide) a coordinated range of services to a specific population.

Centralized management helps provide maximum utilization of human and materiel resources. This eliminates the costly duplication of processing equipment, utilities, space and personnel. Educated and skilled CS technicians must be knowledgeable about the complexities, precautions and techniques required for their job. They must carry out tasks in a manner that protects the welfare and safety of patients, co-workers, themselves, and their community. Proven material handling techniques are employed to provide high levels of efficiency.

When services are centralized, when the most effective processing equipment is used and when a better educated and prepared work force is available, staff can process a greater volume of materials in less time. This helps to meet the demands of increased workloads in today's healthcare environment.

The "Service" In Central Service

The term "service" is the key to what CS is all about. In most cases, the services delivered by CS personnel assist direct patient care providers by providing the items that are essential for proper patient treatment. Other departments (customers) within the healthcare facility depend on CS for processed sterile supplies, instruments, equipment and/or ready-to-use products provided by medical suppliers. CS personnel must remember that they are an integral part of quality patient care.

Central Service by Many Names

The title "Central Service" is the accepted name for this department in many healthcare facilities and professional organizations. In some facilities, the title "Central Service" is changed to reflect the scope of service or other needs. Not all CS departments provide the same services to their customers. Some departments only provide services to surgery, while others may provide services to many other departments in addition to surgery. No matter how many departments are served, the services provided are always guided by the same principles and standards of operation.

Common names for the department include: Central Processing; Sterile Processing and Distribution; Central Sterile Supply; and Surgical Supply and Processing.

Note: The U.S. Department of Labor uses the name "Medical Equipment Preparers" when discussing this field.

CENTRAL SERVICE WORK FLOW

Because the CS department is the central location for the delivery of soiled (used) medical devices and the distribution of clean and sterile items, proper work flow is important to help ensure safety. Soiled materials must be isolated from their clean counterparts to ensure acceptable processing conditions. A one-way flow of materials from the soiled area to the clean processing area, and on to the sterile storage area is required. (See **Figure 1.4**)

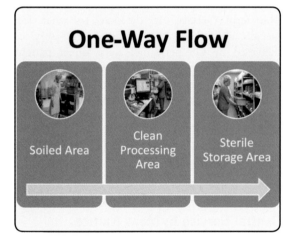

Figure 1.4

To facilitate one-way flow of goods and maintain distinction between soiled and clean work areas, physical barriers or walls are used to segregate the functional areas of CS. These areas include decontamination, preparation and packaging (prep and pack), sterilization and sterile storage/distribution.

Decontamination

The **decontamination** area is where all soiled instruments and other items are received from user departments. Decontamination is the physical or chemical process that renders an inanimate object, such as a medical device that may be contaminated with harmful microbes, safe for further handling. It involves a thorough cleaning process that may be accomplished with manual and/or mechanical cleaning. Cleaning is the first step in the sterilization process. All items returned to this area are considered contaminated and potentially infectious, and items cannot be considered sterile or high-level disinfected if they are not effectively cleaned. CS technicians must have an in-depth knowledge of the items to be cleaned in this area, and must select the appropriate method of decontamination as recommended by the device manufacturer. Medical devices must then be properly sorted, disassembled and cleaned using the established protocols. (See **Figure 1.5**)

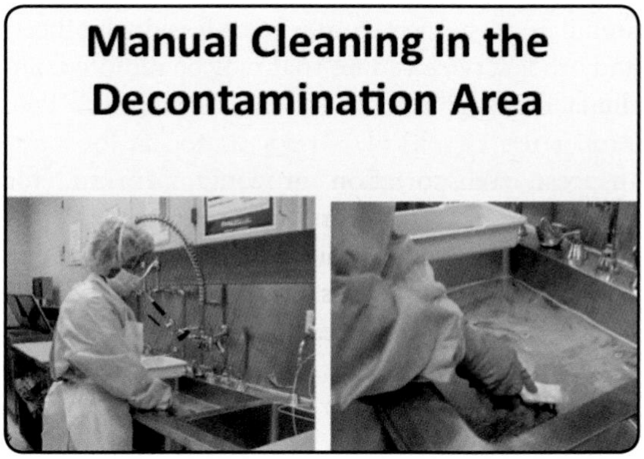

Figure 1.5

> **Decontamination** To make safe by removing or reducing contamination by infectious organisms or other harmful substances; the reduction of contamination to an acceptable level.

Working in the decontamination area requires a thorough knowledge and understanding of microbiology and the decontamination process. CS staff must be able to identify and clean a wide variety of medical devices. Knowledge

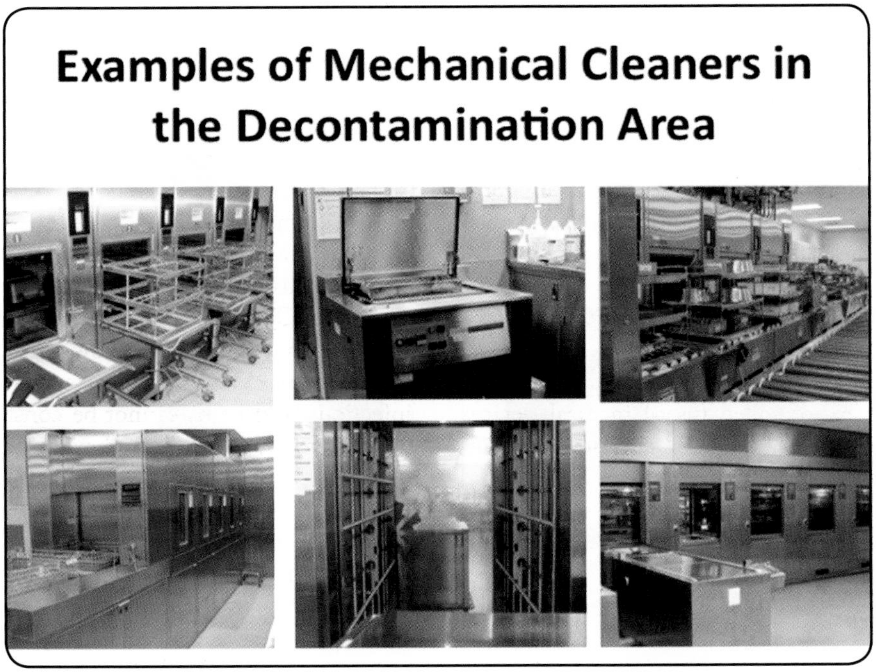

Examples of Mechanical Cleaners in the Decontamination Area

Figure 1.6

about cleaning and disinfecting agents and their proper use is critical. Proper protocols for waste disposal, transportation of contaminated items, and operation of equipment used in the cleaning process, including washer-disinfectors, ultrasonic cleaners, cart washers, steam guns and specialty washers, are also required. (See **Figure 1.6**)

CS technicians working in the decontamination area must be protected from the environment. The physical layout of this area, as well as cleaning equipment used in it, must meet the appropriate standards of governmental agencies and the recommendations of professional organizations. Policies and procedures must be developed and followed to ensure that work practices minimize employee injury and exposure to pathogens. To meet the facility's and the Occupational Safety and Health Administration's (OSHA's) safety requirements, CS technicians must wear special attire, called **personal protective equipment (PPE)**. PPE minimizes exposure to bloodborne pathogens and other contaminants. PPE includes fluid-resistant facemask, eye protection, a fluid-resistant

cover gown, general purpose utility gloves, and fluid-resistant shoe covers.

Personal protective equipment (PPE) A part of standard precautions for all healthcare workers to prevent skin and mucous membrane exposure when in contact with blood and body fluid of any patient. PPE includes fluid fluid-resistant protective clothing, disposable gloves, eye protection, face masks and shoe covers.

Preparation and Packaging

After items are safe for handling, they are delivered to the prep and pack area of the CS department. Each item is carefully inspected for cleanliness, proper function and possible defects. Instruments and other devices are assembled, packaged and labeled in preparation for sterilization.

CS technicians must be able to identify hundreds of surgical instruments. They must understand how instruments are manufactured, how they are constructed, how to test them and how to best maintain them. They must be able to inspect devices for cleanliness, proper condition and function. It is essential that CS professionals have the knowledge and training to maintain instruments properly, consistently and safely. (**Figures 1.7** and **1.8** provide examples of inspection and assembly activities.)

Instrument Inspection Processes

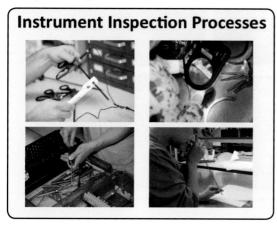

Figure 1.7

Instrument Assembly Processes

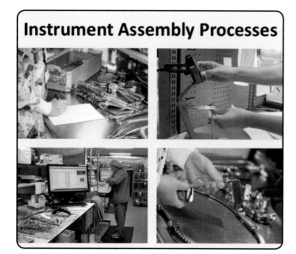

Figure 1.8

Surgical specialty instruments, equipment and implants also require special knowledge and expertise. CS technicians must be able to select the proper packaging system and use proper techniques for wrapping and packaging items for sterilization. (See **Figure 1.9**)

Packaging Processes

Figure 1.9

Sterilization

Items to be sterilized must be properly identified, and the correct methods and parameters for sterilization must be followed according to the manufacturer's **Instructions for Use (IFU)**. The principles necessary to achieve sterilization must be understood and applied. Sterilizers must be loaded and operated properly, and sterilization quality assurance measures must be followed to help ensure that sterilization parameters have been met. Records must be maintained, and factors that can compromise sterile packaging must be understood, prevented and detected. (See **Figure 1.10**)

Instructions for Use (IFU) Information provided by a device manufacturer that provides detailed instructions on how to properly use and process the device.

Examples of Sterilization Activities

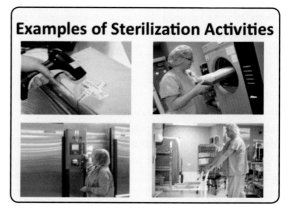

Figure 1.10

Personnel working in the preparation, packaging and sterilization areas of CS must wear facility-restricted attire, such as a scrub suit and hair coverings. It is essential that CS professionals diligently adhere to dress codes and safe work practices to protect the environment from contamination.

Sterile Storage and Distribution

The supply area of CS is dedicated to the storage of sterile instruments and clean or sterile supplies. A separate area for removing supplies from shipping cartons and containers should be provided. The major portion of the work in this area involves receiving, storing, and dispensing supplies and sterile instruments. (See **Figure 1.11**)

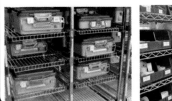

Sterile Storage Areas

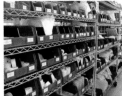

Figure 1.11

While items may be dispensed to almost all departments within a healthcare facility, the major focus of this area is servicing the OR. This is usually accomplished through the use of a **case cart system**. The bulk of surgical supplies may be stored in a central location (the CS department). A dependable system must be in place to supply items to surgery from the sterile storage area. (See **Figure 1.12**)

Examples of Case Cart Systems

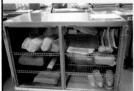 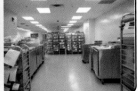

Figure 1.12

Surgical procedures are usually scheduled through a surgery scheduling office using a special computer program. When surgical procedures are scheduled, authorized personnel assign a **case cart** or **doctor's (physician's) preference card** to each procedure. This generates a **case cart pull sheet (pick list)** that identifies items specific to the doctor and procedure. CS technicians use this sheet to place supplies from the sterile storage area storage shelves onto the case carts that transport these items to the appropriate OR/surgical suite. Personnel working in this area usually gather instruments and supplies needed for all scheduled surgical procedures during the day or evening before they will be used.

Other areas within the healthcare facility may be supplied from the sterile storage area. Also, hospital personnel from different departments frequently require items that are only available from CS. Those working in the sterile storage area must be familiar with all supplies within the location in order to provide fast and accurate customer service.

Open lines of communication must be maintained between those in CS and sterile storage areas to help ensure that an adequate stock of sterile items is always available. Also, the **Materiel Management department** is an important link in the supply process; therefore, effective communication and effective problem solving skills must be fostered between personnel in these two important departments.

Personnel working in the sterile storage area must have thorough knowledge of every item, how it is used, where it is located and the process for obtaining it. Other knowledge and skills include those needed for:

- Inventory control and supply distribution.

- Surgical specialties and procedures.

- Sterile storage and handling requirements.

- Computer systems relating to inventory and case carts.

- Acquisition and disposition of supplies.

- Resolution of supply problems.

All CS areas must exercise careful environmental control conditions. Each work area should be restricted to assigned and authorized personnel who consistently follow the facility's dress code policies. Strict traffic control patterns must control the movement of people and goods through the department. Air pressure levels must be maintained to control air movements. Proper air pressure control helps to prevent the flow of bacteria-laden particulates and dust from the soiled to the clean areas.

Case cart system An inventory control system for products/equipment typically used in an Operating Room that involves use of an enclosed or covered cart generally prepared for one surgical case, and not used for general supply replenishment.

Case cart A cart prepared for an individual procedure. Case carts usually contain all instruments, supplies and utensils needed for a specific procedure.

Doctor's (Physician's) preference card A document that identifies a physician's needs (requests and preferences) for a specific medical procedure. Preference cards usually contain information regarding the instruments, equipment, supplies and utensils used by a specific physician. They may also include reminders for the staff of the physician's preferences regarding patient draping, instruments and supplies.

Case cart pull sheet (pick list) A list of specific supplies, utensils and instruments for a specific procedure. Central Service technicians use these lists to assemble the items needed for individual procedures.

Materiel Management department The healthcare department responsible for researching, ordering, receiving, and managing inventory (consumable supplies).

THE PROCESSING CYCLE

Work performed in CS usually follows the following processing cycle. (See **Figure 1.13**) After use, items that can be reprocessed are returned to the decontamination area to start the process all over again. It is important to note that at each step in the process, items are inspected to ensure that they are clean, in good repair, assembled and processed correctly. It is also important to ensure that packaging materials are not damaged, which could compromise sterility.

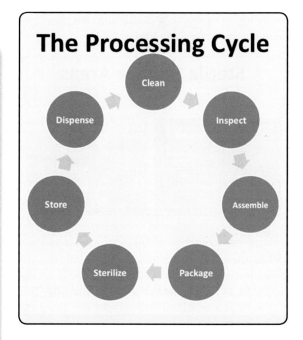

Figure 1.13

CS technicians must not only master specific skills in each work area to perform the job, but they must also learn new ones as technologies, regulations, standards, and best practices evolve. **Figure 1.14** provides some examples of skills CS technicians may routinely perform.

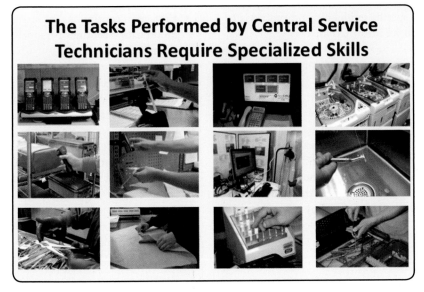

The Tasks Performed by Central Service Technicians Require Specialized Skills

Figure 1.14

A Basic Educational Foundation Is Needed

Numerous dimensions of knowledge and skills are required for Central Service technicians to be successful in their jobs. A basic educational foundation is necessary to form the base for more specialized knowledge and skills. Examples of this education foundation include the ability to:

- Read and write, including the use of reports, manuals and Instructions for Use.

- Communicate with inter- and intra-departmental team members.

- Interpret technical materials used for CS practices and procedures.

- Understand concepts of microbial transmission and infection prevention.

- Understand and use surgical and medical terminology.

- Operate tracking and other CS-related computer systems.

BASIC JOB KNOWLEDGE AND SKILLS

CS professionals require significant knowledge and skill sets to perform effectively on the job. Knowledge and skill sets should include the following:

Communication Skills

CS technicians must know alternative methods of providing and obtaining information; they must be effective oral and written communicators. To do so, they must be able to:

- Assess the ability of other people to understand what is being communicated.

- Adapt communication style to individual needs.

- Apply active listening skills using reflection, restatement and clarification techniques.

- Interact appropriately and respectfully with diverse groups in numerous employment situations.

- Communicate in a straightforward, understandable, accurate and timely manner.

- Use facility-specific guidelines and methods to send and receive information.

- Access and use electronically-produced information.

Facility Systems

CS technicians must understand how their role fits into their department, their organization and the overall healthcare environment. They must be able to identify how key systems affect the services they perform and the quality of care they provide. To do so requires that they:

- Are aware of the range of services offered to customers.

- Prevent unnecessary waste and duplication.

- Participate in quality improvement activities.

- Use resources, including other staff members, manuals and training opportunities.

Employability Skills

Successful CS technicians practice employability skills to enhance their employment opportunities and job satisfaction, and they maintain and upgrade those skills as required. Examples include:

- Maintaining appropriate personal skills, such as attendance and time management, and assume individual responsibility for their actions.

- Maintaining professional conduct standards.

- Using analytical skills to solve problems and make decisions.

- Formulating solutions to problems using critical thinking skills (analyze, synthesize, evaluate), independently and in teams.

- Adapting to changing situations.

- Practice personal integrity and honesty.

- Engage in continuous self-assessment and goal modification for their personal and professional improvement.

- Exhibit respectful and empathetic behavior as they interact with peers, superiors, subordinates and customers in one-on-one and group situations.

- Listen attentively to verbal instructions, requests and other information to verify accuracy.

- Understand various career options and the preparation required for them.

Legal Responsibilities

CS technicians must understand and maintain an awareness of the legal responsibilities and limitations, and the implications of their actions within the healthcare delivery setting. To do so, they must:

- Solve problems relating to legal dilemmas or issues.

- Comply with established risk management factors and procedures.

- Determine when an incident must be reported.

- Maintain confidentiality.

- Operate within the required scope of practice.

- Follow mandated standards for workplace safety.

- Apply mandated standards for harassment, labor and other employment laws.

- Comply with legal requirements for documentation.

Ethics

Ethics relates to knowing the difference between "right" and "wrong." In the healthcare environment, it means conforming to accepted and professional standards of conduct. Ethical behavior is "doing the right thing in the right way." Ethics should govern and guide the way CS technicians act and make decisions. They must always:

- Respect patient rights.

- Promote justice and the equal treatment of all individuals.

- Recognize the importance of the patient's needs over other considerations.

- Exhibit loyalty to fellow workers and the healthcare facility.

- Report any activity that adversely affects the health, safety or welfare of patients, visitors or fellow workers.

- Comply at all times with pertinent regulatory guidelines, facility policies, departmental policies and procedures.

- Respect interdisciplinary differences among team members.

- Differentiate between ethical and legal issues.

- Demonstrate professionalism when interacting with co-workers and customers.

Safety Practices

Successful CS technicians understand existing and potential hazards to patients, co-workers, and themselves. They prevent injury or illness through safe work practices, and they consistently follow health and safety policies and procedures. They do so as they:

- Practice infection control procedures.

- Use **standard precautions** to control the spread of infection.

- Practice appropriate cleaning, disinfecting and sterilizing processes.

- Apply principles of body mechanics, including use of proper lifting techniques.

- Recognize and correct fire and electrical hazards.

- Use equipment as directed.

- Manage hazardous materials.

- Use safety data sheets (SDS).

- Follow emergency procedures and protocols.

- Comply with pertinent regulatory guidelines, including OSHA standards.

Standard precautions Method of using appropriate barriers to reduce the risk of transmission of bloodborne and other pathogens from both recognized and unrecognized sources. It is the basic level of infection control to prevent transmission of infectious organisms from contact with blood and all other body fluids to non-intact skin, and mucous membranes. This standard applies to all patients, regardless of diagnosis or presumed infectious status.

Teamwork

CS technicians must understand the roles and responsibilities of individual members as part of the healthcare team, including their ability to promote the delivery of quality healthcare. They must interact effectively and sensitively with all members of their team, and do so when they:

- Practice team membership skills, such as cooperation, leadership and anticipation of their co-workers' needs.

- Respect diversity within their team.

- Interact with others in a manner consistent with the healthcare team's structure and lines of authority.

- Manage conflict within the workplace by considering the points of view of others.

- Respect and value the expertise and contributions of all team members.

- Accept compromise as necessary to ensure the best outcomes.

Resource Management

CS technicians must understand and practice principles and techniques of resource management. CS technicians manage resources effectively when they:

- Control costs and reduce waste.

- Provide quality service.

- Practice time management skills.

- Identify and solve potential problems and anticipate customers' needs.

- Know and use inventory appropriately.

- Practice recycling and sustainability, whenever possible.

Other Skills

Other skills are also required by CS technicians. For example, they must:

- Practice prescribed techniques to prevent **healthcare-associated infections (HAI)**.

- Keep departmental work areas in good repair.

- Keep their work environment clean and organized.

New healthcare roles demand higher levels of skill than ever before for those working in CS. The complexities created by technology continue to grow and a new breed of healthcare professional is emerging.

> **Healthcare-associated infection (HAI)** An infection that is not present when a patient is admitted to a hospital or healthcare facility. If the infection develops in a patient on or after day three of admission to the hospital or healthcare facility, the infection is referred to as a hospital-acquired or healthcare-associated infection.

BASIC JOB RESPONSIBILITIES

CS technicians are accountable for many tasks. **Job descriptions** are used to define and communicate job duties and requirements to employees within an organization. They are intended to be overviews that capture the general purpose and major accountabilities of a job, and they are used for the following reasons:

- To evaluate positions and determine compensation. They can be used in conjunction with other resources to establish a pay range for a given position.

- To clarify expectations. Job descriptions outline key job duties, which can be reviewed at the time of hire to clarify performance standards and expectations. They should be reviewed regularly (usually annually) by both the supervisor and those who occupy the position.

- To review performance. Job descriptions can be used during annual performance reviews.

- To recognize exceptional performance, restate performance expectations, determine growth opportunities and establish goals.

Because CS departments vary in size and scope of service, and because jobs within the CS department vary, there is no single job description that applies to all situations. When seeking a new position, it is important to review the job description to determine if the duties and expectations are a fit for your skills and abilities.

> **Job description** A human resources tool that identifies the major tasks performed by individuals in specific positions.

Career Growth and Professional Development

Many CS departments still use on-the-job training to fulfill job demands; however, as CS has developed more fully into a profession, formal education and **certification** of CS technicians is frequently becoming a requirement for working in the department. Some states require certification to work in CS, and many healthcare facilities require it as a condition of employment.

Formal CS technology training courses are becoming readily available through post-secondary education systems. Many healthcare systems are developing their own training courses for teaching CS technology. Long-distance learning courses are also available for those who do not have an organized training course readily available in their area.

Career growth and professional development opportunities for CS professionals typically depend on their individual motivation to achieve departmental and personal goals. Many facilities offer career progression with more work responsibilities and higher compensation levels within the role of CS technician. As knowledge and responsibilities increase, a qualified and high-performing technician can advance. *Note: Additional information about professional development is discussed in Chapter 24.*

Certification Association/industry recognition attained by individuals with educational and/or work experience requirements who successfully complete an examination process demonstrating their knowledge of pertinent, job-related subject matter.

Education and Experience Are Critical

To survive in today's dynamic and complex environment, it is necessary to be prepared, and education and experience become absolutely critical to do so. Qualified and educated professionals are in demand to meet the new challenges in Central Service departments.

Upward mobility to supervisory and management positions requires experience, education and skills.

Compensation

Compensation, including benefits, is influenced by many factors, such as job descriptions, scope and span of responsibility, size of facility, organizational structure, job market and geographic location. At the department head level, the CS director should be fairly compensated relative to organizational peers. As previously mentioned, there are a growing number of healthcare facilities that compensate CS staff members with pay increments based on experience, high performance, additional education and training, and upon certification.

CONCLUSION

The Central Service environment is dynamic and fast paced. The work is challenging, highly technical and complex. The performance of this vital department has a major impact on the successful operation of the many departments to which it provides products and services.

Inefficiencies in productivity, errors that create the need for rework, and poor quality performance are costly to hospitals. With the ever-increasing costs of healthcare, CS professionals must conserve resources and minimize expenses. More important is the safety and welfare of patients who have entrusted the facility with their care. Negligence and carelessness in CS could cost a patient's life.

CS is an evolving occupational discipline. Over the years, there have been dramatic changes (ranging from the increased use of technology and support services provided to the job skills, training and educational requirements) needed to fulfill these job responsibilities. Changes continue at a rapid pace.

Conscientious CS professionals will find great satisfaction in knowing their efforts, service, special skills and due diligence are a part of every surgical procedure, every patient's recovery and every positive outcome.

RESOURCES

U.S. Department of Labor. *Medical Equipment Preparers*, http://www.bls.gov/oes/2006/may/oes319093.htm. Accessed September 2014.

Colbert BJ. *Workplace Readiness for Health Occupations*. Second Edition. Thomson Delmar Learning. 2006.

Booth KA. *Health Care Science Technology: Career Foundations*. McGraw-Hill Companies Inc. 2004.

U.S. Department of Education. *National Health Care Skill Standards*. The National Consortium on Health Science & Technology Education.

CENTRAL SERVICE TERMS

Minimally invasive surgery (MIS)

Integrated delivery network (IDN)

Decontamination

Personal protective equipment (PPE)

Instructions for Use (IFU)

Case cart system

Case cart

Doctor's (Physician's) preference card

Case cart pull sheet (pick list)

Materiel Management department

Standard precautions

Healthcare-associated Infection (HAI)

Job description

Certification

Chapter 2

Medical Terminology for Central Service Technicians

Learning Objectives

As a result of successfully completing this chapter, readers will be able to:

1. Explain the importance of medical terminology for Central Service technicians

2. Identify the various elements used in medical terminology including prefixes, roots and suffixes

3. Discuss how medical terminology can refer to the human anatomy, disease processes, surgical instruments and surgical procedures

4. Understand medical terminology used to refer to surgical procedures in surgery schedules

5. Understand the importance of medical terminology for service quality in the Operating Room

INTRODUCTION

Central Service (CS) technicians require knowledge of medical terms to help them succeed on the job. The special terminology used to describe parts of the body, diseases, instruments and surgical procedures will be addressed in this chapter.

IMPORTANCE OF MEDICAL TERMINOLOGY

The Healthcare Profession

The Association of periOperative Registered Nurses (AORN) specifically states that "skilled and competent allied health care providers and support personnel are valued members of the perioperative care team, contributing to safe patient care and positive patient outcomes." As such, CS technicians must have a grasp of the medical terminology that is used by healthcare customers, as well as by fellow CS professionals. The American National Standards Institute (ANSI) and the Association for the Advancement of Medical Instrumentation (AAMI), in ANSI/AAMI ST79, 4.2.2, specifically states that CS technicians must be "knowledgeable and competent" to adequately perform the vital tasks that they perform. Indeed, The Joint Commission (TJC) states that in order to maintain a reliable system for medical device processing, institutions must place an emphasis upon the "orientation, training and competency of health care workers" responsible for this task. Understanding medical terminology is part of the training and competency that CS technicians should possess.

Understanding the Operating Room

CS professionals must provide Operating Room (OR) personnel with the instruments and supplies needed for surgical procedures. As these needs are conveyed, CS technicians must also understand the terminology/language spoken to them in order for them to provide quality customer service and contribute to positive patient outcomes.

For example, if the OR calls for instrumentation needed for an emergency pericardial window, a knowledgeable CS technician will know that this is a cardiac procedure that involves cutting into the pericardium (a membranous sac that surrounds the heart) in order to drain fluid from the pericardial space into the pleural cavity. Also, if the OR calls for a case cart for a **STAT** Repair of an Abdominal Aortic Aneurysm (AAA), this request will be responded to immediately as the CS technician will understand that the patient is at risk of losing his/her life. If the OR issues a request for a case cart for a routine Laparoscopic Cholecystectomy, the CS technician will know that this is not an emergency case. The case cart will still be picked and the instruments and supplies will still be prepared and organized; however, this is usually not an emergency situation.

> **STAT** Abbreviation for the Latin "statim" meaning immediately or at once.

Providing Quality of Service to the Patient

It is through knowing and understanding medical terminology that CS technicians are able to understand what is being asked of them. This knowledge of medical terminology enables the CS technician to react in an appropriate manner when the OR or medical staff makes a request; however, the opposite is also true. If the OR makes a request that is not understood, the productivity of the OR is compromised. This interruption of the perioperative process will compromise the quality of service rendered to the patient and may cause a delay in treatment. Nothing is more important than quality. For this reason, TJC and the Centers for Disease Control and Prevention (CDC) recommend that all healthcare institutions provide comprehensive and intensive training for all staff involved in the processing of medical instrumentation.

ANATOMY OF A MEDICAL TERM

CS technicians frequently encounter specialized medical terms in their daily work activities, and each of those terms contains key elements to help staff better understand the words' origin and meaning. As technicians learn the meanings of these names, they will have a greater understanding of what their work involves, and their competency and job satisfaction will increase.

Word Elements

The majority of medical terms are of either Greek or Latin origin. The word "pericardium," for example, is composed of two Greek **word elements:** peri (meaning around), and kardia (meaning heart). Hence, the term is used to refer to the membranous sac that surrounds the heart, as well as the roots of the great vessels of the heart. The term "rigor mortis" is composed of two Latin word elements: rigor (stiffness) and mortis (meaning "of death"); hence, the term is used to refer to the stiffening of the body that occurs after death. Many terms combine both Greek and Latin word elements to form a single medical term. For example, the term "claustrophobia" (meaning fear of enclosed spaces) joins the Latin word element "claustrum" (enclosed space) to a Greek word element "phobia" (fear). Another example of this blending of Greek and Latin in the formation of medical terms can be seen in the term "autoclave" (a term that is very important for CS). The term "auto" (Greek) refers to self while the term "clavis" (Latin) refers to a key; hence, an autoclave is a type of self-locking device (a sterilizer is designed to not open until its cycle is finished).

At first, medical terminology may seem daunting and overwhelming; however, after a working knowledge of these word elements is gained, it becomes easier to analyze and use the words effectively.

Medical terminology changes with the dynamics of evolving technology in healthcare. New terms, abbreviations and words are constantly being created to meet the needs of this new technology. Through word association and memorization of basic medical terms and word elements, CS professionals can establish a solid foundation upon which to build an extensive vocabulary. A CS professional's vocabulary must be in a constant state of growth, evolution and development.

Prefixes, Roots and Suffixes

The anatomy of a medical word may (but will not always) consist of three types of word elements:

- **Root word element** Tells the primary meaning of a medical term, which can then be modified by either a prefix, suffix or both. Many roots signify a procedure, disease or body part. Again, let's use "cardio," the medical term for "heart" as an example. The term "cardiology" features the root "cardio" in combination with the suffix "ology," which, in this instance, refers to the study of things related to the heart. The term "endocarditis" also features the root "cardio," but here the root is modified by a prefix "endo" (meaning within), as well as a suffix "itis" (meaning inflammation); therefore when the entire word is analyzed, the word means inflammation of the inner portion of the heart. The term "Cardiothoracic" features two roots: "cardio" (meaning heart), and "thoracic" (meaning chest); hence, a Cardiothoracic surgeon performs surgery on the heart, its major vessels, and the lungs. The term "electrosurgery" also features a combination of two roots. While the root "electro" refers to the use of electrical current, the root "surgery" refers to the act of performing surgery (the use of electrical current to cut and cauterize during surgery).

- **Prefix word element** Comes before the root. When added to a root (at the beginning of a word), the prefix can alter or modify its meaning. For example, the medical term for the prefix "around" is "peri"; therefore, the term "pericardial" means "around the heart." The term "perioperative" refers to the entire process surrounding a surgical procedure: before (preoperative), during (intraoperative), and after (postoperative). The prefix "peri" is also found in the surgical instrument called periosteal elevator. Here, the prefix "peri" (around) is attached to the root "osteo" (bone); hence, a periosteal elevator is an instrument used to remove tissue from around a bone (the periosteum). Even the term "abnormal" functions in this way. The "ab" functions as a prefix to negate the meaning of the root "normal"; hence, the meaning of the word is not "normal."

- **Suffix word element** Comes after the root. When added to the root (at the end of a word), the suffix can also alter or modify its meaning. For example, the medical term for the suffix that means inflammation is "itis"; therefore, the term "pericarditis" refers to inflammation (itis) around (peri) the heart (cardio). Most of us are acquainted with the term "tonsillitis" as referring to the inflammation of the tonsils. Bronchitis refers to the inflammation of the bronchi, which are the tubes extending from the trachea into both sides of the lungs; hence, whenever the suffix "itis" is found at the end of a medical term (modifying a root word preceding it), a meaning of inflammation will be present.

Of special note with the term "pericarditis" is that the "o" in the root "cardio" is dropped in the word "pericarditis." This reflects something called a **combining vowel**. In many cases, a combining vowel (usually an "o") is either added to a root or removed from it to ease the pronunciation of the word. The use of combining vowels can result in some rather long medical words. The linguistic effect of this addition or elimination of the combining vowel is to ease the pronunciation of the word. For example, the term "herniorraphy" which refers to the suturing/repairing (-rrhaphy) of a rupture/hernia (herni), contains an "o" which has been added as a combining vowel (herni-o-rrhaphy). Conversely, the term "proctitis," which refers to inflammation of the rectum, features the dropping of the combining vowel "o" (procto/rectum

+ itis/inflammation = proctitis). While the addition or elimination of a combining vowel is common in medical terminology, it is important to understand that not all medical terms have combining vowels.

Word elements Parts of a word.

Root word element Tells the primary meaning of a word; also called base word element.

Prefix word element The word element that comes before the root word element.

Suffix word element The word element that comes after the root word element.

Combining vowel A letter (usually an "o") that is sometimes used to ease the pronounciation of a medical word.

An easy way to remember the difference between prefix (which comes before the root) and suffix (which comes after the root) is to put the words in alphabetical order: prefix, root and suffix. This tells you that prefix is the first word element and suffix is the last word element.

Note: Not all medical terms consist of all three word elements. A medical term may be formed by a root alone, by combining two roots, a root and suffix, or a prefix and root. Some medical terms can even be formed by combining three roots together.

The best way to learn the meaning of a medical term is to analyze and understand its components, so that the word can be taken apart. Begin with the suffix (if present) since it most often gives a clue and meaning about the root, and how it is being used. Then consider the root and prefix (if present). In other words, consider the overall relationship between each word element in the term. Medical terms can be a lot like building blocks; if one can figure out how they fit together, one can determine what they mean.

Prefix	Root	Suffix	Word
hemi- (half)	arthro (joint)	-plasty (surgical restoration)	hemiarthroplasty (surgical restoration of half of a joint, the femoral portion of the hip joint, the proximal femur, a form of hip replacement surgery)
hemi- (half)	gastro (stomach)	-ectomy (surgical removal)	hemigastrectomy (removal of half of the stomach) *Note: The combining vowel "o" is dropped in this word.*
hemi- (half)	colo (colon)	-ectomy (surgical removal)	hemicolectomy (removal of half of the large intestine) *Note: The combining vowel "o" dropped from this word.*
para- (beside, near)	thyroid (thyroid)	-ectomy (surgical removal)	parathyroidectomy (surgical removal of parathyroid glands)
septo- (dividing wall)	rhino (nose)	-plasty (surgical restoration)	septorhinoplasty (surgical restoration of the nose) *Note: Two roots combined with a suffix.*
chole- (bile)	cyst (fluid-filled sac)	-ectomy (surgical removal)	cholecystectomy (surgical removal of the gallbladder) *Note: Two roots combined with a suffix.*
electro- (electrical activity)	cardio (heart)	-gram (written record of)	electrocardiogram (written record of the electrical activity of the heart) *Note: Two roots combined with a suffix.*
electro- (electrical activity)	encephalo (brain)	-gram (written record of)	electroencephalogram (EEG) (the tracing of brain wave activity) *Note: Two roots combined with a suffix.*

Figure 2.1 Combined Word Elements

Figure 2.1 shows additional examples of how word elements are combined to form medical terms. Sample words shown here contain a prefix, a root and a suffix. While not all medical terms feature all three word elements in the same word, it is important to understand that many medical terms do feature all three word elements.

When analyzing medical terms, several suffixes meaning "pertaining to" may be encountered. **Figure 2.2** provides several examples of suffixes, words in which they are used, and the meaning of the words.

Figure 2.2 Suffixes that Mean "Pertaining To"

Suffix	Example	Meaning
-ac	cardi-ac	pertaining to the heart ("o" in cardio is dropped)
-al	derm-al	pertaining to the skin
-ic	hem-ic	pertaining to blood
-eal	esophag-eal	pertaining to the esophagus
-ary	pulmon-ary	pertaining to lungs
-ous	cancer-ous	pertaining to cancer

Just as with the English language, certain rules of grammar apply to medical terminology. Making medical terms conform to the basic rules of spelling and pronunciation may result in letters in the word element being changed, dropped or added. **Figure 2.3** shows some examples.

Figure 2.3 Letters in Word Elements May Be Dropped or Added

Prefix	Root	Suffix	Word	Letters Changed
	procto (rectum)	-itis (inflammation)	proctitis	"o" is dropped
	broncho (bronchus)	-itis (inflammation)	bronchitis	"o" is dropped
	endo (within)	-oscopy	endoscopy	"o" is dropped
	artery (artery)	-ectomy (removal)	endarterectomy	"o" and "y" are dropped
	fascia	-otomy	fasciotomy	"a" is dropped
	chir (hand)	-plasty (surgical repair)	chiroplasty	"o" is added
	herni (rupture)	-rrhaphy (to suture)	herniorrhaphy	"o" is added
	hyster (uterus)	-pexy	hysteropexy	"o" is added

As noted above, when analyzing a medical term, it is sometimes best to start with the meaning of the suffix. In this way, one can readily identify if the word relates to a surgical procedure, a medical condition or a portion of the human anatomy. **Figures 2.4** and **2.5** list some common medical and surgical suffixes. Suffixes are word elements that come after the root word, and may be one or two syllables.

Figure 2.4 Common Medical Suffixes

Suffix	Meaning	Example	Combined Meaning
-algia	pain	neuralgia	nerve pain
-cide	kill	bactericide	a substance that kills bacteria
		virucide	a substance that kills viruses
		fungicide	a substance than kills fungi
-emia	blood	hyperglycemia	high blood sugar
		hypoglycemia	low blood sugar
-genic	origin	osteogenic	originating in the bones
		iatrogenic	an adverse effect or complication originating from a physician
-gram	record/image of	mammogram	a radiographic image of the breast for early detection of breast cancer
		cholangiogram	a radiographic image of the bile ducts using contrast medium to check for blockage (frequently done during a cholecystectomy)
		arthrogram	a radiographic image of a joint after injection of a contrast medium
		angiogram	a radiographic image of the inside, or lumen, of blood vessels and organs of the body using a contrast agent
-itis	inflammation	tonsillitis	inflammation of the tonsils
		hepatitis	inflammation of the liver
		arthritis	inflammation of a joint
		bronchitis	inflammation of the bronchi
		meningitis	inflammation of the meninges (the membranous layer surrounding the brain and spinal cord)
-megaly	large or enlargement	cardiomegaly	enlargement of the heart
-necrosis	death of tissue	arterionecrosis	tissue death of an artery
-ology	study of	bacteriology	the study of bacteria
		oncology	study of cancer
		neurology	study of the nervous system
		cardiology	study of the heart
		nephrology	study of the kidney
-oma	tumor	carcinoma	malignant tumor
		myoma	tumor consisting of muscular tissue
		meningioma	tumor of the meninges (the membranous layer surrounding the brain and spinal cord)
		fibroadenoma	a breast lump composed of fibrous and glandular tissue
		papilloma	a benign tumor which grows on the skin or mucous membrane, can be caused by a virus
-pathy	disease	encephalopathy	disorder or disease of the brain
		cardiomyopathy	disorder or disease of the heart
-rrhage	flow	hemorrhage	uncontrolled flow of blood

Figure 2.5 Common Surgical Suffixes

Suffix	Meaning	Example	Combined Meaning
-cise	cut	excise	to cut out
		incise	to cut into
-ectomy	surgical removal	cystectomy	removal of a cyst
		tonsillectomy	removal of the tonsils
		pneumonectomy	removal of a lung
		laminectomy	removal of a portion of a lamina (part of the vertebra in the spine)
		hysterectomy	removal of the uterus
		appendectomy	removal of the appendix
		thrombectomy	removal of a blood clot
		orchiectomy	removal of a testicle
		nephrectomy	removal of a kidney
		vitrectomy	removal of some or all of the vitreous humor from the eye
		hemorroidectomy	removal of swollen or inflamed vascular structures in the anal canal
		bunionectomy	removal (realignment) of a misaligned bone in the big toe
		discectomy	removal of a herniated disc in the spine
		microdiscectomy	minimally invasive removal of a herniated disc in the spine
		thyroidectomy	removal of the thyroid gland
-oscopy	visual examination and possible treatment of an organ or joint	laparoscopy	visual examination of organs in the abdomen
		arthroscopy	visual examination of a joint
		cystoscopy	visual examination of the bladder
		bronchoscopy	visual examination of the bronchi
		colonoscopy	visual examination of the large intestine
		thoracoscopy	visual examination of the thoracic cavity
		fluoroscopy	an imaging technique which provides live images (motion included) of a surgical site during surgery, referred to as C-Arm due to its shape
-ostomy	creation of an opening	colostomy	creation of new opening to colon
		tracheostomy	creation of new opening to trachea
		urostomy	creation of new opening for the urinary system
		nephrostomy	creation of a new opening to the kidney for the urinary system

Suffix	Meaning	Example	Combined Meaning
		ventriculostomy	creation of an opening within a cerebral ventricle for drainage
		ileostomy	creation of a new opening to the ileum (a portion of the small intestine near the colon/large intestine)
-otomy	incision into an organ	craniotomy	incision into the skull
		thoracotomy	incision into the pleural space of the chest
		arthrotomy	incision into a joint
		osteotomy	incision into a bone
		fasciotomy	incision into the fibrous membrane (fascia) which covers a muscle
		urethrotomy	incision into the urethra
		fistulotomy	incision into a fistula (an abnormal connection between two organs or vessels)
		sternotomy	incision into/splitting of the sternum (breastbone)
-pexy	surgical fixation	orchiopexy	surgical fixation of an undescended testicle to the correct location
		hysteropexy	abdominal fixation of the uterus
-plasty	surgical restoration	rhinoplasty	surgical repair of the nose
		arthroplasty	surgical repair of a joint
		cranioplasty	surgical repair of the skull
		tympanoplasty	surgical repair of the ear drum
		urethroplasty	surgical repair of the urethra
		kyphoplasty	surgical repair of a fractured vertebra by percutaneous (through the skin) injection of bone cement
-rrhaphy	to suture	myorraphy	to suture a muscle wound
		herniorraphy	to suture a hernia
-tome	a cutting instrument	dermatome	an instrument used for cutting skin
		osteotome	an instrument used for cutting bone

As can be seen by the brief listing of suffixes in **Figures 2.4** and **2.5**, medical terms can be complex and can mean entirely different things depending on how they are composed. For example, while the word "tonsillitis" means inflammation of the tonsils, the word "tonsillectomy" refers to the surgical removal of the tonsils. Herein lies the adventure of building a medical terminology vocabulary: words can mean entirely different things depending on how the root is used in concert with a prefix, suffix or both. **Figures 2.6** and **2.7** contain a listing of common roots found in medical terminology. Roots are base word elements that refer to the main body of a medical word.

Figure 2.6 Common Medical Roots

Root	Meaning	Example	Meaning
adeno	gland	adenoma	glandular tumor
aero	air	aerobic	requiring oxygen for growth
		anaerobic	not requiring oxygen for growth
arthro	joint	arthritis	inflammation of a joint
broncho	bronchus	bronchoscope	endoscope used to visualize the bronchi
cardio	heart	endocarditis	inflammation of the inner layer (endocardium) of the heart
		cardiomyopathy	heart muscle disease
		cardiopulmonary resuscitation (CPR)	emergency efforts to revive a person in cardiac arrest by means of chest compressions and rescue breaths
		myocardium	cardiac/heart muscle
cerebro	brain	cerebrospinal	referring to the brain and spinal cord
chole	bile	cholecyst	gallbladder
chondro/io	cartilage	chondroma	cartilaginous tumor
costo	rib	intercosto	between the ribs
cysto	bladder	cyst	any fluid-filled sac
cyto	cell	erythrocyte	red blood cell
derma	skin	dermopathy	skin disease
gastro	stomach	gastrointestinal	pertaining to the stomach and intestines
gyne	woman	gynecology	the study of diseases affecting the female
hema or hemat	blood	hemophilia	inability of the blood to clot
		hemostat	instrument used to control bleeding
		hematoma	collection of blood in tissue
		hemodialysis	filtration of the blood mechanically, occurring outside the body
hepat	liver	hepatitis	inflammation of the liver
leuko	white	leukocyte	white blood cell
		leukemia	a form of cancer of the blood or bone marrow involving abnormal white blood cells
nephros	kidney	nephritis	inflammation of the nephrons in the kidneys
		nephrosis	degenerative disease of the kidneys
thrombus	blood clot	thrombosis	formation of a blood clot inside a blood vessel obstructing the flow of blood (DVT= deep vein thrombosis)

Figure 2.7 Common Surgical Roots

Root	Meaning	Example	Meaning
arthro	joint	arthroscopy	visual examination of a joint
		arthrocentesis	joint puncture for the aspiration of synovial fluid
		arthrodesis	surgical fusion of a joint
colo	colon	colectomy	removal of part of the large intestine
cranio	skull	craniotomy	surgical opening into the skull
herni	rupture	herniorrhaphy	surgical repair of a rupture
hyster	uterus	hysteropexy	abdominal fixation of the uterus
		hysteroscopy	visual examination of the uterus
lipo	fat	liposuction	aspiration of fat cells
litho	stone	lithotripsy	crushing of a stone
mast	breast	mastectomy	surgical removal of a breast
oopher	ovary	oophorectomy	surgical removal of an ovary
osteo	bone	osteosynthesis	surgical reduction and fixation of a bone fracture
rhino	nose	rhinoplasty	surgical repair of the nose
tracheo	trachea	tracheostomy	creation of new opening to trachea
stoma	opening	anastomosis	a connection or reconnection of two separate tubular structures; for example, blood vessels or portions of intestines

Figures 2.6 and **2.7** above list common roots that show how medical terms can mean a variety of things depending on how they are constructed. Roots can be modified by prefixes, suffixes or both. Roots can also be combined to form their own words, or they can be modified by prefixes/suffixes. Meanwhile, the terms themselves can refer to either a portion of the human anatomy, a disease process or a surgical procedure. While this might seem difficult at first, it becomes much easier when one learns how to identify the suffixes and prefixes (if present) attached to the root/roots involved. By learning common suffixes and prefixes, the reader can identify whether the term is referring to the human anatomy, a disease process, a surgical procedure or a surgical instrument. **Figures 2.8** and **2.9** provides a listing of common prefixes used in medical terminology. Prefixes are word elements that are placed before the root to alter or modify its meaning.

Figure 2.8 Common Medical Prefixes

Prefix	Meaning	Example	Combined Meaning
a, an-	without	asepsis	without infection; sterile
		anesthesia	without sensation (local or general)
		atraumatic	not inflicting injury or wound
		analgesia	without pain
		atrophy	a reduction in size of a part of the body (wasting away) due to poor circulation, poor nutrition or a disease process.
ad-	toward (in the direction of)	addiction	toward dependence on a drug
ante-	before	antepartum	before the onset of labor
anti-	against	antiseptic	preventing sepsis (infection)
dis-	apart, away	hip dislocation	displacement of femur from pelvic joint
		disinfectant	chemical used to kill microorganisms
dys-	painful	dysentery	painful inflammation of the intestine
endo-	within	endotracheal	within the trachea
		endoscope	instrument used to visualize a joint or organ in the body
		endoscopy	visualization within, and possible treatment of, a part of the body using an endoscope and endoscopic instrumentation
extra-	outside	extracorporal	outside of the body
hyper-	above, excessive	hyperacidity	excessive acid in the stomach
		hypertensive	high blood pressure
		hypertrophy	excessive growth/size of a part of the body due to cellular enlargement
hypo-	below, deficient	hypoglycemia	low sugar content in the blood
		hypotensive	low blood pressure
inter-	between	intercellular	between, or among, cells
		interstitial	an empty space
		interdepartmental	between departments
		intercostal	between the ribs
intra-	within, inside	intravenous	in, or into, a vein
		intramuscular	located in, or injected into, a muscle
		intraabdominal	within the abdomen
		intraoperative	during surgery
		intraarticular	within a joint
		intraocular	within the eye
		intracranial	within the skull
neo-	new	neonatal	newborn
per-	through	percutaneous	through the skin
post-	after	postpartum	after delivery of a baby
		postoperative	after surgery
pre-	before	preoperative	before surgery
sub-	under, beneath	subcutaneous	beneath the skin
		subclavian	located under the clavicle
		subdural	located under the dura mater (the outermost membrane surrounding the brain)
supra-	above	suprapubic	above the pubis
		supracondylar fracture	fracture of the distal humerus above the elbow joint

Figure 2.9 Common Surgical Prefixes

Prefix	Meaning	Example	Meaning
bi-	two/both sides	bilateral total hip reconstruction (THR)	two (both) total hip reconstructions
		bilateral myringotomy with tubes	incision into (both) ear drums (tympanic membrane) in order to place drainage tubes
		bilateral salpingo-oophorectomy	surgical removal of both fallopian tubes and ovaries
		bilateral strabismus repair	surgery performed on the extraocular muscles to correct eye misalignment
hemi-	half	hemigastrectomy	surgical removal of half of the stomach
		hemiarthroplasty	a form of hip replacement surgery
		hemicolectomy	removal of half of the large intestine
para-	beside, near	parathyroidectomy	surgical removal of parathyroid glands
		paratracheal	beside the trachea
peri-	around, about	periosteal elevator	instrument used to remove tissue around the bone (the periosteum)
		perioperative	all aspects of the surgical process (before, during and after)
		pericardium	the serous (fluid emitting) membrane that stretches around the heart and lines the mediastinum
		peritoneum	the serous (fluid emitting) membrane that stretches around the abdominal cavity and is its lining
post-	after	postoperative	after surgery
trans-	across, through	transanal	through the anus
		transoral	through the mouth
		transesophageal	through the esophagus
		transurethral	through the urethra

Understanding Usage

Learning medical terminology can be an almost endless process, which multiplies as various body parts, procedure types and disease processes are combined to mean different things. As new surgical procedures are created (utilizing new approaches, instruments and technologies), new medical terminology will also be created to refer to these procedures. CS technicians must understand the language spoken to them by the OR and medical staff in order to provide them with the goods and services they need for their procedures. Language frequently used by the OR utilizes abbreviations or acronyms to refer to various types of surgeries. **Figure 2.10** contains a brief listing of some surgical procedure abbreviations or acronyms.

Figure 2.10 Abbreviations/Acronyms for Surgical Procedures

Abbreviation	Surgical Procedure	Meaning
AAA	Repair of abdominal aortic aneurysm	Surgical repair of a weakening/ballooning area of the abdominal portion of the aorta (the largest artery in the body).
ACL	Anterior cruciate ligament	Reconstruction or repairing of the anterior cruciate ligament. In an ACL reconstruction a graft is used to replace the ligament, and in an ACL repair the torn ligament is put back together.
ACF	Anterior cervical fusion	Surgical fusion of vertebrae in the cervical spine, approached from the front side of the patient's body.
ALIF	Anterior lumbar interbody fusion	Spinal surgery in which bone grafts/implants are used to fuse vertebrae in the lumbar spine, approached from the front side of the patient's body.
AKA	Above the knee amputation	Surgical removal of the leg above the knee.
AV Graft	Arteriovenous graft	A surgical connection is made between an artery and a vein to allow hemodialysis access.
BMT	Bilateral myringotomy with tubes	Incision into the eardrum (tympanic membrane, both sides) for drainage via tube placement.
BSO	Bilateral salpingo-oopherectomy	Surgical removal of both fallopian tubes and ovaries.
BKA	Below the knee amputation	Surgical removal of the leg below the knee.
CABG	Coronary artery bypass graft	Creation of a new blood supply to an area of the heart with a clogged/blocked artery using the patient's own blood vessel to function as the graft (frequently harvested from the leg).
CR	Closed reduction	Treatment of a fractured bone without a surgical incision.
D&C	Dilation and curettage	Dilation of the uterine cervix and scrapping of the inner lining of the uterus (endometrium) with a uterine curette.
EGD	Esophagogastroduodenoscopy	Endoscopic procedure that visualizes the upper portion of the gastrointestinal tract up to the duodenum (where the stomach connects to the small intestine).
ESS	Endoscopic sinus surgery	Use of endoscopic instrumentation to operate on the nose.
EUA	Exam under anesthesia	The use of anesthesia to conduct a surgical examination of a sensitive part of the body such as the eye or rectum.
I&D	Incision and drainage	Incision into and removal (drainage) of pus/fluid from an abscess, boil or infected wound/area of the body.
ICD	Implantable cardioverter-defibrillator	Insertion/implantation of a battery-powered device that can deliver a jolt of electricity to treat cardiac arrhythmia (dangerous irregular heartbeats, frequently performed in cardiac catheterization labs).

Abbreviation	Surgical Procedure	Meaning
IMN	Intramedullary nail	Insertion/implantation of a nail or rod, into the medullary cavity (center) of a long bone, such as the femur or tibia.
IOL	Intraocular lens	Insertion/implantation of a lens within the eye to treat cataracts (clouding of the lens of the eye) or myopia (nearsightedness).
IORT	Intraoperative radiation therapy	Use of therapeutic levels of radiation to treat exposed cancer tumors during surgery, frequently done during breast surgery.
LAVH	Laparoscopic-assisted vaginal hysterectomy	A visualization and treatment of pelvic organs (laparoscopy) followed by removal of the uterus through the vagina.
L&B	Laryngoscopy and bronchoscopy	A visual examination of the larynx and the bronchi.
LP	Lumbar puncture	A collection of cerebrospinal fluid (CSF) for diagnostic or therapeutic purposes. Commonly referred to as a spinal tap (not a surgical procedure, but frequently done in surgery for children).
MIDCAB	Minimally invasive direct coronary artery bypass	Use of a small incision in the ribs (mini-thoracotomy) to access the heart to bypass diseased coronary arteries. This is done "off-pump" without the assistance of the heart-lung machine.
MIS	Minimally invasive surgery	A type of surgery that uses endoscopic techniques and instrumentation in order to reduce trauma to the body during surgery (this technique reduces not only trauma to the patient's body, but reduces recovery time and reduces infection risks, as well).
ORIF	Open reduction internal fixation	Treatment of a fractured bone with an incision and the use of plates and screws or pins to hold the fragments together.
PAL	Power assisted liposuction	Aspiration (suction) of fat cells by means of a motorized hand piece and cannula (tube).
PCI	Percutaneous coronary intervention	Coronary angioplasty; a procedure to open narrowed coronary arteries, normally performed in cardiac catheterization labs.
PDA	Patent ductus arteriosus	Repair of a congenital heart disorder in a neonate (a child less than one month old).
PEG	Percutaneous endoscopic gastrostomy	Insertion of a feeding tube (PEG tube) into the stomach through the abdominal wall.
PICC	Insertion of peripherally inserted central catheter	An intravenous catheter inserted in a peripheral vein (such as the arm) for long-term IV access (a sterile procedure, not a surgery).
PLIF	Posterior lumbar interbody fusion	Spinal surgery in which bone grafts/implants are used to fuse vertebrae in the lumbar spine—approached from the back side of the patient's body.

Abbreviation	Surgical Procedure	Meaning
STSG	Split thickness skin graft	Healthy skin is taken from a place on the body, called the donor site, and used as a skin graft elsewhere on the body.
TAH	Total abdominal hysterectomy	Surgical removal of the uterus through an incision in the abdomen.
TEE	Transesophageal echocardiogram	Obtaining an ultrasound image of the heart by means of a probe/transducer inserted into the esophagus (frequently done in connection with cardiac surgery).
THA	Total hip arthroplasty	Hip joint reconstruction by removing the bone and placing a plastic/metal component in the hip socket (the acetabulum), as well as the femoral head (the proximal femur), resulting in a completely rebuilt joint.
TKA	Total knee arthroplasty	Knee joint reconstruction by placing implants on the end of the femur and the top of the tibia, as well as on the knee cap (the patella), resulting in a completely rebuilt joint.
TURP	Transurethral resection of the prostate	Surgical removal of part of the prostate gland by inserting instruments across the urethra to reach the prostate internally.
VATS	Video assisted thoracoscopic surgery	Use of endoscopic instruments to access the chest cavity/lungs/thorax.
VP Shunt	Ventriculo-peritoneal shunt	Surgical placement of a drain (shunt) to transfer excess cerebrospinal fluid (CSF) from the brain (ventricle) to the abdominal lining (peritoneum).
Wound VAC	Wound vacuum assisted closure	Application of a device/dressing that provides negative pressure (vacuum) to facilitate wound closure.
XLIF	Extreme lateral interbody fusion	Spinal fusion surgery approaching from the side of the patient using special instrumentation to reduce trauma on the patient's body.

ANATOMY OF A SURGICAL PROCEDURE

Once CS professionals understand medical terminology with its numerous prefixes, roots and suffixes, they will also be able to better understand the surgical procedures referred to in surgery schedules and the instruments and supplies that will be requested. Challenges arise when the OR is supplied with incorrect instrumentation and supplies for a surgical procedure. When the OR receives a case cart for a scheduled procedure from CS with the incorrect instrumentation and supplies, their attention is diverted away from the patient and onto getting the correct items in the room.

FROM MINIMALLY INVASIVE SURGERY TO OPEN PROCEDURES

The current practice in surgery is always to use a minimally invasive procedure when possible. Over the last 100 years, the vast majority of surgical procedures performed on patients have been "open" procedures. These procedures feature an incision to "open" the patient's body in order to perform whatever the surgical procedure requires. For example, if a patient needed an appendectomy, an incision would be made in order to remove the appendix. Similarly, if the patient needed a cholecystectomy, an incision would be made to remove that patient's gallbladder. Even open heart surgery has been handled in the same manner. If the patient had a diseased heart, the only way to operate on the heart was to split the patient's sternum open in order to access the patient's heart. This is no longer the only way to do surgery.

In today's high-technology surgical climate, many procedures start with some kind of a minimally invasive surgery (MIS) approach (developed during the 1960-1970s). This means that instead of simply cutting the patient's body open to access an organ or body part, some kind of special instruments will be used in order to perform the surgery. For example, some orthopedic procedures begin with something called a closed reduction (treatment of a fractured bone without an incision) prior to attempting an open reduction internal fixation

(implantation of plates/screws, etc.). If a closed reduction is not possible/successful, the surgeon might attempt a percutaneous pinning, which means that the surgeon might be able to access the broken bone through the skin (percutaneous) in order to reduce that fracture and stabilize it by insertion of a Steinmann pin/K-wire. If these approaches are unsuccessful (or not possible given the patient's condition), the surgeon will perform an open reduction internal fixation of the fracture (plates and screws will be used internally to stabilize the fracture).

Similarly, if the patient needs their gallbladder removed, in most cases the procedure will be booked as laparoscopic versus an open cholecystectomy. This means that the surgeon will start by attempting to remove the patient's gallbladder using endoscopic/laparoscopic instrumentation, as this technique is less traumatic to the patient's body. The surgeon will only convert to an open procedure (using a larger incision to access the involved organ) if the laparoscopic approach is unsuccessful. This is also very common in thoracic surgery as many surgical procedures involving the chest start with what is called a thoracoscopic surgery (use of endoscopic instruments to access the lungs) and only convert to an open thoracotomy (incision into the thorax/chest) if the thoracoscopic approach is unsuccessful.

Other surgical procedures are following a less-invasive approach in an effort to reduce trauma to the patient. In the case of breast surgery, for example, treatment will start with a minimally-invasive biopsy, followed by a lumpectomy, if indicated. If a mastectomy is required (surgical removal of a breast), the procedure will be booked in a manner that reduces trauma to the patient's body, while still effectively treating the disease. Therefore, a partial mastectomy can be performed (removal of a portion of the breast), or a radical mastectomy can be performed (complete removal of the breast). The same is also true for prostate surgery in men. If possible, the surgeon will attempt a transurethral resection of the prostate (TURP) using special instrumentation to reduce patient trauma. Only if the patient cannot be treated adequately using an endoscopic technique will the surgeon perform an open procedure called a radical prostatectomy. In today's world of surgical technology, it is even possible to have a total joint replacement (arthroplasty) using some kind of MIS technique, such as a unicompartmental knee arthroplasty.

Not all patients are candidates for MIS. Some illnesses and injuries are not remedied by such an approach. For example, if a patient's cancer has grown significantly inside an organ or another area of the body, that cancer will need to be resected (removed) by means of an open procedure. Also, if a patient has a severely broken femur, this patient will require the introduction of a trochanteric (intramedullary) nail to stabilize that fracture (a form of open reduction internal fixation). If a patient's gallbladder is about to rupture, the surgeon might elect to perform an open cholecystectomy without attempting a laparoscopic approach.

CS technicians must understand that contemporary surgery is always attempted to be minimally invasive to the patient as these approaches cause less trauma to the patient's body, reduce pain, reduce recovery time, and shorten length of hospital stay. When reading surgery schedules, it is vital that CS professionals understand that, in many cases, a laparoscopy will precede a laparotomy, an arthroscopy will precede an arthrotomy, or a thoracoscopy will precede a thoracotomy. The CS professional must know that minimally invasive procedures utilize a different assortment of instruments and supplies than open procedures. In some cases, the OR will only require the endoscopic instrumentation and supplies. In other cases, OR personnel will require both "set ups," one for the endoscopic procedure and one for the open procedure.

As important as endoscopic procedures are in reducing patient trauma, new advances in surgical techniques have evolved, which can be even less invasive than traditional MIS. Whether it is the removal of the gallbladder (cholecystectomy), removal of the uterus (hysterectomy) or the removal of the prostate (prostatectomy), these procedures can now be done using robotic technology. Even

open heart procedures can now be done by means of robotic technology. These procedures utilize a complex blend of highly-specialized instrumentation and supplies. This is the least invasive and most technologically-advanced form of surgery in history. CS professionals have the responsibility of processing these complex devices.

PROCEDURE APPROACH AND PURPOSE

When reading surgery schedules and interacting with OR staff, CS technicians need to understand how procedure approach and purpose are identified. When a surgical procedure is referred to in a surgery schedule, the suffix attached to the primary medical term will indicate the purpose of the procedure. For example, "oscopy" will refer to visual examination of and possible treatment, "otomy" will refer to an incision into, "ectomy" will refer to removal of, and "plasty" will refer to repair/reconstruction of.

Another key element in how a procedure can be understood relates to the approach that the surgeon will use in performing the surgery. The approach or method typically comes at the beginning of the surgical procedure term. A laparoscopic cholecystectomy will remove the patient's gallbladder using laparoscopic instrumentation and techniques. A robotically-assisted prostatectomy will remove the patient's prostate by using robotic instrumentation and techniques. A bilateral myringotomy will make incisions for drainage into the patient's eardrum/tympanic membrane on both sides. An anterior cervical fusion will fuse some of the patient's cervical vertebrae approaching from the front of the patient's body. A posterior lumbar interbody fusion will fuse some of the patient's lumbar vertebrae approaching from the back of the patient. A vaginal hysterectomy will remove the patient's uterus via the vaginal canal. A total abdominal hysterectomy will remove the uterus through an open incision in the abdomen. All of these procedures utilize completely different instrument sets and supply packs.

CASE CARTS AND INSTRUMENT TRAYS

In the past, the surgical team took responsibility for "picking" the needed instrumentation and supplies for their scheduled procedures. Some facilities still function in this manner; however, in recent years it has become more common for CS professionals to perform this function. Therefore, CS technicians may be responsible for reading the OR surgery schedule in order to print pick lists, obtain the needed instrumentation, and even find/obtain instrumentation that is already "in use" in another surgical procedure.

Surgery schedules are prioritized according to patient needs, which allows the OR to schedule procedures for the next day or following week. If a case is booked as a thoracoscopy (possible thoracotomy), for example, pick lists may be required (one for the endoscopic portion and another for the possible open procedure). **Figure 2.11** provides a basic example of a surgery schedule.

Many procedures in today's surgical climate require what is called "loaner" instrumentation. These are sets of instruments (frequently multiple sets of instruments) that are shipped to the hospital specifically for use by a specific physician on a specific patient. These instruments may be used one time and then returned to the vendor. To keep surgical procedures on schedule, it is also essential that CS professionals anticipate the need for loaner instrumentation. This helps ensure that devices are delivered well in advance to allow for safe, effective reprocessing and prompt delivery to the OR. More information on loaner instrumentation is discussed in Chapter 11.

Sample Surgery Schedule

Understanding Medical Terms can help CS Technicians better understand procedural needs.

Room	Start Time	Patient	Surgeon	Procedure	Comments
1	7:00	John Doe	Dr. Wells	Cystoscopy with Left Retrogrades, Left Stent Insertion	C-Arm
	TF	Tom Smith	Dr. Wells	Transurethral Resection of the Prostate	
2	7:00	Jon Williams	Dr. Green	Septoplasty, Possible Endoscopic Sinus Surgery	
	TF	Tammi Jones	Dr. Green	Tonsillectomy	
3	7:00	Mary Smith	Dr. Clark	TAH with BSO	
	TF	Jane Doe	Dr. Clark	D & C	
4	7:00	Bill Williams	Dr. Jones	TKA Right – Revision	Loaner Instruments
	TF	Sally Sims	Dr. Jones	ORIF – Left Ankle	
	TF	Bob Roberts	Dr. Jones	CR, Possible Pinning Right Thumb	Possible ORIF

Figure 2.11

THE VALUE OF MEDICAL TERMINOLOGY IN THE OPERATING ROOM

Awareness within the Operating Room

Knowledge of medical terminology and language is essential for ensuring that CS professionals have a clear understanding of what the OR and other healthcare customers require for their procedures. Prefixes, roots and suffixes discussed in this chapter are not mere items to remember or memorize. Instead, they are vital tools that will allow CS professionals to become more proficient in the department, improve communication with the OR and other healthcare customers, and provide safe, consistent, high-quality service that drives positive patient outcomes.

CONCLUSION

Medical and surgical staff members appreciate when everything goes smoothly with their patients/cases. The patient's needs are the motivating factor of every Central Service professional. CS professionals must respond to Operating Room staff in a timely, effective way. It is the responsibility of the CS department to assist the surgical and medical staff to deliver the highest quality of care to each and every patient. Communicating effectively and successfully meeting the needs of the OR and other healthcare customers requires CS professionals to possess a functional, ever-evolving understanding of medical terminology and language.

RESOURCES

Association for the Advancement of Medical Instrumentation. ANSI/AAMI ST79, A4 2013, Section 2. *Comprehensive Guide to Steam Sterilization and Sterility Assurance in Health Care Facilities.*

The Joint Commission. *Hospital Accreditation Standards, IC-10.* 2014.

Centers for Disease Control and Prevention. *Guideline for Disinfection and Sterilization in Healthcare Facilities.* 2008.

Leiken JB, Lipsky MS, Eds. *American Medical Association Complete Medical Encyclopedia.* Random House. 2003.

Stedman TL. *Stedman's Medical Dictionary 28th Ed.,* pp. 1047-1048. Lippincott Williams & Wilkins. 2005.

CENTRAL SERVICE TERMS

Case cart

STAT

Word elements

Root word element

Prefix word element

Suffix word element

Combining vowel

Chapter 3

Anatomy for Central Service Technicians

Learning Objectives

As a result of successfully completing this chapter, readers will be able to:

1. Review the structure, function, activities and role of cells, tissues and organs in the body

2. Identify and describe the structure and roles of each major body system and identify common surgical procedures that involve each system:
    - Skeletal
    - Muscular
    - Nervous
    - Endocrine
    - Reproductive
    - Urinary and excretory
    - Respiratory
    - Digestive
    - Circulatory

3. Explain how knowledge of anatomy can help with surgical instrument identification

INTRODUCTION

Many surgical interventions have been developed to treat the human body and enable it to heal. Central Service (CS) technicians play an important role in the surgical support process by providing the instruments and supplies needed to perform specific surgeries. As members of the surgical team, developing a basic understanding of the human body can aid in communication with the Operating Room (OR) and can help facilitate requests.

The study of the human body requires an understanding of **anatomy** and **physiology**. Our study begins by considering cells, tissues and organs.

> **Anatomy** The study of the structure and relationships between body parts.
>
> **Physiology** The study of the functions of body parts and the body, as a whole.

CELLS, TISSUES AND ORGANS
Cells

Here are some facts about **cells**:

- They are the basic living unit of life. The human body is made up of more than one hundred trillion of these tiny structures.

- They vary in size, shape and function, depending upon their location in the body.

- They are so small that they can only be seen with a microscope.

- Within each cell are still smaller structures called organelles: microscopic organs within a cell that perform specific functions.

- Functions of the cell include respiration, nutrition, energy production, waste elimination, and reproduction.

- Living cells come only from other living cells.

Regardless of their size and shape, each human cell consists of three main parts:

- The **cell membrane** is porous and flexible, and surrounds the cell to keep it separated from the outside environment. The cell membrane surrounds the cytoplasm and allows and controls the passage of materials in and out of the cell. Examples include the absorption of oxygen and food and the elimination of waste products produced by the cell. (See **Figure 3.1**)

- The **cytoplasm** is a clear jelly-like substance that surrounds the nucleus and contains the cell fluid and organelles.

- The **nucleus** is surrounded and protected by the cytoplasm. This oval structure acts as the brain center of the cell to direct and control all activities, including duplication into two new cells.

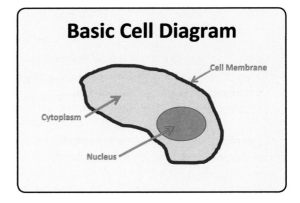

Figure 3.1

> **Cell** The basic unit of life; the smallest structural unit of living organisms capable of performing all basic functions of life.
>
> **Cell membrane** The outer covering of a cell that regulates what enters and leaves it.
>
> **Cytoplasm** Clear, jelly-like substance of a cell between the cell membrane and nucleus.
>
> **Nucleus** The functional center of a cell that governs activity and heredity.

Tissue

- Two or more cells that are similar in structure and function are joined together to form **tissue**.

The four primary tissues of the human body are:

- Epithelial tissue – This tissue covers the body's external surface (skin) and the linings of body cavities (the mouth, ears, nose and throat).

- Connective tissue – This tissue provides support, stores energy and connects other tissues and parts. Examples of connective tissue include bone, fat, blood and cartilage. Bones provide protection, support and shape to the body, and storage for calcium. Fat keeps the body warm, cushions organs and stores nutrients. Blood transports food and oxygen to all body parts and removes all waste products. A final example of connective tissue is cartilage, which provides framework and support to the human body.

- Muscular tissue – This tissue shortens as it contracts. When attached to bone, these contractions make body movement possible. Muscle tissues also line the inner walls of organs that contract to help food pass through the digestive system. As cardiac muscles contract, blood is pumped through the body.

- Nervous tissue – This tissue is located throughout the body. When stimulated, nervous tissue carries messages back and forth between the brain and every part of the body.

Organs

Organs are formed when two or more different types of tissues are grouped together to perform a specific function.

Examples of organs include the:

- Brain – An organ in the central nervous system that is the primary receiver, organizer and distributor of information in the body.

- Heart – The organ that pumps blood throughout the body.

- Stomach – An organ that is part of the digestive system and helps digest food by mixing it with digestive juices and converting it into a liquid.

- Skin – The largest organ of the body that serves as the body's outer covering.

> **Tissue** A group of similar cells that perform a specialized function.
>
> **Organ** A part of the body containing two or more tissues that function together for a specific purpose.

BODY SYSTEMS

A **system** is a group of organs that work together in the body to carry out a particular activity.

While each body system provides a specific bodily function, none are independent of any other. Each system must work together to help the body function as a total organism. With the exception of the reproductive system, each body system and its organs work together to help maintain life. The remainder of this chapter will provide details about the body's major systems and common procedures performed to treat issues that can occur in those systems.

Skeletal System

Without the skeletal system (See **Figure 3.2**), the body would just be an immovable mass. There are approximately 206 bones that, collectively, comprise the body's skeletal system. They are arranged in an orderly manner and are fastened together by tough connective tissue known as **tendons** and **ligaments**. The five main functions of the skeletal system are to:

- Give the body shape and support.

- Allow movement.

- Protect vital organs.

- Produce blood cells.

- Store calcium.

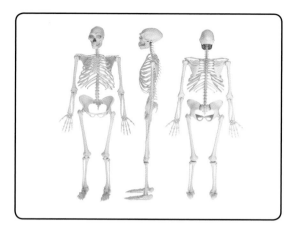

Figure 3.2

Most bones are made from **cartilage**, but through a process known as **ossification**, cartilage is sometimes replaced by bone. Cartilage is a flexible connective tissue that provides framework to the body; its purposes include:

- Supporting body structures, such as the ears and nose.

- Connecting the ribs to the sternum.

- Serving as a cushion between bones to prevent them from rubbing together at junctures and joints.

System A group of organs that work together to carry out a specific activity.

Tendon A cord of fibrous tissue that attaches a muscle to a bone.

Ligament A band of connective tissue that connects a bone to another bone.

Cartilage A type of flexible connective tissue.

Ossification The process by which cartilage is replaced by bone.

Joint Any place where two bones meet.

A **joint** is any place where two bones meet. Some are immovable, such as those found in the skull, and others, such as the knee and elbow joints, are movable and allow the bones that they connect to move. **Figure 3.3** shows the location of some joints in the body.

There are several types of joints:

- Gliding joints – Allow the head to lower as the vertebrae (bones in the spinal column) of the neck slide over one another.

- Ball and socket joints – Allow movements like swinging one's arm around in a circle. Ball and socket joints consist of a bone with a rounded head that fits into a rounded cup (hip and shoulder joints) socket of another bone.

- Pivot joints – Allow a turning motion, such as the palm of the hand rotating from up to down when a bone rotates on another ring-shaped bone.

- Hinge joints – Allow backward and forward bending motions, like a door hinge (knees, knuckles and elbows).

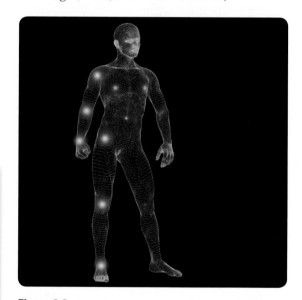

Figure 3.3

The overall covering or lining of a joint is called a synovial membrane. It secretes a fluid, called synovial fluid, to lubricate joint surfaces. (See **Figures 3.4** and **3.5**)

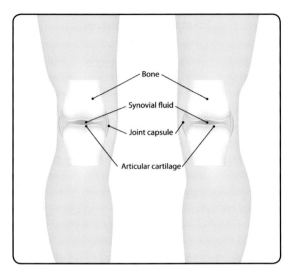

Figure 3.4

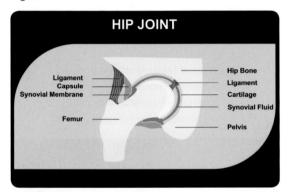

Figure 3.5

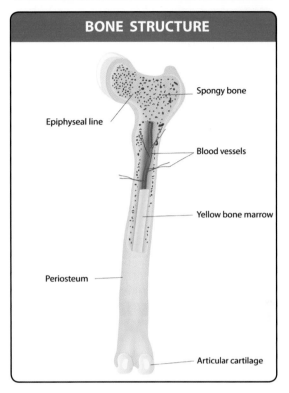

Figure 3.6

Examples of surgical procedures that involve the skeletal system:

- Craniotomy – Making an opening into the skull bone to access the brain.

- Anterior cervical fusion – Removal of disc tissue pressing on a nerve in the neck area by inserting a piece of bone between the vertebrae and fusing this area with plates and screws.

- Posterior lumbar interbody fusion (PLIF) – Removing disc tissue pressing on the lower spine area by inserting a piece of bone between the vertebra and fusing this area with plates and screws.

- Open reduction internal fixation (ORIF) – Making an incision in the skin, realigning a fractured bone, and inserting screws and plates to ensure the bone ends do not move, so healing can be promoted. (See **Figure 3.7**)

Bones are comprised of living tissue, and their strength and hardness comes from chemical substances, called minerals. Bone consists of two principal materials:

- A hard outer material called cortical or compact bone, that is dense and strong and consists of calcium and phosphorous. This hard outer surface is surrounded by the periosteum, a tough membrane that contains bone-forming cells and blood vessels.

- The inner section, called spongy or cancellous bone, is porous.

Bones are filled with a material called marrow. A pipeline of blood vessels and nerves runs through the middle of thick bones. (See **Figure 3.6**)

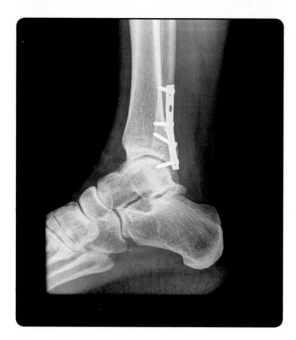

Figure 3.7

- Total knee arthroplasty (TKA) – Removing the bone at the distal (farthest) end of the femur and the bone at the proximal (nearest) end of the tibia, and replacing them with metal/plastic components. (See **Figure 3.8**)

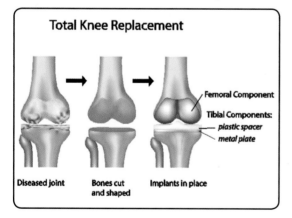

Figure 3.8

- Total hip arthroplasty (THA) – Removing the head of the femur and the socket where it fits in the hip bone, and replacing these structures with metal, ceramic and plastic components. (See **Figure 3.9**)

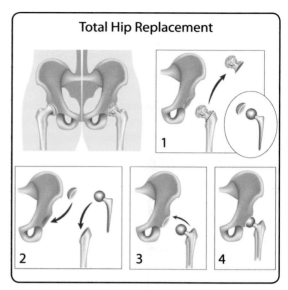

Figure 3.9

- External fixation – Treating fractures with extensive tissue damage with either an optimal frame (placing pins with connected tubes to create a frame) or modular external fixator (rod to rod construction) to hold the bones together. (See **Figure 3.10**)

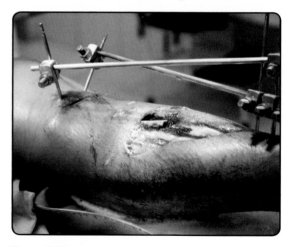

Figure 3.10

- Hip pinning – Stabilizing broken hip bones with surgical screws, nails, rods or plates. Also known as internal fixation of the hip. (See **Figure 3.11**)

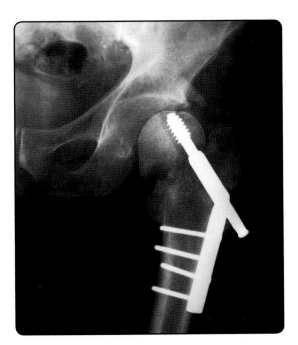

Figure 3.11

- Trigger finger release (stenosing tenosynovitis) – Making a small incision in the palm, then cutting the tendon sheath tunnel to widen it and allow the tendon to slide through it more easily.

- Tibial osteotomy – A procedure to realign the knee by wedging open the upper shin bone (tibia) to reconfigure the knee joint. The weight-bearing part of the knee is shifted from degenerative or worn tissue onto healthier tissue.

Muscular System

The muscular system works with the skeletal system to enable movement of the body or of materials through the body. (See **Figure 3.12**) Even as one sleeps, many of the more than 600 muscles in the body, including 400 which are skeletal, are actively at work to keep us alive. For example:

- Heart muscles contract to pump blood throughout the body.

- Chest muscles contract to move air in and out of the lungs.

- Muscles in the digestive tract move food and fluid through the body.

- Muscles throughout the body contract to produce heat and maintain the body's core temperature.

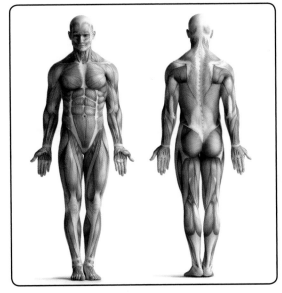

Figure 3.12

Muscles are made of up long, thin cells or fibers that run parallel to one another, and they are bundled together by connective tissue, called **fascia**. Muscle fibers have the ability to contract (shorten), and this contraction causes body movements.

> **Fascia** Band or sheet of fibrous connective tissues.

There are three types of muscle tissue: skeletal, smooth and cardiac. (See F**igure 3.13**)

- Skeletal muscles – are attached to bones by tendons. As skeletal muscles contract, the arms, legs, head or other body parts to which they are attached move. We consciously control skeletal muscles; they move only when we want them to move.

- Smooth muscles – are organized into thin, flat sheets of tissue. Smooth muscles are called involuntary or visceral muscles because they contract and function without our conscious control. They control breathing and the movement of food and fluid in the digestive system, movement of blood throughout the circulatory system and the movement of urine through the urinary system.

- Cardiac muscle – is similar to woven mesh fibers that branch out through the heart to give it more strength to pump blood. These involuntary durable muscle fibers contract and make the heart beat. In a healthy heart, they do not normally tire.

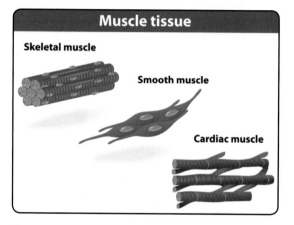

Figure 3.13

To function properly, these muscle fibers require energy (derived from consumed food) and oxygen (derived from the environment when we breathe). Their functions include movement and support, the maintenance of posture and body position and the production of body heat.

Examples of procedures involving the muscular system:

- Fasciotomy – Making an incision into the fibrous membrane covering a muscle, usually to relieve pressure from an injured or swollen muscle.

- Herniorrhaphy – Repairing a cavity wall/muscle layer that is allowing all or part of an organ to project through the opening.

- Rotator cuff repair – Repairing the muscles and ligaments of shoulder joints depend on the size and shape of the tear. Frequently-used methods are the Bankart, Putti-Platt and Bristow procedures. (See **Figure 3.14**)

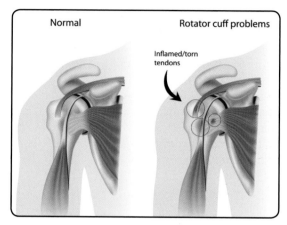

Figure 3.14

- Anterior cruciate ligament (ACL) repair – Rebuilding the ligament in the center of the knee with a new ligament from the patient's own body, or from a deceased donor, usually by knee arthroscopy. In some cases, ACL repair is done by making an incision into the knee (open procedure). (See **Figure 3.15**)

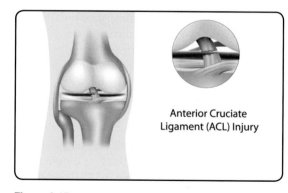

Figure 3.15

- Muscle biopsy – Removing a small sample of muscle tissue for testing in a laboratory using either a needle biopsy (inserting a needle into the muscle) or open biopsy (making a small cut in the skin and into the muscle).

- Tendon repair – Treatment that retrieves a torn tendon and reattaches it (tenodesis) to soft tissue or bone with either a small incision or arthroscopic techniques.

Nervous System (Including Sense Organs)

The nervous system is a vast communication network. It coordinates and carries messages between all parts of the body and enables us to be aware of changes in the environment—and to react accordingly. A complex series of nervous tissues, somewhat like electrical wiring, runs from the brain and spinal cord throughout the entire body. (See **Figure 3.16**)

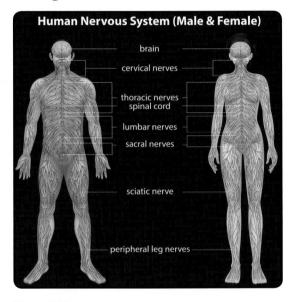

Figure 3.16

The nervous system controls all body activities and allows us to respond to stimuli. Many reactions are automatic, such as blinking when a foreign object approaches the eye. Nerve tissue carries electrical messages from the brain and spinal cord that signal muscles to contract. Other actions are more conscious and involve emotion, reason and memory. Like a computer, the brain stores information based on past experiences that can later be communicated to the body by the nervous system.

Anatomically, the nervous system is divided into two parts: **central nervous system (CNS)** and the **peripheral nervous system (PNS)**.

The CNS consists of the brain and spinal cord, which are covered by protective membranes called meninges. The CNS is the body's control center and is the storehouse for information about what is happening or has happened within or outside the body.

The **brain**, a spongy and complex organ, is the main control unit of the CNS. It is comprised of more than 100 billion nerve cells.

The brain is divided into three parts, each carries out a specific function: **cerebrum**, **cerebellum** and **brain stem**. (See **Figure 3.17**)

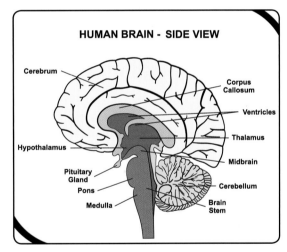

Figure 3.17

The cerebrum is the largest part of the human brain. It functions to:

- Manage the nerve impulses that allow us to think, speak and remember.

- Control most voluntary muscle contractions.

- Interpret information gathered by the senses.

- Influence the foundation of personality, emotions and attitudes.

Central nervous system (CNS) The part of the nervous system that includes the brain and spinal cord.

Peripheral nervous system (PNS) All nerve tissue outside the central nervous system.

Brain The main control unit of the central nervous system.

Cerebrum The largest part of the brain. It controls mental activities and movement.

Cerebellum The second largest part of the brain. It controls muscle coordination, body balance and posture.

Brain stem This controls many automatic body functions, such as heartbeat and breathing.

The cerebrum is divided into two halves (hemispheres). Each half controls different mental activities and movement on the opposite side of the body. A series of nerve pathways run between each half to facilitate communication.

The cerebellum is located inferior (below) and posterior (behind) the cerebrum. It is the second largest part of the brain, and its role is to adjust the motor impulses that control muscular coordination, body balance and posture.

The brain stem is located at the base of the brain and is formed by bundles of nerves that extend from the cerebrum and cerebellum. The lowest part of the brain stem (the medulla oblongata) joins the brain to the spinal cord. It contains nerve centers that control many automatic body functions, including heartbeat and breathing.

PNS involves the network of nerves and sense organs that branch out of the CNS and connect the CNS to other parts of the body. One part (the autonomic nervous system) controls all involuntary body processes, like heartbeat and peristalsis (the rippling motion of muscles in the digestive tract that mixes food with gastric juices to form a thin liquid). Other nerves are under direct control of the conscious mind. When we tell our hand to wave, for example, a message is sent from the brain down the spinal cord through a peripheral nerve to our hand.

The Sense Organs

The sense organs (eyes, ears, nose, tongue and skin) are accessory structures of the nervous system that provide an impression of all that surrounds us. They house special sensory receptors that are message-carrying structures. Most sense organs respond to stimuli from outside the body, while others keep track of the body's internal environment. They respond to light, sound, taste, chemicals, heat and pressure.

Eyes

Eyes (See **Figure 3.18**) are the organs of vision. They produce images by focusing light rays that are interpreted by the brain. The eyes consist of three layers of tissue:

- The sclera is the white portion of the eye and serves as an outer coat to provide protection. At the center front of the sclera is a transparent protective shield, called the cornea.

- The choroid is the middle layer of the eye that furnishes nourishment to the eye via blood vessels. The choroid layer includes the iris, a muscle that is the colored portion of the eye. A circular opening, called the pupil, is found at the center of the iris. It controls the amount of light entering the eye as it narrows or widens. Between the cornea and eye lens is the aqueous humor: a watery-like fluid that fills the anterior (front) compartment of the eye.

- The retina is the eye's third layer. It is located on the back surface of the eyeball. The eye lens focuses light onto the retina, which contains light-sensitive cells (receptors) that receive and transmit impressions to the brain through the optic nerve. The vitreous humor is a fluid-filled compartment of the eye that gives the eyeball its round shape.

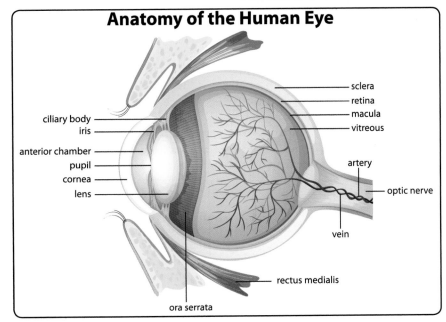

Figure 3.18

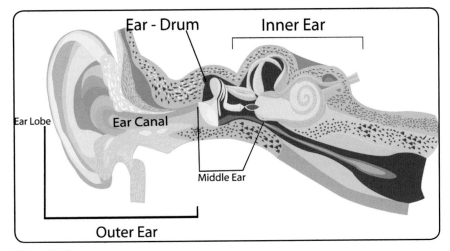

Figure 3.19

Ears

Ears are the organs of hearing. They are made of up three parts: the external, middle and inner ear. (See **Figure 3.19**) Sound waves travel through the ear to the auditory nerve that transmits nerve impulses to the brain. Here's how the ear allows us to hear:

- The external ear serves as a funnel that gathers sound waves and passes them through the ear canal to the tympanic membrane (also known as the eardrum).

- The eardrum consists of a tightly-stretched membrane that separates the outer ear canal from the middle ear. Vibrations of the eardrum enter the middle ear, which contains three tiny bones: the malleus, incus and stapes.

- The sound vibrations are then passed through these bones into the fluid-filled inner ear. There, vibrations are channeled through the fluid into a spiral-shaped tube called the cochlea, which contains the receptors or nerve endings that transmit nerve impulses to the brain.

The inner ear also contains semi-circular canals consisting of three curved tubes filled with fluid. Body balance is regulated by this fluid as it shifts with body movement. As the fluid shifts, it presses against tiny hairs stimulating nerve impulses that travel to the brain. The brain responds to these impulses by coordinating muscle movement.

Nose

The nose is the organ of smell and consists of many sensory receptors or cells. These receptors are located in the mucous membranes of the nasal cavity and are sensitive to chemicals carried through the air. The olfactory nerve endings extend to the receptors and are stimulated by different odors. Olfactory bulbs are the enlarged portion at the ends of the olfactory nerves.

Tongue

The tongue is the organ of taste and is covered with taste buds (sensory receptors). The sense of taste, like smell, is a chemical sense. Chemicals are carried by the saliva throughout the mouth. Taste buds located in different areas of the tongue can distinguish four kinds of taste: sweet, sour, bitter and salty. There are 80 different types of chemical odors, and the combination of taste and odors produces flavors.

Skin

The skin is the largest body organ. It contains many nerve endings at and below its surface. The skin, therefore, acts as an important sensory organ. Touch receptors near the skin's surface allow us to distinguish textures and to respond to heat and cold. Further below the skin surface are receptors that respond to touch and pressure. The sense of pain stimulates nerves and sends messages of potential danger to the brain.

There are numerous surgical procedures involving the nervous system:

- Craniotomy – Creating an opening in the skull to expose the brain to facilitate procedures, such as the removal of tumors and clots.

- Carpal tunnel repair – Removal of tissue or displaced bone in the wrist area to release pressure on the median nerve. (See **Figure 3.20**)

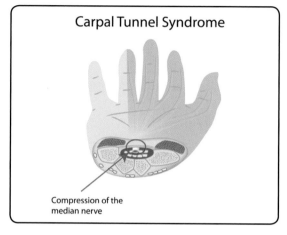

Figure 3.20

- Ulnar nerve transposition – Making an incision at the elbow area, allowing the ulnar nerve to be moved to an area that provides protection and comfort.

- Cataract extraction with implant – Removing a clouded eye lens and replacing it with a clear, artificial lens replacement. (See **Figure 3.21**)

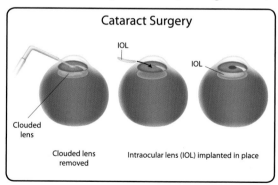

Figure 3.21

- Corneal transplant – Grafting corneal tissue from a donor eye to another to improve vision when the cornea is damaged or scarred.

- Bilateral myringotomy with tubes (BMT) – Making an incision into the tympanic membrane (eardrum) to permit fluid to drain. Small tubes are placed in the membrane to allow continuous drainage. The tubes fall out as the membrane heals.

- Stapedectomy – Removal of the stapes (an ear bone) when it has thickened and no longer transmits sound waves. It is replaced with an artificial implant to improve hearing.

- Tympanoplasty – Reconstructing the eardrum, so sound waves can be sent to the middle and inner ear.

- Split-thickness skin graft (STSG) – Cutting the skin (graft) from a donor site and using a graft mesher to expand the graft. The graft is then transplanted onto the surgical area.

Endocrine System

The endocrine system adapts to changes in the environment. During times of excitement, stress or when one feels threatened, how does the body react? Chances are, muscles tensed, the heartbeat quickened and breathing rhythm changed. These rapid changes in bodily functions are set in motion by the **hormones** or secretions produced by the glands of the endocrine system. (See **Figure 3.22**) These glands and the substances they produce have a profound influence on bodily functions, such as **metabolism**, growth and personality.

Since hormones are distributed throughout the body, the endocrine glands that produce them are not necessarily next to the organs they control. Regardless of where hormones enter the bloodstream, they continue their journey through the circulatory system until they reach their targeted organ. Tissue cells and organs recognize and accept hormones made for them and reject others that are not.

The nervous system and endocrine system work together. When the brain interprets information as a threat, it rapidly sends out nerve impulses that trigger certain endocrine glands to release their

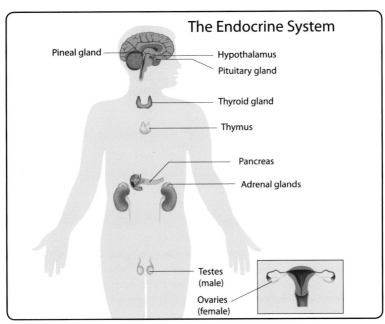

The Endocrine System

Pineal gland
Hypothalamus
Pituitary gland
Thyroid gland
Thymus
Pancreas
Adrenal glands
Testes (male)
Ovaries (female)

Figure 3.22

hormones into the bloodstream. In a fearful situation, the hormones cause the heartbeat to accelerate and prepare muscles for action. In this state, one is ready for fight or flight (to defend or run).

The major glands of the endocrine system include:

- Pituitary gland – A small, pea-shaped gland located at the base of the brain. It is considered the master gland because it helps control the activities of all other endocrine glands. Its secretions also stimulate skeletal and body growth, development of sex organs, regulation of blood pressure, the reproductive process and muscle development.

- Thyroid gland – Located at the base of the neck just below the larynx (voice box), its hormones help regulate the rate of metabolism and maintain the body's levels of calcium and phosphorous.

- Parathyroid gland – Four pea-shaped glands located on (or sometimes in) the thyroid that control the blood's calcium level.

- Adrenal glands – During sudden stress these glands, which are located on top of each kidney, release adrenalin that increases our heart rate and physical strength. Adrenalin also enhances our ability to think and to respond more quickly than usual in emergency situations.

- Pancreas – Located just below the stomach, this gland contains cells organized into groups, known as the Islets of Langerhans. Two primary hormones are produced by the pancreatic islets: **insulin**, which reduces the level of sugar in the bloodstream, and **glucagon,** which can increase the blood's sugar level.

- Ovaries (female sex glands) – Produce two hormones: estrogen and progesterone. Estrogen is responsible for the development of female characteristics, and progesterone, together with estrogen, regulates the menstrual cycle.

- Testes – Male sex glands that produce the hormone testosterone that stimulates the development of masculine characteristics.

> **Hormones** Chemical messengers that travel through the blood and act on target organs.
>
> **Metabolism** The total chemical changes by which the nutritional and functional activities of an organism are maintained.
>
> **Insulin** A hormone that reduces the level of sugar in the blood.
>
> **Glucagon** A hormone that can increase the blood sugar level.

Examples of surgical procedures involving the endocrine system:

- Thyroidectomy – Removal of all or part of the thyroid gland.

- Oophorectomy – Removal of an ovary.

- Orchiectomy – Removal of a testicle.

- Pituitary tumor resection – Removal of a tumor on the pituitary gland, which is located at the bottom of the skull.

- Thyroid excision – Removal of nodules and/ or goiters (enlargements) on the thyroid.

- Adrenalectomy – Removal of one or both (bilateral adrenalectomy) adrenal glands.

Reproductive System

Everyone begins life as a single cell, formed when two other cells join together in a process called fertilization. The male sex cell is produced by the male reproductive system and is called **sperm**. The female sex cell (egg) is called **ovum** (plural: ova) and is produced by the female reproductive system. Both sperm and ovum contain rod-shaped structures called **chromosomes** that are responsible for inherited characteristics passed on from parent to child. Each sex cell contains 23 chromosomes; therefore, a fertilized egg consists of 46 chromosomes, receiving 23 from the sperm and 23 from the ovum.

The male reproductive system consists of two **testes**. These oval-shaped glands are located in a skin-covered, pouch-like structure called the **scrotum**. Two tube structures are also in the scrotum. The **epididymis** is a tube that carries sperm cells from the testes to the **vas deferens** (a thick-walled tube structure approximately 18 inches long) where they mature. The vas deferens then carries sperm to a hollow chamber, called the **seminal vesicle**, located behind the bladder.

The seminal vesicle joins with the vas deferens to form the ejaculatory duct. The secretions of the seminal vesicle are called **semen**, which bathes and nourishes the sperm cells. In the **ejaculatory duct**, the semen-containing sperm, upon ejaculation, enter the **urethra**, a membranous canal running through the **penis**, which transfers the sperm to the female's body.

The **prostate gland** is a partly glandular and partly muscular gland surrounding the neck of the bladder. It secretes a fluid, which is part of the semen, and stimulates sperm motility (movement).

The female reproductive system consists of the **vagina**, a muscular canal approximately 4 ½ inches long through which a baby passes during birth. It extends from an external opening to the **cervix** (neck of the uterus). The **uterus** is located between the rectum and urinary bladder, and is a hollow, pear-shaped organ. It is lined with a fluffy vascular layer of tissue called **endometrium**. The fertilized ovum embeds itself into the endometrium, which sloughs off (separates) during menstruation if the ovum is not fertilized.

The **fallopian tubes** (oviducts) extend from two openings on each side of the anterior portion of the uterus. The distal (farthest) ends of the fallopian tubes are funnel-shaped, and finger-like projections, called **fimbriae**, extend from them. They are located near, but not attached to, the **ovaries**. The fimbriae draw the ovum into the fallopian tube where it travels to the uterus.

Sperm The male sex cell.

Ovum The female sex cell.

Chromosomes Rod-shaped structures responsible for inherited characteristics passed on from parent to child.

Testes Male reproductive gland that forms and secretes sperm and several fluid elements in semen.

Scrotum Sac in which testes are suspended.

Epididymis A tube that carries sperm cells from the testes to the vas deferens.

Vas deferens A duct that transfers sperm from the epididymus to the seminal vesicle.

Seminal vesicle A gland that produces semen.

Semen Mixture of sperm cells and secretions from several male reproductive glands.

Ejaculatory duct A duct formed by the joining of the seminal vesicle with the vas deferens, through which semen moves during ejaculation.

Urethra A tube that discharges urine.

Penis Male organ of urination and intercourse.

Prostate gland Produces a fluid element in semen that stimulates the movement of sperm.

Vagina The muscular canal in a female that extends from an external opening to the neck of the uterus.

Cervix Lower end (neck) of the uterus.

Uterus A female organ within which the fetus develops during pregnancy.

Endometrium Lining of the uterus.

Fallopian tubes Slender tubes that convey the ova (eggs) from the ovaries to the uterus.

Fimbriae Finger-like projections extending from the fallopian tubes that draw ova (eggs) into the fallopian tube.

Ovaries Female reproductive organs.

Examples of surgical procedures involving the reproductive system:

- Orchiopexy – Relocating a non-descended testicle to the correct location in the scrotum.

- Transurethral resection of the prostate (TURP) – Removal of part of the prostate gland through the insertion of instruments across the urethra to reach the prostate internally.

- Radical prostatectomy – Removal of the prostate gland using an incision in the abdomen, and also the urinary bladder. Frequently, additional tissue is biopsied for invasion of cancer cells.

- Hysterectomy – Removal of the uterus.

- Bilateral salpingo-oophorectomy (BSO) – Removal of fallopian tubes and ovaries.

- Endometrial ablation – Scarring or removal of the inner lining of the uterus to treat abnormal bleeding.

- Dilation and curettage (D&C) – Widening of the cervix (opening of the uterus) to permit evacuation of the contents or scraping of the lining of the uterus.

- Ectopic pregnancy – Removal of a fertilized ovum growing in the fallopian tube to prevent complications, such as hemorrhage, shock and scarring of the fallopian tube.

- Pelviscopy – Visualization of the pelvic cavity (lower abdomen) using an endoscope for medical diagnosis or treatment of female reproductive organs.

- Tubal ligation – Cutting, burning, tying or applying a clip on the fallopian tubes to prevent future pregnancies. (See **Figure 3.23**)

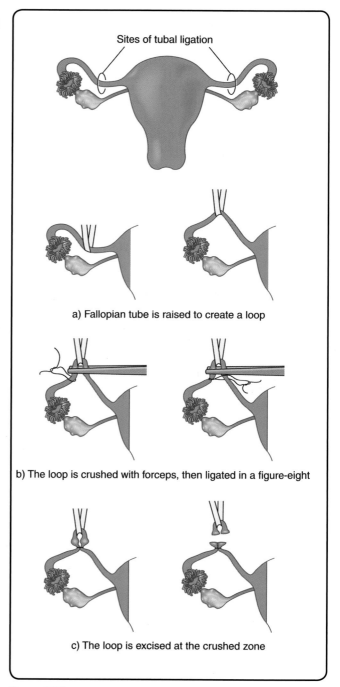

Sites of tubal ligation

a) Fallopian tube is raised to create a loop

b) The loop is crushed with forceps, then ligated in a figure-eight

c) The loop is excised at the crushed zone

Figure 3.23

- Vasectomy – A surgical procedure for male sterilization and/or birth control. (See **Figure 3.24**)

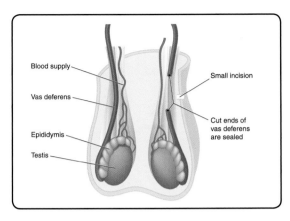

Figure 3.24

Urinary and Excretory Systems

The urinary system provides "pollution control" by eliminating body waste. This process takes place as blood is filtered by the urinary system. Urine is a water solution consisting of various waste substances that are products of metabolism. It obtains its color from excreted bile pigments and may be a shade of amber, pale or clear. Depending on the amount of liquid intake or loss through perspiration, an average adult may excrete between 1000cc to 1800cc of urine during a 24-hour period. In males, the urinary and reproductive systems are closely related and comprise the genitourinary system. In the female, however, the two systems are not interrelated.

Organs of the urinary system in both sexes include: (See **Figure 3.25**)

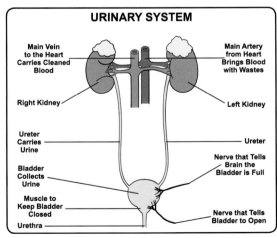

Figure 3.25

- **Kidneys** – Two bean-shaped organs containing a vast network of vessels and tubules, called nephron, that act as a filter to remove excess water and waste substances (including salts and minerals) from the blood to produce urine.

- **Ureters** – Two tube-like structures that extend from each kidney and connect them to the urinary bladder. The peristaltic (automatic constriction and relaxation) action of the ureters moves urine from the kidneys to the urinary bladder.

- **Urinary bladder** – Serves as a reservoir for urine. It is a muscular, membranous sack located in the pelvis just anterior (front) of the sigmoid colon and posterior to (behind) the pubis. The bladder is flexible and its size depends upon the amount of urine present. The average capacity ranges from between 300cc to 500cc in adults. As the amount of urine in the urinary bladder increases, it applies pressure on the bladder walls, sending an impulse to the central nervous system. As the bladder wall contracts, the sphincter muscle at the junction of the urethra relaxes and urine is released.

- Urethra – A membranous canal or tube that connects the urinary bladder to outside the body to eliminate urine. In the male the urethra is approximately 20cm long. It passes through the prostate gland and pelvic wall, and extends through the penis. The female urethra is about 4cm long. It runs from the bladder through the sphincter muscles to the external meatus (opening) located at the anterior (front) of the vagina.

Kidneys Organs that remove excess water and waste substances from the blood in a process that yields urine.

Ureters Tube-like structures extending from the kidneys to the urinary bladder that move urine between these organs.

Urinary bladder The reservoir for urine.

The excretory system removes toxic (poisonous) waste substances. The kidneys (urinary system) and lungs (respiratory system) also perform excretory functions, as do the **liver** and **skin**.

The liver is another filter for the blood. It removes amino acids and can neutralize some harmful toxins. It can also convert hemoglobin from worn-out blood cells into substances the body requires.

Skin contains sweat glands, oils, hair and nails. Dead skin cells form hair and nails. Sweat glands remove excess water, salt and other bodily wastes. These are located in the dermis (inner layer of skin) and consist of coiled tubes connected to pores in the skin's surface. The sweat glands, through the process of perspiration, produce and excrete sweat. Perspiration rids the body of waste and also helps to regulate the body's temperature by cooling its outside surface. The excretion of oil by the sebaceous glands keeps the skin soft and prevents hair from becoming too dry or brittle.

> **Liver** An organ that filters the blood to remove amino acids and neutralize some harmful toxins.
>
> **Skin** This organ contains sweat glands that, through the process of perspiration, produces and eliminates sweat.

Examples of surgical procedures involving the urinary system:

* Nephrectomy – Removal of the kidney.

* Lithotripsy (kidney stone shock wave treatment) – Serves to crush stones that form in the kidney and become stuck in an ureter. The procedure involves decreasing the size of the stones with a laser or shock waves or removing them using a long, flexible instrument called a stone basket. (See **Figure 3.26**)

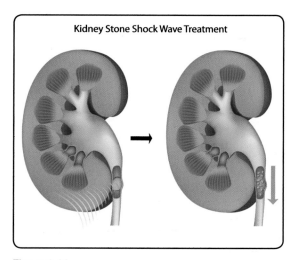

Kidney Stone Shock Wave Treatment

Figure 3.26

* Cystoscopy – Viewing the urinary bladder using an endoscope.

The Respiratory System

The respiratory system (See **Figure 3.27**) supplies the body with oxygen and removes carbon dioxide.

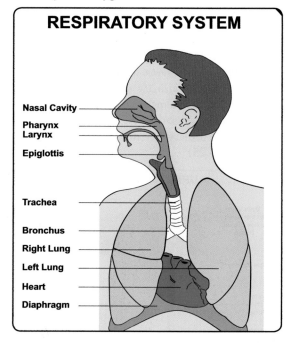

RESPIRATORY SYSTEM

Nasal Cavity
Pharynx
Larynx
Epiglottis
Trachea
Bronchus
Right Lung
Left Lung
Heart
Diaphragm

Figure 3.27

This exchange of gases is accomplished automatically as one breathes in a two-step process: inspiration (inhaling air into the lungs) and expiration (exhaling air from the lungs). Air contains impurities, such as dirt, dust and microorganisms, and these are filtered out by the respiratory system.

The primary organs of the respiratory system are:

- **Nose** (nasal cavity) and **mouth** – During inspiration, air enters the nostrils (nasal openings) and mouth. Air in the nose is filtered, moistened and warmed.

- **Pharynx** – Air passes to the pharynx (throat), which is the crossroads of the nose, mouth, voice box, and **esophagus**. Food continues down the esophagus, while air passes through the **larynx** (voice box) to the **trachea**.

- Trachea (windpipe) – The trachea divides into two tube-like structures, the right and left **bronchi**, that extend into the **lungs**.

- Lungs – Air continues through the bronchi to the bronchioles, a series of many smaller tubes extending from each bronchus (somewhat like branches of a tree). At the end of each bronchiole are small clusters of air sacs, called alveoli, that comprise the lungs' tissue. Alveoli and each alveolus are covered by a thin wall surrounded by a vast network of capillaries (tiny blood vessels). There the blood picks up oxygen from the inspired air and releases the waste gas, carbon dioxide, during expiration.

Nose Organ of smell; also filters the air we breath.

Mouth Opening through which air, food and beverages enter the body; beginning of the alimentary canal.

Pharynx Throat.

Esophagus Connects the throat to the stomach.

Larynx Voice box.

Trachea Windpipe.

Bronchi The main passageway for air to travel from the trachea to the lungs.

Lungs Main organs of the respiratory system whose function is transporting oxygen into the blood and removing carbon dioxide from the blood.

The right lung consists of three lobes. The left lung consists of two lobes to allow space for the heart.

The lungs are located in the thoracic cavity (chest), where they are covered by thin membranes, called pleura, and protected by the skeletal rib cage and sternum. The pleura secrete a lubricating fluid that permits smooth movement of the lungs during the respiratory cycle.

The diaphragm is a muscle located below the lungs. It contracts and causes the chest cavity to expand to allow more space for air. During expiration, the diaphragm relaxes and air is forced out of the lungs.

Examples of surgical procedures involving the respiratory system:

- Thoracotomy – Making an opening into the thoracic cavity (chest) to give surgeons access to the lungs and heart.

- Thoracoscopy – Viewing the thoracic (chest) cavity with an endoscope for diagnosis or treatment.

- Pneumonectomy – Removal of a lung.

- Tracheotomy – Making an incision into the trachea. (See **Figure 3.28**)

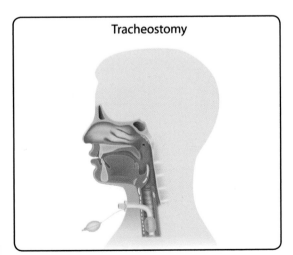

Tracheostomy

Figure 3.28

- Lobectomy - Removal of a lobe of an organ, usually referring to the brain, the lung or the liver.

- Laryngectomy – Removal of the larynx (voice box).

- Bronchoscopy – Visualizing the bronchus with an endoscope.

- Septoplasty – Straightening or removing cartilage and/or bone in the nose when the nasal septum is deformed, injured or fractured.

- Endoscopic sinus surgery (ESS) – Removal of bone defects or inflamed tissue of the paranasal sinuses to allow the sinuses to drain.

The Digestive System

The human body, like any other complex piece of machinery, requires a source of energy or fuel to keep it functioning. The body gets its fuel from the chemicals (nutrients) in food.

The function of the digestive system (See **Figure 3.29**) is to convert food into energy for the body. The human body requires six basic categories of nutrients: proteins, carbohydrates, fats, water, minerals and vitamins. A well-balanced diet is important to keep the body healthy and strong.

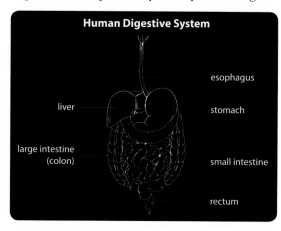

Human Digestive System

esophagus

liver

stomach

large intestine (colon)

small intestine

rectum

Figure 3.29

The process of digestion breaks food down mechanically and chemically so it can be absorbed by body cells or discharged as waste. The pathway that food takes through the digestive system is called the **alimentary canal** (digestive tract).

The alimentary canal is approximately 30 feet long, and consists of the mouth, esophagus, **stomach**, **small intestine**, **large intestine**, **rectum** and **anus**.

The liver, gallbladder and pancreas are accessory organs of the digestive system.

The salivary, gastric and intestinal glands are accessory structures to the digestive system that contribute to the process of digestion.

A review of the components of the alimentary canal allows us to study the digestive process.

- Mouth – The digestive process begins in the mouth. There, food is softened by saliva secreted by salivary glands located throughout the mouth. The teeth tear and grind the softened food into smaller particles that allow it to be easily swallowed. The food then passes through the esophagus.

- Esophagus – A somewhat flexible, muscular tube that produces peristaltic contractions, which move food into the stomach.

- Stomach – An elongated and muscular J-shaped pouch that serves as a reservoir for food as gastric gland secretions (mucin, hydrochloric acid, and enzymes) convert the food into a semi-liquid material, called chyme.

- Small intestine – From the stomach, the liquified food enters the small intestine (an organ approximately 20 to 23 feet long). This is where the greatest amount of digestion and absorption of nutrients into the body cells occurs. The small intestine is divided into three portions: duodenum, jejunum and ileum. Bile (produced by the liver and stored in the gallbladder), along with pancreatic and intestinal juices, facilitates digestion in the small intestine.

- Large intestine (colon) – Material that is not absorbed by the small intestine enters the large intestine (colon), which is approximately five to six feet long. The first few inches of the large intestine are called the cecum, from which the appendix extends. The large intestine consists of six portions: ascending colon, transverse colon, descending colon, sigmoid colon, rectum and anus. Peristaltic action moves food through the large intestine where the absorption of water and electrolytes or salt occurs.

- Rectum and anus – The rectum is the last several inches of the large intestine where the remaining waste (feces) becomes dehydrated and is eliminated through the anus.

Alimentary canal The pathway that food takes through the digestive system; also called digestive tract.

Stomach A pouch that serves as a reservoir for food that has been consumed.

Small intestine The organ in the digestive system where the greatest amount of digestion and absorption of nutrients into the body cells occurs.

Large intestine (colon) The digestive organ that dehydrates digestive residues (feces).

Rectum The last several inches of the large intestine.

Anus The lower opening of the alimentary canal.

Examples of surgical procedures involving the digestive system:

- Appendectomy – Removal of the appendix.

- Parotidectomy – Removal of a salivary gland (parotid) because of tumor formation.

- Gastrectomy – Removal of the stomach. Other procedures include removal of portions of the stomach [e.g., hemi (half) gastrectomy or gastric sleeve]. (See **Figure 3.30**)

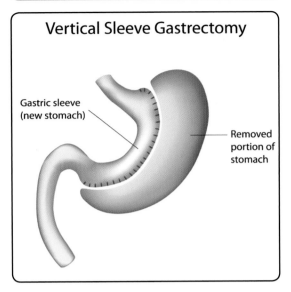

Figure 3.30

- Gastric bypass – Isolating a small portion of the stomach and suturing part of the small intestine to it to treat morbid obesity. Food intake is then limited to the small part of the stomach. (See **Figure 3.31**)

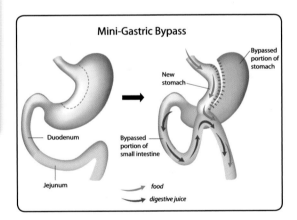

Figure 3.31

- Gastric banding – An inflatable silicone device placed around the top portion of the stomach to treat obesity. (See **Figure 3.32**)

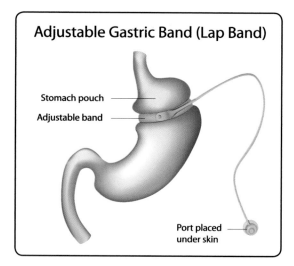

Figure 3.32

- Cholecystectomy – Removal of the gallbladder with a surgical incision or by endoscopic surgery, called laparoscopic cholecystectomy. (See **Figure 3.33**)

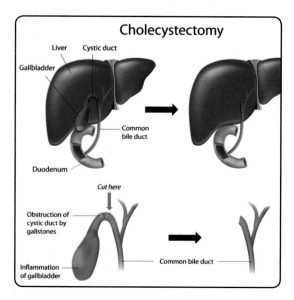

Figure 3.33

- Colectomy – Removal of all or part of the large intestine.

- Laparoscopic cholecystectomy– Removal of the gallbladder with endoscopic instrumentation.

The Circulatory System

The circulatory system (See **Figure 3.34**) is the body's primary transportation network. It delivers nutrients and oxygen to body cells, and carries away carbon dioxide and other harmful waste products from them. This is accomplished as blood is pumped through 60,000 miles of blood vessels in the body.

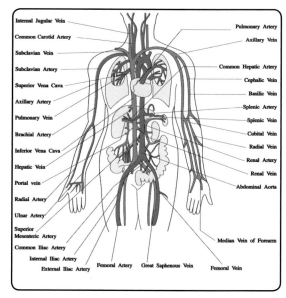

Figure 3.34

The lymphatic system (See **Figure 3.35**) is a subsidiary of the circulatory system and serves a vital role in the body's defense against disease.

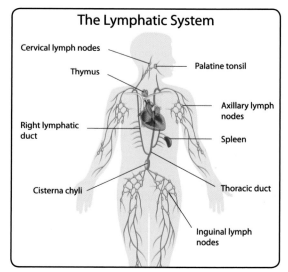

Figure 3.35

The lymphatic system consists of a series of tiny vessels located throughout the body that carry clear liquid fluid (lymph) that originates from blood plasma. Large numbers of lymph nodes (tissue masses containing special cells called lymphocytes) that filter bacteria and other harmful materials out of the lymph are located in the lymph and blood vessels. Lymph flows from the lymph vessels into two veins located in the neck region to return lost fluid back into the bloodstream.

Tonsils are one type of a lymph node, and they are located on both sides of the base of the tongue in the throat. (See **Figure 3.36**)

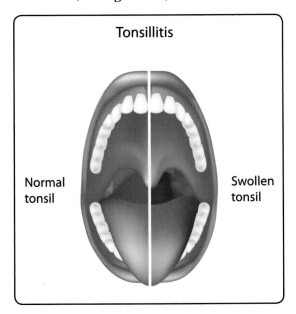

Tonsillitis

Normal tonsil

Swollen tonsil

Figure 3.36

Sentinal lymph nodes are frequently identified during cancer surgery. The surgeon tries to find the first (sentinal) lymph node where the cancer cells have started to spread.

Blood is a type of connective tissue fluid that moves throughout the circulatory system and transports many important substances. The body contains an average of five to seven liters of blood. Blood is a mixture of plasma, red blood cells (erythrocytes), white blood cells (leukocytes) and platelets:

- **Plasma** – More than 55% of blood is made up of plasma, a yellowish liquid that is composed of water (92%) and proteins. Plasma serves as the vehicle of transportation for dissolved nutrients, enzymes, waste and other substances through the body.

- **Red blood cells** – These structures have thin centers that allow them to be pliable when moving through narrow capillaries. Red blood cells are rich in hemoglobin (an iron protein) that picks up oxygen in the lungs, transports it to all the body cells and then transports carbon dioxide back to the lungs. These cells are produced in the bone marrow and have a life span of approximately 120 days. Worn out or damaged red blood cells are broken down in the liver and destroyed by the spleen.

- **White blood cells** – Some white blood cells are twice as large as red blood cells, and their life span can range from hours to years. White blood cells are also produced by bone marrow and their purpose is to attack, destroy and digest disease-producing organisms that enter the body.

- **Platelets** – These tiny cell fragments detach from bone marrow and enter the bloodstream. They have no color or nucleus, and last for a maximum of 10 days. Enzymes released by the platelets act on other blood components to create fibrin. This chemical weaves across cells in blood vessels, and traps blood cells and plasma that will harden and clot.

Blood A type of connective tissue fluid that transports many substances throughout the circulatory system.

Plasma The largest component of the blood. Plasma transports nutrients throughout the body and helps remove wastes from the body.

Red blood cells Blood cells that carry oxygen throughout the body.

White blood cells Blood cells that circulate in the blood and help defend the body against infection or foreign invaders.

Platelets Blood cells whose function is to help the blood to clot.

Circulation in the body is a continuous process, traveling the same route throughout the body all the time. Blood moves from the heart to the lungs and then back to the **heart** where it is pumped to all the cells of the body through a system of vessels. Blood then returns back to the heart to be recurculated.

The vessels that carry blood away from the heart are called **arteries**. **Veins** are the vessels that carry blood back towards the heart. **Capillaries** are the tiny vessels abundant throughout the body that serve as connections between veins and arteries.

The heart (See **Figure 3.37**) is a muscular organ, about the size of a fist, that pumps five liters of blood through the body every minute, while resting only between beats. Located in its upper right side is a "pacemaker" that signals the heart muscle to contract; this controls the heartbeat. Here's how the heart works:

- The heart consists of four hollow chambers: two on each side.

- A thick tissue wall, called the septum, separates the right and left sides of the heart.

- The upper chambers of the heart are called **atria** and the lower chambers are called **ventricles**.

- Deoxygenated blood (blood that has had oxygen removed by the cells) returns to the heart and enters the right atrium.

- As the right atrium becomes full, a tissue flap (called a heart valve) opens. It allows blood to flow into the right ventricle.

- When the right ventricle is full, the valve closes to prevent backflow of blood.

- As the right ventricle contracts, blood is forced out of the heart through the pulmonary artery into the lungs where it is oxygenated.

- The oxygenated blood leaves the lungs through the pulmonary veins and enters the left atrium.

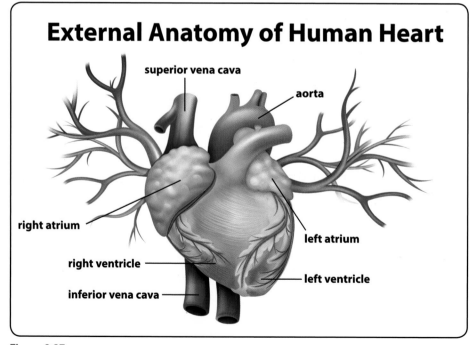

External Anatomy of Human Heart

superior vena cava

aorta

right atrium

left atrium

right ventricle

left ventricle

inferior vena cava

Figure 3.37

- As the left atrium becomes full, the left atrium heart valve opens and the blood flows into the left ventricle. As the left ventricle becomes full, the left atrium valve closes, the left ventricle contracts, and oxygenated blood leaves the heart.

As the heart contracts, blood is forced out of the left ventricle through the aortic valve into the **aorta**, the largest blood vessel in the body. The aorta is an artery that carries blood away from the heart, and it branches out into a vast network of smaller arteries throughout the body. The left ventricle pumps blood throughout the entire body, working about six times as hard as the right ventricle, which only pumps blood a short distance.

> **Heart** The muscular organ that pumps blood throughout the body.
>
> **Arteries** Vessels that carry blood away from the heart.
>
> **Veins** Vessels that carry blood back to the heart.
>
> **Capillaries** Vessels that serve as connections between veins and arteries.
>
> **Atria** The two upper chambers of the heart.
>
> **Ventricles** The two lower chambers of the heart.
>
> **Aorta** The largest blood vessel in the body.

Examples of surgical procedures involving the circulatory system:

- Tonsillectomy – Removal of lymph tissue in the pharynx (throat).

- Adenoidectomy – Removal of tonsil tissue at the end of the soft palate (roof of the mouth).

- Arteriovenous (AV) fistula – Suturing the radial artery and cephalic vein together in the lower arm to allow the dilated (enlarged) vein to be used for large bore needle insertion for renal dialysis.

- Aneurysm repair – Abdominal aortic aneurysm (AAA) – Removing a weakened, balloon-like area in the aorta and replacing it with a synthetic product. (See **Figure 3.38**)

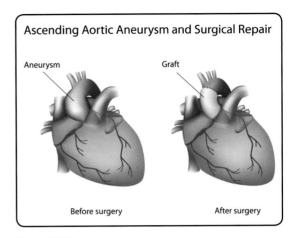

Figure 3.38

- Pacemaker insertion - A small electrical medical device implanted in a patient to make the heart beat regularly. (See **Figure 3.39**)

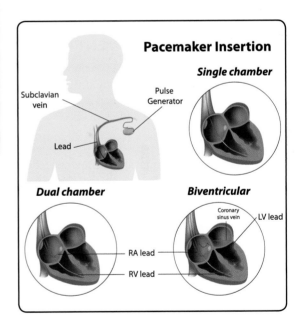

Figure 3.39

- Hemorrhoidectomy – Removal of swollen inflamed veins from the anus.

- Coronary artery bypass graft (CABG) – Removal of a vein, usually from a lower limb, to bypass the blocked section of the coronary arteries. (See **Figure 3.40**)

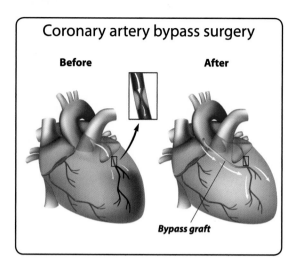

Coronary artery bypass surgery

Before   **After**

Bypass graft

Figure 3.40

- Carotid endarterectomy – A procedure to reduce the risk of stroke by removing plaque from the carotid artery that causes lack of brain oxygenation.

ANATOMY AND INSTRUMENT NAMES

CS professionals who familiarize themselves with common aspects of human anatomy and physiology may find it easier to understand the need for specialized instruments to address a specific body system.

The names of many surgical instruments reflect the anatomical region for which they have been designed. For this reason, taking the time to learn how the body works will help CS professionals better understand the purpose of a particular instrument, and help remember its name.

Here are just a few examples of the hundreds of instruments that reflect the anatomical area from which their names are derived:

- Aortic compressor

- Vaginal speculum

- Adenotome

- Eyelid retractor

- Urethratome

- Bowel forceps

- Anal retractor

- Lacrimal duct probes

- Hip skid

- Uterine sounds

- Brain spatula

CONCLUSION

While Central Service technicians do not provide direct patient care, an understanding of basic anatomy and common surgical procedures can help improve communication with surgery and other procedural units and, therefore, improve patient outcomes. A basic understanding of anatomical terms can also increase instrument knowledge. Both enhancements make it easier to function in the role of surgical support.

The human body is incredibly sophisticated. With its many parts, networks and functions, it is amazing to contemplate how these various systems must work together in a grand orchestral maneuver, and how disease or injury can disrupt the symphony. By gaining a basic understanding of how the body works and the common surgical procedures that are performed to treat certain conditions, CS technicians can become more knowledgeable about the instruments and devices in their care, and improve their ability to communicate with the surgical team.

RESOURCES

Brooks M. *Exploring Medical Language: A Student-Directed Approach. Fifth Edition.* Mosby Inc. 2002.

Davies J. *Essentials of Medical Terminology. Third Edition.* Delmar Publishers Inc. 2002.

Fremgen B. *Medical Terminology: An Anatomy and Physiology Systems Approach.* Prentice-Hall Inc. 1997.

Gylys B. *Medical Terminology Simplified: A Programmed Learning Approach by Body Systems.* F. A. Davis Company. 1995.

Gylys B, Wedding M. *Medical Terminology: A Systems Approach. Third Edition.* F. A. Davis Company. 1995.

Isler C. *The Patient's Guide to Medical Terminology. Third Edition.* Health Information Press. 1997.

Lillis C. *A Concise Introduction to Medical Terminology. Fourth Edition.* Appleton & Lange. 1997.

McCann Schilling J. *Medical Terminology Made Incredibly Easy.* Springhouse Corp. 2001.

CENTRAL SERVICE TERMS

Anatomy

Physiology

Cell

Cell membrane

Cytoplasm

Nucleus

Tissue

Organ

System

Tendon

Ligament

Cartilage

Ossification

Joint

Fascia

Central nervous system (CNS)

Peripheral nervous system (PNS)

Brain

Cerebrum

Cerebellum

Brain stem

Hormones

Metabolism

Insulin

Glucagon

Sperm

Ovum

Chromosomes

Testes

Scrotum

Epidilymis

Vas deferens

Seminal vesicle

Semen

Ejaculatory duct

Urethra

Penis

Prostate gland

Vagina

Cervix

Uterus

Endometrium

Fallopian tubes

Fimbriae

Ovaries

Kidneys

Ureters

Urinary bladder

Liver

Skin

Nose

Mouth

Pharynx

Esophagus

Larynx

Trachea

Bronchi

Lungs

Alimentary canal (digestive tract)

Stomach

Small intestine

Large intestine (colon)

Rectum

Anus

Blood

Plasma

Red blood cells

White blood cells

Platelets

Arteries

Veins

Capillaries

Heart

Atria

Ventricles

Aorta

Chapter 4

Microbiology for Central Service Technicians

Learning Objectives

As a result of successfully completing this chapter, readers will be able to:

1. Define the term "microbiology" and explain why it is important for Central Service professionals to have a basic understanding of its science

2. Restate basic facts about microorganisms

3. Identify common ways to identify and classify microorganisms by:
    - Shape
    - Color change
    - Need for oxygen

4. Explain environmental conditions necessary for bacterial growth and survival

5. Provide basic information about non-bacterial organisms:
    - Viruses
    - Protozoa
    - Fungi
    - Prions

6. Review basic procedures to control and eliminate microorganisms

INTRODUCTION

Central Service (CS) professionals are sometimes daunted by microbiology because much of its terminology is unfamiliar and because it deals with a world that cannot be seen without a microscope; however, we can see the effects that microorganisms have on us. For example, we have all become sick with infections like colds or the flu and, even though we didn't see the microorganisms that infected us, we felt their effects.

Microscopic invaders can enter our bodies and cause serious illness and even death. How can something so small have such massive power over the human body? Why can anyone, even the strongest and healthiest person, become infected by microorganisms? Why does the risk of infection increase in people whose immune systems or natural body defenses are compromised? CS technicians must have a clear understanding of basic information about microorganisms. This chapter will help answer these and related questions about how these unseen organisms impact everyone in the healthcare facility.

OVERVIEW OF MICROBIOLOGY

Most people have some understanding of microbiology. They know that it is not wise to eat food that falls on the floor, touch a sick person's soiled facial tissues or share eating utensils. They know they should wash their hands before eating and after using the restroom. They understand that taking these precautions helps to protect against germs. For the average person, this limited understanding of the world of microbes is typically enough; however, CS technicians must have a better understanding about **microbiology** for two reasons:

- They have the responsibility to protect patients from microorganisms in the healthcare environment.

- The nature of their job duties places them and their co-workers in harm's way for exposure to harmful microorganisms.

Microorganisms are tiny organisms that can only be seen with a microscope. Examples of how small they are can be seen in **Figures 4.1** and **4.2** that show magnified photos of a contaminated needle.

> **Microbiology** The study of microorganisms. The scientific study of the nature, life and action of microorganisms.

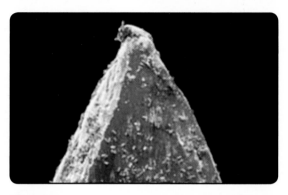

Figure 4.1

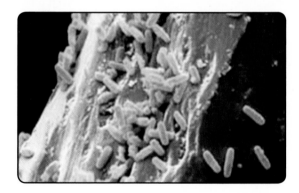

Figure 4.2

CS technicians should be able to recognize the conditions that favor the growth of microorganisms and recognize that even though we cannot see microorganisms with the naked eye, they are present in our environment. The surgical instruments, equipment and utensils processed by CS personnel every day are **contaminated** with microorganisms that pose a threat to patients, CS professionals and other facility personnel.

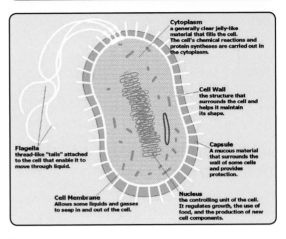

Figure 4.3

Contamination The state of being soiled by contact with infectious organisms or other material.

In this chapter, we will provide a broad overview of microbiology, including:

- Basic facts regarding microorganisms.

- Beneficial vs. dangerous microorganisms.

- How microorganisms are identified and classified.

- The conditions microorganisms need to grow and reproduce.

- How microorganisms are transmitted.

- How microorganisms can be controlled and eliminated.

Basic Facts Regarding Microorganisms

Cells are the basic units of all living organisms (plants, animals, protozoa and bacteria), and they are the smallest unit that can live, grow and reproduce. Cells differ in size and shape, but they all have: (See **Figure 4.3**)

- A nucleus (the controlling unit of the cell).

- Cytoplasm (the material that fills the cell).

- Cell membrane (the outer membrane that allows some liquids and gasses to seep in and out of the cell).

Bacterial cells differ from both plant and animal cells because they have no membrane to separate the nucleus (one strand of DNA) from the cytoplasm. Plants and animals have a nuclear membrane surrounding many strands of DNA.

BENEFICIAL VS. DANGEROUS MICROORGANISMS

Many microorganisms, or microbes, are harmless. In fact, 95% of bacteria are beneficial and essential to our lives. They are everywhere in nature and are necessary for the existence of all plants and animals. For example, microorganisms maintain the balance of chemical elements in the natural environment by breaking down dead matter and recycling carbon, nitrogen, sulfur and other elements. Microorganisms are useful in sewage treatment to convert waste materials into soluble, odorless compounds for disposal. Harmless microorganisms are also found in people: on the skin and hair, in the intestinal tract and in some bodily discharges.

Microorganisms can cause infections when introduced into a body site where they are not normally found. Microorganisms that can cause illness are called **pathogens**. Pathogens cause disease by producing powerful toxins that interfere with how body systems work. Their uncontrolled reproduction can overwhelm body systems or cause tissues to degenerate.

Pathogens are a specific concern for CS professionals, as disease-causing organisms can reside on the instruments and devices used in patient care, leading to healthcare-associated infections (HAIs). It is estimated that 722,000 patients every year acquire infections in the healthcare facility that have nothing to do with their illness.

> **Pathogen** Capable of causing disease (disease-causing microorganism).

HOW MICROORGANISMS ARE IDENTIFIED AND CLASSIFIED

There is a prescribed method for naming microorganisms. The first word in a microorganism's name (always capitalized) is the genus, or tribe, (family) of the microorganism; the second word is the specific name of the organism, also called the species. Microorganisms, like all living things, are identified and classified according to certain characteristics. We will break these organisms into two camps: bacteria and non-bacteria.

Bacteria

Characteristics

Bacteria are incredibly small; so small, in fact, that a microscope that can magnify at least 900 times is necessary to view them. Bacteria are measured by **microns** and most bacteria are one to two microns in size.

The most common ways to identify and classify bacteria are by shape, by color change and by need for oxygen (**aerobic** or **anaerobic**).

> **Micron** 1/25,000 of an inch or 1/1,000 of a millimeter.
>
> **Aerobic** Requiring the presence of air or free oxygen.
>
> **Anaerobic** Bacteria that can live in the absence of atmospheric oxygen.

Shape

One of the properties used to identify and classify bacteria is by shape, which is determined by cell wall structure. The common shapes of bacteria are:

- Spherical – These bacteria are shaped like a circle or sphere (coccus) such as *Staphylococcus aureus* and *Streptococci*. (See **Figure 4.4**)

- Rod – These bacteria are shaped like rods or bricks (bacillus). Examples include *Pseudonomas aeruginosa* and *Enterobacteria*. (See **Figure 4.5**)

- Spiral – These bacteria are shaped like spirals (spirilla). *Helicobacter pylori* is a spiral bacteria. (See **Figure 4.6**)

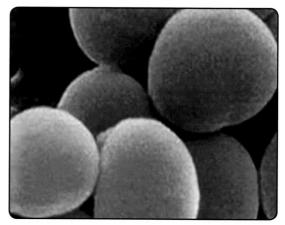

Figure 4.4

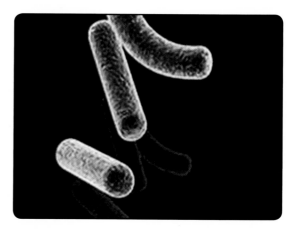

Figure 4.5

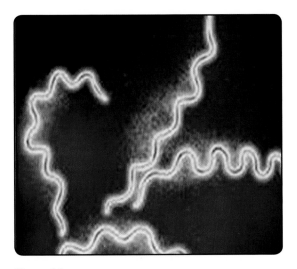

Figure 4.6

Certain bacteria can change into a different form called **endospores (spores)** by developing a thick coat around the cell's nucleus when conditions required for growth are not adequate. These spores can become infectious and produce toxins once inside the body. For example, some spores (such as *Bacillus anthracis* that causes anthrax and the *Clostridium* species that cause tetanus, botulism and severe diarrhea) are found in the soil, air and all over the body. (See **Figures 4.7** and **4.8**) Spores are very resistant to disinfection and other conditions, such as heat, making them very difficult to kill.

Examples of Spores

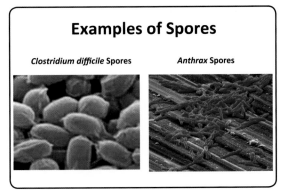

Figure 4.8

Color Change

Bacteria are normally clear and colorless organisms, and they cannot be seen, even when viewed under the microscope, unless they are dyed with a stain so the shape of each individual organism can be seen. There are two main types of staining processes used to identify the shapes and characteristics of bacteria.

Gram staining is used most frequently. Gram staining is a multi-step process using several stains and rinses. The specimen is affixed to a slide that is first stained purple, with crystal violet. It is then stained with iodine, discolored using alcohol or acetone, and, finally, stained with safranin.

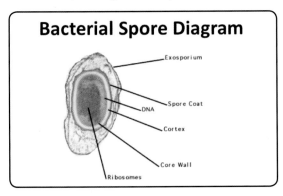

Figure 4.7

> **Endospores (spores)** Microorganisms capable of forming a thick wall around themselves enabling them to survive in adverse conditions; a resistant form of bacterium.

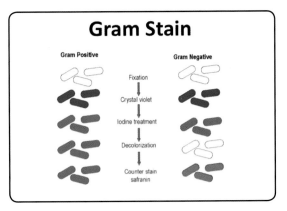

Figure 4.9

Gram-negative bacteria have an outer membrane that will not retain the purple stain after treatment with iodine; they will stain pink. Gram-negative bacteria include *Pseudonomas aeruginosa* that causes urinary tract infections, *Escherichia coli (E. coli)* and *Salmonella* species that cause intestinal disease, and *Klebsiella* species that cause pneumonia. (See **Figure 4.10**)

Gram-positive bacteria have no outer membrane and will retain the purple stain, even if a decolorizer is used. Gram-positive bacteria include *Staphylococcus aureus* that effects skin and mucous membranes, *Bacillus anthracis* that causes anthrax, and *Clostridium difficile* that causes diarrhea. (See **Figure 4.11**)

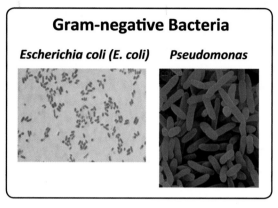

Figure 4.10

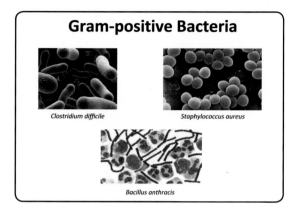

Figure 4.11

Gram Stain Chart

Gram Stain Classification		
Bacteria	**Shape**	**Gram stain**
Staphylococcus	Cocci	Gram-positive
Streptococcus	Cocci	Gram-positive
Enterococcus	Cocci	Gram-positive
Mycobacterium tuberculosis	Bacillus	Gram-positive
Mycobacterium leprae	Bacillus	Gram-positive
Clostridium tetani	Bacillus	Gram-positive
Clostridium botulinum	Bacillus	Gram-positive
Clostridium perfringes	Bacillus	Gram-positive
Bacillus anthracis	Bacillus	Gram-positive
Geobacillus species	Bacillus	Gram-positive
Neisseria meningitis	Cocci	Gram-negative
Neisseria gonorrheae	Cocci	Gram-negative
Acinetobacter	Cocci	Gram-negative
Escherichia coli (E. coli)	Bacillus	Gram-negative
Proteus	Bacillus	Gram-negative
Klebsiella	Bacillus	Gram-negative
Pseudomonis	Bacillus	Gram-negative
Salmonella typhi	Bacillus	Gram-negative
Shigilla dysenteriae	Bacillus	Gram-negative

Figure 4.12

Acid Fast (Ziehl-Neilson Stain)

Some acid-fast bacilli are rod-shaped and are very difficult to stain, but once stained and heat or other agents are used, the bacteria will resist decolorization with a dilute acid-alcohol solution. (See **Figure 4.13**) This group includes mycobacteria, such as *M. tuberculosis*, which causes tuberculosis (TB), and *M. leprae*, which causes leprosy. (See **Figure 4.14**)

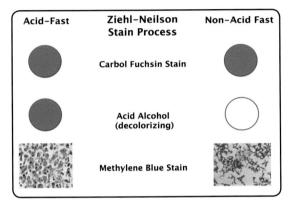

Figure 4.13

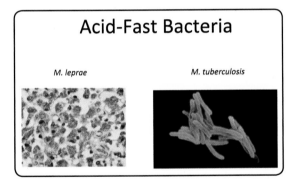

Figure 4.14

Need for Oxygen

Bacteria can also be classified according to whether they need oxygen to grow.

Aerobic bacteria require oxygen, just as humans do. They may grow in liquids; however, the liquid must have oxygen dissolved in it because oxygen is needed for respiration and metabolism.

On the other hand, anaerobic bacteria, such as *C. tetani*, which causes tetanus, and *C. botulinum*, which causes botulism, must have oxygen

eliminated from the environment for them to grow. (See **Figure 4.15**) For example tetanus (lockjaw), bacteria are introduced deep into the flesh by a nail or similar object. Then, when it is removed, the tissue and tissue juices close the wound, oxygen is removed from the environment, and the anaerobic bacteria can grow.

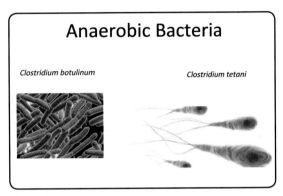

Figure 4.15

The Conditions Microorganisms Need to Grow and Reproduce

Groups of microbes have specific requirements for growth and survival. This tends to limit where they may be found. Suitable environments for bacteria are as diverse as the bacteria themselves. For example, a microbe that lives and thrives in the soil may not grow well in the vital organs of humans, and vice versa. The suitable environments for bacteria can be broken down into nutritional needs, temperature, moisture/humidity, **pH** and light.

Pathogenic bacteria are most likely to thrive where their specific nutritional needs can be met. Some, like *Staphylococci*, can grow on and in many areas of the body, skin, blood and hair follicles. Others, such as *Neisseria gonorrhoeae*, are more delicate and require a special environment, such as the mucous membranes of the reproductive system where they can live and invade deeper tissue.

Temperature requirements vary widely among bacteria, as well. **Psychrophile** bacteria like cold temperatures (59°F to 68°F); **mesophiles**, which are bacteria most pathogenic to humans, like moderate temperatures, such as 68°F to 113°F; and **thermophiles** like warm temperatures of 122°F to 158°F. (See **Figure 4.16**)

---

pH Measure of alkalinity or acidity on a scale of 0 to 14; pH of 7 is neutral (neither acid or alkaline); pH below 7 is acid; pH above 7 is alkaline.

Psychrophiles (bacteria) Bacteria whose optimum temperature for growth is 59°F to 68°F (15°C to 20°C) or below.

Mesophiles (bacteria) Bacteria that grow best at moderate temperatures: 68°F to 113°F (20°C to 45°C).

Thermophiles (bacteria) Bacteria which grow best at a temperature of 122°F to 158°F (50° to 70 °C).

Vegetative stage State of active growth of microorganisms (as opposed to the resting or spore stages).

Angstrom A unit used to measure the length of light waves.

Moisture and relative humidity play a major role in the growth and survival of microorganisms. Those which inhabit our skin, other bacteria that produce spores and the TB bacillus can survive for years in a dry state. Other species, like gonorrhea bacteria, cannot survive for more than 30 seconds when subjected to complete dryness.

Except for bacteria used in the fermentation process (such as vinegar and sauerkraut), most species will not grow in an acid pH of 4.4 or lower. Pathogenic microorganisms have an optimum pH range of 7 to 7.8, the same pH as blood.

Dark conditions are favorable to the growth of bacteria, while sunlight is lethal to organisms in their actively growing or **vegetative stage**. When spores of gram-positive bacilli are in a resting stage, they are most resistant to sunlight. The most lethal light is ultraviolet light in the range of 2537 **angstrom**, which can be used to disinfect air and purify the environments in the OR setting. Both ultraviolet light and sunlight kill bacteria by causing breaks in the nuclear DNA.

Bacteria are transmitted primarily by the droplet route (diphtheria and strep throat), by contaminated water or food (food poisoning by *Staphyloccocus* or *Salmonella* species), by direct contact (gonorrhea), through wounds (tetanus), by airborne mode (tuberculosis) and by disease-carrying animals (bubonic plague).

How Bacteria Grow

Under optimal conditions, most bacteria and other microorganisms reproduce approximately every twenty minutes in a process called **binary fission**, in which the original "mother" cell divides into two "daughter" cells.

Binary fission The typical method of bacterial reproduction in which a cell divides into two equal parts.

Temperature Requirements for Bacteria

Name	Description	Optimum Temperature for Growth
Psychrophiles	Cold Temperature	59° F to 68° F (15° C to 20° C)
Mesophiles	Moderate Temperature	68° F to 113° F (20° C to 45° C)
Thermophiles	Warm Temperature	122° F to 158° F (50° C to 70° C)

Mesophiles are the bacteria most pathogenic to humans

Figure 4.16

Multiple-Drug Resistant Organisms

In some cases, microorganisms adapt and change as a means of survival. For example, multiple drug-resistant organisms (MDRO) have become resistant to antibiotics used to treat bacterial infections. MDRO are increasingly found in hospitals, nursing homes and healthcare facilities of all sizes, and are eliminating the effectiveness of our best antibiotics, leaving us with more and more infections that cannot be treated. Resistant pathogens can produce many types of infection in almost any body site, including urinary tract, wound, blood infections and pneumonia. The most common drug-resistant bacteria today are:

- Methicillin-resistant *Staphylococcus aureus* (MRSA) lives on the skin and is known for causing severe infections, especially on the skin. Staph infections are spread by direct contact with someone with the infection or by touching contaminated surfaces. (See **Figure 4.17**)

Methicillin-resistant *Staphylococcus aureus* (MRSA)

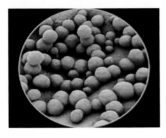

Figure 4.17

- Vancomycin-resistant *Enterococci* (VRE) lives in the bowels. This bacteria is transmitted when hands become contaminated from feces, urine or blood that is infected. It is also contracted by touching contaminated environmental surfaces. (See **Figure 4.18**)

Vancomycin-resistant *Enterococci* (VRE)

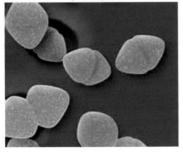

Figure 4.18

- Vancomycin-resistant *Streptococcus pneumoniae* lives asymptomatically in the nose and pharynx of healthy carriers. This bacteria causes pneumonia in susceptible humans. Strep is transmitted through direct contact with infected droplets from coughing or sneezing or from contact with other infected fluids. (See **Figure 4.19**)

Vancomycin-resistant *Streptococcus pneumoniae*

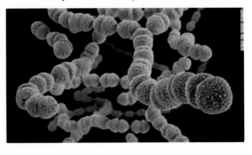

Figure 4.19

- *Klebsiella* is found on the hands and in the intestinal tract. This bacteria causes pneumonia, nasal infections, urinary tract, wound and bloodstream infections. *Klebsiella* is usually transferred from infected patients or surfaces through hand contact. (See **Figure 4.20**)

Klebsiella

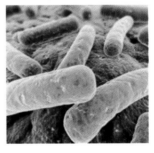

Figure 4.20

- *Acinetobacter* is found normally in soil. This bacteria can cause various illnesses ranging from pneumonia to serious blood or wound infections, and the symptoms vary depending on the disease. Acinetobacter can be resistant to many of today's antibiotics. It is transmitted by person-to-person contact or by contact with contaminated surfaces. (See **Figure 4.21**)

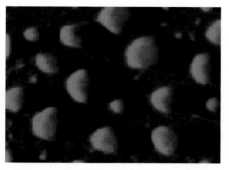

Acinetobacter

Figure 4.21

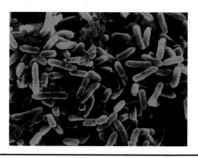

Pseudomonas aeruginosa

Figure 4.22

• *Carbapenem-resistant Enterobacteriaceae* are a family of germs that are difficult to treat because they have high levels of resistance to antibiotics. Klebsiella species and Escherichia coli (E. coli) are examples of Enterobacteriaceae, a normal part of the human gut bacteria that can become carbapenem resistant. CRE infections have been associated with devices, such as flexible endoscopes, ventilators, urinary catheters or intravenous catheters. Some CRE bacteria have become resistant to most available antibiotics. CRE infections are very difficult to treat and can contribute to death in up to 50% of patients who become infected.

• *Pseudomonas aeruginosa* is sometimes called the water bug because it is frequently found in water; however it is also found naturally in soil. *Pseudomonas* may not necessarily be drug-resistant, but is a pathogen commonly acquired in both hospitals and the community. *Pseudomonas* infections include urinary tract infections, respiratory system infections, dermatitis, soft tissue infections, bacteremia, bone and joint infections, gastrointestinal infections and a variety of systemic infections. These infections can occur particularly in patients with severe burns, and in cancer and AIDS patients who are immunocompromised. *Pseudomonas* is transmitted through hand to hand contact or contact with contaminated surfaces. (See **Figure 4.22**)

Even though the above bacteria are known to cause severe infections in humans and may be highly resistant to today's antibiotics, they require no special cleaning protocols. Following manufacturer's Instructions for Use (IFU), cleaning policies and procedures, and paying careful attention to the process is all that is required to clean items contaminated with these microbes.

Non-Bacterial Microorganisms

Viruses

Viruses are the smallest microorganisms and are about 1,000 times smaller than bacteria.

A virus enters a living plant or animal cell and reproduces itself within the cell. It usually destroys the cell, then enters another cell to survive. The virus itself has no means of movement and depends on air, water, insects, humans or other animals to carry it from one host to another. Some viruses contain envelopes: membrane structures that enclose the nuclear capsid (protein coat) that contain viral-specified proteins that make it unique. Herpes simplex, chickenpox and infectious mononucleosis are among the envelope viruses. (See **Figure 4.23**)

In the healthcare setting, there are several bloodborne viral pathogens of significance: human immunodeficiency virus (HIV), hepatitis B virus (HBV) and the most prevalent chronic bloodborne infection today, hepatitis C virus (HCV). (See **Figures 4.24** and **4.25**)

Viruses that are transmitted primarily by the airborne or droplet route include chickenpox (varicella), shingles (zoster), measles (rubeola), influenza and the common cold.

Ebola virus or Ebola hemorrhagic fever is a viral disease caused by the filovirus species. This virus is contracted by contact with blood or body fluids of an infected animal or human. The incubation period ranges from two to 21 days after exposure. The World Health Organization (WHO) states that ebola has a mortality rate of approximately 50%, as of April 2015. (See **Figure 4.26**)

Viruses transmitted by contaminated water or food include those that cause acute viral gastroenteritis such as rotavirus, Norovirus and noro-like virus. These often have symptoms similar to bacterial infections and spread through the four Fs: food, feces, fingers and flies. Another virus spread by food or water is hepatitis A that is contracted by eating raw or improperly cooked shellfish.

Viruses that spread primarily by direct contact include cold sores (herpes labialis), genital herpes, genital warts, infectious mononucleosis and rabies.

Like bacteria, some viruses can survive away from the host for many hours or days when in organic material, such as scabs, blood and bodily waste. Some viruses, like the herpes simplex virus (HSV), can survive in a dry state for 1¹/₂ to four hours on toilet seats, up to 72 hours on cotton gauze and 18 hours on plastic.

Standard cleaning protocols with careful attention to cleaning processes are usually sufficient to control these microorganisms.

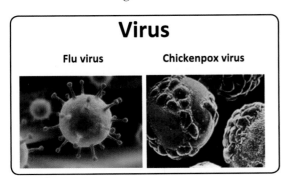

Figure 4.23

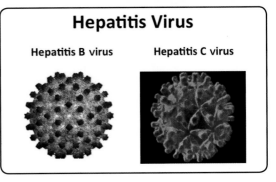

Figure 4.24

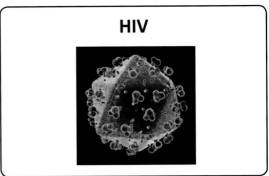

Figure 4.25

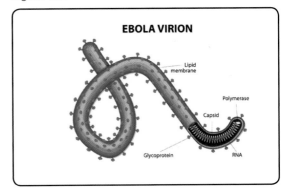

Figure 4.26

Protozoa

Protozoa are one-celled animal organisms that vary widely in size and shape and contain no cell walls.

Most protozoa live in moist habitats and are aerobic, but some species found in the human intestines are anaerobic. While most protozoa reproduce asexually, some species have sexual reproduction. They are known for their ability to move independently. The cells move by first becoming longer and then retracting (called amoeboid movement) on false feet, called blunt pseudopodia. Protozoa consume food by flowing around a particle and taking it into itself. During their life cycle, all protozoa have a feeding stage, called trophozoite. Some protozoa can form cysts and become pathogenic. Some protozoa are spread by insects or by direct contact.

The most frequently encountered pathogenic protozoa is *Entamoeba histolytica*. It is found in feces, intestinal ulcers and liver abscesses of infected persons. *Cryptosporidium* is another protozoan that can cause diarrhea and abdominal pain. This organism causes severe, life-threatening diarrhea in AIDS or cancer patients, and organ transplant recipients. (See **Figure 4.27**)

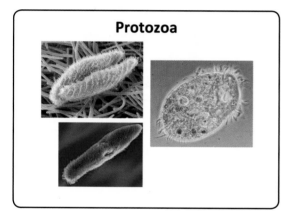

Protozoa

Figure 4.27

Fungi

Fungi are a large group of plant-like organisms that include molds, mushrooms and yeasts. Fungi and bacteria are often found together in nature. While some fungi, such as yeast, occur as single cells that require a microscope to see, others, such as mushrooms, are quite large.

The vegetative structure of a fungus (thallus) can vary widely in size, shape and complexity. Their shape and distribution of reproductive structures is how fungi are identified and classified (except for yeasts). Fungi can reproduce sexually, asexually or both. Fungi are mostly aerobic and require a carbohydrate or some reduced carbon source for carbon, electrons and energy.

Molds are composed of many-celled organisms that usually grow in compact masses of intertwining, branching and hair-like filaments. They reproduce in a variety of ways, including the formation of spores, fruiting bodies and binary fission.

Fungi have three major roles: to turn dead organic matter into usable substances through decay and mildew; to have a mutually symbiotic relationship with other organisms; and to be parasitic or pathogenic to plants or animals.

Fungi live by feeding on living or dead organisms and this process can be both beneficial and harmful. For instance, fermentation by fungi has been used for years to preserve food where refrigeration is unavailable. Fungi are necessary to produce bread, cheese, wine and beer, while other fungi, such as mushrooms, are used as food. Some fungi are used to produce pharmaceuticals, such as cortisone, the mold *Penicillium notatum* that produces penicillin, as well as the immunosuppressive agent cyclosporine. On the other hand, mold can produce toxins, such as aflatoxins, and can spoil food and create illness. (See **Figure 4.28**)

Several species of fungus can cause respiratory diseases in humans who acquire infections by inhaling spores from dust, bird droppings, soil and other sources, and these pathogenic fungi can be isolated to certain regions or widespread. For example, histoplasmosis, caused by the *Histoplasma capsulatum* fungus, occurs around the world, but has a relatively high incidence in certain countries. Histoplasmosis is generally mild, may affect more than one organ and can be difficult to diagnose since symptoms can vary from mild to severe disease; it can also cause chronic pulmonary diseases.

Some fungi target the skin, hair, nails and mucosal surfaces, and are called superficial fungi. Common examples are ringworm of the scalp (*Tinea capitis*), athlete's foot (*Tinea pedis*) and candida, such as thrush and vulvovaginitis.

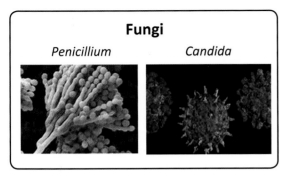

Fungi

Penicillium   *Candida*

Figure 4.28

Prions

Prions are abnormal, pathogenic agents that are transmissible and able to induce abnormal folding of specific normal cellular proteins, called prion proteins (found most abundantly in the brain). (See **Figure 4.29**) The abnormal folding of the prion proteins leads to brain damage and the characteristic signs and symptoms of prion disease.

Prion diseases or transmissible spongiform encephalopathies (TSEs) are a family of rare progressive neurodegenerative disorders that affect both humans and animals. They are distinguished by long incubation periods, characteristic spongiform changes associated with neuronal loss and a failure to induce inflammatory response. Prion diseases are rapidly progressive and always fatal.

Creutzfeldt-Jakob Disease (CJD) is a specific type of prion disease. It is rare that CS professionals in the U.S. receive instrumentation exposed to CJD, but when they do, they must know and apply proper processing procedures.

This section considers processing concerns for instruments and medical devices that have been exposed to patients known or suspected to have CJD. The processing of this instrumentation requires a shift from the use of standard precautions where all items are processed in the same manner.

CJD is a neurological disease believed to be caused by prions, pathogenic agents that are smaller than viruses, and are extremely resistant to inactivation by heat and disinfecting agents. The incubation period can be many years long and death is almost certain within a year after initial onset of symptoms.

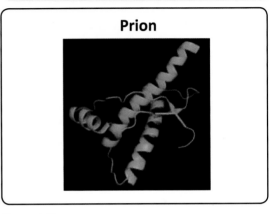

Prion

Figure 4.29

CJD is named after the German psychiatrists who first described the disease in the 1920s. It, along with other similar diseases, is classified as a TSE. Under a microscope, infected tissue, generally the brain, has a sponge-like appearance.

The CJD affects about one person per million worldwide with approximately 200 cases seen in the U.S. each year.

CJD has a relatively long incubation time (up to 30 years) during which the disease is unnoticed. Therefore, patients with CJD who have brain or spinal surgery may contaminate instruments with the infectious agents. This makes plans and policies for control of CJD very important.

In infected patients, prions are most frequently found in the brain, dura mater (the tough membrane that encases the nerves of the spinal cord), and eyes. They are also detected less frequently in cerebrospinal fluid, spleen, lymph nodes, kidney and liver. Seldomly, they are located in blood, urine, skin, muscle, bone, adrenal gland, heart, feces, peripheral nerves, nasal mucous, gingival, saliva, sputum and tears. When a suspected CJD patient undergoes a procedure, all healthcare professionals involved with that patient must be notified and the facility's CJD policies and procedures must be followed.

Cleaning and sterilization of items contaminated with prions is a challenge as prions are difficult to remove or deactivate and standard cleaning/sterilization procedures are ineffective against prions. Whenever a suspected CJD case is scheduled for an invasive procedure the following actions should be taken:

Information:

- Inform department manager as soon as notification of a prion or potential prion procedure is received.

- Immediately contact Infection Prevention and Control to determine which cleaning and sterilization guidelines will be followed at your facility. Currently recommended guidelines are published by the WHO, the Centers for Disease Control and Prevention (CDC), and the Society for Healthcare Epidemiology of America (SHEA). Current guidelines are reviewed and updated as new knowledge regarding prions is gained.

- Ensure the most current cleaning and sterilization information is available in the facility.

Instrumentation:

- Due to the difficulty in cleaning and sterilization, disposable instruments should be used whenever possible. All current guidelines suggest disposing of reusable instruments that have become contaminated with high-risk tissue (brain tissue, dura mater, spine and eye tissue). Reusable instruments will likely be damaged or completely destroyed during the stringent cleaning and sterilization protocols.

- Heat- and moisture-sensitive items should not be used as they would probably be destroyed during cleaning and sterilization.

- Some facilities will quarantine instruments used on suspected CJD cases. This is done as a precaution while awaiting a diagnosis.

Environmental surfaces:

- Surfaces, such as countertops, that have become contaminated with prion material should be cleaned following the most current published protocols.

- Contaminated non-critical equipment should be cleaned following the most current published guidelines.

Prion-contaminated instruments pose a special challenge to CS professionals. Careful attention to the most current published guidelines for cleaning and sterilization is the most important factor for your safety, and the safety of patients and co-workers.

Note: Additional information about CJD can be found on the WHO and SHEA websites, in AAMI ST79, Annex C, and from the CDC website (www.cdc.gov/ncidod/dvrd/cjd/qa_cjd_infection_control.htm#reprocessed).

CONTROLLING AND ELIMINATING MICROORGANISMS

To prevent the spread of the microorganisms that can cause disease, healthcare settings must practice microbial control. The departments of Infection Prevention and Control and CS, in particular, are vital to microbial control and patient safety. Every time an instrument or device enters a patient's body during an invasive or minimally invasive procedure, there is a risk of infection. This risk is increased because many items used in patient care and treatment are processable: they are used on one patient, processed and then are used on another patient. It is up to the CS department to control the spread of microorganisms from one patient to another through proper instrument cleaning, disinfection and sterilization.

It is important to remember that even if you cannot see these microorganisms they can pose a significant threat to humans. Let's compare microorganisms to seeds and draw some comparisons. There are many varieties of seeds, and each produces a different plant. Seeds must have the right conditions to grow and continue living. Those in a paper envelope at the store will not germinate and grow (See **Figure 4.30**); however, when they are placed in the right conditions with proper soil, water, fertilizer, warmth and sunlight, they grow and develop. In the same manner, there are many varieties of microorganisms, and each can produce a specific effect (an infection or disease) when they have the right conditions for growth and reproduction.

Like microorganisms, seeds need the right conditions to grow.

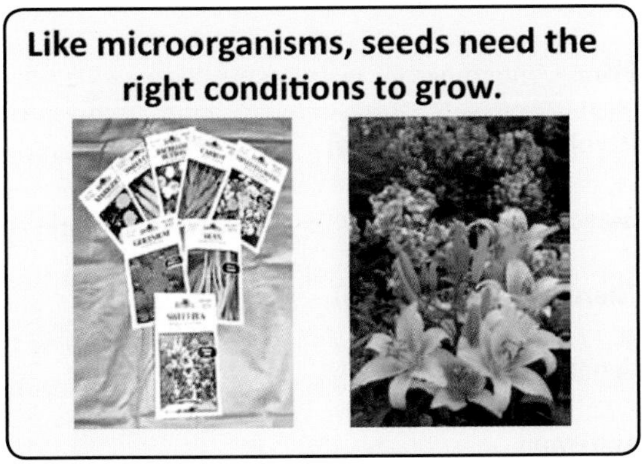

Figure 4.30

CS professionals should be able to recognize the conditions that favor the growth of microorganisms, and learn to "see" microorganisms in the workplace. For example, the decontamination work station in the left-side image in **Figure 4.31** looks safe to the untrained eye; however, if microorganisms were as easy to see as plants, that same workstation might look like the photo on the right.

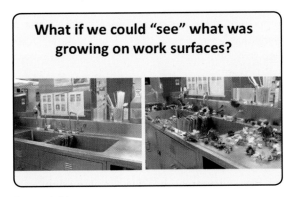

What if we could "see" what was growing on work surfaces?

Figure 4.31

Microbial control is a complicated endeavor. Just as microorganisms differ in their needs for growth and reproduction, they also die at different rates. The type of microbial control used against an organism varies according to how susceptible the microbes are. Some pathogens are more difficult to kill than others and that is one reason why disinfection and sterilization processes are so complex. Microbial control can also depend on whether the goal is to kill a pathogen-causing infection through antibiotics, inactivate or kill microorganisms on the skin through antisepsis, or in the case of CS, kill pathogens on medical instruments or devices that will be used on patients. In addition to microbial susceptibility, the vast array of items that must be processed is another reason why no single disinfection or sterilization process can kill all microorganisms.

A Common Question:

You receive a case cart from the OR to the decontamination area with a note stating instruments are contaminated with hepatitis B or MRSA. How will you handle the instruments?

Answer:

All instruments, except those contaminated with prions, are to be cleaned following the manufacturer's instructions and the facility's cleaning procedures. Items contaminated with prions have special cleaning and handling requirements.

CONCLUSION

Having a basic understanding of the principles of microbiology and learning about bacterial and non-bacterial organisms and how they can be transmitted helps Central Service professionals understand the important role they play in preventing disease.

RESOURCES

Needham C, Hoagland M, McPherson K, Dodson B. *Intimate Strangers: Unseen Life on Earth.* ASM Press. 2000.

Huys J. *Sterilization of Medical Supplies by Steam.* Vier-Turme GmbH Benedict Press. 2004.

Tierno P. *The Secret Life of Germs.* Pocket Books. 2003.

Centers for Disease Control and Prevention. *Guideline for Isolation Precautions: Preventing Transmission of Infectious Agents in Healthcare Settings.* 2007.

Alcamo E. *Cliffs Quick Review: Microbiology.* Hungry Minds Inc. 1996.

McCall D, Stock D, Achey P. *Introduction to Microbiology.* Blackwell Science Inc. *2001.*

Association for the Advancement of Medical Instrumentation ANSI/ AAMI ST79, Annex C. Comprehensive guide to steam sterilization and sterility assurance in health care facilities. 2013.

Chess B. *Foundations in Microbiology: Basic Principles, 9th Edition.* 2014.

CENTRAL SERVICE TERMS

Microbiology

Contamination

Pathogen

Micron

Aerobic

Anaerobic

Endospores (spores)

pH

Psychrophiles (bacteria)

Mesophiles (bacteria)

Thermophiles (bacteria)

Vegetative stage

Angstrom

Binary fission

Prion

Chapter 5

Regulations and Standards

Learning Objectives

As a result of successfully completing this chapter, readers will be able to:

1. Explain the difference between regulations, voluntary standards and regulatory standards

2. Provide basic information about the U.S. Food and Drug Administration and other government and regulatory agencies

3. Explain the roles and responsibilities of the regulatory agencies that impact how the Central Service department functions

4. Discuss how organizations and associations that develop regulations and standards affect Central Service

INTRODUCTION

Statutes, **regulations** and voluntary **standards** impact every healthcare professional, including those working in Central Service (CS). These laws and guidelines establish minimum levels of quality and safety. When these laws and guidelines are not followed, the results can vary from legal consequences to poor patient outcomes. This chapter will explain regulatory requirements that must be followed, as well as voluntary guidelines that are recommended.

> **Statute** A written law adopted by a legislative body that governs a city, county, state or country.
>
> **Regulation** Rules issued by administrative agencies that have the force of law.
>
> **Standard** A uniform method of defining basic parameters for processes, products, services and measurements.
>
> **Regulatory standards** A comparison benchmark that is mandated by a governing agency. Noncompliance with regulatory standards may lead to citations and legal penalties.
>
> **Voluntary standards** Guidelines or recommendations for best practices to provide better patient care. Industry, nonprofit organizations, trade associations and others develop these.
>
> **Best practice** A method or technique that has consistently shown results superior to those achieved by other means.

Standards may be regulatory or voluntary. **Regulatory standards** are those with requirements imposed by government agencies. These standards can yield legal penalties if not followed. **Voluntary standards** are strongly suggested for better patient care, but are not mandated with legal consequences for non-compliance. Statutes and regulations are laws that must be followed. Statutes are created by legislative bodies or by the electorate. Regulations are rules issued by governmental administrative agencies. Violations of statutes and regulations may have legal penalties.

Industry, nonprofit organizations, trade associations and others develop voluntary standards. Generally, voluntary standards are not law; however, they may be incorporated into law by governmental bodies and then they would become a statute or regulation, which would make them law.

CS professionals are affected by statutes, regulations and voluntary standards. CS professionals must be familiar with applicable regulations and statutes for the following reasons:

- Statutes and regulations must be followed and failure to comply with them may result in legal consequences to the healthcare facility.

- Regulations and voluntary standards may include workplace safety issues, which may help protect CS professionals from exposure to infectious agents and toxic substances.

- Regulations and voluntary standards may include disinfection and sterilization practices. These standards and regulations may be helpful in pre-purchase product evaluation.

- By careful compliance with statutes, regulations and voluntary standards, patient safety is at its highest level of quality of care.

Regulations and regulatory and voluntary standards are issued by federal, state and local governing agencies. Voluntary standards are also issued by professional organizations. Voluntary standards provide significant assistance to healthcare personnel because they are developed according to **best practice**.

The remainder of this chapter will provide information on government and regulatory agencies, the impact of regulatory agencies on CS, and how organizations develop voluntary standards.

REGULATORY AGENCIES

U.S. Food and Drug Administration

The U.S. Food and Drug Administration (FDA) is the federal agency responsible for ensuring that foods, cosmetics, human and veterinary drugs, biological products, medical devices,and electronic products that emit radiation are safe and effective for public use.

The FDA functions within the Public Health Service of the U.S. Department of Health and Human Services. The FDA regulates the manufacture of all medical devices and requires premarket clearance of new medical devices. It also regulates the sterilants and high-level disinfectants (HLDs) used to process critical and semi-critical devices. Rigorous testing with a broad range of microorganisms is required prior to marketing these chemicals. Packaging materials, sterilizers and quality monitors, such as biological indicators, are also regulated by the FDA.

Medical Device Classification

The level of regulation placed on any device depends upon how the FDA classifies that device:

- Class I Devices – These include low-risk devices, such as most hand-held surgical instruments and ultrasonic cleaners. These items are subject to "general controls," which include registration and device listing, medical device reporting, and quality system regulation and labeling. Most Class I devices are exempt from a premarket notification approval [501(k)]. *Note: 510(k) submission requirements are discussed in the next section of this chapter.*

- Class II Devices – These are devices considered to pose potential risks great enough to warrant a higher level of regulation. Class II devices include most types of sterilization equipment, and biological and chemical indicators. Manufacturers are required to submit a premarket notification application 510(k) before they can sell these products. Class II

devices are usually subject to performance standards, postmarket surveillance studies, and specific guidelines or special labeling.

- Class III Devices – These are the most stringently regulated devices and include heart valves, pacemakers and other life-sustaining devices. Manufacturers of new Class III devices must obtain a premarket approval (PMA) from the FDA to demonstrate product safety and efficacy.

Pre- and Postmarket Requirements

Unless a device is listed as exempt from regulation, a 510(k) submission is required for Class I and II devices. Class III devices may require either a 510(k) or a PMA. A 510(k) application is a comprehensive package of information designed to demonstrate that the new product is "substantially equivalent" to one or more medical devices already being marketed. By contrast, a PMA is required for most Class III devices that are new to the healthcare market. A PMA is more complicated to complete because it must prove the device has a reasonable assurance of safety and effectiveness for its intended use, based on valid scientific evidence. Sometimes, submission of clinical data is also necessary to prove safety and efficacy. The FDA requires a satisfactory inspection of the manufacturing facility before the PMA application can be approved.

A postmarket surveillance may be required by the FDA on some critical products. This is a process of collecting data about the product's use and function, while in actual use. This data is submitted and reviewed annually by the FDA. The purpose of this process is to verify that assumptions made during design and manufacturing of a device are accurate, and that the device continues to work as planned throughout its useful life.

FDA regulations help to ensure medical devices are safe for patients and healthcare workers, including CS technicians, as the agency requires the manufacturer to provide Instructions for Use (IFU) with the product. The IFU should contain detailed instructions on how to properly process and use the product. This includes disassembly, cleaning, assembly, disinfection and sterilization instructions. (See **Figure 5.1**)

Medical Device Reporting Requirements

The Safe Medical Devices Act of 1990 requires healthcare facilities to report medical device malfunctions to the FDA. Before the passage of this Act, only medical device manufacturers were required to notify the FDA whenever they learned of a patient death or serious injury that may have been caused by, or was attributed to, their devices—and whenever they learned of a device malfunction that, if it recurred, could cause a death or serious injury. Medical device reporting regulations require user facilities (hospitals, ambulatory surgical facilities, nursing homes and outpatient treatment facilities) to report suspected medical device-related deaths to the FDA and device manufacturers within 10 days of the event. User facilities must report medical device-related serious injuries only to the manufacturer within 10 days of the event. If the manufacturer is unknown, the injury should be reported to the FDA.

A serious injury is defined as "an injury or illness that is life-threatening; resulting in permanent impairment of a body function or permanent damage to body structure; or necessitates medical or surgical intervention to preclude permanent impairment of a body structure." A semi-annual report of deaths and serious injuries must also be submitted to the FDA on January 1 and July 1 of each year. This act is important to CS departments because certain sterilization failures may have to be reported if they can be linked to patient illness.

The FDA **MedWatch** program is designed for the voluntary reporting of device-related problems. It provides a vehicle by which healthcare professionals can notify the FDA about medical device malfunctions, labeling inadequacies and other problems, including ineffective IFU.

In recent years, the FDA has used both voluntary and mandatory reporting programs to collect information about specific potential problems. Forms to report either voluntary or mandatory device issues may be obtained from the FDA website at www.fda.gov/safety/medwatch.

Manufacturer Instructions for Use

Hard Copy

Online Access

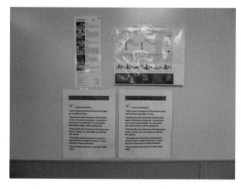 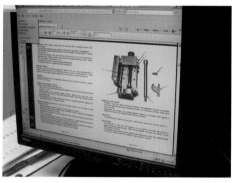

Figure 5.1 IFU

> **MedWatch** A safety information and adverse event reporting system that serves healthcare professionals and the public by reporting serious problems suspected to be associated with the drugs and medical devices they prescribe, dispense or use.

Medical Device Recalls

A recall is an action taken to address a problem with a medical device. This action can be initiated when a device is defective and/or poses a health risk. Recalls can be instituted voluntarily by the manufacturer, distributor or other interested party, or they can be mandated by the FDA. A recall does not always mean the affected product can no longer be used. Instead, it could mean that the product must be checked or repaired. For example, if an implant, such as a pacemaker, is recalled, it may not have to be removed from the patient; however, the risks of the removal decision should be discussed with the patient. The FDA monitors all mandated recalls to ensure the actions taken by the manufacturer are adequate to protect the public.

There are three categories of FDA recalls:

- Class I: High Risk – There is a reasonable chance the product will cause serious health problems or death. The manufacturer must notify customers and direct them to notify the product recipients. The notification must include the name of the device being recalled, the lot or serial numbers, the reason for the recall, and instructions to correct, avoid or minimize the problem. The manufacturer must also issue a press release to notify the public. In addition, the FDA may also issue its own press release or public health notice. The FDA posts applicable information on its medical device recalls website: www.fda.gov/safety/recalls.

- Class II: Less Serious Risk – There is a possibility that the product will cause a temporary or medically reversible adverse health problem, or there is a remote chance that the device will cause serious health problems. The manufacturer must

notify customers and, sometimes, ask them to inform the product's recipients. Generally, neither the FDA nor the manufacturer issues a press release.

- Class III: Low Risk – Use of a product is not likely to cause adverse health consequences. Because the product violates FDA law, there is a need to take an action to address the problem. The manufacturer must notify customers, and neither the FDA nor the manufacturer will issue a press release.

> ## Medical Device Recalls
>
> Product recalls in 2014 included the following items:
>
> - Infusion pumps
>
> - Ventilators
>
> - Defibrillator electrodes
>
> - Deep brain stimulation lead kits
>
> - Endotracheal tubes
>
> To learn about recently-recalled items, including the manufacturer and the product status, visit the FDA website (www.fda.gov/safety/recalls).

FDA Labeling Document

The FDA has expressed concern about the potential for the transmission of infectious diseases caused by improperly reprocessed medical devices. The FDA released a document, "Labeling Reusable Medical Devices for Reprocessing in Healthcare Facilities." This document provides guidance for FDA reviewers who evaluate premarket approval applications for medical devices. This document requires manufacturers to comply with certain criteria, mostly involving reprocessing instructions, when they submit medical device applications to the FDA for evaluation. The FDA places the responsibility for safe and effective reprocessing of medical devices with both the manufacturer and the user. This is because reprocessing requires the manufacturer to provide IFU that the healthcare facility must follow.

The manufacturer is responsible for:

- Supporting the claim of reuse with adequate labeling and ensuring the labeling has sufficient instructions on how to prepare the device for the next patient.

- The validation and documentation of tests, which show that the instructions are adequate, and can be reasonably executed by users.

The users are responsible for:

- Confirming they have the facilities and equipment to execute the instructions.

- The verification of manufacturer's instructions and ensuring the instructions are followed.

This is a major step toward providing healthcare professionals with manufacturers' reprocessing IFU, which are necessary resources that have often been difficult to obtain. These recommendations are useful for users as they select equipment needed to successfully reprocess the devices used in their facility. For example, this information allows facilities to purchase equipment, such as ultrasonic cleaners, washers and sterilizers, with the proper cycles necessary to process the devices within their department.

The FDA continues to refine the process of maintaining medical device safety by addressing any area that can affect patient safety, such as technology and human factors.

FDA Enforcement Requirements for Hospitals Reprocessing Single-Use Devices

In August 2000, the FDA released its guidance document, *Enforcement Priorities for Single-Use Devices (SUD) Reprocessed by Third Parties and Hospitals.*

As of August 2002, all hospitals and third-party reprocessors who reprocessed SUD were required to be in compliance with the premarket and postmarket requirements outlined in the enforcement document. These requirements state that facilities (including hospitals) must obtain and comply with FDA 510(k) directives to reprocess SUD.

Faced with the FDA regulatory requirements, hospital administrators may consider outsourcing their SUD reprocessing to a third-party reprocessor. While outsourcing does relieve the hospital of the burden of the actual work, it does not relieve the facility of legal and ethical responsibilities applicable to the reprocessing of SUD. It is necessary to provide safe and effective medical devices, regardless of who does the processing or where the processing takes place.

As previously stated, facilities that choose to reprocess SUD must obtain a 510(k) to do so. To obtain approval, the facility must prove it can properly clean and sterilize the product to the original manufacturer's standards each time the product is reprocessed. The facility must also show it is able to test the product to prove the standards have been met in all reprocessing areas, including decontamination, disinfection and sterilization. For more information, visit: www.fda.gov.

Centers for Disease Control and Prevention

The Centers for Disease Control and Prevention (CDC) is a federal agency organized within the U.S. Department of Health and Human Services. It works to promote health and quality of life by preventing and controlling disease, injury and disability, and by responding to health emergencies.

CDC personnel developed the first practical recommendations for isolation techniques and guidelines for infection control. Although CDC guidelines are not considered regulatory, other agencies rely heavily on them and review healthcare facilities for compliance.

Many CDC guidelines are incorporated into the policies and procedures of healthcare facilities, including their protocols for instrument processing following exposure to prions (see www.cdc.gov/ncidod/dvrd/cjd/qa_cjd_infection_control.htm).

In 2008, the CDC released its document "Guideline for Disinfection and Sterilization in Healthcare Facilities." This document "presents evidence-based recommendations on the preferred methods for cleaning, disinfection and sterilization of patient care medical devices, and for cleaning and disinfecting the healthcare environment." This document is widely used by other agencies and healthcare facilities, including CS departments. CS departments use this document to help develop their standards, practices, policies and procedures for cleaning, disinfection and sterilization of medical devices. This document can be downloaded free of charge at: http://www.cdc.gov/hicpac/pdf/guidelines/Disinfection_Nov_2008.pdf.

For more information about the CDC, visit www.cdc.gov.

U.S. Department of Transportation

The U.S. Department of Transportation (DOT) is a federal government agency dedicated to ensuring a fast, safe and efficient transportation system. (See **Figure 5.2**) Laws relating to healthcare include those concerning the transportation of minimally-processed instrumentation for repair, reprocessing and the transportation of hazardous and radioactive wastes. The DOT inspects and cites organizations for statute violations.

When CS departments transport soiled instrumentation between healthcare and repair facilities, DOT regulations for labeling and packaging must be followed. These requirements include proper biohazard labeling and containment. CS departments should contact their state's DOT for specific requirements.

Note: State or local regulations may be more restrictive than federal regulations and, in all cases, regulations with the most stringent provisions apply.

For more information about the DOT, visit www.dot.gov.

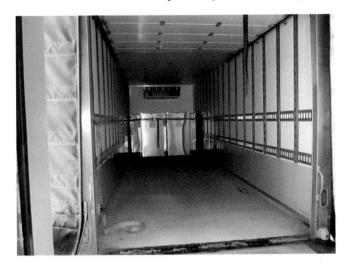

Soiled instruments secured for transport to another facility for processing.

Figure 5.2 Carts in truck for transport

U.S. Environmental Protection Agency

Congress created the U.S Environmental Protection Agency (EPA) as a regulatory agency in 1970 for the purpose of protecting human health and the environment by writing and enforcing regulations based on laws passed by Congress. The EPA is responsible for minimizing **greenhouse gases** and toxic emissions, regulating the reuse of solid wastes, controlling indoor air pollution, and developing and enforcing pesticide regulations.

The EPA administers two acts that are important to CS technicians: the Federal Insecticide, Fungicide and Rodenticide Act (FIFRA), and the 1990 Clean Air Act Amendments.

FIFRA regulates pesticide safety and effectiveness, and it impacts all antimicrobial products, including disinfectants, sanitizers and ethylene oxide (EtO). Every disinfectant and sanitizer manufacturer must obtain an EPA registration number for every covered product. The manufacturer must submit data relating to labeling claims, effectiveness and safety data to a division of the EPA's Office of Pesticide Program. If the data is approved and accepted, a registration number is issued. All EPA approved products must contain the following label information:

- Product ingredients.

- Directions for use.

- Product precautions and warnings.

- Directions for storage and disposal.

- EPA registration number.

- Expiration date (if applicable).

CS technicians must always read and consistently follow the information provided on all chemical labels.

The EPA also administers the 1990 amendments to the Clean Air Act Amendments, which created a regulatory program achieve air quality goals. In 1996, the production of chlorofluorocarbons (CFC), an ozone-depleting chemical used in the 12/88 mixture of EtO sterilant, was phased out. The EPA approved an alternate mixture using hydrochloroflurocarbons (HCFC).

As of December 14, 2014, the Clean Air Act bans the sale of most HCFC products. This leaves 100% EtO as the only option for healthcare facilities.

The 1990 Clean Air Act Amendments also established National Emission Standards for Hazardous Air Pollutants (NESHAP). These regulations established emission standards for industrial EtO sterilization facilities. Several states have developed standards for the allowable amount of ethylene oxide a facility may emit into the atmosphere. To date, there are no national emission standards for EtO sterilization within the healthcare industry.

Since the EPA regulates disinfectants, all disinfectants used in the CS department must be EPA-approved.

For more information about the EPA, visit: www.epa.gov.

> **Greenhouse gases** Any of the gases that absorb solar radiation are responsible for the greenhouse effect, including carbon dioxide, methane, ozone and fluorocarbons.

Occupational Safety and Health Administration

Created in 1971, the Occupational Safety and Health Administration (OSHA) operates under the U.S. Department of Labor. Its primary role and responsibility is to protect workers from occupationally-caused illnesses and injuries.

Many of OSHA's regulations and standards are represented in laws passed by U.S. Congress. CS professionals should be aware of OSHA regulations pertaining to their work areas.

The Occupational Exposure to Bloodborne Pathogens Standard

This comprehensive guideline outlines employee safety in all areas of the facility as they relate to potential exposure from bloodborne pathogens. This guideline is addressed in depth in Chapter 6. *Note: Non-compliance with this standard, such as not following the guidelines for transportation of contaminated instruments or not complying with the personal protective equipment (PPE) requirements, carry heavy fines.*

Guidelines for the Use of Ethylene Oxide Sterilization

Guidelines for the safe use of EtO is addressed in Chapter 15.

General Duty Clause of the Occupational Safety and Health Act

This act requires that each employer furnish each employee a place of employment which is free from recognized hazards that are causing, or are likely to cause, death or serious physical harm to his employees.

This means that OSHA may intervene in a matter of worker protection even if there is no specific regulation that covers the situation. OSHA personnel conduct announced and unannounced facility inspections. The need for inspections is based on complaints through the OSHA Whistle Blower Program, the rate of workplace accidents, high hazard targets, referrals, and follow-ups of previous visits. Some of the OSHA penalties are as follows:

- An employer who "willfully or repeatedly violates the requirements of section five of this Act" or rules promulgated under section six of this Act may be assessed a penalty "of not more than $70,000 for each violation, but not less than $5,000 for each willful violation."

- An employer who received a citation for a serious violation under section five of this Act or rules promulgated under section 6 shall be assessed a "penalty up to $7,000 for each such violation."

- An employer who received a citation for violating section five or six and is not one of "a serious nature" may be assessed a penalty up to $7,000 for each violation.

- Repeat - A violation of any standard, regulation, or rule where, upon reinspection, a substantially similar violation is found.

- Failure to abate - Failure to correct a prior violation may result in high financial penalties.

OSHA representatives may enter a facility for a specific reason; however, once inside the facility, they have the right and obligation to investigate any violation in any department they may find.

Recent penalties and citations may be viewed by accessing the OSHA website at www.osha.gov/oshstats/ and listing search criteria, such as zip code, facility size or citation type.

For more information about OSHA, visit www.osha.gov.

The Centers for Medicare & Medicaid Services

The Centers for Medicare & Medicaid Services (CMS) operates under the U.S. Department of Health and Human Services. CMS is responsible for the operation of **Medicare**, **Medicaid** and the State Children's Health Insurance Program. CMS is also one of the agencies that administers the standards of the **Health Insurance Portability and Accountability Act (HIPAA)**. HIPAA is the act that established national standards to protect patients' medical records and other personal health information. CMS is important to CS technicians because the agency performs both announced and unannounced surveys of hospitals, long-term care facilities, ambulatory surgery centers and laboratories. Failing to follow CMS standards may result in the loss of all federal funding to a facility, including Medicare and Medicaid payments. In 2008, CMS stopped reimbursing hospitals for patients that acquired any of the specific infections/events while in the hospital. These infections/events include:

- Foreign object retained after surgery.

- Air embolism.

- Blood incompatibility.

- Stage III and IV pressure ulcers.

- Falls and trauma.

- Manifestations of poor glycemic control.

- Catheter-associated urinary tract infection (UTI).

- Vascular catheter-associated infection.

- Surgical site infection, mediastinitis, following coronary artery bypass graft.

- Surgical site infection following bariatric surgery for obesity.

- Surgical site infection following certain orthopedic procedures (spine, neck, shoulder, elbow).

- Surgical site infection following cardiac implantable electronic device (CIED).

- Deep vein thrombosis (DVT)/ Pulmonary embolism (PE) following certain orthopedic procedures (total knee replacement, hip replacement).

- Iatrogenic pneumothorax with venous catheterization.

Non-payment for the amount of time the patient is in the hospital due to healthcare-associated infection (HAI) means less operating funds for the facility. This loss of funds may result in fewer instrument and equipment purchases that could impact the CS workload. Violating HIPAA rules may result in loss of employment.

For more information on CMS visit www.cms.gov.

Medicare A federal medical insurance program that primarily serves those over age 65 years of age (regardless of income), and people under 65 with certain disabilities and people of all ages with end-stage renal disease.

Medicaid A federal and state assistance program that pays covered medical expenses for low-income individuals. It is run by state and local governments within federal guidelines.

Health Insurance Portability And Accountability Act (HIPAA) The HIPAA Privacy Rule provides federal protections for individually identifiable health information held by covered entities and their business associates, and gives patients an array of rights with respect to that information. www.hhs.gov

State Regulatory Agencies

State agencies may also be involved in the regulation of healthcare facilities and the CS departments within them.

- Department of Health Services (DHS) Many states look to their DHS to establish local health safety standards that may mirror federal standards or be more stringent. A few states include DHS surveyors in the TJC survey process. DHS surveys are often random and unannounced.

- Department of Transportation (DOT) Several states have their own regulations for transporting healthcare wastes from the facility to landfills or other final disposal sites. The regulations of this state agency may affect CS technicians working in the decontamination area.

- Environmental Protection Agency (EPA) Some states have EPA offices that regulate issues that concern their jurisdiction. State regulations regarding biohazardous waste and drain discharge are important to CS technicians. State EPA offices monitor chemicals poured into the main sewer lines, and there may be regulations against pouring blood and disinfectants into drains in CS decontamination areas.

- Occupational Safety and Health Administration (OSHA) Approximately 25 states and two territories have state OSHA offices. These offices typically follow the same penalty criteria as those at the federal level.

Standards and regulations of state agencies may be more restrictive than, but cannot be less restrictive than, those of their federal counterparts. In other words, the requirements of the most restrictive agency always apply.

CS professionals must be aware of and consistently comply with applicable state and other localized standards and regulations.

PROFESSIONAL ASSOCIATIONS

Professional associations may develop and promote voluntary standards that provide a foundation for processes and practices performed in the CS functions.

Association for the Advancement of Medical Instrumentation (AAMI)

Founded in 1967, the Association for the Advancement of Medical Instrumentation (AAMI) is a nonprofit voluntary consensus organization whose membership is comprised of healthcare technology professionals, many of whom sit on one or more technical committees and working groups. These healthcare professionals may be manufacturers, scientists, healthcare organizations, independent healthcare personnel, or members of another organization, such as the FDA, with an interest in the development, management and use of safe and effective medical technology. These committees and workgroups research and develop new **standards** and **Technical Information Reports (TIRs)** that address the use, care and processing of devices and systems, or revise existing standards and TIR. Committees also develop standards for manufacturers, which recommend the labeling, safety and performance requirements for the products they produce.

> **Standards (AAMI)** Voluntary guidelines representing a consensus of AAMI members that are intended for use by healthcare facilities facilities and manufacturers to help ensure that medical instrumentation is safe for patient use.
>
> **Technical Information Reports (TIRs)** Reports developed by experts in the field that contain valuable information needed by the healthcare industry. TIRs have not undergone the formal approval system that standards are submitted to and may need further evaluation by experts. TIR may be revised or withdrawn at any time because they address a rapidly-evolving field or technology.

AAMI publishes many standards and TIRs. Many of these address functions that affect the CS department, including cleaning, sterilization, packaging and equipment testing.

In 2010, AAMI released its best-selling healthcare document, ANSI/AAMI ST79: *Comprehensive guide to steam sterilization and sterility assurance in health care facilities.* This document quickly became one of the most widely used documents in CS. ST79 is used to write policies and procedures and serve as a reference for best practices. Although the title states the document is related to steam sterilization, many sections of this document address processes that affect all types of sterilization, such as cleaning, packaging, indicators, product verification, education, and departmental work flow and design. This document became more important to CS departments in 2011 when TJC surveyors began referencing ST79 during facility surveys.

Although AAMI is a voluntary organization, AAMI standards are considered a key resource for healthcare guidelines, as many of their documents have been approved by the American National Standards Institute (ANSI). Noncompliance with these standards is cited by regulatory organizations that inspect healthcare facilities. CS technicians should be familiar with current AAMI standards that address many of these processing and sterilization practices.

For more information about AAMI, visit www.aami.org.

American National Standards Institute

Founded in 1918, the American National Standards Institute's (ANSI's) primary mission is to "enhance the global competitiveness of U.S. business and the American quality of life by promoting and facilitating voluntary consensus standards and ensuring their integrity." ANSI represents the interests of more than 125,000 companies and 3,500,000 individuals. ANSI does not develop American standards; however, it provides a neutral arena for interested parties to work toward agreement. ANSI's committee membership is similar to that of AAMI. Standards are submitted to ANSI for approval from other organizations, such as AAMI. Examples of ANSI-approved standards include the standards developed by AAMI. ANSI is the sole U.S. representative to the International Standards Organization (ISO).

Note: ISO is discussed later in this section.

For more information about ANSI, visit www.ansi.org.

Association of periOperative Registered Nurses

The Association of periOperative Registered Nurses (AORN) is a professional organization consisting of perioperative nurses and others who are dedicated to providing optimal care to the surgical patient. AORN's committees are comprised of AORN members and allied association members who develop nationally-recognized, evidence-based standards, recommended practices, and guidelines. AORN's Guidelines for Perioperative Practice currently have several sections devoted to topics directly affecting the CS department. These include sections on cleaning, disinfection, packaging, endoscope processing and sterilization. Although the standards are reprinted annually, most standards are on a five-year review cycle. AORN, like the other professional associations being discussed in this chapter, is not a regulatory agency; however, regulatory officials look for compliance with AORN recommended practices. CS technicians should be aware of AORN recommended practices and guidelines that relate to instrument processing, as many of them are incorporated into departmental policies and procedures. These documents are also utilized by surveying agencies when reviewing the CS area.

For more information about AORN, visit www.aorn.org.

The Association for Professionals in Infection Control and Epidemiology

The Association for Professionals in Infection Control and Epidemiology (APIC) is a voluntary international organization whose members work to prevent HAIs in healthcare facilities. APIC members work in conjunction with other agencies, such as the CDC, to adopt standards for infection/disease prevention. Examples include the "Bioterrorist Readiness Plan and Guidelines for Infection Prevention" and "Control in Flexible Endoscopy." CS technicians may interact with their facility's infection preventionist when they conduct departmental surveys to ensure compliance with APIC standards, practices and guidelines. Infection preventionists may also be in the CS department to collect and analyze health data relating not only to HAI, but regarding employee health issues and trends within the department, or to provide inservice education on infection prevention topics. TJC holds the Infection Prevention department, in conjunction with the CS management staff, responsible for cleaning and sterilization outcomes within the CS department.

For more information about APIC, visit www.apic.org.

International Standards Organization

The International Standards Organization (ISO) ISO is a non-government organization with a network of National Standards Institutes representing 163 countries. International standards give state-of-the-art specifications for products, services and good practice, helping to make the industry more efficient and effective. ISO standards are voluntary and the organization has no legal enforcement authority; however, many ISO standards have been adopted by some countries or are referred to in legislation, which makes them regulatory in these jurisdictions. Proposed standards are submitted from members, such as AAMI, to the general membership, and are granted ISO status based on consensus of the entire membership. It is a growing trend within the healthcare industry to become ISO-certified. Once certified, CS departments may be part of an annual survey that is similar to CMS surveys; however, the ISO focus is more results- and problem resolution-oriented.

For more information about ISO, visit www.iso.org.

The Joint Commission

The Joint Commission (TJC) is a private, independent, nonprofit organization that develops standards for healthcare facilities. TJC personnel evaluate healthcare organizations and programs in the U.S. by conducting on-site surveys at least every three years. TJC teams will arrive unannounced at a facility and spend two to five days studying virtually every aspect of care within the facility. TJC-accredited healthcare facilities are recognized as those that are dedicated to quality practices. TJC standards are voluntary; however, they carry significant weight. Failure to comply with these standards as evaluated through the TJC survey process may result in loss of accreditation by federal and state governments. This, in turn, may result in the forfeiture of millions of dollars in Medicare and Medicaid program payments.

CS technicians must understand and cooperate with their facility's procedures to comply with TJC. They must know and promote the hospital's mission and consistently comply with all safety standards, including those specific to their department. They must attend all mandatory hospital inservice sessions, assist with quality improvement tactics for their specific functions and follow all directives of Infection Prevention personnel. TJC emphasizes continuous quality improvement for patient care, and CS professionals play a key role

in improved patient outcomes. TJC standards may be incorporated by reference into federal, state and/or local statutes, and then become binding on healthcare facilities.

For more information about TJC, visit www.jointcommission.org.

National Fire Protection Association

The National Fire Protection Association (NFPA) is an international organization that works to reduce the burden of fire and other hazards around the world. NFPA members represent nearly 100 nations and organizations, and use a consensus process to develop codes and standards that influence building safety in the U.S. and in other countries. NFPA is important to CS technicians because of the fire safety standards used for the buildings in which they work. NFPA standards address the fire burden of all disposable packaged items, such as surgical drapes and gauze sponges, stored and used within the facility; the fire standards for patient drapes utilized in the OR; and wrappers utilized in the CS processing area.

For more information about NFPA, visit www.nfpa.org.

United States Pharmacopoeia – National Formulary

The United States Pharmacopoeia-National Formulary (USP-NF) creates and revises standards for the purity of medicines, drug substances and dietary supplements. These standards are published in the USP National Formulary (NF). Standards are set for packaging, labeling, bacteriological purity, pH and mineral content. The USP is important to CS technicians who work with purified water or sterilizing water for irrigation.

For more information about USP-NF, visit www.usp.org/uspnf.

World Health Organization

The World Health Organization (WHO) is an agency of the United Nations that was established in 1948 to further international cooperation in improving health conditions. Its major task is to combat disease, especially key infectious diseases, and to promote the general health of people worldwide. WHO staff members coordinate international efforts to monitor outbreaks of infectious diseases, such as Severe Acute Respiratory Syndrome (SARS), malaria, Acquired Immune Deficiency Syndrome (AIDS), and Creutzfeldt-Jakob Disease (CJD).

This agency provides a central clearing house for research services and international standards. Agencies, such as the CDC, base many standards on the research and direction provided by WHO. For example, the standards healthcare facilities follow for processing items contaminated with CJD are from WHO.

For more information about WHO, visit www.who.org.

Society of Gastroenterology Nurses and Associates

The Society of Gastroenterology Nurses and Associates (SGNA) is a nonprofit organization of nurses and associates dedicated to the safe and effective practice of gastroenterology and endoscopy nursing. SGNA collects information and establishes standards and guidelines relating to the processing of flexible endoscopes. In 2013, SGNA released its "Guideline for the Use of High Level Disinfectants and Sterilants for Reprocessing of Flexible Gastrointestinal Endoscopes," followed by "Standard of Infection Control in Reprocessing of Flexible Gastrointestinal Endoscopes" in 2012. Both of these documents may be downloaded free of charge at www.sgna.org/Education/ StandardsandGuidelines.aspx.

For more information about SGNA, visit www.sgna.org.

Canadian Standards Association

The Canadian Standards Association (CSA) is a nonprofit organization that develops standards for industry, government and healthcare for all Canadian providences. The CSA has developed many standards for the processing of surgical instrumentation.

For more information about CSA, visit www.csa.ca.

European Committee for Standardization

The European Committee for Standardization (CEN) sets the standards for Europe in much the same way that AAMI sets standards for the U.S. The 33 member countries have adopted CEN standards exclusively. U.S. companies that sell products for instrument processing in Europe must follow CEN standards for the products sold in member countries.

CONCLUSION

Standards and regulations are designed to keep both patients and employees safe. Central Service technicians should become familiar with the agencies and organizations that develop the requirements that impact their jobs and should strive to keep abreast of changes as they happen; doing so creates an environment of safety and competency.

FOR FURTHER READING

Premarket requirements are found in the Food, Drug and Cosmetic Act (the Act), Sections 510, 513 and 515, and in 21 CFR Parts 807 and 814. Note: "The Act" provides the regulation; the CFR indicates the classification and tells what is needed to comply with the regulation. Information concerning the substantial equivalence decision-making process can be found online at www.fda.gov/cdrh/k863.html.

Information for successfully completing a 510(k) notification is available at: www.fda.gov/cdrh/devadvice/314.html.

PMA information is contained in Sections 513 and 515 of the Act, and 21 CFR Part 814. Guidance for preparation of a PMA may be obtained at www.fda.gov/cdrh/ode/448.pdf.

Additional information about each postmarket requirement is available through the CDRH homepage: www.fda.gov/cdrhl/; select "Postmarket requirements." Guidance documents are also available on these postmarket requirements by accessing the CDRH homepage and selecting "Device Advice"; www.fda.gov/cdrh/devadvice/.

Healthcare personnel who wish to voluntarily report device problems or potential hazards may call Medwatch (800.FDA.1088) or visit www.fda.gov/medwatch/report/hcp.htm to report online, or to obtain additional information and/or forms.

Labeling Reusable Medical Devices for Reprocessing Health Care Facilities: FDA Reviewer Guidance, Office of Device Evaluation, Page 2. April 1996.

Current FDA reuse information is found at: www.fda.gov/cdrh/reuse/index.shtml.

Current FDA reuse information is found at: www.fda.gov/chrh/reuse/index.shtml.

OSHA Employer Responsibilities is found at www.osha.gov/as/opa/worker/employer-responsibility.html.

RESOURCES

U.S. Food and Drug Administration. Code of Federal Regulations, Title 21, Part 813 — Medical Device Reporting, Subparts A, B, C. U.S. Government Printing Office. 2000.

U.S. Environmental Protection Agency. Data Requirements for Registration. Federal Register 49, No. 207: 42881-42905. October 24, 1984.

U.S. Environmental Protection Agency. Clarification of HIV (AIDS Virus) Labeling Policy for Antimicrobial Pesticide Products. Federal Register 54, No. 26:6288-6290. February 9, 1989.

U.S. Environmental Protection Agency. National Emission Standards for Hazardous Air Pollutants for Source Categories, Code of Federal Regulations, Title 40, Part 63, Subpart 0 (Updated 1996). Washington, D.C. 1994.

Centers for Disease Control and Prevention. Guidelines for Disinfecting and Sterilizing in Healthcare Facilities. Guidelines for Hand-washing and Hospital Environmental Control. 2008.

Occupational Safety and Health Administration. Occupational Exposure to Formaldehyde. Federal Register 52, No. 233:46168-46312. Code of Federal Regulations, Title 29, Part 1910. 1987.

Occupational Safety and Health Administration. Occupational Exposure to Ethylene Oxide. Federal Register 49, No. 122: 25734-25809. Code of Federal Regulations, Title 29, Part 1910.1047. 1984.

Occupational Safety and Health Administration. Occupational Exposure to Ethylene Oxide. Federal Register 53, No. 66: 53:11414-11438. Code of Federal Regulations, Title 29, Part 1910.1047. 1988.

Occupational Safety and Health Administration. Hazard Communication Standard. Code of Federal Regulations, Title 29, Part 1910.1200.

Occupational Safety and Health Administration. Occupational Exposure to Blood-borne Pathogens: Final Rule. Federal Register 56, No. 235: 56:64004. Code of Federal Regulations, Title 29, Part 1910.1030. 1991.

Occupational Safety and Health Administration. Occupational Exposure to Bloodborne Pathogens: Final Rule. 29 CFR Part 1910.1030. 1992.

Occupational Safety and Health Administration. Occupational Exposure to Bloodborne Pathogens; Needlestick and Other Sharp Injuries; Final Rule. Amended and effective April 18, 2001; and 29CFR 1910.1035 Occupational Exposure to Tuberculosis, Proposed Rule. October 17, 1997.

CENTRAL SERVICE TERMS

Statute

Regulation

Standard

Regulatory standard

Voluntary standards

Best practice

MedWatch

Greenhouse gases

Medicare

Medicaid

Health Insurance Portability and Accountability Act (HIPAA)

Standards (AAMI)

Technical Information Reports (TIRs)

Chapter 6

Infection Prevention

Learning Objectives

As a result of successfully completing this chapter, readers will be able to:

1. Explain the role of Central Service in the prevention of healthcare-associated surgical infections

2. Explain the principles, practice and importance of personal hygiene and attire, including personal protective equipment

3. Identify the hazards of bloodborne pathogens and how the Occupational Safety and Health Administration's requirements impact personal safety

4. Explain the rationale for the separation of clean and dirty, and the environmental requirements for maintaining that separation

5. Discuss the chain of infection and the technician's role in breaking that chain

INTRODUCTION

The Central Service (CS) professional plays a significant role in the prevention of surgical site and healthcare-associated infections (HAIs). When the importance of this role is understood, technicians recognize that their work practices can mean the difference between a patient's successful surgery or hospital stay, and a negative outcome that could lead to infection or possibly death.

CENTRAL SERVICE PROCESSES

Every step or process in the CS department is carefully designed to prevent poor patient outcomes. Poor outcomes can be traced to many factors; including the condition of instruments, trays and other medical devices that are processed in CS.

In the most simplistic terms, CS supports infection prevention by:

- Cleaning contaminated medical devices to make them safe for handling and prepare them for a **biocidal** process.

- Inspecting instruments to help ensure they are safe and functional.

- Assembling and packaging instruments in a manner that facilitates the method of sterilization chosen and provides a barrier after sterilization.

- Selecting and properly using the sterilization or high-level disinfection (HLD) method for each medical device.

- Safely storing items until they are needed and delivering them using methods that protect the integrity of the sterile packages.

While those tasks may appear easy, there are several steps to each process. Each requires attention to detail, understanding of specific protocols and process parameters, an understanding of each medical device's manufacturer Instructions for Use (IFU) and dedication to processing each item exactly as stated in the IFU. Every medical device not processed according to the manufacturer's IFU has the potential to cause infection in both the patient and healthcare worker.

Cause for Concern

In 2011, the Centers for Disease Control and Prevention (CDC) reported that approximately one of every 25 hospitalized patients, or 722,000, contracted an HAI. Of those approximate 722,000, about 75,000 patients died during their hospitalizations. Many of these infections may have been preventable. A **surgical site infection (SSI)** is an infection that occurs after surgery in the part of the body where the surgery took place. As many as three of every 100 surgical patients develop these infections per year, according to the CDC.

Approximately 51.4 million surgical procedures are performed in the U.S. annually, the CDC reports. Each involves the use of medical devices or instruments that have contact with a patient's sterile tissues or mucous membranes. Infection is a major risk in all of these procedures. Additionally, a growing number of microorganisms are becoming resistant to antibiotics or are naturally difficult to control. Many of these microorganisms may be easily transferred to other surfaces and people. Controlling these microorganisms and preventing their transmission is the number one responsibility of the CS department.

Infection prevention principles and practices are based on knowledge of the nature and characteristics of disease-producing microorganisms. This includes an understanding about how they are transmitted in the healthcare environment, and their place in the **chain of infection**. The more CS technicians know about microorganisms, the better equipped they are to prevent the spread of these organisms. **Figure 6.1** identifies the top HAI-causing pathogens, as identified by the CDC.

> **Biocidal** Process or ability to kill or control the growth of living organisms.

CDC Top HAI Causing Pathogens	
Acinetobacter	*Burkholderia cepacia*
Clostridium difficile	*Clostridium sordellii*
Enterobacteriaceae (Carbapenem-resistance)	Hepatitis
Human immunodeficiency virus *(HIV)*	Influenza
Methicillin-resistant *Staphylococcus aureus*	*Klebsiella*
Norovirus	*Mycobacterium abscessus*
Staphlococcus aureus	*Pseudomonas aeruginosa*
Vancomycin-intermediate *Staphylococcus aureus*	Tuberculosis (TB)
Vancomycin-resistant *Enterococci (VRE)*	Vancomycin-resistant *Staphlococcus aureus*

Source: http://www.cdc.gov/HAI/organisms/organisms.html

Figure 6.1

Surgical site infection (SSI) An infection that occurs after surgery in the part of the body where the surgery took place.

Chain of infection A way of gathering the information needed to interrupt or prevent an infection. Each of the links in the chain must be favorable to the organism for the infection to continue. Breaking any link in the chain can disrupt the infection. Which link is most effective to target will depend on the organism.

Protection from Pathogens

The origins of isolation precautions date back to the days of quarantine, a control measure used in infectious disease epidemics of earlier times. In the early 1970s, the CDC established the first practical recommendations for the isolation technique. The new recommendations categorized infections and communicable diseases based upon the likely mode of transmission. To protect healthcare staff and patients from infectious diseases, Standard Precautions were adopted; the basis of this is to treat all human blood, bodily fluids and other potentially infectious materials as infectious.

Standard precautions drive the infection prevention and control procedures that CS technicians must use because they are exposed to contaminated instrumentation and equipment. Failure to wear the appropriate personal protective equipment (PPE) increases the individual's risk of acquiring an infection.

The primary purpose of the CS department is to stop the spread of disease-producing microorganisms to patients from instruments and other medical devices. CS technicians must ensure that items used in patient care, including instruments, utensils, supplies and equipment, are made safe by either disinfection or sterilization. Chapter 4 addressed microorganisms: how they live, grow and are transmitted from person to person and place to place. This chapter addresses how CS professionals control the spread of microorganisms and prevent infection. Understanding **asepsis** in healthcare is an important piece of the basic knowledge required to work in CS.

PRINCIPLES OF ASEPSIS

Asepsis can be defined as the absence of microorganisms that cause disease. **Aseptic technique** includes any activity or procedure that prevents infection or breaks the chain of infection.

There are two types of aseptic techniques:

- **Medical asepsis** (clean technique) - Procedures performed to reduce the number of microorganisms to minimize their spread. Examples include handwashing and decontamination of equipment.

- **Surgical asepsis** (sterile technique) – Procedures to eliminate the presence of all microorganisms, and/or prevent the

---

introduction of microorganisms to an area [e.g., sterilization of instrumentation and techniques performed in the Operating Room (OR) prevent contamination of sterile instruments and supplies].

Asepsis The absence of microorganisms that cause disease.

Aseptic technique Any activity or procedure that prevents infection or breaks the chain of infection.

Asepsis (medical) Clean technique; procedures performed to reduce the number of microorganisms and minimize their spread.

Asepsis (surgical) Surgical technique; procedures performed to eliminate the presence of all microorganisms, and/or prevent the introduction of microorganisms to an area.

There are five basic principles of asepsis:

- Principle one: know what is dirty. Items that have been used for patient care are considered contaminated. An item is considered to be either contaminated or not contaminated. For the CS technician, the terms "dirty" and "contaminated" mean the same thing. Microbial contamination cannot be seen with the naked eye; however it can be present even when it is not seen. Examples of contaminated items include opened surgical instrument trays, IV pumps and suction machines.

- Principle two: know what is clean. Cleanliness is the basis of aseptic technique. Mechanical cleaning removes soil and most microorganisms. Any item that has been properly cleaned via manual or mechanical means is considered clean. If that item has been cleaned with a detergent disinfectant or a thermal decontamination process, it is considered clean and decontaminated. The physical task of washing/cleaning removes soil and most microorganisms.

- Principle three: know what is sterile. Sterility is defined as the absence of all microbes. Sterility is impossible to see with the naked eye; one cannot look at a specific item and determine its sterility. Absence of microbes can only be achieved by use of steam, ethylene oxide (EtO) or other sterilization methods.

- Principle four: keep the three conditions separate. There must be separation between dirty, clean and sterile areas to allow a margin of safety. Clean or decontaminated items must not come in contact with dirty items. If they do, they must again be considered dirty. If sterile items come in contact with non-sterile items, they must also be considered non-sterile. Sterile items should not be stored near sinks or in any location where there is a risk that they will become wet or soiled. The presence of moisture allows the passage of microorganisms through wrappers, resulting in contamination of sterile supplies.

- Principle five: remedy contamination immediately. When dirty, clean and sterile areas or items have not been separated, the situation must be corrected immediately. One who observes a procedure has as much responsibility for maintaining proper aseptic technique as the person who performs the procedure. There are times when only a CS technician will know or suspect that something may be contaminated (e.g., when something is dropped on the floor). Even though processing the item may result in more work, this must be done to protect the patient.

A careless attitude may lead to an increased risk of infection, so CS professionals must always be aware of their actions. By adhering to the principles of asepsis, the risk of infection will be reduced for patients and the facility's employees. The responsibility of CS technicians to provide safe items for use should never be compromised.

CS professionals must assume several important responsibilities in their facility's infection prevention and control efforts. The infection prevention and control goals of the CS department are to:

- Eliminate and/or destroy all potentially infectious contaminants present on reusable instruments and equipment.

- Safely distribute reusable and single-use items required for the delivery of patient care.

- Establish and enforce standards for decontamination, disinfection and sterilization in various healthcare settings.

The importance of these responsibilities is clear. The use of medical devices that have not been properly handled, disinfected or sterilized can cause infections in patients and staff. CS professionals are responsible for providing safe items that support good patient outcomes.

PERSONAL HYGIENE AND ATTIRE

Preventing the spread of microorganisms and maintaining appropriate environments for clean and sterile items requires good self management skills. Hygiene and adherence to dress code protocols are critical components of infection prevention in the CS department.

Personal Hygiene

Hand hygiene is a term that means either handwashing, or using an approved antiseptic hand rub (such as an alcohol-based product). Hand hygiene is considered the single most important factor in reducing infections.

Handwashing refers to the use of soap, water and friction to wash one's hands. Effective handwashing consists of wetting, soaping, lathering and vigorously rubbing one's hands together, making certain to lather between fingers and around nails for at least 20 seconds. Washing should be followed by rinsing with running water and thoroughly drying with a disposable towel. (See **Figure 6.2**)

Hand sanitizing refers to the use of an alcohol-based gel or foam. Alcohol does not kill some highly-infectious bacteria, like *C. difficile,* and some food borne pathogens; therefore, handwashing is critical before and after any meal, and before and after using the restroom.

> **Hand hygiene**   The act of washing one's hands with soap and water or using an alcohol-based hand rub.

Handwashing should be done prior to starting work, upon entering or leaving the work area, before and after eating or using the restroom or whenever hands become soiled or contaminated. Infection control and prevention experts recommend that hands be washed immediately and thoroughly if they become soiled with blood, bodily fluids, secretions or excretions. After coming in contact with contaminated items without visible soil or after gloves are removed), an alcohol-based hand rub should be used according to the manufacturer's recommendations. Approved hand lotions may be used after handwashing to keep the skin healthy, and to minimize skin irritation and excessive drying.

CS departments are equipped with handwashing sinks conveniently located for easy access. CS technicians should wash their hands only in dedicated handwashing sinks (not in those used for decontamination purposes).

Because fingernails harbor microorganisms, they should be kept clean and not extend beyond the fingertips. Long nails also increase the risk of tearing gloves. Fingernail polish should not be worn in the CS department because nail polish may chip and fall onto an instrument set. Artificial nails should not be worn in CS because they also harbor microorganisms and may detach and fall into a tray unnoticed.

Infection prevention begins at home. Personal hygiene is important for the prevention of infections. Bathing and shampooing regularly, wearing clean clothing and practicing good hand hygiene prepares CS professionals to continue this practice in the healthcare facility.

Personnel with open or weeping wounds or excessive skin irritations should refrain from handling any patient care equipment until the condition is resolved or medically evaluated.

Attire

CS professionals must wear attire specific for the area in which they work. This protects the employee and other staff members, patients and the public.

Attire should be clean, provided by the facility, and not worn outside the facility. Technicians should change out of their street clothing (clothing worn at home) and shoes, and into scrubs and shoes kept at the facility. Usually, there will be a locker space for personal belongings. At the end of the workday, scrubs will be left behind in the facility's laundry, protecting employees from infecting anyone at home or in the community. Necklaces, rings or other jewelry should not be worn because they can harbor microorganisms.

Lanyards, if used, should be left at the facility and cleaned on a regular basis.

Basic attire should be worn in every area of the department and by everyone working in or visiting the department. (See **Figure 6.3**)

- Scrub attire should be changed daily, anytime it becomes soiled or as soon as it may have become contaminated. Scrub attire should consist of at least clean pants and a top. Some facilities provide long-sleeve jackets. T-shirts, if worn, should be completely covered by the scrub top. No part of the T-shirt should be visible outside the scrub attire. *Note: Some facilities allow outside visitors to wear disposable cover clothing, such as jump suits, instead of scrub attire.*

Handwashing Procedure
1. Remove all jewelry
2. Turn on faucet using a paper towel
3. Wet hands and apply liquid soap
4. Work soap into a lather and scrub hands for at least 20 seconds*
5. Keep hands at a lower angle than elbows to prevent dirty water from running back onto arms
6. Interlace fingers to clean between them
7. Dry hands with clean disposable towels
8. Turn off the faucet using a clean disposable towel

* Source: Centers for Disease Control & Prevention

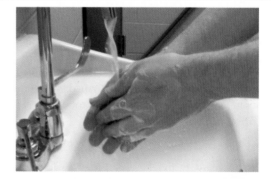
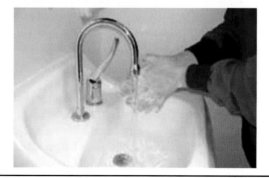

Figure 6.2

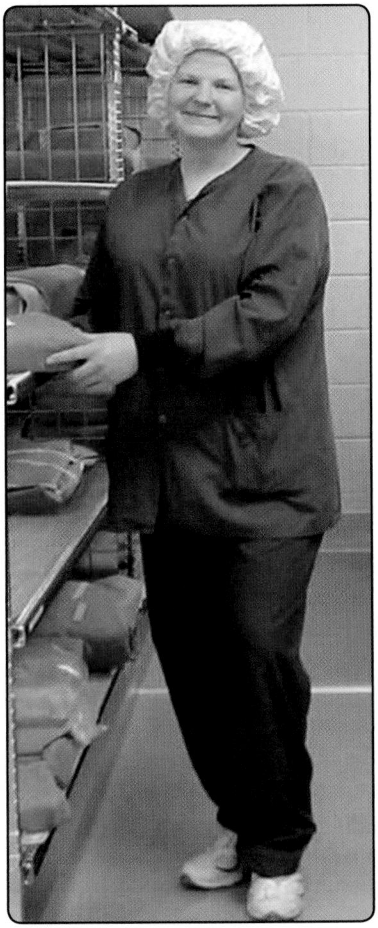

Figure 6.3

Scrub attire should always be donned (put on) just prior to starting work and doffed (removed) before leaving work.

- A disposable bouffant-type head covering should be worn in all areas of the department. Head covers should cover all head hair, except eyelashes and eyebrows. Reusable head covers, if allowed in the facility, should be covered with a bouffant cover to keep from contaminating the area with outside bacteria or with bacteria that may have multiplied on the caps due to improper cleaning. Skull-type caps are no longer suggested for use because they do not always cover all head hair. Beards and mustaches should be covered with an approved cover to prevent facial hair from shedding onto the items being processed.

- Sturdy shoes with non-skid soles should be worn in the department. Shoes should be able to protect the feet from items that may inadvertently fall from work areas. It is good practice to have shoes dedicated to the area and not worn out of the facility.

- A cover gown/lab coat may be used to protect the scrub attire when leaving the department for another area of the same facility (this depends on facility policy). *Note: Cover gown/lab coats are not meant to protect departmental attire while outside the building.*

Decontamination attire: All individuals working in the decontamination area must comply with dress code requirements for PPE. This is required by the Occupational Safety and Health Administration (OSHA), and was established to help ensure workers are protected from potential pathogens.

Risk of exposure to pathogenic microorganisms can be reduced by diligently following dress codes in decontamination areas. For example, fluid-resistant gowns provide protection from splashes that may soak into and contaminate regular scrub attire. (See **Figure 6.4**)

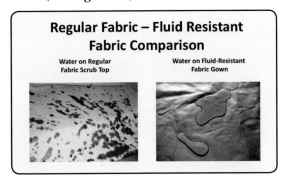

Figure 6.4

All of the basic attire outlined previously, except the cover gown, should be worn in the decontamination area. Because of the nature of the work in the decontamination area (soiled and contaminated devices, water and chemicals) additional attire is required. **Figure 6.5** provides examples of PPE worn in the decontamination area. Decontamination PPE includes:

- Gloves approved for the decontamination area. These gloves are thicker than examination gloves to protect the hands. They also have longer cuffs (some are elbow length), so they can be placed over the gown cuff to keep fluids from flowing into the glove or up the gown sleeve.

- Mask that fits around the ear or ties on the head to protect the nose and mouth.

- Fluid-resistant gown or jumpsuit to protect clothes and skin. Fluid-resistant materials will keep fluids away from the skin, while standard fabrics will absorb fluids allowing the skin beneath the fabric to become wet and contaminated.

- Goggles or face shield to protect the eyes (face shield will also protect the face, mouth and nose). *Note: Wearing a face shield does not replace the need to also wear a face mask.*

- Shoe covers protect the shoes from contamination. Shoe covers should be worn even if the shoes are dedicated to department use only. Using boot length covers (not required) will help protect the leg area, as well.

Figure 6.6 provides a recap of basic PPE requirements and the reason each component is important. There is a proper way to don and doff PPE. **Figures 6.7** and **6.8** give the proper sequence for donning and doffing PPE.

MANAGING THE ENVIRONMENT TO PREVENT THE SPREAD OF BACTERIA

The first step in maintaining environmental integrity is to control the traffic that enters and passes through the CS department. The aforementioned dress codes apply to all who enter the CS department. Department dress standards for visitors (e.g., sales representatives, maintenance personnel and clinical engineering staff) vary between facilities. In some facilities, they must change into surgical scrubs; in others, coveralls (worn over street clothes) are required. CS technicians must protect the integrity of the environment by enforcing traffic control guidelines. This may sometimes mean educating visitors about dress code and traffic control protocols.

Dress code requirements may change as CS technicians move from one area to another. For example, surgical scrubs and hair coverings may be appropriate for the clean assembly area,

---

Examples of PPE

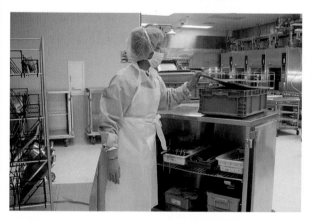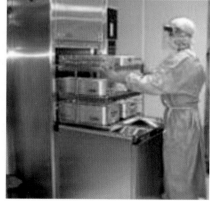

Figure 6.5

Types of PPE

Type of PPE	Protects	Why
Fluid-resistant gown, apron, jumpsuit	Protects skin and scrubs	Provides a barrier against splash or spray
Mask	Protects mouth, nose, chin	Protects respiratory tract from airborne infectious aerosols
Goggles	Protect the eyes	Protects eyes from infectious aerosols
Face shield-full length	Protects eyes, nose, mouth, face	Protects eye, nose, mouth, face from spray and infectious aerosols
Shoe covers	Protect shoes (boot length will protect calf to knee)	Protects the shoes (lower leg) from spray
Gloves	Protect hands	Protects hands from contaminated instruments

Figure 6.6

How to Don (Put on) on PPE

*	Before beginning	Don surgical scrubs, a head cover and appropriate shoes.
1.	Gown or jumpsuit	Don the impervious gown or jumpsuit. Tie, snap or zip completely
2.	Mask	Secure the ear pieces around the ears or tie the strings on the head area. Fit the mask over the nose area, ensure the nose and mouth areas are completely covered.
3.	Goggles or face shield	Don goggles or face shield and adjust to fit properly (goggles should wrap around the side of the face).
4.	Shoe covers	Don shoe covers and ensure shoes are completely covered.
5.	Gloves	Don gloves and ensure gloves are over the gown cuff.

Figure 6.7

CDC Recommendations for Doffing (Removing) PPE

1.	Remove shoe covers
2.	Remove gloves
3.	Remove goggles or face shield
4.	Remove gown
5.	Remove mask
6.	Remove head cover
7.	Wash hands

Figure 6.8

but OSHA-required PPE is necessary for the decontamination area. (See **Figure 6.9**) Dress codes are an important part of traffic control; therefore, CS technicians must understand what attire is appropriate in different areas. *Note: If in an unfamiliar area and unsure of the attire requirements, ask before entering.*

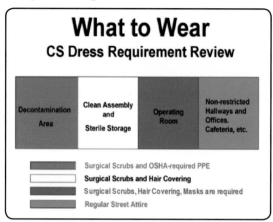

Figure 6.9

Areas that CS technicians routinely travel through may have three separate traffic control/dress code requirements:

- Restricted – Areas where sterile surgical procedures are performed. Surgical scrub attire, hair coverings and masks are required in restricted areas. Those working within the sterile field (including surgeons, surgical technologists and nurses) are also required to wear a sterile surgical gown and gloves. *Note: Semi-restricted areas in the OR, such as access corridors to surgical suites, must follow restricted dress code.*

- Semi-restricted – These areas include peripheral support areas to the OR, CS clean assembly, and sterile storage areas. Surgical scrub attire and hair coverings are required in these areas.

- Unrestricted – These areas include normal traffic areas, such as hospital corridors, most offices, locker rooms and general public areas (e.g., cafeteria and waiting rooms). Street clothes may be worn in unrestricted areas.

CS departments use signage to assist in traffic control. All restricted and semi-restricted areas also have signage that informs people entering the area about the need for specific dress codes. (See **Figure 6.10**)

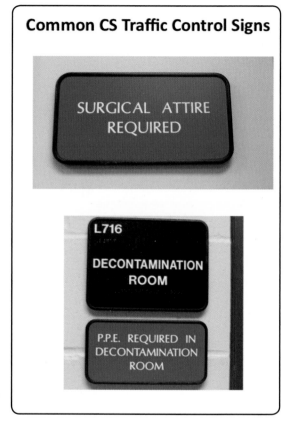

Figure 6.10

OCCUPATIONAL SAFETY AND HEALTH ADMINISTRATION 29 CFR 1910.1030

OSHA is the primary federal agency charged with the enforcement of occupational safety and health legislation. In response to concerns, OSHA published the Bloodborne Pathogens Standard, recognizing the potential for occupational exposure to bloodborne diseases (hepatitis B and C and HIV). The standard places the responsibility for providing a safe work environment on the employer, and contains several key elements:

- A written exposure control plan (ECP) that summarizes the employer's program for the protection of workers from occupational exposure to bloodborne diseases. The ECP must be reviewed annually and updated whenever new tasks or procedures affecting occupational exposures are instituted. An ECP contains the following provisions:

› Determination of employee exposure.

› Implementation of various methods of exposure control, including:

  - Standard precautions (also known as universal precautions).

  - Engineering and work practice controls: The use of engineering controls to physically remove the hazard, and development of work practice controls (policies and procedures) to prevent occupational exposure and transmission of bloodborne pathogens.

  - Use of PPE.

  - Housekeeping: Provision of a clean and sanitary working environment including scheduled cleaning using hospital germicides (disinfectants) approved by the U.S. Environmental Protection Agency (EPA).

  - Hepatitis B vaccination: The facility must offer the hepatitis B vaccine at no cost. Employees who choose not to take the vaccine must sign a declination (refusal) form, and they may reconsider at any time during their employment.

  - Post-exposure evaluation and follow-up: Provision for medical evaluation and treatment when an employee experiences an exposure incident.

  - Communication of hazards to employees and training regarding those hazards.

  - Recordkeeping: Proof of training upon initial hire and annually thereafter. If significant changes are made to the ECP, additional training is required to address the changes. Medical records regarding any exposure must be maintained.

  - Procedures for evaluating circumstances surrounding an exposure incident.

› The use of fluorescent orange or orange red "BIOHAZARD" labels to identify contaminated items or regulated waste that may be stored or transported in refrigerators, freezers or other containers. (See **Figure 6.11**) Labels are not required when using red bags or marked containers. (See **Figure 6.12**)

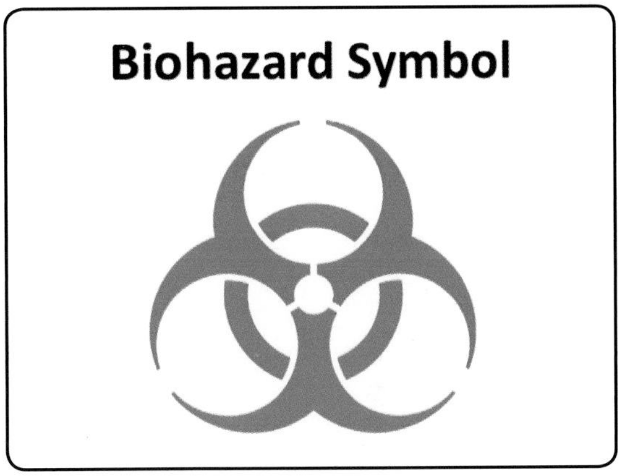

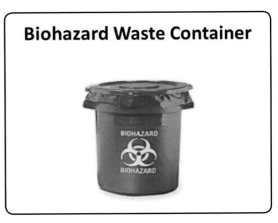

Figure 6.11

Figure 6.12

› Disposal of all sharp items in rigid, puncture-proof containers that are covered, properly labeled or color-coded. (See **Figure 6.13**)

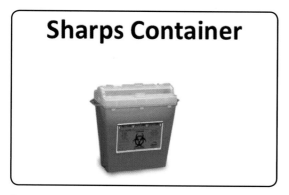

Figure 6.13

Reusable sharps should be transported in enclosed carts or hard-sided containers to prevent injury. (See **Figure 6.14**)

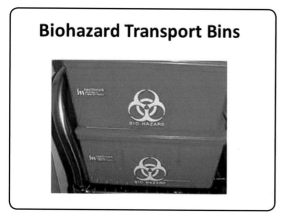

Figure 6.14

ENVIRONMENTAL CONCERNS IN CENTRAL SERVICE AREAS

In addition to specific guidelines for dress codes and standard precautions, there are environmental tools designed to help CS technicians promote infection prevention. Some tools are evident. Others, while not as evident, still play an important role in maintaining an environment that is safe for patients and employees.

Physical Design

CS departments' physical design should incorporate a clear separation of clean and dirty, and workflow patterns should be designed that create a one-way flow of goods from dirty to clean.

In addition to walls separating the decontamination area from the rest of the department, the area is designed to reduce the likelihood that airborne bacteria can be transmitted from the decontamination area to the clean area. This is accomplished with use of positive and negative air pressure. The decontamination area has negative (lesser) air pressure. This means that when a door or window is opened between the separate work areas, air flows from the clean (positive pressure) area to the dirty (negative pressure) area. This minimizes the risk of airborne bacteria in the decontamination area being carried to the clean area. **Figure 6.15** illustrates the airflow created by the use of positive and negative air pressure. To maintain the balance necessary for air pressure systems to function correctly, windows and doors between the decontamination and clean areas must remain closed when not in use.

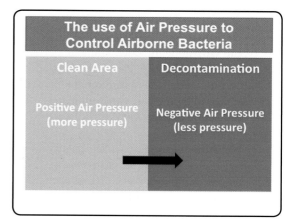

Figure 6.15

In addition to the air pressure requirements, CS areas must meet specific temperature, humidity and air exchange requirements. These vary by work area and CS technicians must be familiar with the requirements for each specific area, and ensure that policies designed to manage airflow, temperature and humidity are followed at all times. In many departments, CS technicians may be responsible

CS Department Temperature, Humidity, and Air Exchange Requirements

Central Service Department Temperature, Humidity, and Air Exchanges			
Work Area	**Temperature**	**Humidity***	**Air Exchanges**
Decontamination	60°F to 65°F (16°C to 18°C)	30% to 60%	10
General work areas	68°F to 73°F (20°C to 23°C)	30% to 60%	10
Sterile storage	75°F or lower	Not to exceed 70%	4
Sterilization equipment room	75°F to 85°F (24°C to 29°C)	30% to 60%	10

Figure 6.16

Some facilities may choose to use 20% for the lower humidity level. CS departments should check with their supply and equipment manufacturers to ensure that the lower humidity is acceptable for items stored in the area.

for collecting data, such as temperatures and humidity, and recording that data as part of their department's formal documentation system. **Figure 6.16** provides temperature, humidity and air exchange requirements for CS work areas.

Use of fans should not be permitted in any CS work area. Fans create highly turbulent air flow, which recirculates dust and microorganisms from the floor and work surfaces, and interferes with air flow.

Work Area Cleanliness

The cleaner the work area, the more likely that the products prepared in CS will be safe for use in a sterile environment. Dust and lint particles not only carry bacteria, but, in some cases, lint remaining in a sterile set may enter the patient's body during surgery and cause infection. CS technicians must minimize the amount of contaminants, such as dust, lint and bacteria in these work areas.

Bacteria can be transmitted by contact with contaminated items. Items in the decontamination and clean assembly areas can also be contaminated, which may be transmitted to other objects. Inanimate objects that can transmit bacteria are called **fomites**. Common fomites that become contaminated in CS areas include door handles, computer pads and keyboards, telephones, work surfaces and other items routinely handled by multiple people. CS technicians should know that by routinely cleaning these items and their general work areas (workstations), they can control the unwanted spread of bacteria within their workplace.

Fomite An inanimate object that can transmit bacteria.

Food and beverages should not be allowed in CS work areas. This standard is well understood for decontamination areas; however, this rule is also necessary in clean areas of the department for the following reasons:

- Beverages should not be allowed because they may spill and contaminate sterile items, or they may spill onto items that need to be sterilized and impact sterilization outcomes. Spilling may also contaminate items being assembled for sterilization or damage count sheets, reference books and other items on the work station.

- Foods should not be allowed because it may also contaminate items. CS technicians should not eat food in their work areas because their hands may become soiled and they could transmit bacteria. Snack foods leave oily residue on hands that can adhere to instruments being packaged for sterilization. This oil may impede the contact of the sterilant with the entire surface of the instrument. Food and beverages also attract insects and may increase the chance of insects invading the work area.

Environmental cleaning (housekeeping) is a vital component in the department's overall infection prevention and control process. CS departments are routinely cleaned to ensure that the microbial population is minimized. Basic housekeeping procedures used in CS should be the same as those used in the OR and delivery rooms. Cleaning guidelines include:

- Floors should be cleaned (wet mopped) at least daily. Floors should never be swept or dust mopped because dust will rise and fall on items, such as instruments, in the area. When sterile packages are opened, the dust that has accumulated on them may fall onto the package contents.

- The decontamination area should have separate and dedicated cleaning equipment, such as mops and buckets. Items used to clean the decontamination area should not be used elsewhere.

- Horizontal work surfaces, such as counters and work tables should be cleaned at least daily and, preferably, every shift.

- Light fixtures or their covers, and air vents should be cleaned at least every six months or as necessary. This function is usually performed by another department such as Environmental Services or Plant Maintenance.

- Other surfaces (including walls, cabinets and racks) should be cleaned on a regularly scheduled basis.

Many CS housekeeping functions are performed by Environmental Services personnel; however, routine cleaning of sterile storage cabinets, carts and racks is usually the responsibility of CS technicians who have been trained to properly handle sterile items, and who know specific product names and locations.

Other Environmental Cleaning Requirements

Fixtures and furniture in CS departments must be constructed of materials that can be washed, and they must be cleaned on a regularly scheduled basis.

The area designated for sterile storage may consist of either open (rack) or closed (cabinet) storage units. The decision about the type of storage used is based on the types of items to be stored, and the amount of traffic in the area. For example, closed cabinets may be used in high traffic areas, and open shelving (racks) may be used in more controlled, low traffic areas. Open rack systems should have a solid bottom, so items stored on the lower shelves are protected from contamination during housekeeping tasks. *Note: Specific information about sterile storage will be covered in Chapter 16.*

CS technicians work with items at all stages of the decontamination, sterilization, storage and distribution processes, so they must be well versed in basic infection control principles. To ensure the workflow is maintained, and items are handled appropriately at each stage in the processing cycle, staff must understand and practice the principles of asepsis.

An Important Concern

As discussed in Chapter 4, some microorganisms are becoming resistant to antibiotics or are naturally very hard to control. Many of these resistant microorganisms can be transferred to other surfaces and people very easily. Controlling these microorganisms and preventing their transmission is the number one responsibility of the CS department.

Understanding the way microorganisms can be transmitted is the key to helping stop cross-contamination.

ELEMENTS OF TRANSMISSION AND THE CHAIN OF INFECTION

Infection transmission is a complicated process that involves many factors in order for a pathogenic microorganism to result in disease or illness. According to the CDC *Guideline for Isolation Precautions: Preventing Transmission of Infectious Agents in Healthcare Settings, 2007*, the transmission of infectious agents in a healthcare setting requires six elements: a **causative agent**, a **reservoir**, a **portal of exit**, a **mode of transmission**, a **portal of entry** and a **susceptible host**. This infectious disease process is better known as the chain of infection. (See **Figure 6.17**)

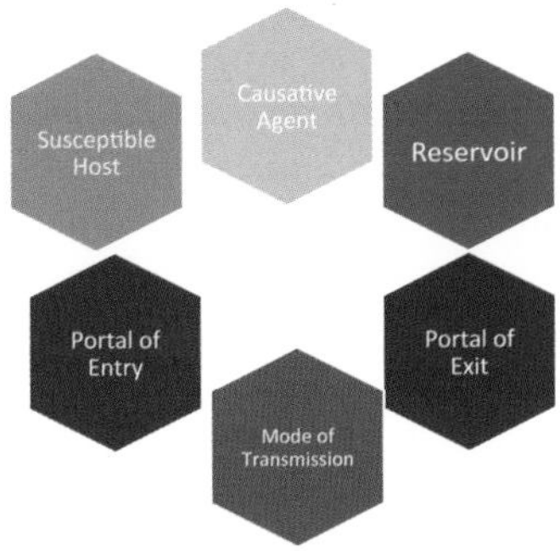

The Chain of Infection

Figure 6.17

> **Causative agent** (chain of infection) The microorganism that causes an infectious disease.
>
> **Reservoir** (chain of infection) The place where an infectious agent (microorganism) can survive.
>
> **Portal of exit** (chain of infection) The path by which an infectious agent leaves the reservoir.
>
> **Mode of transmission** (chain of infection) The method of transfer of an infectious agent from the reservoir to a susceptible host.
>
> **Portal of entry** (chain of infection) The path used by an infectious agent to enter a susceptible host.
>
> **Susceptible host** (chain of infection) A person or animal that lacks the ability to resist infection by an infectious agent.

Causative Agent

The first link is the causative agent, meaning the pathogenic microorganism: bacteria, virus, fungi, protozoa or prions. The characteristics that make the organism capable of causing disease include:

- Invasiveness – the ability of an organism to invade the host and cause damage.

- Pathogenicity – the ability of an organism to gain entry into the host and cause disease.

- Virulence – the degree of pathogenicity.

- Infectious dose – the quantity of organisms required to cause disease.

- Viability in a free state – the ability of the organism to survive outside the host.

- Ability to develop resistance to antimicrobial agents.

The only way to interrupt the transmission of a causative agent is to eliminate it. This can be done by promptly initiating the appropriate processes, such as using aseptic technique to avoid cross contamination, physically removing the contaminated substances through cleaning, and using effective disinfection and sterilization processes.

Reservoir/Source

The second link is the reservoir or source of the agent, a place in which an infectious agent can survive. In the healthcare setting, the most common reservoirs are human sources, such as patients, healthcare personnel, family, and visitors. However, inanimate objects, such as environmental surfaces, surgical instruments and devices, have also been implicated, as have contaminated food, water or intravenous fluids.

Those with active infections, but without obvious symptoms, and those who are **carriers**, represent the greatest risk to other patients and healthcare workers because the presence of disease-producing organisms may go undetected.

> **Carrier** A person or organism infected with an infectious disease agent, but displays no symptoms. Although unaffected by the disease themselves, carriers can transmit it to others.

Good personal hygiene and health habits, the use of appropriate housekeeping measures, and the proper cleaning, decontamination, disinfection and sterilization of hospital equipment can eliminate reservoirs.

Portal of Exit

The third link is the portal of exit, or the path by which an infectious agent leaves the reservoir. Portals of exit associated with humans and animal reservoirs include:

- Respiratory tract (coughing and sneezing).

- Genitourinary tract (urine, vaginal secretions or semen).

- Gastrointestinal tract (vomit or stools).

- Skin/mucous membrane (mucous or wound drainage).

- Blood (blood transfusions or contact with blood).

- Transplacental (through the placenta from mother to baby).

Common ways CS technicians can block the portal of exit include covering nose/mouth when sneezing/coughing, disposing facial tissues immediately after use, performing proper hand hygiene, disposing of trash and effectively using PPE.

Mode of Transmission

The fourth link is the mode of transmission, or how a pathogenic organism is spread. This can vary by the type of organism, and by its route.

Direct contact occurs when microorganisms are transferred directly from one infected person to another via blood or other blood-containing bodily fluids. Indirect contact occurs through a contaminated object or person such as through inadequately cleaned or sterilized instruments, the hands of healthcare personnel, or contaminated PPE. Some infections transmitted by contact include herpes simplex virus (HSV), *Staphylococcus aureus*, respiratory syncytial virus and *Clostridium difficile*.

Droplet transmission occurs when an infected person coughs, sneezes or talks during procedures, such as endotracheal intubation or suctioning. Infectious droplets can travel short distances to the susceptible person's mucous membranes of the eyes, nose and mouth. Some of the diseases spread in this manner include influenza virus, group A Streptococcus, adenovirus and some types of meningitis.

Airborne transmission occurs when very small droplet particles are dispersed in the air over long distances by air currents and are then inhaled by susceptible individuals. Infectious agents transmitted by this route include Mycobacterium tuberculosis (TB), spores of Aspergillus spp, and varicella-zoster virus (chickenpox).

Common vehicle transmission occurs when infectious agents are present in a vehicle, such as food (salmonella), blood (HIV) or water (pseudomonas).

Vector-borne transmission rarely occurs in U.S. hospitals. Agents can be carried on insects (e.g., on the feet or wings of flies) or by the bites of insect or arthropods (mosquitoes, ticks and fleas).

Pathogenic transmission can be interrupted through proper hand hygiene, cleaning, decontamination, disinfection and sterilization, Standard and Isolation Precautions, as well as proper food handling, proper water treatment, and proper maintenance of heating and air conditioning systems.

Portal of Entry

The fifth link is the portal of entry, or the path used by an infectious agent to enter a susceptible host.

Patients are particularly vulnerable to transmission in areas where the usual defense mechanisms are bypassed. Portals of entry associated with a human host include:

- Respiratory tract

- Genitourinary tract

- Gastrointestinal tract

- Skin/mucous membranes

- Transplacental

- **Parenteral**

> **Parenteral** Something that is put inside the body, but not by swallowing (e.g., an injection administered into the muscle).

Safe protocols include maintaining clean or sterile techniques during patient care procedures. Proper hand hygiene can alter access of an infectious agent to a susceptible host. Other practices involve using only properly disinfected/sterilized equipment for invasive procedures, and safe handling and disposing of sharps. *Note: Caregivers and their patients rely on CS to provide medical devices that are safe from infectious microorganisms.*

Susceptible Host

Most of the factors that influence whether a person gets an infection are related to the sixth and final link: whether the individual is a susceptible host and lacks the ability to resist infection Some who are exposed to an infectious agent will become severely ill and die, while others never develop symptoms at all. Some may progress from **colonization** to symptomatic disease right after exposure to the pathogen, while others will become temporarily or chronically colonized and never have symptoms.

> **Colonization** Occurs when microorganisms live on or in a host organism, but do not invade tissues or cause damage.

Whether or not an individual becomes susceptible to a microorganism can be influenced by various factors:

- Age (very young or very old).

- Disease history/underlying disease, such as cancer, diabetes and heart disease.

- Medications and treatments that can compromise immune systems, including chemotherapy, radiation and steroids.

- Trauma (the injury itself and the treatment of the injury can increase the risk of infection).

Some measures to boost the ability to fight disease include treating the primary disease (e.g., keeping blood sugar under control in diabetics), administering vaccines (such as pneumonia and influenza) and recognizing that patients are at high risk for infection.

From a CS perspective, there are many opportunities to interrupt the chain of infection and play an active and important role in preventing and controlling infectious diseases. **Figure 16.18** provides an example of how the chain of infection can be impacted by the CS department.

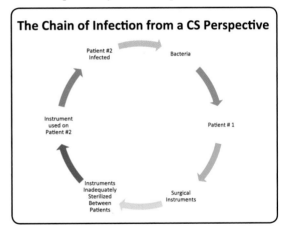

The Chain of Infection from a CS Perspective

Figure 6.18

CONCLUSION

Central Service technicians face the ongoing challenge of ensuring that the instruments and equipment they process are safe for patient use. Advances in technology and the emergence of new microbiological challenges have increased the difficulty in meeting this challenge. Every CS professional must appreciate the importance of infection control and prevention, and thoroughly understand their role in the process.

RESOURCES

Centers for Disease Control and Prevention. www.cdc.gov/nchs/fastats/insurg.htm.

Centers for Disease Control and Prevention. http://www.cdc.gov/HAI/organisms/organisms.html.

Association of periOperative Registered Nurses. *AORN Perioperative Standards and Recommended Practices 2013, Recommended Practice: Surgical Attire.*

Association for the Advancement of Medical Instrumentation. *NSI/AAMI ST79:2013, Section 3.*

Occupational Safety & Health Administration. *Bloodborne Pathogens (29 CFR 1910.1030).*

CENTRAL SERVICE TERMS

Biocidal

Surgical site infection (SSI)

Chain of infection

Asepsis

Aseptic technique

Asepsis (medical)

Asepsis (surgical)

Hand hygiene

Fomite

Causative agent

Reservoir

Portal of exit

Mode of transmission

Portal of entry

Susceptible host

Carrier

Parenteral

Colonization

Chapter 7

Decontamination: Point-of-Use Preparation and Transport

Learning Objectives

As a result of successfully completing this chapter, readers will be able to:

1. Review the four main goals of soiled item preparation and transport

2. Identify the sources of contaminated items

3. Explain point-of-use preparation procedures

4. Review basic procedures to transport soiled items from user areas to the Central Service decontamination area

5. Discuss safety guidelines for transporting soiled items to the Central Service decontamination area

6. Identify basic sources for education and training information applicable to the transport of contaminated items

INTRODUCTION

Reusable instruments and other medical devices processed in the Central Service (CS) department are transported to patient care and treatment areas where they are used in a wide variety of procedures and applications. After use, they must be transported back to the CS decontamination area to be processed for reuse. Sometimes, the transport distance is only a few feet, but other items may need to be transported a few miles (or more) between facilities. Whether the distance is only a few feet from the user department and CS, or several miles between facilities, consistant handling of soiled instruments is a must. This chapter reviews recommended protocols and requirements for these transportation activities.

GOALS OF POINT-OF-USE PREPARATION AND TRANSPORT

Regardless of transport distance, soiled item transport must fulfill four main goals:

- Removal of **gross soil**: Gross soil left on instruments not only makes them more difficult to clean but can damage the instrumentation. (See **Figure 7.1**)

- Prevention of damage: Soiled items must be prepared for transport in a manner that will prevent damage during return to the decontamination area of the CS department.

- Prevention of cross contamination: Soiled items must be safely transported from point of use to the decontamination area without cross contaminating the environment between those areas.

- Keeping others safe: Soiled items must be contained and labeled to help ensure that all individuals who may come in contact with contaminated items remain safe during the transportation process.

Gross soil Tissue, body fat, blood and other body substances.

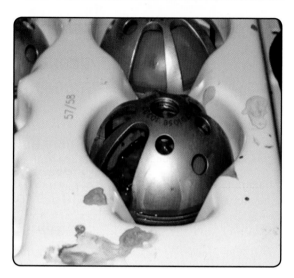

Figure 7.1 Gross soil

SOURCES OF CONTAMINATED ITEMS

Reusable medical devices, such as instruments and equipment, are used in numerous locations throughout the healthcare facility. The surgery department generates high volumes of contaminated items, but other areas such as Labor & Delivery, the Emergency Department, Endoscopy, Cardiac Care Services and any procedure-based areas also generate contaminated items.

In many facilities, the CS decontamination area is located close to the Operating Room (OR). That is the logistical choice because surgery is the source of the majority of soiled items transported to CS. Enclosed carts filled with contaminated instruments, equipment and utensils can be easily, quickly and safely transported to the decontamination area through a connecting hallway. If the CS department is located on another level of the facility, items can be transported between floors using a dedicated elevator or dumbwaiter system that is used exclusively to transport contaminated items (See **Figure 7.2**).

Example of a dedicated elevator used to transport contaminated items.

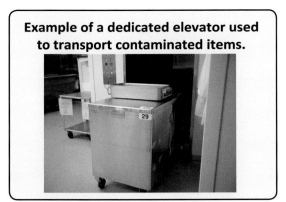

Figure 7.2 Dedicated soiled elevator

Contaminated items may be returned to the CS decontamination area during scheduled soiled pick up rounds or upon request from a user department. Sometimes, soiled items may be delivered to the decontamination area by employees of the user department. For example, surgical staff return case carts to the decontamination area after surgical procedures. Generally, however, contaminated items are placed in a designated holding area to be picked up by CS technicians at designated times. (See **Figure 7.3**)

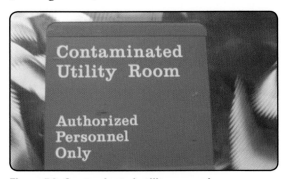

Figure 7.3 Contaminated utility room sign

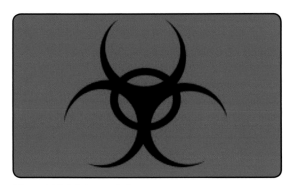

Figure 7.4 Biohazard signage

Holding Items until Return to Central Service

All departments that use and store reusable items for later transport to the Central Service department need a designated holding area for contaminated items until they can be retrieved. These areas should be clearly designated with **biohazard signage** (See **Figure 7.4**) and should not be accessible to visitors or other unauthorized personnel. The contaminated holding area should have contaminated trash and linen receptacles, and a dedicated handwashing sink. Areas where liquid waste, including blood and suction canister contents, may be an issue will also need a shielded flush-type commode for liquid waste disposal.

Biohazard signage Notices posted in easily-seen locations that alert persons in the area about the presence of harmful bacteria, viruses or other dangerous biohazardous agents or organisms.

POINT-OF-USE PREPARATION

Instrument decontamination begins at the point of use. When the procedure is complete, instruments should be prepared in a manner that will help to ensure that they can be transported safely to the CS decontamination area for complete cleaning. CS professionals must enlist the help of user departments to ensure that instruments and equipment are correctly prepared for the decontamination process immediately after use. Some facilities have CS technicians assigned to the OR to assist with instrument set up and breakdown, so it is important to know proper point-of-use instrument handling.

Reasons for Point-of-Use Preparation

There are three important reasons that the preparation process should begin in the user department at the point of use:

- Point-of-use preparation helps prolong the life of instruments. Common substances to which instruments are exposed during procedures, such as blood and saline, can break down devices' protective finish and accelerate decomposition.

- Dry soil and debris, especially in instruments with lumens and hard-to-reach crevices, are much more difficult to remove than moist soil and debris.

- Soil and excess moisture promote the formation of biofilm colonies. **Biofilm** is highly resistant to cleaning and disinfecting chemicals, so removing the causes of biofilm is essential.

> **Biofilm** A collection of microorganisms that attach to surfaces and each other and form a colony. The colony produces a protective gel that is very difficult to penetrate with detergents and disinfectants.

When soil dries, instruments require more aggressive cleaning methods and instruments with dried soil also take longer to clean. This can increase processing time and that delay may impact instrument availability for subsequent use.

The proper care and handling of instruments and equipment is the responsibility of everyone who comes in contact with them, and that begins with personnel at the point of use.

Personnel responsible for handling instruments at the point of use must keep in mind that those instruments are precision devices that can have a negative impact on patient care if not managed properly. Instruments should be handled with care throughout the procedure and be properly prepared for transport according to facility policy. **Figure 7.5** provides an example of an instrument set-up in an OR.

Point-of-Use Preparation Guidelines

Point-of-use preparation does not replace the cleaning process; instead, its purpose is to begin the cleaning process. The following guidelines should be followed when users prepare items for transport to the CS decontamination area:

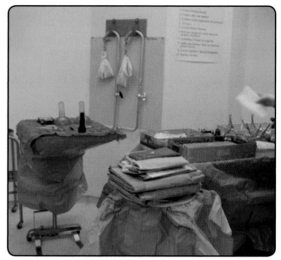

Figure 7.5 Instrument set up

- Remove gross soil from instruments. Wear appropriate personal protective equipment (PPE) while preparing instruments for transport.

- Follow the manufacturer's instructions for point-of-use cleaning and preparation. For example, flexible fiberoptic endoscope manufacturers typically suggest that water and enzymatic solution be suctioned through the scope's suction channel at the end of a procedure to preclean the suction channel. They also state the shaft should be wiped to remove gross soil.

- Separate reusable **sharps** from other instruments. Place instruments with sharp points or edges, such as reusable needles, cutting edges and skin hooks, in a separate container, so they can be easily identified and to reduce the risk of injuries from sharps.

> **Sharps** Cutting instruments, including knives, scalpels, blades, needles and scissors of all types. Other examples include chisels and osteotomes, some curettes, dissectors and elevators, rongeurs and cutting forceps, punches, saws and trocars.

- Separate reusable linen. Reusable linen should be removed and placed into an appropriate bag or container. Users should take extra caution to ensure that small instruments are not mistakenly included with the linen.

- Remove disposable components, such as blades, disposable tubing and canisters. Sharp items should be placed in a hard-sided container labeled "Biohazard." Separating disposable from reusable components reduces the amount of contaminated items that must be transported, and it also reduces the risk of injury from sharps, such as knife blades and needles. When separating disposable items, watch closely to ensure that reusable items are not removed and discarded with disposable components. (e.g., metal drape clamps are sometimes left attached to disposable drapes).

- Open hinged instruments, disassemble multi-part instruments and place instruments in the appropriate instrument tray in an orderly manner. **Figure 7.6** provides an example of instruments that have not been properly prepared for transport. Place heavy instruments on the bottom of the tray with lighter instruments on top. Handle cords, scopes and cameras with care. Do not place any items on top of them. Notify the CS department if some instruments are not being returned with the set for any reason.

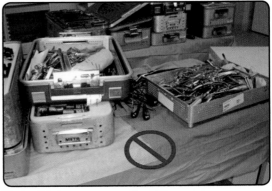

Figure 7.6 Improper case breakdown

- Keep items together. Instrument sets or multi-part items should be kept together for their transport to the CS decontamination area. If items are separated or left behind, reassembly will be delayed. Failure to keep items together also increases the risk that components will be misplaced or lost.

- Keep instruments moist to prevent soil from drying on their surface. (See **Figure 7.7**) This can be accomplished by using commercial foams, gels or spray products, or placing a moist towel over them. *Note: If instruments are placed in a soak basin or solution, they should not be exposed to the solution for an extended period of time because this may damage the instruments' surface. The soak solution must be discarded before transport to reduce the risk of spills. Care should be taken not to contaminate the outside of the tray or container.*

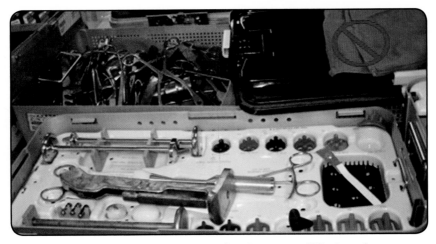

Figure 7.7 Dried blood on instruments makes them more difficult to clean

- Empty fluids from containers. If a contaminated device has a reusable fluid container, bottle or receptacle, the fluid should be removed and disposed of according to the facility's protocols. Disposable fluid containers should also be handled according to required facility procedures.

- Third-party reprocessing items should be removed and properly contained, or separated and sent to CS, per facility protocols.

- If reusable instruments were used during a case with suspected or known Creutzfeldt-Jakob Disease (CJD), notify CS and Infection Prevention and Control. Follow hospital procedures for initial cleaning and containment for transport to the CS decontamination area.

- Notify the CS department about items needing repair. If instruments or equipment are in need of repair, tag them so they can be removed from the system for repair or refurbishing. (See **Figure 7.8**)

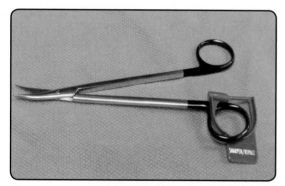

Figure 7.8   Tagged instrument

- Notify the CS department about items requiring **turnover/turnaround** for another case; do not automatically assume the department has this information.

> **Turnover/turnaround**   Term used to describe instruments or equipment that must receive priority processing in order to be made available for another procedure.

CS professionals must work together with end users to ensure that point-of-use preparation is carried out according to manufacturers' Instructions for Use (IFU) and any specific requirements. In many cases, departments will need to develop joint procedures for the handling of used items to ensure that everyone involved understands their role in the process.

TRANSPORT OF SOILED ITEMS

Contaminated items should be contained before transport through the facility to minimize airborne or contact spread of microorganisms and reduce the risk of cross contamination and infection. The best way to transport soiled instruments is in enclosed carts. (See **Figure 7.9**) If an open transport cart is used, the cart must have a solid bottom shelf to prevent drips and spills, and the cart must be covered during transport. Smaller numbers of instruments from other departments can be transported in dedicated transport containers or in plastic bags that are clearly labeled Biohazard. (See **Figure 7.10**) Large items, such as suction units and other types of patient care equipment, can be transported in special carts designed for soiled item transport. (See **Figure 7.11**)

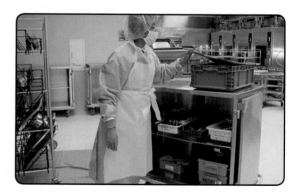

Figure 7.9   Enclosed cart

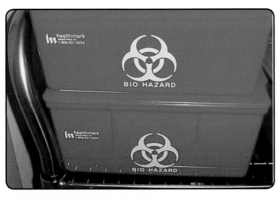

Figure 7.10 Transport containers

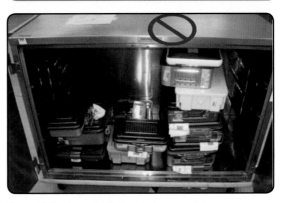

Figure 7.12 Incorrectly loaded case cart

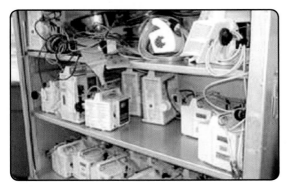

Figure 7.11 Large item transport cart

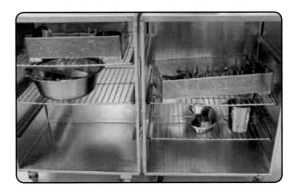

Figure 7.13 Cart correctly loaded for transport

The goal of all soiled transport is to transfer the contaminated items to the CS decontamination area while minimizing the risk of cross contamination. All transport devices must be free from external gross contamination, such as blood, before transport to reduce the risk of environmental contamination and personnel exposure. Contaminated items should be handled as little as possible to reduce the risk of exposure to employees and patients.

Place instrument sets securely in the cart. Sets should be placed so they do not slide or fall during transport. Metal trays and containers should not be placed on top of more fragile plastic trays and containers. (See **Figure 7.12**) Do not mix unopened sterile and soiled instruments in the same cart because this will contaminate sterile items.

Personnel transporting contaminated items should be trained and must consistently follow safe handling procedures. These include methods to safely load transport devices to avoid spillage and to ensure items are securely contained. (See **Figure 7.13**)

The transport of contaminated items should be kept physically separate from the transport of their clean and sterile counterparts. Containers and carts used for transporting contaminated items should not be used to transport and deliver clean items, unless they are thoroughly decontaminated between use (e.g., surgical case carts used to transport soiled instruments from surgery to the decontamination area must be decontaminated before they can be used to transport sterile packages back to surgery). (**Figure 7.14** provides an example of a cart washer that can be used for this purpose.)

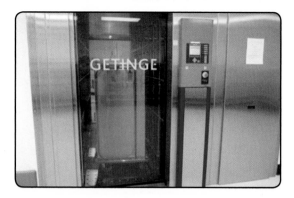

Figure 7.14 Cart washer

Ideally, soiled devices will be transported to the CS decontamination area immediately after use. This reduces the opportunity for soil to dry on the instruments. The longer instruments are damp and unclean the greater the chance biofilm will begin to form. Returning instruments quickly allows the items to be returned to service in a timely manner.

Contaminated items from other departments are often placed in a holding area for pick up on a scheduled basis by CS technicians who then return them to the decontamination area for processing. These soiled pick up rounds should be conducted as scheduled because failure to perform soiled item pick-ups can lead to equipment and instrument shortages. All healthcare facilities have limited numbers of instrument sets and patient care equipment. The instrument and equipment replenishment system relies on items moving through the system (from storage to use to processing and back to storage) in a timely manner to maintain an adequate supply of available instruments and equipment.

SAFETY GUIDELINES FOR SOILED ITEM TRANSPORT

All instruments, utensils and equipment used in patient care and treatment processes should be considered contaminated. CS technicians who transport contaminated items should also wear gloves to handle the items as they are picked up and placed into the transport cart. Gloves should then be removed and hands should be washed before leaving the pick-up location.

Whenever there is a danger of splashes, spills or aerosol exposure, CS technicians should wear the appropriate PPE required by the Occupational Safety and Health Administration (OSHA). CS technicians who clean and decontaminate the soiled items must also follow OSHA regulations for PPE.

Transporting equipment and carts through corridors can pose significant safety concerns. CS technicians must maintain control of transport carts at all times and should not move them at excessive speeds. Patients, visitors, healthcare providers and movable equipment share the same hallways as transport carts, and excessive speed or inattention could lead to accidents. CS technicians should maintain control of their carts and pay particular attention to hallway intersections and doors that may open into the path of the cart. Many facilities install safety mirrors at hallway junctions to help prevent accidents. (See **Figure 7.15**) Carts containing soiled items should never be left unattended.

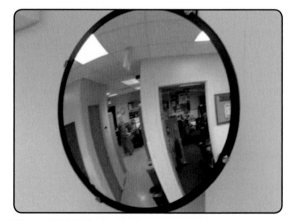

Figure 7.15 Safety mirror

In addition to maintaining safe control of their transport carts, CS technicians should always yield to patients and visitors in hallways and at elevators. In any healthcare facility, the routine transport of soiled items never takes precedence over the transport of patients.

OFF-SITE PROCESSING

Sometimes, contaminated items may need to be transported between buildings or to a central off-site processing center. When it is necessary to transport contaminated items using a truck or van, facility personnel must consult U.S. Department of Transportation (DOT) guidelines and follow applicable state and local requirements for the safe transport of biohazard materials.

When preparing items for off-site transport, care should be taken to protect the instruments from damage during transport. Instruments should be placed in their containers in a manner that will shield the instruments from movement that could lead to damage. Instrument trays should be placed securely in a transport cart, which can then be secured inside the transport vehicle. Instruments should be transported as soon as possible after the procedure to reduce the risk of the soil drying, which makes instruments more difficult to clean.

EDUCATION AND TRAINING

When performed improperly, the transport of contaminated items can pose a threat to the safety of patients, visitors and employees. Carefully thought-out procedures must be developed to help ensure that all contaminated items are appropriately handled. The development of these procedures should be done with the input and/or support of the facility's Infection Prevention and Hazardous Materials committees.

Recommended practices for contaminated item transport are provided by the Association for the Advancement of Medical Instrumentation (AAMI). Procedures should also reflect OSHA regulations. Additional information regarding soiled instrument preparation and transport can be obtained from the Association for periOperative Registered Nurses (AORN).

Everyone who may have contact with contaminated items must be educated about the dangers associated with biohazardous items. In addition to education and training for CS technicians, this includes Environmental Service employees, courier and transport technicians and drivers. Their education should include proper handling of biohazardous items, and the correct application and use of PPE.

CONCLUSION

Instrument preparation at the point of use and proper transport to Central Service requires interdepartmental teamwork. Good communication and training can help personnel in all departments protect their facility's instruments and better serve patients. By understanding and following the recommended guidelines for the preparation and transport of contaminated items, CS technicians help protect patients, visitors and healthcare workers.

RESOURCES

Association for the Advancement of Medical Instrumentation. *ANSI/AAM ST79: Comprehensive Guide to Steam Sterilization and Sterility Assurance in Health Care Facilities.* 2013.

Association of periOperative Registered Nurses. *Guidelines for PeriOperative Practice: Instrument Cleaning.* Guidelines for PeriOperative Practice. 2015.

Occupational Safety and Health Administration. *CFR 1910.1030. Bloodborne Pathogens Standard.*

Phillips N. *Berry & Kohn's Operating Room Technique, 11th Ed.* 2007.

CENTRAL SERVICE TERMS

Gross soil

Biohazard signage

Biofilm

Sharps

Turnover/turnaround

Chapter 8

Cleaning and Decontamination

Learning Objectives

As a result of successfully completing this chapter, readers will be able to:

1. Define cleaning and identify challenges to cleaning medical devices

2. Discuss the purpose and set up of the decontamination area

3. Identify the importance of personal protective equipment and standard precautions

4. Explain the role of common cleaning tools

5. Discuss mechanical cleaners

6. Discuss the use of chemicals in the decontamination area

7. List steps in the cleaning process

8. Explain manual cleaning processes

INTRODUCTION

Cleaning is the cornerstone of instrument processing. Items that have not been cleaned properly cannot be sterilized or made safe for patient use. The cleaning processes performed in Central Service (CS) are very different than the cleaning processes carried out in other situations. When cleaning is performed outside the healthcare facility (for example, in home settings), the definition of clean can vary with the individual. When cleaning is performed in the healthcare facility, it must be performed to the highest level and it must be performed with consistency. Improper cleaning can cause infections and even death. This chapter will examine the cleaning process—from the tools required to perform cleaning to the basic steps necessary to carry out a successful process.

WHAT IS CLEAN?

Cleaning is defined as the removal of all visible and non-visible soil and other foreign material from medical devices being reprocessed. When faced with the complex configurations of today's medical devices, the cleaning process becomes quite challenging. Some soils are easy to see and remove; others are not. The goal of every cleaning process in the decontamination area is to remove all soils, not just the ones that are easy to see and remove.

Proper cleaning requires the right tools, the right technique, and attention to detail. A medical device may appear clean at first glance, but may harbor soils that are not readily visible. The following photos (**Figures 8.1** through **8.4**) provide some examples of the challenges associated with cleaning medical devices. **Figure 8.1** provides a look at the inside of a bulb syringe that was mistakenly assumed to have been cleaned. It is extremely difficult, if not impossible, to properly clean any area that cannot be seen. Lumens and other areas that do not provide good access for cleaning pose a significant challenge to CS technicians. **Figure 8.2** provides a look inside an arthroscopic shaver using a flexible inspection scope. The configuration of this instrument makes it impossible to see all areas for cleaning.

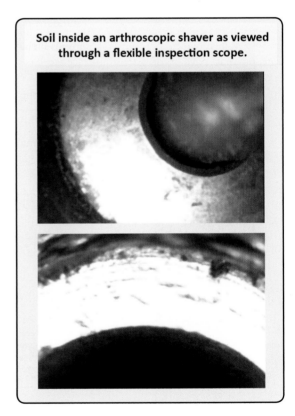

Dried soil inside a bulb syringe

Figure 8.1

Soil inside an arthroscopic shaver as viewed through a flexible inspection scope.

Figure 8.2

Even when item surfaces are clearly visible, inadequate cleaning can occur. **Figure 8.3** provides a look at a common clamp that has undergone fluorescence-based protein detection testing to detect residual protein soils. Although the clamp appeared visibly clean, several areas of concern were identified. The yellow and orange areas indicate residual soil.

Residual protein soils detected by fluorescence-based protein detection testing

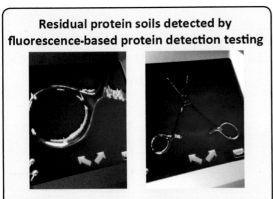

Figure 8.3

Figure 8.4 provides a look at common biopsy forceps that have undergone fluorescence-based protein testing to detect residual protein soil.

These examples illustrate that even simple instruments can pose a significant cleaning challenge. Every item that passes through the decontamination process has the potential to harm a patient or present a danger to healthcare workers. That is why CS technicians assigned to the **decontamination area** must have the proper cleaning tools, must understand the correct cleaning technique for every item, and must always pay close attention to detail as they perform their duties.

Cleaning The removal of all visible and non-visible soil, and any other foreign material from medical devices being processed.

Decontamination area The location within a healthcare facility designated for the collection, retention and cleaning of soiled and/or contaminated items.

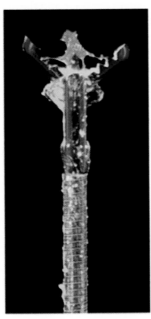 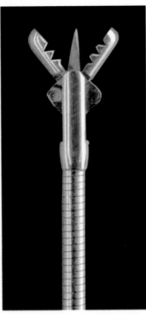 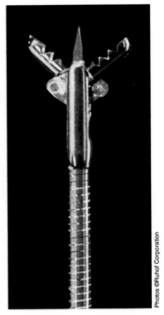

Biopsy forceps prior to reprocessing. Bioburden can clearly be seen in this laboratory photo.

After reprocessing, this same instrument appears to be clean to the naked eye.

In some cases residual bioburden still remains after reprocessing, as seen in this laboratory photo.

Photos ©Ruhof Corporation

Figure 8.4

INTRODUCTION TO THE DECONTAMINATION WORK AREA

This section provides an overview of the decontamination area, and the equipment and processes needed to accomplish thorough cleaning.

Design and Location of the Decontamination Area

The process of cleaning and decontamination begins long before even one soiled instrument arrives in the decontamination area. A great deal of planning and preparation goes into the design and set up of the work area and the acquisition of cleaning equipment, tools and supplies. CS technicians assigned to the decontamination area should be aware of the processes and safeguards used to facilitate the cleaning of soiled items, reduce the spread of microorganisms and ensure the safety of patients and employees.

Decontamination areas are unique because of their purpose and design. Soiled instruments should only be cleaned in a designated decontamination area. The decontamination area serves as a receiving area for soiled instruments and, in many cases, other medical devices and equipment from surgery and other areas of the healthcare facility. Several design-related factors must be considered as the decontamination area is planned. It is more cost effective to centralize the decontamination function to one area of the healthcare facility. If the decontamination area is not centralized, additional expenses will be incurred for duplicate equipment and space.

The location of the decontamination area should consider the need to transport contaminated devices from the point of use. Proper transportation of contaminated devices is necessary to reduce the risk of cross contamination and exposure to bloodborne pathogens. (See **Figure 8.5**) In many cases, the decontamination area is located near the Operating Room (OR) because the majority of soiled instruments are generated there.

Floors and walls in the decontamination area should be constructed with materials that can tolerate cleaning chemicals. Walls should not be constructed of particulate or fiber-shedding materials. Spills and splashes are a common occurrence in the decontamination area and can create a need for frequent cleaning/disinfecting of surfaces.

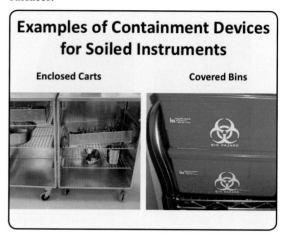

Examples of Containment Devices for Soiled Instruments

Enclosed Carts   Covered Bins

Figure 8.5

The ventilation system should allow for no less than 10 air exchanges per hour, and the area should be under negative pressure in relation to other areas adjacent to the decontamination area. Temperature should be regulated between 60°F and 65°F (16°C and 18°C). The low temperature is needed because CS technicians working in the decontamination area must wear fluid-resistant attire that, when worn for extended periods of time, can become uncomfortable and hot. A low temperature also helps inhibit the growth of microorganisms. **Relative humidity** is also important and should range from 30% to 60%.

> **Relative humidity** Amount of water vapor in the atmosphere; expressed as a percentage of the total amount of vapor the atmosphere could hold without condensation.

Lighting is essential to a safe work environment, and is a key element in the cleaning process. Instrument cleaning requires attention to detail, and lighting must enable technicians to perform inspections associated with the cleaning process.

Traffic should be restricted to personnel working in the area, and access to the area should be controlled. (See **Figure 8.6**)

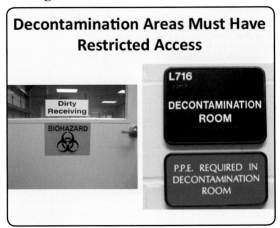

Figure 8.6

Emergency eyewash/shower equipment should be placed so these safety stations are accessible within 10 seconds or 30 meters of areas of potential chemical exposure. (See **Figure 8.7**)

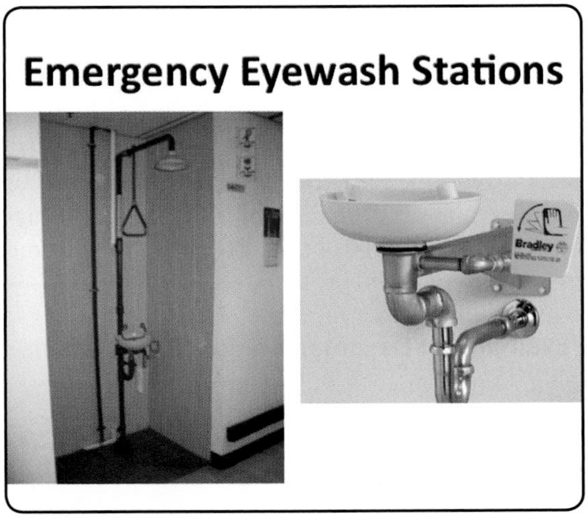

Emergency Eyewash Stations

Figure 8.7

The decontamination area is the central point for handling contaminated devices, and a high microbial count will be present in the environment. The first line of defense for reducing contaminates is maintaining as clean a work area as possible. Special attention should be given to the cleaning procedures in the work area. For example:

- Horizontal work surfaces should be cleaned and disinfected at least at the beginning and end of each shift.

- Spills should be spot-cleaned immediately.

- Floors should be cleaned and disinfected daily.

- **Biohazardous waste** should be removed at frequent intervals.

Adequate storage for equipment used to clean the decontamination area should be available and tools, such as mops, used in this area should not be used in other areas of the department.

> **Biohazardous waste** Waste containing infectious agents that present a risk or potential risk to human health, either directly through infections or indirectly through the environment.

Dress Code and Personal Behaviors

Employee safety is an important concern at all times during instrument cleaning and decontamination. Since CS technicians do not know the origin of the contamination, they must assume that every item received in the decontamination area can pose a potential risk to them. For these reasons, following personal protective equipment (PPE) requirements is essential. (See **Figure 8.6**)

Developing and adhering to good work practices and personal safety habits can reduce the risk of potential exposure to pathogens.

Handwashing and frequent use of appropriate hand germicidal agents is required. Whenever CS technicians remove PPE, they should properly wash their hands. A sink dedicated to hand hygiene should be provided within the decontamination area, and it should be separated from sinks used to sort and prepare instruments for processing.

Personal protective equipment (PPE)

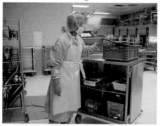

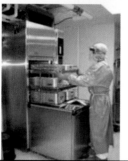

- Hair covering.

- Eye protection, such as goggles or eyeglasses with solid side shields, or a chin-length face shield.

- Fluid-resistant face mask.

- A gown with reinforced cuffs and a front that acts as a barrier to fluids.

- Strong general-purpose utility gloves that cover the cuffs of the reinforced gown and can resist cuts and tears.

- Skid-resistant decontamination shoe covers.

- Employer-provided cloth scrub attire that is changed at the end of each shift, or when wet or soiled.

Figure 8.8

Effective, ongoing education and training is critical to the safe processing of medical devices. Safety training is the ongoing responsibility of both the employer and the CS technician.

Before any new staff member is assigned to the decontamination area, he/she must receive a thorough and comprehensive orientation.

Traffic Control and Environmental Management

Technicians assigned to the decontamination area should be constantly vigilant of their surroundings. Traffic control is imperative due to the potential for exposure to bloodborne pathogens and hazardous chemicals.

Work Area Set Up

Preparation of the work area is an essential first step in promoting safety and efficacy in the decontamination area.

Sinks - Ideally, each workstation will have three sink bays for washing, intermediate rinsing and final rinsing. If three bays are not available, the cleaning process must be modified to accomplish the cleaning process as if there were three sink bays. (See **Figure 8.9**) Regardless of the configuration, the workflow should always be from dirty to clean. (See **Figure 8.10**)

Examples of Decontamination Workstations

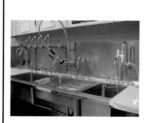

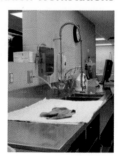

Figure 8.9

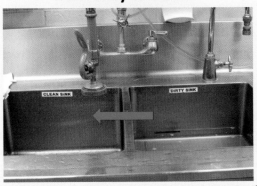

All soiled items should flow from dirty to clean.

Figure 8.10

A three-sink arrangement used for manual cleaning should consist of:

- A wash sink with water and detergent or enzymatic solution. This sink should be filled with warm water with a temperature range of 80°F to 110°F [27°C to 44°C]. The temperature of the solution should be monitored. (See **Figure 8.11**) Water hardness, pH, temperature and the type of soil present on instrumentation impact the effectiveness of enzyme cleaners and detergents. *Note: The detergent manufacturer's Instructions for Use (IFU) must be consulted for specific instructions.*

All cleaning chemicals must be mixed per manufacturer's instructions. Marking the sink to indicate gallon levels can help ensure that solutions are mixed to the proper dilution. (See **Figure 8.12**) Cleaning solutions should be changed frequently for maximum cleaning.

- A second sink (intermediate rinse) that contains plain or softened water. After cleaning, devices should be thoroughly rinsed to further assist in removing debris and detergent residues. This rinse water should be changed frequently, so the cleaning chemicals do not build up and reattach to the instruments being rinsed.

- A third sink (final rinse) with **distilled**, **deionized** or **reverse osmosis (RO)** water. This helps prevent instrument spotting, rinse off cleaning chemical residues and **pyrogens**, and prevent the redeposit of minerals, microbes and pyrogens.

Deionized (DI) water Water that has had all minerals removed through an ion exchange process.

Distilled water Water that is heated to steam, then allowed to cool and condense. Distillation removes impurities, like gases and organic material; it also removes some bacteria.

Reverse osmosis (RO) A water purification process by which a solvent, such as water, is removed of impurities after being forced through a semipermeable membrane.

Pyrogen A substance, typically produced by a bacterium, that produces fever when introduced/released into the blood.

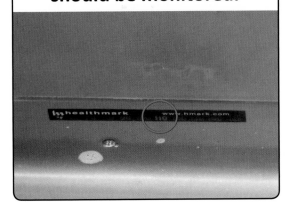

Temperature of solutions should be monitored.

Figure 8.11

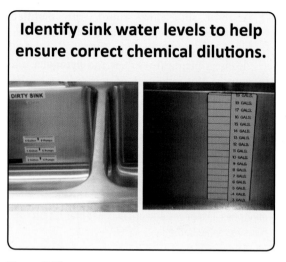

Identify sink water levels to help ensure correct chemical dilutions.

Figure 8.12

Adequate cleaning and rinsing should result in low bioburden, which is essential to the effectiveness of terminal sterilization.

Cleaning Tools

Water

Although it is often taken for granted, and not often considered to be a tool, water quality makes a big difference in instrument/equipment cleaning outcomes. Poor water quality can impact the performance of chemicals used for cleaning and disinfection, and it can also affect the rinse phase by leaving deposits on items that have been cleaned.

Regardless of where the water originates, a natural aquifer, or in surface water, it must be purified to provide the proper quality for the instrument cleaning process. There are many impurities in water, even in tap water treated at a municipal water treatment plant. Water from any source typically contains minerals, dissolved solids, particles, gases, and organic and non-organic chemicals. Some water sources also contain bacteria, algae and parasites. These contaminants may impede cleaning and biocidal processes and, in some cases, contaminates may shorten the life of instruments by harming their finish.

Water used as a final rinse in any cleaning process should be purified to reduce or eliminate these elements. Water sample tests should be made at each site where it is used as a final rinse in manual and mechanical (ultrasonic, cart washer and washer-disinfector) processes. Tests can be performed by facility personnel. Alternatively, manufacturers and distributors of cleaning products, cleaning machines and water treatment products often provide these tests free of charge. Knowing the pH and what is in the water used to process instruments allows facilities to make wise choices in the selection of cleaning and disinfecting chemicals used, and the type of water purification system needed. Many chemicals used in the decontamination process require specific pH ranges, and final rinse water must be free of impurities. **Figure 8.13** provides a comparison of pH levels to common household items.

CS departments must ensure that the water used for the cleaning process meets the requirements for the specific use.

Manual Cleaning Tools

Decontamination requires a combination of manual and mechanical cleaning processes; therefore, the area will have equipment for both types of cleaning.

The following section provides information about manual cleaning tools.

Brushes

Brushes are available in many diameters and lengths. Some must be rigid and others must be flexible to properly clean the many different lumens, channels and crevices in instruments. (See **Figure 8.14**) Brushes used for cleaning usually have nylon bristles; however, metal varieties, brushes with plastic wands and sponge tips are also available. Some brushes are impregnated with enzymatic detergents that can help with the cleaning process.

pH Level Comparison

14	Liquid drain cleaner, Caustic soda
13	bleaches, oven cleaner
12	Soapy water
11	Household Ammonia (11.9)
10	Milk of magnesium (10.5)
9	Toothpaste (9.9)
8	Baking soda (8.4), Seawater, Eggs
7	"Pure" water (7)
6	Urine (6) Milk (6.6)
5	Acid rain (5.6) Black coffee (5)
4	Tomato juice (4.1)
3	Grapefruit & Orange juice, Soft drink
2	Lemon juice (2.3) Vinegar (2.9)
1	Hydrochloric acid secreted from the stomach lining (1)
0	Battery Acid

Figure 8.13

Examples of cleaning brushes

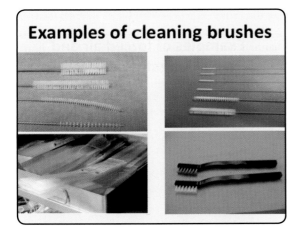

Figure 8.14

Ideally, disposable brushes should be used. If reusable brushes are used, they should be decontaminated at least daily and when visibly soiled to ensure they are not a source of contamination. Abrasive brushes should never be used because they can scratch the surface of the instrument and accelerate corrosion. Metal or wire brushes should only be used if indicated in the instrument's IFU.

Correct brush size is also critical. Consider lumen cleaning, for example. If the brush is too large, it will not fit into the lumen. If the brush is too small, it will not have complete contact with the lumen walls, and will not thoroughly clean them. The brush must also be long enough to extend through the lumen. (See **Figure 8.15**) Brushes that are worn should be discarded. (See **Figure 8.16**)

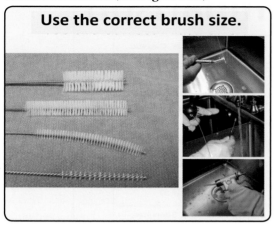

Use the correct brush size.

Figure 8.15

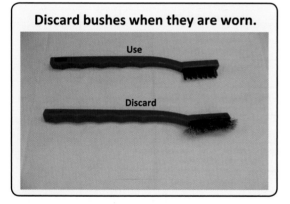

Discard bushes when they are worn.

Use

Discard

Figure 8.16

Cleaning Cloths

Most cleaning cloths are made of textiles. Some have lint and others are low-lint or lint-free. Use of a lint-free or low-lint cloth reduces the risk of fibers being left on instruments. Cloths should be changed regularly, or when visibly soiled or stained.

Sponges

Sponges can be used to clean some medical devices. Some sponges are impregnated with detergents and should be used according to the manufacturer's IFU. Unfortunately, the sponge's structure makes them virtually impossible to completely clean and sterilize for reuse, so they must be discarded and replaced at least daily or after each use, according to the manufacturer's IFU. (See **Figure 8.17**)

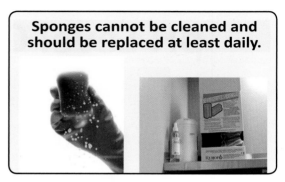

Sponges cannot be cleaned and should be replaced at least daily.

Figure 8.17

Water Irrigators and Forced Instrument Air Devices

Water irrigation devices (See **Figure 8.18**) and instrument air devices should be checked to ensure they are in working order and have all the necessary attachments. Care should be used to direct air and water spray away from employees.

What Is Instrument Air?

Instrument air is compressed air that has had dust, dirt and other pollutants removed. In healthcare, instrument air is used to power medical devices, such as pneumatic drills and saws, and calibrate medical equipment. Instrument air is also used to dry medical devices after cleaning and decontamination. To qualify as instrument, air must be free of oil, water, hydrocarbons and other contaminates that could cause infection.

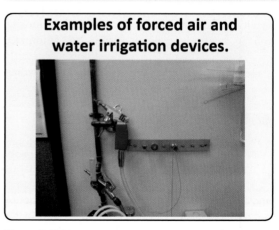

Examples of forced air and water irrigation devices.

Figure 8.18

Floor Drains and Spray Nozzles

Many decontamination areas are equipped with a spray nozzle and floor drain/grate that provides drainage when manually cleaning bulkier items that do not fit in the cleaning sinks. The spray nozzle system is also used for cleaning the wheels of mobile equipment that cannot be sent through an automatic process. (See **Figure 8.19**)

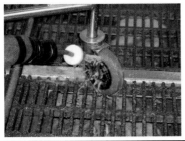

Example of a spray nozzle system for cleaning mobile equipment and cart wheels.

Figure 8.19

Additional Tools

Specific instruments may require specific tools to perform cleaning and decontamination. For example, flexible endoscopes may require leak testing devices. Specific cleaning tools should be purchased at the same time as the instrument(s) and replaced, as necessary. All CS technicians assigned to the decontamination area should be trained in the proper use of special cleaning tools.

MECHANICAL CLEANERS

Several mechanical options are available to assist with decontamination. Mechanical cleaning facilitates the decontamination process by removing soil and microorganisms using an automated cleaning process. When functioning correctly, these machines function consistently and reduce time and labor for CS professionals. *Note: The use of mechanical cleaners does not completely replace the need for manual cleaning.*

Some units reduce microbial contamination through a multi-step approach using a combination of cleaning solutions, hot water, rinsing, lubrication and drying, while others provide a cleaning function only. Mechanical devices commonly found in the decontamination area include ultrasonic cleaners, irrigating sonics, washer-disinfectors, cart washers, pasteurizers and automated endoscope reprocessors (AER).

CS technicians should not use any type of mechanical equipment without receiving proper training and competency review.

The following is an overview of common equipment found in the decontamination area.

Ultrasonic Cleaners (Sonics)

Ultrasonic cleaners are used for fine cleaning, not for disinfection or sterilization. They are used to remove soil from joints, crevices, lumens and other areas that are difficult to clean by other methods.

The term "ultrasonic" is an appropriate name for this type of mechanical cleaner. "Ultra" means beyond and "sonic" means sound. When an ultrasonic wave passes through a liquid, it makes the liquid vibrate. Hospital sonic cleaners produce from 20,000 to 38,000 vibrations per second. The vibrations are transmitted through the detergent bath and create **cavitation**. With this process, ultrasonic waves pass through a cleaning solution, the molecules of the solution are set in very rapid motion, and small gas bubbles develop. As the bubbles grow larger, they become unstable until they implode (not explode). (See **Figure 8.20**) This creates a vacuum in the solution that draws minute bits of foreign matter (including microorganisms) from cracks and crevices, such as hinges and serrations on instruments. This vacuum action results in cleaning of hard-to-reach areas.

After cavitation, rinsing is necessary to remove any residue, including detergents that remain on the instruments. Since the ultrasonic cleaning process lifts proteins, starches and lipids from instruments, it is important to routinely clean the tank according to the manufacturer's instructions.

Cavitation The process used by an ultrasonic cleaner in which low-pressure bubbles in a cleaning solution burst inward and dislodge soil from instruments.

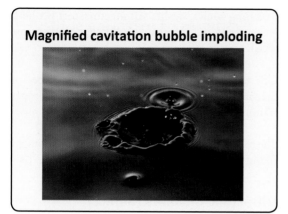

Magnified cavitation bubble imploding

Figure 8.20

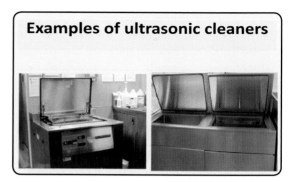

Examples of ultrasonic cleaners

Figure 8.21

Instruments to be processed must be pre cleaned to remove gross soil, such as blood and tissue debris. In addition, protein absorbs sound and reduces the cleaning action in the sonic cleaner. Bath temperatures for cleaning instruments should be between 80°F and 109°F (27°C and 43°C), unless otherwise specified by the equipment or detergent manufacturer. Temperatures above 140°F (60°C) will coagulate protein, making it more difficult to remove. Water should be changed when it is visually soiled, or at regularly scheduled intervals, to prevent soiled particles from redepositing on instruments. The unit's tank should be cleaned and the drain should be checked for debris at each water change.

An ultrasonic unit may have one, two or three chambers. The first chamber is for the detergent bath, the second is for rinsing and the third is for drying. (See **Figure 8.21**) Some single-chamber sonics may only provide a cleaning process, while other single- chamber units perform both cleaning and rinsing functions. When using a single-chamber unit, it is necessary to know if the rinsing function is automatic. If the unit does not have a rinse cycle, it is important to manually rinse instruments after removing them from the sonic cleaner.

Water must be degassed each time it is changed in the sonic cleaner. Excess bubbles in the water are formed during filling, and these gas bubbles reduce the energy released during implosion. To de-gas a unit, fill the sonic cleaner, close the lid and run it for five to 10 minutes. Degassing should only be done after the tank is filled (not while it is being filled) to avoid damaging the equipment. Some ultrasonic cleaners will automatically de-gas the solution when the chamber is filled. The lid of the sonic cleaner should be closed at all times when the unit is operating to prevent aerosols from being dispersed.

When using ultrasonic cleaners there are some important factors to remember:

- Instruments must be precleaned prior to placing them in a sonic.

- Instruments should be placed in trays designed for use in the machine. They are typically of small wire construction with at least eight openings per inch to allow transmission of sonic energy.

- All lumens must be completely filled with fluid, so the cavitation process can be effective inside the lumen.

- All instruments must be completely submerged in the solution, so they are exposed to the cavitation process.

- Hinged instruments placed in the sonic cleaner should be opened.

- Trays must not be overloaded. Check the ultrasonic IFU for load limitations. (See **Figure 8.22**)

Do not stack or overload instruments.

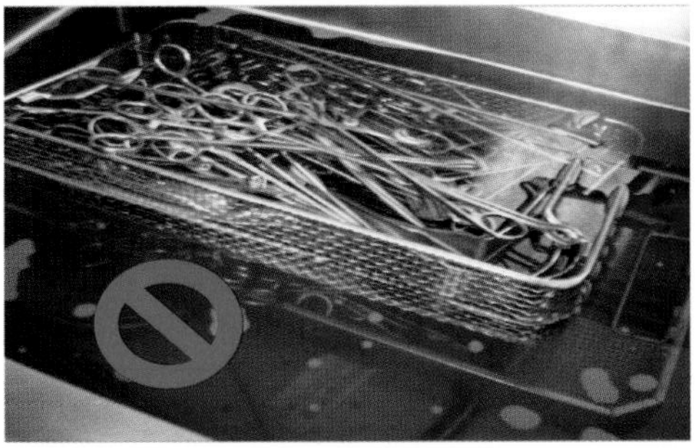

Figure 8.22

Ultrasonic energy can loosen the tiny screws of delicate instruments and degrade the glues or amalgam in other devices. Items that should not be placed in a sonic cleaner include:

- Chrome-plated and ebonized instruments, and those made of plastic, cork, glass, wood, chrome and rubber.

- Needles, unless approved for the process by the needle manufacturer's IFU.

- Instruments that contain fiber optic components.

Stainless steel instruments should not be mixed with aluminum, brass or copper instruments in a sonic cycle. Users should be aware that some sonic detergents may change or dull the color of anodized aluminum.

Irrigating Sonics

Some sonics are equipped with irrigating ports or connections to help facilitate cleaning of long lumened devices, such as laparoscopic or robotic instrumentation. (See **Figure 8.23**) It is important to check the flow of the solution through these connections to ensure they are not clogged.

Examples of irrigating sonics

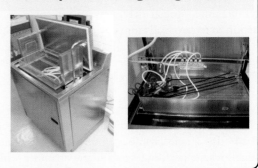

Figure 8.23

As with all processing equipment, the sonic cleaning equipment manufacturer's operating and maintenance recommendations should always be carefully followed.

Detergents for Ultrasonic Cleaners

Only detergents that have been specially formulated for ultrasonic cleaners should be used. Detergents must be low-foaming to prevent interference with the cleaning process.

Washer-Disinfector

Washers have been used for many years in CS departments, and they are effective to clean instrumentation, instrument containers, basins and graduates. Most are designed to perform multiple cleaning functions automatically. *Note: Automated mechanical washers are not appropriate for washing electrical, battery or pneumatic devices, unless otherwise stated in the device's IFU.*

Washers work on the principle of **impingement**. They are an effective means for cleaning and disinfecting instruments because of their spray force and thermal action.

Impingement The spray-force action of pressurized water against instruments being processed to physically remove bioburden.

In some ways, impingement washers work like a dishwasher; they rely on a combination of water temperature, special detergent and a spray force action to remove soil from devices being processed. To clean effectively, items must be properly prepared and positioned in a manner that facilitates the mechanical cleaning process.

Mechanical washer-disinfectors may be a single-chamber model or an indexed model. (See **Figure 8.24**) In single-chamber models, all cleaning functions are performed in a single chamber while the index model moves the instrument trays into separate chambers for each function. Many washer models have multiple types of cycles, including gentle, orthopedic instrument and glass, as well as the regular instrument cycle. Mechanical impingement washers typically use several successive steps during the wash cycle.

- The first step is a cool prerinse to wet the instruments and prepare them for the detergent cycle. The prerinse may be cool water or an enzymatic solution. The cool temperatures helps prevent coagulation of proteins.

- The second step is a detergent cycle with water at a higher temperature to maximize the effectiveness of the detergent action.

- The third step is rinsing, followed by a pure rinse cycle to remove any remaining detergents and debris. *Note: Some washers also provide a lubrication cycle during the rinse cycles.*

Examples of washer-disinfectors

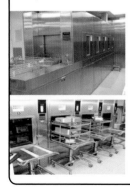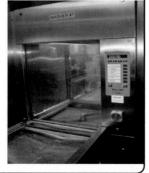

Figure 8.24

Washers are only effective when used and serviced according to the manufacturer's recommendations. Operator manuals and detailed instructions about the basic operation and loading of instrument racks should be provided. CS technicians should understand and comply with these instructions. Important factors to remember when using a washer-disinfector:

- Washer racks should never be overloaded, and spray arms should move freely during operation. Instruments that are sticking up and/or out of their perforated baskets must be relocated away from the spray arms travel paths.

- Instruments should be disassembled, and their small parts placed inside an approved containment device (part holder) for processing in the washer. (See **Figure 8.25**)

Examples of small part holders

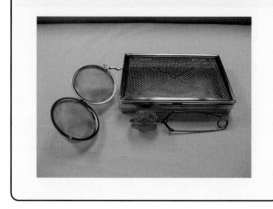

Figure 8.25

- Hinged instruments should be opened to permit direct contact of the water and detergent. (See **Figure 8.26**)

Open hinged instruments and make certain all instruments will be contacted by the washer spray.

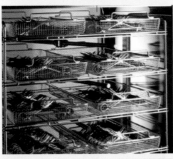

Figure 8.26

- Trays or sets with multiple levels should be opened, and each tray should be placed separately on the washer's rack. Failure to separate multi-level trays can cause the wash process to fail because tray layers impede contact between the spray action and the items within the tray. (See **Figure 8.27**)

- Trays with lids/covers should be opened so contents may be exposed to the washer spray.

- Delicate instruments may be dislodged from the racks due to the blunt force of the spray action. These instruments should be confined in small perforated baskets with approved lids.

Make certain washer spray can make contact with tray contents.

Remove lids from trays   Do not stack trays

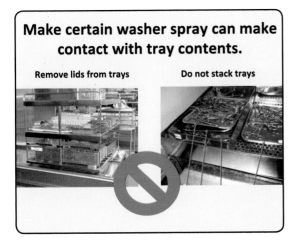

Figure 8.27

Instrument washer racks and conveyor systems should be inspected daily. Routine cleaning of washers should include inspection and cleaning of spray arms and washer jets. Mineral build up will hinder spray action and disrupt cleaning efficacy. Washer traps/screens need special attention and should be inspected for debris at least daily (See **Figure 8.28**), and cleared of any obstructions. Washer detergent levels should be frequently monitored. If detergent drums are allowed to run dry, a column of air may enter the detergent feed lines and impact the delivery of replacement detergent.

Debris should be removed from washer traps daily.

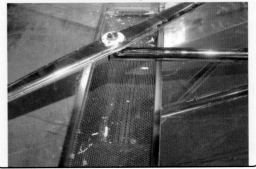

Figure 8.28

It is important to keep the chamber walls clean, so the washer can perform at maximum efficiency. If a white scale is seen in the chamber, it should be removed immediately with an approved descaler because scale can fall on instruments and clog pumps, motors and spray arms. (See **Figure 8.29**)

Example of a Washer with Scale

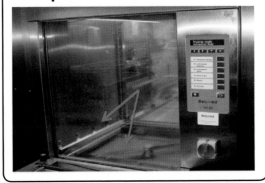

Figure 8.29

Automated washers have preset, factory-installed cycles for use with different cleaning situations. Instrument cycles generally are the longest cycle because they have multiple rinse, wash, lubrication and drying times to meet the instruments' cleaning needs. Basins and containers are generally run on a utensil cycle. Some washer manufacturers offer special cycles for delicate instruments. When running a mixed load of containers and instruments, the instrument cycle should normally be utilized for maximum cleaning. CS technicians should be familiar with different washer cycles, and should be able to select the appropriate cleaning cycle for the items to be processed.

Some washer racks (manifolds) are equipped with irrigation lines that can be connected to certain complex instruments to add a channel flush to the mechanical cleaning process. (See **Figure 8.30**)

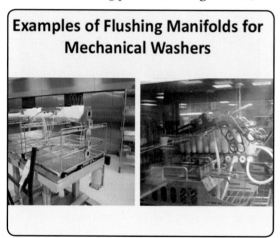

Examples of Flushing Manifolds for Mechanical Washers

Figure 8.30

Automated Cart Washers

Cart washers were originally designed to clean carts used for transport of various supplies and instruments. (See **Figure 8.31**) Some cart washers are designed to process rigid containers and other miscellaneous items. Some models have programmed instrument cycles. Several manufacturers offer cart washers with design features and special washer racks to facilitate the processing of basins, pans, bedside commodes and surgical stainless steel tables. Processing rigid

containers, basins and other transport containers in a cart washer can yield operational speed and efficiency. (See **Figure 8.32**)

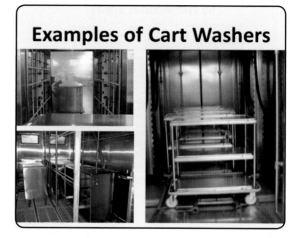

Examples of Cart Washers

Figure 8.31

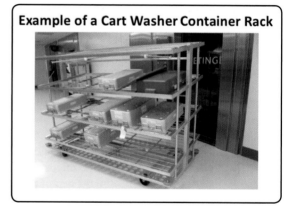

Example of a Cart Washer Container Rack

Figure 8.32

Cart washers operate in a manner similar to automated instrument washers, but on a larger scale. Spray arms deliver high-temperature water and detergent, and successive steps provide rinse water and hot air drying cycles. Cart washers resemble automated car washes in their cleaning process. Most cart washers do not have multiple phase cycles like washer-disinfectors, but include a high-temperature process to reduce bacteria and facilitate drying. Detergents selected for cart washing should be formulated for use in cart washers. Important factors to remember when using a cart washer include:

- When cleaning enclosed carts, ensure they are approved to be cleaned by a cart washer. Older enclosed carts are not designed to allow water to drain from the interior, so the cart may be damaged by the lingering moisture.

- Do not process instruments in a cart washer that is not designed for that purpose.

- Do not process items inside carts. The walls of the cart will keep cleaning solution and rinse water from reaching the items inside.

As with the other equipment, it is important to test the cleaning ability of cart washers on a regular basis. Commercial testing products are available.

Automated Endoscope Reprocessors

Some AERs have cleaning cycles, as well as a disinfection process. This equipment will be discussed in depth in Chapter 9. It is important to note the following when using the cleaning cycles:

- Only process items approved for processing in this type of equipment.

- All items must be manually cleaned prior to placing them in these units.

- Only use cleaning chemicals that have been approved by the equipment manufacturer.

- The equipment must be tested on a regular basis.

EQUIPMENT TESTING

ANSI/AAMI ST79, 10.2, recommends a quality assurance program to ensure that the mechanical equipment is working properly. Commercially-prepared products can be obtained to verify the cleaning effectiveness of the equipment. (See **Figure 8.33**)

If the mechanical cleaner has a printout, the printout should be reviewed and initialed after each cycle to ensure the cycle reached the expected parameters.

Mechanical cleaners can save time and labor, while producing a consistent process; however, remember that human factors play a significant role in mechanical cleaning. In other words, mechanical cleaners are only as good as their operators. CS technicians must understand how to properly prepare items for cleaning and use each piece of equipment according to instructions.

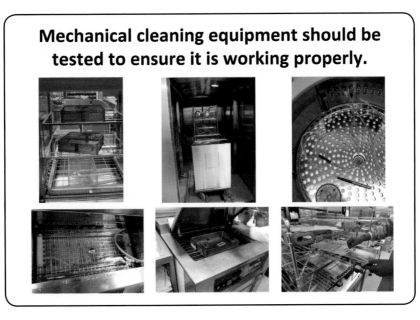

Mechanical cleaning equipment should be tested to ensure it is working properly.

Figure 8.33

CLEANING CHEMICALS AND LUBRICANTS

Many types of soil can be present on reusable devices. When soil, especially blood, is allowed to dry prior to cleaning, it becomes difficult to remove. (See **Figure 8.34**) Blood flows into instrument joints, hinges, grooves and other difficult to clean locations. It then coagulates and dries to create a significant challenge to cleaning. Soil adheres to microscopic irregularities in the surface of instruments and has to be manually and mechanically scrubbed away, or chemically treated, otherwise it could result in the formation of biofilm. Using proper chemicals in the correct concentrations rehydrates and loosens the soil, and helps to properly clean the devices.

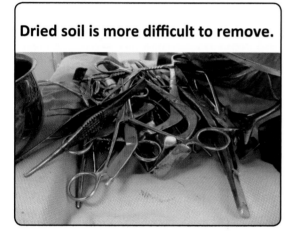

Dried soil is more difficult to remove.

Figure 8.34

Each chemical used should be compatible with both the medical device and the equipment used for cleaning.

Different types of chemicals are used in the cleaning process, including enzymatic products, detergents and presoaks (precleaning agents). Each has a specific purpose in efficiently processing reusable items.

Enzyme Products

Enzymatic cleaners are biodegradable, non-toxic cleaning agents used to break down soils, stains and other debris on heavily-soiled instruments. They are very helpful for processing difficult-to-

clean devices, such as instruments with lumens. They are also used to keep instruments moist and begin breaking down the soil on instruments immediately after a procedure. Enzymes are very specific in their action. For example, a protein enzyme will not affect fat molecules.

There are different types of enzymatic products available. Some can be used at the point of use to moisten and loosen soil on instruments, and others are used in manual or automatic washing processes. Popular enzymes used in CS departments include:

- Protease enzymes (protein) – Break down blood, mucous, feces and albumin.

- Lipase (fat) – Break down fatty deposits, such as bone marrow and adipose tissue.

- Amylase – Catalyzes (changes) starch.

Elements in soil can gradually degrade enzymes during use and reduce their cleaning efficacy. Dried soil on a device must be rehydrated before enzymes that facilitate its removal can be effective. Point-of-use precleaning (keeping the instruments free of gross soil) can reduce these problems. After precleaning, the instrument should remain moist to keep soil from drying and maintain hydration needed to optimize the enzyme's efficacy.

Many enzyme products used in the decontamination area are single enzyme products, so it is important to know the type of soil being cleaned. Multi-enzymatic products contain protease (for soils), lipase (for fats) and amylase (for starches). Detergents take longer to clean if they are not used in conjunction with enzyme products.

Proper temperature is critical when dealing with enzyme-based products. Temperatures should not exceed 140°F (60°C), unless otherwise stated by the enzyme manufacturer.

Detergents

Since water is not an effective cleaning agent, detergents are used to enhance its cleaning ability.

Detergents contain **emulsifiers, surfactants** and **chelating agents** to increase their cleaning efficacy. Chelating agents have an ionic charge that allows soils with the opposite charge to break away and attach to the chelating agent. An emulsifier surrounds these particles to prevent them from reattaching, and they also help break bonds that oils can create to trap soil.

> **Emulsifier** Any ingredient used to bind together substances that normally do not combine, such as oil and water.
>
> **Surfactant** A substance that lowers the surface tension of the water and increases the solubility of organic compounds.
>
> **Chelating agents** Chemicals that hold hard water minerals in solution and prevent soaps or detergents from reacting with the minerals.

When used properly, detergents penetrate and remove soil from instruments and keep soil in suspension, so it does not reattach to the instrument. Remember that detergents do not kill microorganisms (unless they contain a germicide). They help to clean the instrument by removing bacteria-laden soil.

Detergents are designed to perform specific tasks. In the home setting, there are different detergents for washing dishes, washing laundry and cleaning floors. In a similar manner, detergents for decontamination in the healthcare facility are formulated for different applications. Some detergents work in hard water, some are low-foaming, so they do not hinder the operation of the mechanical cleaning equipment, and others are developed specifically for a certain type of equipment, like those formulated for ultrasonic cleaners.

Detergents also come in several forms. Liquid detergents can be purchased in small quantities for use at a sink, or large quantities for use in mechanical washers. Solid forms (blocks) of detergents that mix with water as they are dispensed are also available. (See **Figure 8.35**)

Examples of Different Forms of Detergents

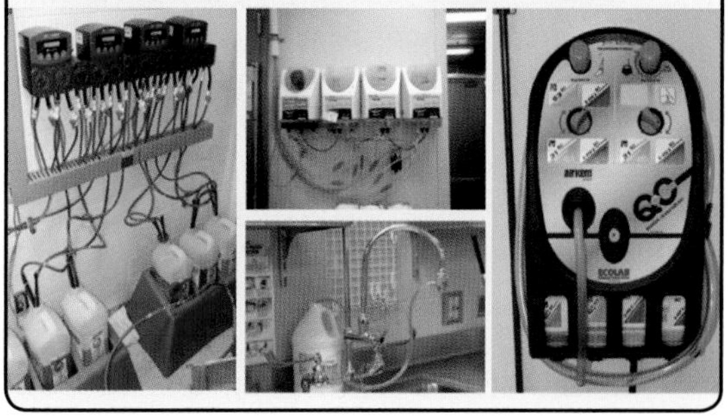

Figure 8.35

Detergents are selected at each facility, based on the item's and facility's specific cleaning needs, the quality of their water, and the types of soils present. There are several types of detergents that can be used for cleaning surgical instruments. Each has its advantages and disadvantages, so it is important to know how each type of detergent functions and how to properly use them.

- Neutral detergents are the most commonly-used type in the U.S. Neutral detergents have a pH value of 6 to 8.

  › Advantages - Neutral-pH detergents are effective on organic and inorganic soils, and are safe to use on aluminum products.

  › Disadvantages - Neutral-pH detergents are not very effective in hard water, produce more foam and are more difficult to rinse than other types of detergents.

- Alkaline detergents are highly effective at removing organic soils (blood, fat and oils). Alkaline detergents range in pH from 8 to more than 11. Prior to using an alkaline detergent, refer to the manufacturer's IFU.

  › Advantages - They remove a wider range of soil than any other type of detergent; they are economical to use and low foaming.

> Disadvantages - Alkaline detergents require thorough rinsing as they can leave a powdery residue on the instrument surface. Alkaline detergents cannot be used on devices made of bronze, copper or aluminum.

• Acid detergents are primarily used to remove mineral deposits, such as hard water, urine, minerals and scale. Acid detergents have a pH of 1.6 to 3.

> Advantages - Excellent for removing mineral deposits and urine. Acid detergents work well on inorganic soils, neutralize alkaline residues and make stainless steel shine.

> Disadvantages - Can damage the surfaces of stainless steel and aluminum, bronze and glass. Disposal into drains and sewer lines may be restricted in some states.

Review of Common Chemicals Used in the Decontamination Area

During the course of any shift, CS technicians must select and properly use several different chemicals. While initial selection of chemicals to be used in the department is done by managers, the technician must select the proper chemical for the job from the chemicals available in the decontamination area. *Note: Each chemical is different and cannot be substituted for another.* (See **Figure 8.36**) Read labels carefully and ask questions if any information is not understood.

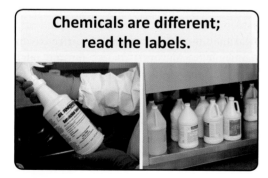

Chemicals are different; read the labels.

Figure 8.36

The following is a review of chemicals commonly found in the decontamination area.

• Precleaning chemicals are used in the first step in the decontamination process. Some commonly-used precleaning agents are detergent solutions, enzymatic detergents and combination enzyme-germicide detergents.

Precleaning should begin immediately after the completion of any invasive procedure. Blood and other visible debris, if left on an instrument, serve as a reservoir for microbial growth, and may damage an instrument's finish. If not removed, the corrosive agents in blood and body tissue can penetrate the protective outer layer of an instrument and cause rusting or pitting of the stainless steel. The manufacturer's directions must be followed when using these precleaning products. Exceeding the time allowed for the instruments to be immersed in the solution can damage and corrode instruments.

Precleaning chemicals are applied at point of use, but they may also be used in the decontamination area to keep soil moist and loosen dried soil.

• Manual cleaning chemicals – These products, when mixed properly, penetrate under the soil and break the bond that attaches the soil to the instruments. Their main function is to remove soil, not kill microorganisms. Low-foaming and free-rinsing manual cleaners should be used. The manufacturer's IFU should be followed for proper dilution and to determine the proper water temperature for their use. Manual cleaners are usually neutral or alkaline products.

• Mechanical cleaners are specially designed for use in mechanical cleaning processes. They are low foaming and designed to work with the specific mechanical cleaning process (for example, an ultrasonic cleaner), so careful attention must be paid to the manufacturer's IFU.

- Descalers are not typically required if the water quality and detergent mixtures are correct, and the equipment is operating properly. Still, problems can go unnoticed until a chalky-powdery, hard to remove substance appears on the walls of equipment and sinks. When this occurs, an acidic detergent or a descaler is needed to remove the scale. It is important to use a descaling product when scale is detected in the cleaning equipment because scale can interfere with the cleaning ability of the equipment.

- Lubricants (often called "instrument milk" because of its milky appearance) are an important part of the instrument maintenance program because they help maintain the integrity of instruments and keep them in good working order. Lubrication is performed after cleaning, as one of the final steps in the mechanical wash process, or it can be applied manually in the clean assembly area using a spray bottle. In the past, instrument baths (pans filled with instrument lubricating solution) were commonly used. This process has been discontinued because of increased risk of contamination. Always use lubrication according to the manufacturer's instructions to ensure the proper contact time and dilution concentration. Ensure the lubricant is designed for use with the instruments to be cleaned and compatible with specific sterilization processes that will follow.

- Stain and rust removers are used when the normal cleaning process does not remove stains on an instrument. Stains and rust usually result from improper care, such as soaking the instruments in saline. Stain and rust remover can be used after instrument cleaning to restore the luster to stainless steel instruments. These chemicals remove hard water deposits, rust scale and discoloration from instrumentation and processing equipment. Most stain and rust removers are acid-based compounds (0 to 6.9 pH) that react with minerals and iron on the instruments. They remove mineral and detergent build up, leaving the surfaces bright and shiny, and the instruments moving freely. Because these chemicals are acid-based, the IFU must be carefully followed to prevent instrument damage. After using a stain remover, the instruments should be recleaned.

When using any cleaning chemical, temperature is an important factor. Most cleaning chemicals deactivate if the temperature is higher than 180°F (82°C). Unless specified by the manufacturer, cleaning chemicals should never be combined with other chemicals.

To prevent instrument damage, the following chemicals should not be used (unless recommended by the device manufacturer) to clean instruments:

- Abrasive cleaning compounds.

- Saline.

- Buffered iodine, such as Betadine.

- Hydrogen peroxide.

- Any chemical not specifically recommended by the medical device manufacturer.

INSTRUCTIONS FOR USE

Knowing and following the manufacturer's IFU is a critical component of the decontamination process. CS technicians must understand how to follow the medical device's IFU, as well as clearly understand the IFU for any equipment and any chemical they use. Failure to follow an IFU can result in a failed decontamination process and damage to instruments and equipment.

The remainder of this chapter will examine basic cleaning and decontamination processes.

STEPS IN THE PROCESS OF DECONTAMINATION

Point of Use

The process of decontamination begins with the end user, at the point of use. OR staff should take the time to ensure that the initial steps of decontamination are performed. The Association for the Advancement of Medical Instrumentation (AAMI) and the Association of periOperative Registered Nurses (AORN) recommend that instrument users take the time to properly prepare instrumentation for transport to the decontamination area.

Soiled Receiving

If soiled items are hand delivered to the decontamination area, the person delivering the items should place them on a cart or counter top designated for receipt of items into the decontamination area. (See **Figure 8.37**)

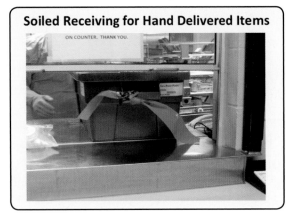

Soiled Receiving for Hand Delivered Items

Figure 8.37

When carts loaded with soiled items are received, proper body mechanics must be used when handling the heavy carts. When loading and unloading carts from dumbwaiters or elevators, check the weight of the cart. Ensure that the wheels are aligned, and that they will roll over door spaces or uneven edges. Unload some items to lighten the cart if it is too heavy to move easily.

If items are in a closed cart or transport container, open the lid or doors carefully, as items may have shifted during transport. (See **Figure 8.38**)

Carefully remove items from the cart or container and place them on a flat surface near a sink.

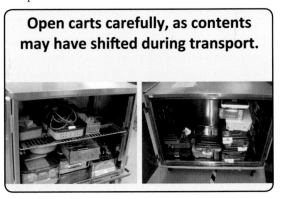

Open carts carefully, as contents may have shifted during transport.

Figure 8.38

Use the following guidelines during the unloading process:

- Fluids should be disposed of or contained at the point of use. If transported, fluids should be in a leak-proof container. Dispose of any fluids, per facility policy.

- If possible, disposable items and reusable textiles should be removed at the point of use. If this is not feasible, these items should be bagged and sent to the decontamination area. They should not be transported unless contained. (See **Figure 8.39**)

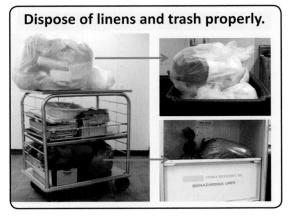

Dispose of linens and trash properly.

Figure 8.39

- Reusable sharps, including scissors and chisels, should be separated and safely contained at the point of use. Disposable sharps, such as scalpel blades and trocars, should be removed and discarded at the point of use. If disposable sharps are found in the transport device or in any tray, they should be removed and discarded in an approved sharps container. (See **Figure 8.40**)

Carefully remove all tray liners, indicators, filters and other disposable items left inside instrument trays.

- Rigid containers:

  › Remove filter retention plates from rigid containers. Containers and lids should be cleaned without the retention plate or reusable filter in place. Discard disposable filters and clean reusable filters per manufacturer's instructions. (See **Figure 8.41**)

  › If the container system has valve-type closures, the valves should be inspected and cleaned following manufacturer's instructions. Improper cleaning of container valves can inhibit the sterilant from reaching the instruments to be sterilized.

Improperly cleaned valves may also lead to contamination of the instruments after sterilization.

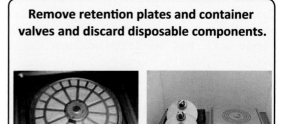

Remove retention plates and container valves and discard disposable components.

Figure 8.41

- Interior baskets should be removed from inside the container. Instruments may be mechanically cleaned inside the interior tray after manual preparation.

- Ensure the transport container or the case cart is completely empty, then clean per the manufacturer's IFU.

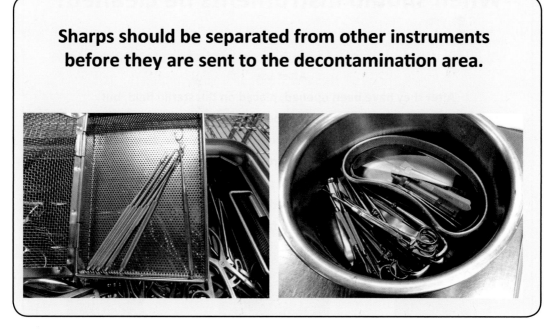

Sharps should be separated from other instruments before they are sent to the decontamination area.

Figure 8.40

Cleaning

The cleaning of instruments and other medical devices is the primary function of the decontamination area. It is obvious that instruments should be cleaned after use; however, there are also other times when instruments should be cleaned. **Figure 8.42** lists some circumstances when instruments should be sent to the decontamination area for cleaning.

Thorough cleaning and adherence to IFU is important because failure of the cleaning process puts patients and staff at risk.

There are several types of cleaning methods:

• Precleaning (this process should occur at the point of use).

• Manual cleaning (also known as cleaning by hand).

• Mechanical cleaning (cleaning items using specialized cleaning equipment).

The method of cleaning selected should follow the device manufacturer's IFU.

Manual Cleaning

Manual cleaning is done to remove soil that was not removed, or was only softened during the precleaning process; this is achieved by the use of friction and appropriate cleaning chemicals.

Manual cleaning may be performed:

• Before the item is mechanically cleaned to ensure blood protein and other soil is removed.

• When the decontamination area does not have a mechanical method of cleaning.

• To clean items that cannot be immersed in water.

• For instruments with lumens.

• For delicate or complex medical devices, such as microsurgical and robotic instruments.

When should instruments be cleaned?

Clean Instruments:

After use.

After they have been opened, placed on the sterile field, but have not been used.

When new instruments are received at the facility.

When used instruments return from repair or refurbishing.

When instruments are pulled from back up stock.

When instruments are inadvertently contaminated.

When loaner instruments are received.

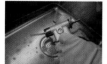 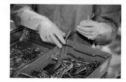

Figure 8.42

- For all items that require manual cleaning as part of their IFU.

Manual Preparation and Cleaning Processes

Set up the work area to accommodate the type of items to be cleaned. For example, for instruments that can be immersed, fill the sink with the appropriate cleaning solution. Place heavier instruments in the sink first, followed by lighter, more delicate items. Gently place the items into the sink. Do not pour them into the sink because instruments can damage easily.

The items should be placed in the sink in the following manner:

- Hinged instruments should be placed in the sink, fully opened.

- Multi-part instruments should be disassembled, following manufacturer's instructions, so all parts of the instrument can be exposed to the cleaning solution. (See **Figure 8.43**) Keep all parts near each other during the cleaning process.

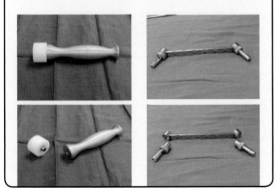

Disassemble Multi-part Instruments

Figure 8.43

- Lumen/cannulated items should be fully submerged then flushed with cleaning solution; this will force the air bubbles out of the lumen and ensure all the inner surfaces

are in contact with the cleaning solution. If available, placing lumened items in a vertical soaking cylinder also helps ensure air bubbles are not inside the lumens.

Ensure detergent can reach every part of the device being cleaned. If the detergent cannot reach every part of the instrument, the instrument cannot be thoroughly cleaned.

Items that cannot be immersed, like power equipment and many cables and cords, should be set aside to process separately. Many CS departments have a sink area designated for cleaning these non-immersable items. Cleaning procedures for these items will be discussed later in this chapter.

Carefully clean all instrument surfaces. Cleaning efforts must be focused and done consistently. Instruments should be brushed in a "to and fro" motion under the surface of the water. Brushing under the surface of the water prevents aerosolization. Aerosolization occurs when ultramicroscopic particles are released into the air. (See **Figure 8.44**) This is a concern because the cleaning solution contains contaminates from the instruments being cleaned. When cleaning, pay special attention to hinges and the tips of the instruments because these areas harbor the most soil. All serrated, toothed and crevice areas should be brushed to ensure the instrument is properly cleaned.

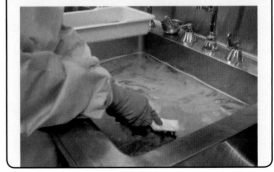

Brush under the surface of the water to prevent aerosols.

Figure 8.44

Lumened instruments (See **Figure 8.45**) should be carefully cleaned with a brush after soaking in the cleaning solution. Select a brush that fits into the lumen and touches all inner surfaces. (See **Figure 8.46**) With the lumened instrument under the surface of the water, gently push the brush through the lumen several times. Check the lumen for cleanliness by using a clean brush or an approved, non-linting pipe cleaner type product.

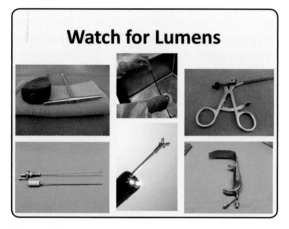

Watch for Lumens

Figure 8.45

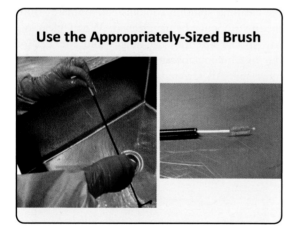

Use the Appropriately-Sized Brush

Figure 8.46

Because curettes, kerrisons, ronguers and other orthopedic instruments can conceal bone and other bioburden, removing material with bristle brushes should be an initial step in the cleaning process. Check all crevices carefully as blood and bone may be in other areas of the instrument besides the biting or cutting section. (See **Figure 8.47**)

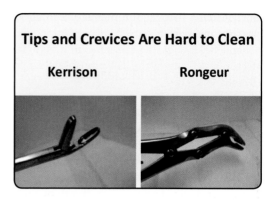

Tips and Crevices Are Hard to Clean

Kerrison   Rongeur

Figure 8.47

Instruments tagged for repair must still be cleaned and decontaminated. When instruments are returned from repair, they must be considered contaminated. (See **Figure 8.48**) They must be cleaned, decontaminated and inspected before being returned to their respective sets.

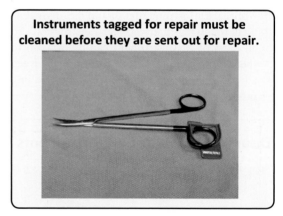

Instruments tagged for repair must be cleaned before they are sent out for repair.

Figure 8.48

Delicate instruments are a cleaning challenge; they must be separated from regular or heavy instruments during cleaning. Devices used for delicate surgical procedures are generally lightweight, with fine points and tips. Mixing them with heavy instruments or placing heavy devices on top of them can cause damage and misalignment. Delicate instruments, such as skin hooks, can slip through perforated baskets and become entangled. Check the IFU to ensure the proper cleaning chemical is being used. Unless otherwise stated by the manufacturer, clean these instruments as one would other surgical instruments, but with more care in handling. Always check the IFU to see if the instrument can be mechanically processed after manual cleaning. If processing in a washer-disinfector, a delicate cycle will probably need to be selected.

Ophthalmic instruments have special cleaning protocols because of the increasing incidents of **toxic anterior segment syndrome (TASS)**. Manufacturer cleaning instructions must be carefully followed. It is recommended that facilities have sufficient instrumentation to allow adequate time for processing between patients.

Toxic anterior segment syndrome (TASS) Acute postoperative inflammatory reaction in which a noninfectious substance enters the anterior segment and induces toxic damage to the intraocular tissues.

TASS Precautions in the Decontamination Area

TASS occurs when contaminants enter the eye during eye surgery. Those contaminants can be the result of inadequate instrument processing. The risk of TASS can be reduced in the decontamination area by:

- Carefully following all manufacturer IFU for cleaning.
- Taking actions to prevent the formation of biofilm on instruments.
- Using only enzymes and detergents recommended by the manufacturer.
- Keeping cleaning tools, such as brushes and syringes, clean.
- Flushing lumens.
- Copious rinsing with the recommended rinse water.

Note: Be sure to follow the facility's specific protocols for processing eye instruments. Pay attention to detail and do not take shortcuts at any step in the process.

Ortho instruments are often loaded with gross soil.

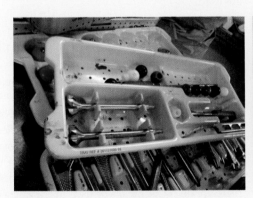 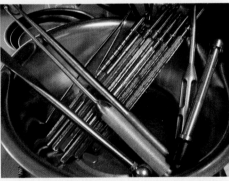

Figure 8.49

There are thousands of instruments on the market and cleaning each one requires specific knowledge. Instruments that are designed to perform the same function, but are made by different manufacturers, may need different cleaning processes. Consult the medical device manufacturer for special considerations, and to determine if these devices can withstand automated washers.

Orthopedic and neurologic surgery has many instrument sets that require extended preparation and inspection prior to and during cleaning. Joint replacement cutting guides, rasps, reamers and broaches hide gross amounts of blood, bone and tissue. (See **Figure 8.49**) This can occur even with the best point-of-use care in the OR, and these instruments must be cleaned with brushes and extensive hand detailing. Presoaking with enzymatic detergents can help remove much of the bioburden from the crevices. Some washer manufacturers have designed special washer racks to hold and flush out these devices.

Laparoscopic and robotic instrumentation can be difficult and time consuming to clean. The instrument manufacturers provide extensive cleaning instructions; these instructions must be carefully followed to ensure the instruments are clean. Always use properly-sized brushes in the lumened areas and carefully follow any flushing instructions provided by the manufacturer. For example, these instruments, especially robotic instruments, can be damaged if too much air and water pressure is used. Some types of mechanical cleaning equipment have special baskets, manifolds or connections to flush these items during mechanical cleaning. These items must still be manually cleaned and flushed, even when using a mechanical method.

Flexible and rigid endoscopes also pose special cleaning concerns. Endoscope cleaning and decontamination is discussed separately in Chapter 11.

New or repaired instruments received in the CS department must be cleaned prior to disinfection or sterilization. Although these instruments may look clean, their surfaces are covered in fine metal dust, oils and other debris from the manufacturing and repair processes. These instruments have also been handled and exposed to outside elements during shipping.

Instruments from back-up stock should be cleaned prior to use because they have been hanging on walls or stored in drawers for some time. These instruments could have been handled multiple times and most likely contain dust and other environmental contaminants. (See **Figure 8.50**)

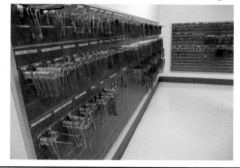

Back up instruments contain dust and other contaminants from storage.

Figure 8.50

Cleaning Instruments That Cannot Be Immersed

Instruments such as power equipment and cameras cannot be immersed in water. The device manufacturer's IFU should be reviewed to ensure proper cleaning chemistries and cleaning methods are used.

Hoses and cords should be carefully wiped down using the approved solution and a clean, soft cloth. Special care should be taken at the ends of the hoses and cords because water will damage these items. Many of these types of instruments are a dark color, which makes it difficult to see dried blood, so meticulous attention must be paid to cleaning these items. (See **Figure 8.51**) Unless approved by the manufacturer, do not rinse these items under running water. Carefully check these items to ensure there are no nicks, breaks or tears in the outer cover. If any damage is noted, mark the item for repair prior to sending it to the assembly area.

Dark-colored hand wash items make it difficult to see blood.

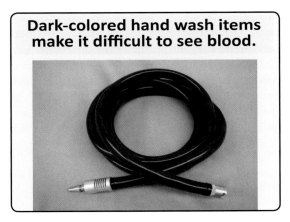

Figure 8.51

Power equipment presents challenges to CS technicians. These devices are powered by batteries, pneumatic air or electricity. Care should be taken to prevent exposure of the connection points and battery contacts to moisture or chemicals. These connection areas can react with chemicals and cause damage and loss of electrical contact with the power source. The use of a battery, hose or cable designated for the decontamination area will help keep these connections dry. (See **Figure 8.52**) *Note: Chapter 11 provides a more detailed discussion on cleaning power instrumentation.*

Powered Surgical Instrument (PSI) Precautions

Moisture can damage a PSI

Prevent moisture from entering connection areas

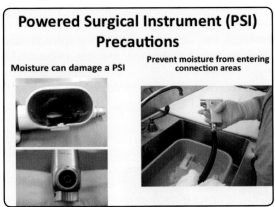

Figure 8.52

Cannulated drills may have their lumens cleaned with running tap water, if approved by the manufacturer, and they should be brushed with a soft brush. (See **Figure 8.53**) A plastic syringe filled with water and enzymatic detergent can assist in delivering cleaning agents to hard-to-reach

areas. If the instrument cannot be cleaned under running water, use a clean soft cloth, appropriately-sized brushes, and syringes filled with cleaning and rinsing solutions.

Cleaning PSI Cannulas

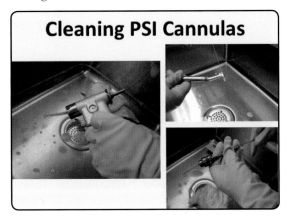

Figure 8.53

Orthopedic saws frequently have residual bone chips and impacted bioburden in their working parts. They must be flushed and brushed clean under running water, if approved by the manufacturer.

Power accessories, such as chucks, can usually be immersed in the cleaning solution; however, some may need to be hand processed without immersion. Drill and saw attachments usually need non-immersion cleaning; consult and follow the manufacturer's IFU for the proper cleaning method.

Cleaning Instrument Containers and Basins

Cleaning rigid instrument containers and basins requires procedures that differ from those used for instruments. A neutral-pH detergent is usually recommended because acidic or alkaline pH detergents will damage aluminum and some composite materials. If processing manually, carefully clean all surface areas while the item is immersed in the cleaning solution. Rinse with softened water, then with pure water. If cleaning these items mechanically, place on the appropriate rack or manifold. When cleaning containers, the filter retention plate should be removed and not processed attached to the container or lid. Handles, locking mechanisms and container rims should be inspected for cracks and missing components. If basins are dented or bent, or if containers are damaged, mark them for repair or removal from service prior to sending them to the assembly area.

Mobile Patient Care Equipment

Mobile patient care equipment has different processing needs than surgical instrumentation. In general, the use of mild cleaning agents and disinfectants can be utilized to clean exterior components of patient care equipment. Use of an incorrect cleaning agent may affect product warranties and device functionality. Some chemicals may cause cosmetic changes in plastic and other materials.

Some devices have access doors and hatches that must be opened to clean intricate parts. (See **Figure 8.54**) Extreme care is needed to avoid damage to these critical parts. Soft materials and applicators may be used to clean these areas. Care must also be taken to thoroughly clean around switches and cords. It is important that the cleaning cloth is not overly wet (dripping), as water may damage the equipment.

CS technicians must clean many pieces of mobile equipment including isolation and special

procedure carts. Carts must be cleaned after each use. Do not empty the inside drawers of these carts while they are in the decontamination area because this would expose the supplies in the carts to the area's bioburden. Carts should be emptied before transport. Transport the empty cart to the decontamination area and clean all surfaces inside and out. Then transport the cart to a clean room and complete the restocking tasks.

Inspection

CS technicians play one of the most important roles in the next step of the decontamination process: inspection. It is a crucial step in the process because this step helps ensure the safety of themselves, their co-workers and the patient. Each item cleaned must be carefully inspected for visible debris. If debris is found, then the item should be cleaned again according to the manufacturer's IFU.

Quality Testing

There are several devices available to inspect instruments for cleanliness; some examples were shared at the beginning of this chapter. (See **Figures 8.2**, **8.3** and **8.4**) Another method commonly used to check instruments for cleanliness is a swabbing process where an item that has been cleaned is swabbed, and the swab is processed to determine if there was residual soil present. **Figure 8.55**

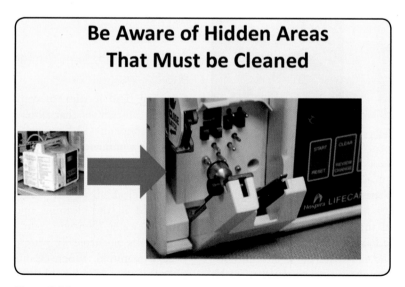

Figure 8.54

provides an example of this process.

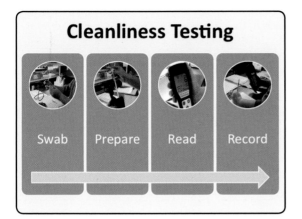

Cleanliness Testing

Swab | Prepare | Read | Record

Figure 8.55

DECONTAMINATION

The decontamination process involves the use of physical or chemical procedures to remove, inactivate or destroy bloodborne pathogens on an item's surface. The purpose of decontamination is to make devices safe for people who are not wearing gloves and to reduce the bioburden to make the next processing steps easier. Some instruments are safe for handling after they have been thoroughly cleaned; however, others require exposure to a microbiocidal process. Thermal and chemical disinfection are discussed in detail in Chapter 9.

CONCLUSION

Cleaning is a complex, multi-step process. The success of disinfection and sterilization processes depends on a successful cleaning process. Central Service technicians must understand the cleaning process for each medical device, and perform it consistently to help ensure the safety of patients, visitors and healthcare personnel.

RESOURCES

Association for the Advancement of Medical Instrumentation. *ANSI/AAMI ST79:2010: & A1 2010: & A2 2011: & A3 2012: & A4, 2013. Comprehensive Guide to Steam Sterilization and Sterility Assurance in Health Care Facilities.*

Occupational Safety and Health Administration, *Regulations Standards CFR 1910.1030, Bloodborne Pathogens.*

Association of periOperative Registered Nurses. *Guidelines for PeriOperative Practice: Instrument Cleaning.* Guidelines for PeriOperative Practice. 2015.

International Association of Healthcare Central Service Materiel Management. *Central Service Leadership Manual,* Chapter 20. 2010.

CENTRAL SERVICE TERMS

Cleaning

Decontamination area

Relative humidity

Biohazardous waste

Deionized (DI) water

Distilled water

Reverse osmosis (RO)

Pyrogen

Cavitation

Impingement

Emulsifier

Surfactant

Chelating agents

Toxic anterior segment syndrome (TASS)

Chapter 9

Disinfection

Learning Objectives

As a result of successfully completing this chapter, readers will be able to:

1. Define the term disinfection and explain how disinfection differs from sterilization

2. Explain disinfection levels as identified in the Spaulding Classification System:

   • Low-level disinfection

   • Intermediate-level disinfection

   • High-level disinfection

3. Provide basic information about the types of disinfectants commonly used in healthcare facilities:

   • Quaternary ammonium compounds

   • Alcohol

   • Phenolics

   • Chlorine

   • Iodophors

   • Glutaraldehyde

   • Ortho-phthalaldehyde

   • Hydrogen peroxide

   • Peracetic acid

4. Identify good work practices for manual disinfection processes

5. Discuss automated equipment utilized for disinfection, and good work practices for working with automated disinfection processes

6. Explain disinfection quality assurance practices

INTRODUCTION

Once an item has been properly cleaned, there are some decisions to make. Is the item safe for its intended use or does it need further processing? If further processing is needed, what type of processing does it need and how can that be accomplished? (See **Figure 9.1**) Central Service (CS) technicians must be able to identify the type of **bactericidal** process needed (**sterilization** or **disinfection**), select the method that will provide that process, and perform that process effectively. (Sterilization processes are examined in later chapters.) This chapter will provide basic information on disinfectants and disinfecting processes that are frequently used in CS departments.

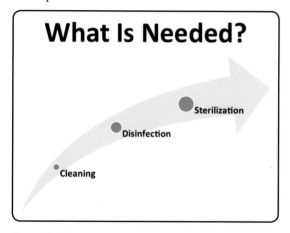

What Is Needed?

Sterilization

Disinfection

Cleaning

Figure 9.1

INTRODUCTION TO DISINFECTANTS

The Spaulding Classification System

The selection of a **disinfectant** must be based, in part, upon the intended use of the device and the degree of disinfection required for that device. The **Spaulding Classification System** divides patient care items into three categories, each based on the degree of risk of infection when the items are used in patient care. The Centers for Disease Control and Prevention (CDC) and the Association for the Advancement of Medical Instrumentation (AAMI) use the Spaulding Classification System in their guidelines and standards. (See **Figure 9.2**) The three Spaulding categories are:

- Critical items – Instruments or objects introduced directly into the bloodstream or into other sterile areas of the body; examples include surgical instruments, cardiac catheters and implants; these items must be **sterilized** before use (disinfection is inadequate).

- Semi-critical items – Although these items come in contact with intact mucous membranes, they do not ordinarily penetrate body surfaces. Examples include non-invasive flexible fiberoptic endoscopes, endotracheal tubes and anesthesia breathing circuits. Semi-critical items should be subjected to a **high-level disinfection** process that can be expected to destroy all microbial organisms, but not necessarily microbial spores.

- Non-critical items – These items usually come into direct contact with the patient's unbroken skin. Examples include crutches and countertops. These items require thorough cleaning, and in some cases, **low-level disinfection** to **intermediate-level disinfection**.

Spaulding's Classification System

Device Classification	Examples	Requires
Critical – Enters sterile tissue or vascular system.	• Implants • Surgical instruments • Needles	Sterilization
Semi-Critical – Touches mucous membranes, except dental.	• Flexible endoscopes • Laryngoscopes • Endotracheal tubes	High-level disinfection
Non-Critical – Touches intact skin.	• Thermometers • Hydrotherapy tanks	Intermediate-level disinfection
	• Stethoscopes • Tabletops • Bedpans	Low-level disinfection

Figure 9.2 Spaulding Classification System

Bactericidal   Relating to the destruction of bacteria.

Sterilization   The process by which all forms of microbial life, including bacteria, viruses, spores and fungi, are completely destroyed.

Disinfection   The destruction of nearly all pathogenic microorganisms on an inanimate (non-living) surface.

Disinfectant   A chemical that kills most pathogenic organisms, but does not kill all spores.

Spaulding Classification System   A system developed by Dr. E. H. Spaulding that divides medical devices into categories based on the risk of infection involved with their use.

Sterile/Sterilization   Completely devoid of all living microorganisms.

High-level disinfection   The destruction of all vegetative microorganisms, mycobacterium, small or nonlipid viruses, medium or lipid viruses, fungal spores and some bacterial spores.

Low-level disinfection   The destruction of vegetative forms of bacteria, some fungi and lipid viruses (but not bacterial spores).

Intermediate-level disinfection   The destruction of viruses, mycobacteria, fungi and vegetative bacteria (but not bacterial spores).

There is no single disinfectant that will work for all situations. That is why every decontamination area has more than one disinfectant to choose from in the work area. CS technicians must be able to select the appropriate disinfectant for the job; to do so, a basic understanding of the different types of disinfectants is needed.

Understanding Chemicals

Central Service professionals work with a wide variety of chemicals every day.

While the disinfectants used in a healthcare facility may all be a type of disinfectant, they all work differently to perform different tasks.

CS technicians understand the different disinfectants they work with and know how to achieve desired results.

TYPES OF DISINFECTANTS

The term "disinfection" is a generic term that is used to describe a process. Within that process are products that perform at different levels. (See **Figure 9.3**)

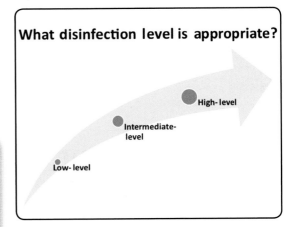

What disinfection level is appropriate?

High-level

Intermediate-level

Low-level

Figure 9.3

The following is a review of common disinfectants used in healthcare facilities and the level (type) of disinfection they are designed to provide.

Low-Level and Intermediate-Level Disinfectants

Items requiring low-level or intermediate-level disinfection only come in contact with intact skin. These items usually only touch the outside of the body (this includes items like crutches and countertops). These disinfectants may also be used on hard environmental surfaces and some mobile equipment. This group of disinfectants commonly includes quaternary ammonium compounds, alcohols, phenolics, chlorines and iodophors.

These low-level to intermediate-level disinfectants have one important thing in common: the germicidal action of each is reduced by the presence of **organic materials**. (See **Figure 9.4**)

Organic materials Compounds containing oxygen, carbon and hydrogen; derived from living organisms. Organic matter in the form of serum, blood, pus or fecal material can interfere with the activity of disinfectants.

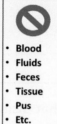

No Soil!
The germicidal action of disinfectants is reduced by the presence of soil.

🚫
- Blood
- Fluids
- Feces
- Tissue
- Pus
- Etc.

Figure 9.4

Quaternary Ammonium Compounds

Quaternary Ammonium Compounds (commonly called "quats") are low-level disinfectants. The most common chemical in most quats is benzalkonium chloride.

Quats are incompatible with soap. Soaps are not recommended for use in the CS decontamination process because of the residues they leave behind.

Some quats are absorbed by materials, such as cotton and filter paper. A quat that is absorbed by cotton should not be used with cotton towels, cloths or mop heads. It is important to consult the specific quat's Instructions for Use (IFU) to determine if cotton and/or paper can be used with them.

Figure 9.5 reviews basic information about quats.

Summary of Quats

Advantages
-Bactericidal, fungicidal and virucidal against lipophilic viruses
-Wetting agents with built-in detergent properties

Disadvantages
-Not sporicidal
-Generally not tuberculocidal or virucidal against hydrophilic viruses, unless multiple compounds are included
-May be inactivated (absorbed or neutralized) by cotton and charcoal
-Not compatible with soap
-Not effective against some gram-negative organisms commonly found in hospitals.
-Deactivated by organic material

Uses
-Environmental sanitation of non-critical surfaces such as floors, walls and furniture
-If multiple compounds in solution (super quat) may be used on instruments if properly rinsed
-Must remain wet on surface to be disinfected six to 10 minutes (or according to Manufacturer's IFU)

Figure 9.5

Summary of Ethyl or Isopropyl Alcohol

Advantages

–Rapid bactericidal agent against vegetative microorganisms; tuberculocidal, fungicidal and virucidal (ethyl isopropyl is not effective against hydrophilic viruses)
–Fast acting; no residue
–Nonstaining

Disadvantages

–Requires wet contact of at least five minutes to achieve a reasonable level of disinfection
–No residual activity
–Volatile; flammable
–Inactivated by organic material
–Can dissolve lens mountings on certain optical instruments
–Tends to harden and swell plastic tubing, including polyethylene
–Non–sporicidal

Uses

–To disinfect fixed equipment after cleaning and for patient–use items, such as ear specula, stethoscopes, etc.
–Can be used as a drying agent

Figure 9.6

Alcohol

Alcohol can be used as both an antiseptic and a disinfectant. Both ethyl and isopropyl (rubbing) alcohol have good disinfecting properties. One of the challenges when using alcohol as a disinfectant is that to achieve a reasonable level of disinfection, the alcohol must remain in wet contact with the surface of the object being disinfected for a minimum of five minutes. Alcohol evaporates quickly and maintaining wet contact for an extended period of time can be difficult.

Figure 9.6 reviews basic information about alcohol.

Antiseptic or Disinfectant?

Antiseptics are used on living tissue (skin); for example, receiving an alcohol prep before an annual flu shot. Disinfectants are used on inanimate objects; for example, disinfecting a piece of equipment between uses.

Phenolics

Phenolics are intermediate-level to low-level disinfectants containing phenol, which has a long history of use. During the 1800s, Dr. Joseph Lister used phenol to develop aseptic surgical techniques. Phenolic compounds have long been the agent of choice for housekeeping services because a residual phenolic film is left after use, and that film can be reactivated later by damp mopping; however, this same residual film can be a problem when left on medical devices. For example, irritation of sensitive skin can occur after exposure to phenolic residues. Like all disinfectants, for maximum disinfectant effectiveness, phenolics require a specific time for wet contact.

Figure 9.7 reviews basic information about phenolics.

Stainless steel instruments should not be subjected to strong phenolics for a prolonged period of time because phenolics can be corrosive. Some plastics also react poorly to phenolics. Follow the

Summary of Phenolic

Advantages

-Broad spectrum of use: bactericidal for gram-negative and gram-positive bacteria, fungicidal and tuberculocidal; active against lipophilic viruses
-Residual activity. *Note: This can also be a disadvantage*

Disadvantages

-Not sporicidal
-Inactivated by organic material (but less than some other disinfectants)
-Corrosive to some plastics

Uses

-Housekeeping usage for walls, floors, countertops and furnishings
-Phenolics are used in the decontamination area for disinfection of hard surfaces
-Copious rinsing is required to eliminate the potential for skin burns

Figure 9.7

Summary of Chlorine

Advantages

-Effective against gram-positive and gram-negative (vegetative) microorganisms; tuberculocidal, fungicidal and virucidal
-Fast acting

Disadvantages

-Inactivated by organic matter
-Corrosive to metals
-Non-sporicidal
-Stains fabrics, plastics and other synthetic materials
-Relatively unstable

Uses

-Widely used for disinfection of dialysis machines, hydrotherapy baths, toilets, lavatories and bathtubs; also used as a bleach for laundry and as a sanitizer for dishwashing
-A 1:10 dilution of 5.25% sodium hypochloride has been recommended by the CDC for cleaning blood spills
-Must remain wet on items to be disinfected one to two-and-a-half minutes (check specific manufacturer's IFU)

Figure 9.8

the device manufacturers' IFU for the types of materials that can withstand disinfection with phenolics.

Chlorine

Chlorine is an intermediate-level disinfectant that is commonly used for the treatment of water and sewage. Chlorine, a member of the halogen family may be found in CS departments as a hypochlorite solution, often recommended for biohazard clean-up procedures; however, chlorine is not considered a disinfectant of choice for CS due to its corrosive qualities. Metal instruments subjected to chlorine may have their finishes damaged by exposure to the chlorine solution.

Figure 9.8 reviews basic information about chlorine.

Iodophors

Iodophors are buffered iodines that are also members of the halogen family. Like alcohol, iodophors are used both as antiseptics and disinfectants. The best-known and most widely used iodophor is povidone-iodine. Iodophors can stain both skin and patient equipment. Iodophors should not be used on surgical instruments.

Figure 9.9 summarizes basic information about iodophors.

High-Level Disinfectants

High-level disinfectants (HLDs) are used to process semi-critical items that may come in contact with mucous membranes of the body. Items, such as flexible fiber optic endoscopes and laryngoscopes, require HLDs. There are several types of disinfectants in this category. Some can be used in a manual (soak) process, and others are used in mechanical processes. (See **Figure 9.10**)

Like their low-level and intermediate-level counterparts, HLDs are inactivated by organic materials; therefore, thorough cleaning is critical to successful outcomes. As with other disinfectants, CS technicians must understand the differences between the HLDs and how to use them effectively. The following section provides some basic information on HLD. As with all disinfectants, consult individual manufacturer's IFU before attempting to process items.

Summary of Iodophores

Advantages

- Bactericidal, virucidal and tuberculocidal
- Rapid action against vegetative bacteria

Disadvantages

- Corrosive to metals unless combined with anti-corrosive agents when formulated
- Detrimental to some plastics
- Stains fabrics and other materiel
- May require long contact time to kill some fungi

Uses

- Used in skin preparations
- Disinfection of some equipment
- The corrosive nature of iodine on metals and some plastics limits its use as a primary disinfectant in Central Service
- Must remain wet on items to be disinfected for at least two minutes (Check Manufacturer's IFU)

Figure 9.9

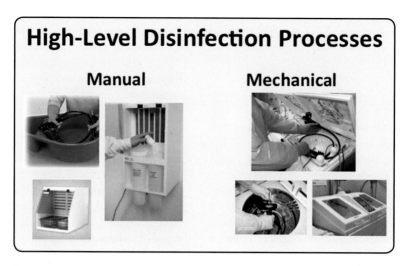

Figure 9.10

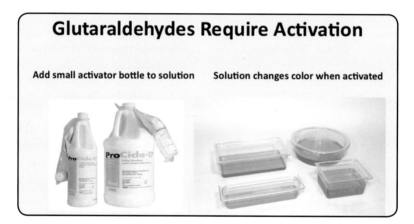

Figure 9.11

Glutaraldehyde

Glutaraldehyde is an HLD used for semi-critical devices, such as endoscopes and ultrasonic probes. Glutaraldehyde is compatible with materials used in many modern medical devices and can be used to process medical devices containing heat-sensitive materials. It kills microorganisms by **alkylation** of protein. Glutaraldehyde is usually a clear liquid that turns color when **activated** (See **Figure 9.11**) and it has a sharp, pungent odor. It is a strong irritant to the skin, eyes and respiratory system. Nitrile or butyl gloves and face/eye protection should be used when working with glutaraldehyde.

Following immersion in a glutaraldehyde solution, instructions for rinsing items should be carefully followed to ensure the chemical is completely removed. Care must be taken to ensure that the item is not recontaminated.

Glutaraldehyde should be used in a separate, designated area. Any room where glutaraldehyde is used should be well-ventilated with a minimum of 10 air exchanges per hour. When a dedicated area is not available, glutaraldehyde disinfection may be performed at an enclosed work station. These self-contained workstations manage air flow and reduce exposure to fumes. **Figure 9.12** shows some examples of these stations.

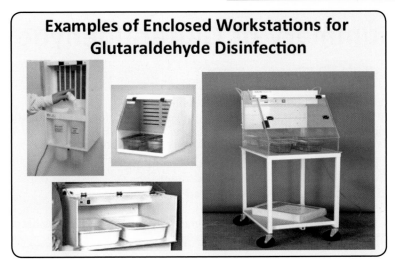

Examples of Enclosed Workstations for Glutaraldehyde Disinfection

Figure 9.12

Unused glutaraldehyde solution should be stored in a cool, secure location and in tightly-closed, properly-marked containers labeled with the activation date.

> **Alkylation** A chemical reaction where hydrogen is replaced with an alkyl group. This causes the cell to be unable to normally metabolize or reproduce, or both.
>
> **Activated (activation)** Process by which a solution is combined with an activating chemical before use. Glutaraldehydes must be activated before initial use.

Glutaraldehyde-based products can be used in automated or manual HLD processes. Most glutaraldehyde-based instrument disinfectants are labeled for reuse for 14 to 28 days. During the recommended reuse period, the concentration of the glutaraldehyde in the solution should be tested with test strips recommended by the manufacturer. If the solution falls below its **minimum recommended concentration (MEC)** level it should be discarded, regardless of how many days the solution has been in use.

Glutaraldehyde vapors increase whenever the solution is agitated, such as when it is poured into or dumped out of a soaking bin. Exposure levels for CS technicians during disposal can be reduced by adding a glutaraldehyde-neutralizing agent to

the solution prior to disposal. Consult state and local requirements and the manufacturer's IFU for proper disposal measures.

> **Minimum effective concentration (MEC)** The percentage concentration of the active ingredient in a disinfectant or chemical sterilant that is the minimum concentration at which the chemical meets all its label claims for activity against specific microorganisms.

Figure 9.13 presents basic information about glutaraldehyde.

Ortho-Phthalaldehyde (OPA)

Ortho-phthalaldehyde (commonly called OPA) is an HLD that provides a fast and effective way to disinfect a wide range of instruments.

The OPA solution may be used and reused within the limitations indicated by the manufacturer for up to 14 or 28 days. The concentration of the OPA solution should be tested with test strips recommended by the manufacturer, before each use. If the solution falls below its MEC level, it should be discarded, regardless of how many days the solution has been in use.

Following immersion in OPA solution, instructions for rinsing items should be carefully followed to

Summary of Glutaraldehyde

Advantages

-Kills vegetative bacteria (within two minutes)
-Bactericidal (gram-positive and gram-negative), tuberculocidal, fungicidal, virucidal and sporicidal. *(For sterilization (killing spores), the soak time is six to 10 hours. The manufacturer's label for recommendations should be consulted.)*

Disadvantages

-Noxious odors; good ventilation is required
-Unstable (14 or 28-day product life)
-Dilution of product reduces the activity necessary for high-level disinfection

Uses

-Semi-critical items, such as laryngoscope blades, flexible scopes, etc.

Figure 9.13 Glutaraldehyde

Summary of OPA

Advantages

- Solution is compatible with a wide range of endoscopes and other medical devices
- Requires no activation or mixing
- 14-day reuse life
- Can be discarded down facility drains in accordance with local regulations

Disadvantages

-Does not have a sterilant label claim

Uses

-Semi-critical items, such as laryngoscope blades, flexible fiberoptic endoscopes, etc.

Figure 9.14

ensure the chemical is completely removed. Care must be taken to ensure that the item is not re-contaminated.

Figure 9.14 provides a summary of basic information about OPA.

Hydrogen Peroxide

Hydrogen peroxide is a broad-spectrum HLD that is available in different concentrations.

As with other HLDs, hydrogen peroxide dilution must be monitored by regularly testing the MEC.

Summary of Hydrogen Peroxide

Advantages

-Broad spectrum HLD. Kills bacteria and viruses including Norovirus, Rotavirus, RSV, MRSA and TB
-Can be used as a sterilant at the right concentrations

Disadvantages

-Corrosive to some materials

Uses

-Disinfection of hard and soft surfaces

Figure 9.15

Summary of Peracetic Acid

Advantages

-Broad spectrum HLD
-May be used as a sterilant in the appropriate AER
-Compatible with many materials

Disadvantages

-Corrosive to some materials

Uses

-HLD of laryngoscope blades, endoscopes

Figure 9.16

Follow the manufacturer's IFU for specific instructions.

Figure 9.15 provides a summary of basic information about hydrogen peroxide.

Peracetic Acid

This chemical achieves HLD in five minutes at room temperature. Some dilutions are designed to be used in a manufacturer-specific automated endoscope reprocessor (AER) as a sterilant only. Peracetic acid is compatible with many materials and can be used to disinfect laryngoscope blades and endoscopes; however, it is also known to be corrosive, so check with the device manufacturer to determine material compatibility. Follow the manufacturer's IFU for specific instructions.

Figure 9.16 provides a summary of basic information about peracetic acid.

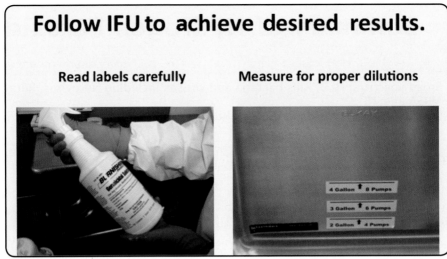

Follow IFU to achieve desired results.

Read labels carefully   **Measure for proper dilutions**

Figure 9.17

Caution!

Before using a chemical disinfectant, be sure to review the manufacturer's IFU. Using the correct chemical the wrong way is just as dangerous as using the wrong chemical.

SAFE WORK PRACTICES WHEN PERFORMING MANUAL DISINFECTION

No matter which disinfectant is chosen, failure to use it properly (according to the manufacturer's IFU) will result in failure of the disinfection process, which puts both patients and staff at risk.

Work Area Set Up

Disinfection processes should be performed only in designated areas separate from the area used for cleaning. The workflow should help ensure that the item(s) being processed are not recontaminated during or upon completion of the disinfection process.

Any accessories needed for the disinfection process, such as measuring devices, soaking bins and timers, should be collected prior to beginning the process.

Labels

Since chemical disinfectants have different capabilities, it is important to read the product labels to ensure they are used appropriately. Check the

IFU of the disinfectant and medical device(s) to be processed to ensure compatibility. (See **Figure 9.17**)

Disinfectants used in healthcare facilities are harsh chemicals. It is important to read and follow all safety precautions.

Preparation Instructions

In addition to choosing the appropriate disinfectant, there are various factors that are vital to the success of chemical disinfection. When preparing disinfectant solutions, check the label for essential preparation instructions, which include:

- Appropriate concentration for use (diluted or full strength?).

- Dilution or mixing requirements.

- Correct temperature required for the disinfectant.

- Water quality and pH requirements.

Important Safety Note
While manufacturers may combine chemicals to create a more effective disinfectant, CS technicians should never mix chemicals on their own. Some common chemicals can be lethal when combined.

Contact

Disinfectants are not effective unless they make direct contact with all surfaces of the device. Improper cleaning will leave organic matter that prevents direct contact. Lack of contact through improper application or because soil remains on a device will result in a failed disinfection process.

Direct contact may also be impeded if items are not disassembled properly, or if they are only partially submerged in a disinfectant soak solution. When disinfecting a lumen, care must be taken to ensure there are no air bubbles in the lumen that prevent the disinfectant from coming in contact with all interior surfaces of the lumen. (See **Figure 9.18**)

Exposure Time

Exposure times vary by type of disinfectant. Many times, the term "wet contact" is stated in the IFU. This means the amount of time the device must remain wet with the disinfectant. Use a timer to ensure the proper exposure time is met.

What Is Wet Contact Time?

Wet contact time means that the item must remain wet with the disinfectant for the entire stated contact time. If the disinfectant evaporates or the item is allowed to dry before the total contact exposure time is met, the disinfectant must be reapplied and the exposure time must start over.

Rinsing

Disinfectants require a rinsing process. Pure water should be used to rinse disinfected instruments, with care being taken to thoroughly rinse all surfaces according to manufacturer instructions.

ACHIEVING DISINFECTION USING MECHANICAL PROCESSES

Sometimes disinfection is performed using a mechanical process. The most common mechanical process is the one carried out in washer-disinfectors. These automated washers provide a cleaning process followed by a **thermal disinfection** process. Thermal disinfection uses heat to reduce the amount of bacteria on items, such as surgical instruments and utensils. (See **Figure 9.19**) Water temperature is the key source of disinfection in any automatic washer that claims to provide thermal disinfection. The exposure time and temperature used to achieve thermal disinfection differs by brand of washer. Check the manufacturer's IFU and the washer operator's manual for specific information.

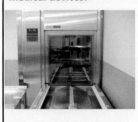
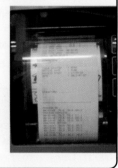

Thermal Disinfection

The use of heat to disinfect medical devices.

Figure 9.19

Thermal disinfection The use of heat to reduce the amount of microorganisms (excluding spores) on a medical device.

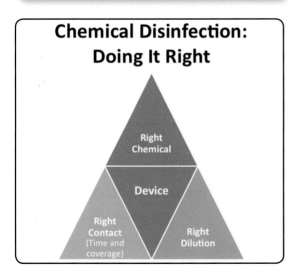

Chemical Disinfection: Doing It Right

Right Chemical

Device

Right Contact (Time and coverage)

Right Dilution

Figure 9.18

Pasteurizers

Pasteurization equipment provides disinfection at water temperatures of 150° to 170°F (65° to 77°C). The temperature is maintained for a minimum of 30 minutes of exposure to the instruments. Items must be able to withstand immersion in solution and be thoroughly cleaned prior to placing them in a pasteurizing unit. Water temperature and exposure time must be closely monitored. **Figure 9.20** is an example of a pasteurizer.

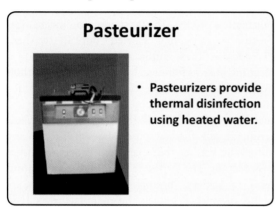

Figure 9.20

Automated Endoscope Reprocessor

The most recent addition to mechanical disinfectors are Automatic Endoscope Reprocessors (AER). These units make the process of disinfecting flexible fiber optic endoscopes simpler and safer.

AERs offer several advantages over manual processing. They reduce personnel exposure to the HLD disinfectant and its vapors. Their use may also increase quality assurance by providing consistent processes and documenting several cycle parameters.

Advantages of most AER include:

- Consistent exposure to the cleaning agent.

- Timed contact with the liquid chemical disinfectant.

- Continuous movement of the HLD.

- Alcohol flush cycle to facilitate drying.

- Use of an air flush cycle to remove excess moisture.

- Use of copious and consistent amounts of water.

- Monitoring of channels during processing.

- Documentation of the cycle parameters.

Endoscope design limitations create the need for some manual reprocessing steps. Refer to the AER's operating manual for information about limitations of automated cycles.

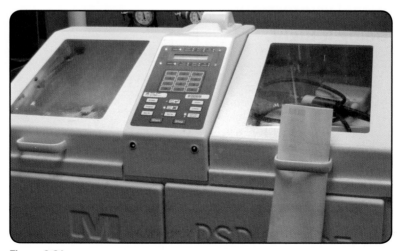

Figure 9.21

When using an AER:

- Follow the scope manufacturer's IFU for proper manual cleaning prior to placing the scope in an AER

- Follow the manufacturer's instructions to connect the endoscope to the AER.

- Place valves and other removable parts in the AER, if possible.

- Follow the manufacturer's IFU for the types of disinfectants and their proper use.

- Set the machine for the recommended cycle time.

QUALITY ASSURANCE PRACTICES FOR DISINFECTION

In addition to reading and following the manufacturer's IFU when performing disinfection processes, other quality assurance practices should be in place. Those practices should help ensure that disinfection processes are performed correctly, safely and according to product-specific requirements.

Education

All technicians who perform disinfection activities should be trained and should meet competencies for each disinfection process they perform. Each time a new product or process is introduced into the work area, training must be performed and competencies established.

Safety

Safety of patients and staff is of concern when performing disinfection processes. Improperly disinfected medical devices pose a risk to patients. The harsh chemicals (and sometimes fumes) associated with chemical disinfection can pose a safety risk to CS technicians, as well. It is important to understand the following recommendations for handling disinfectants:

- Personal protective equipment (PPE) requirements.

- Environmental (ventilation) requirements.

- Spill and leak procedures.

- Storage requirements.

- Disposal requirements.

QUALITY ASSURANCE TESTING FOR HIGH-LEVEL DISINFECTANTS

HLDs are much more complex chemicals than low- to intermediate-level disinfectants, and the items processed in these chemicals are used in semi-critical areas of the body. It is important to monitor these chemicals to assure they are performing as expected, and to document the results of that monitoring.

Minimum Effective Concentration Testing

In order to determine if the HLD can be reused, it is important to routinely test the solution with a chemical indicator. HLDs must be tested prior to each use and the results must be clearly documented. Chemical indicators are developed to be used for specific products. Be certain to use the correct indicator for the solution being tested. **Figure 9.22** provides an example of a chemical test strip. Follow specific manufacturer testing protocol and carefully document all MEC testing. **Figure 9.23** provides an example of an MEC testing log sheet.

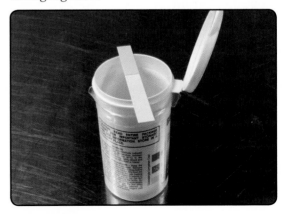

Figure 9.22

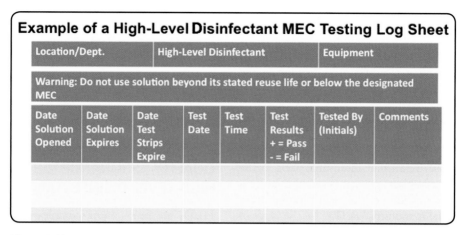

Example of a High-Level Disinfectant MEC Testing Log Sheet

Location/Dept.		High-Level Disinfectant			Equipment		
Warning: Do not use solution beyond its stated reuse life or below the designated MEC							
Date Solution Opened	Date Solution Expires	Date Test Strips Expire	Test Date	Test Time	Test Results + = Pass - = Fail	Tested By (Initials)	Comments

Figure 9.23

HLD LOG SHEET

Date/Time of Test	Pt. ID	Physician/ Procedure	Items processed (include serial numbers)	Technician who cleaned items	Technician performing HLD	HLD Solution	Expiration Date of HLD	Test strip quality test results	MEC Test Results	HLD Equipment Used (include lot number of	Verification of Rinsing (Tech Initials if manually disinfected)	Comments

Figure 9.24

Documentation

In addition to documenting the MEC of the HLD, concise documentation must be kept to enable tracking of the disinfected items to the patient receiving the items. A manual or computerized record should be maintained when using HLD. Documentation should at least contain:

- Lot number of the HLD process, including AER or soak basin number.

- Items being disinfected, including quantities and device serial numbers, if applicable.

- Patient name or identifier.

- Physician's name and procedure.

- HLD solution information including activation or dilution date and the last date the solution may be used (unless MEC testing fails before that date).

- Exposure time and temperature, if manually soaking.

- Date and time of the process.

- Technician identification.

- MEC test strip results.

Figure 9.24 provides an example of a HLD log sheet. *Note: It is not always necessary to have both a MEC and a HLD log sheet. The documentation may be combined on a single document, as long as all required information is documented.*

CONCLUSION

Performing any successful disinfection process is much more difficult than it appears. Careful attention to detail from the initial cleaning process through the completion of the disinfection process is critical to achieve desired results.

Central Service technicians must select the appropriate disinfectant designed for the job they want to do, prepare the items properly and use the disinfectant as directed to ensure the safety of staff and patients.

The success or failure of any disinfection process depends on the knowledge of the CS technician and their attention to detail. (See **Figure 9.25**)

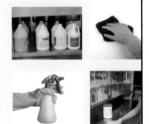
Disinfectants:
- are not all the same.
- must be appropriate for the job.
- are only effective when used according to direction.

Figure 9.25

RESOURCES

Block S. *Disinfection, Sterilization and Preservation, 5th Ed.* 2001.

Society of Gastroenterology Nurses and Associates. *Guideline for Use of High-Level Disinfectants & Sterilants for Reprocessing Flexible Gastrointestinal Endoscopes.* 2013.

Centers for Disease Control and Prevention. *Guideline for Disinfection and Sterilization in Healthcare Facilities.* 2008.

Association for periOperative Registered Nurses. *Guidelines for PeriOperative Practice: High Level Disinfection.* Guidelines for PeriOperative Practice. 2015.

Association for the Advancement of Medical Instrumentation. *Chemical Sterilization and High-Level Disinfection in Health Care Facilities.* 2013.

CENTRAL SERVICE TERMS

Bactericidal

Sterilization

Disinfection

Disinfectant

Spaulding Classification System

Sterile/sterilized

High-level disinfection

Low-level disinfection

Intermediate-level disinfection

Organic materials

Alkylation

Activated (activation)

Minimum effective concentration (MEC)

Chapter 10
Surgical Instrumentation

Learning Objectives

As a result of successfully completing this chapter, readers will be able to:

1. Discuss the importance of surgical instruments and the role of the Central Service technician in instrument care and handling

2. Review basic steps in the surgical instrument manufacturing process

3. Define basic categories of surgical instruments based upon their functions and identify the points of inspection, anatomy and procedures to measure the following types of instruments:
    *   Hemostatic forceps
    *   Needle holders
    *   Tissue forceps
    *   Dressing forceps
    *   Retractors
    *   Scissors
    *   Suction devices
    *   Single- and double-action rongeurs
    *   Kerrison/laminectomy rongeurs
    *   Nail nippers
    *   Graves and Pederson vaginal speculums

4. Identify solutions that can damage stainless steel instruments

5. Explain procedures to test instruments for sharpness and identify (mark) them

6. Emphasize the importance of instrument lubrication and review tray assembly safeguards

INTRODUCTION

Approximately 51.4 million inpatient procedures are performed in the U.S. each year. Procedures performed in ambulatory surgery centers and clinics significantly increase the total number of procedures performed in the U.S. Add in procedures from dental centers and other facilities, and it is easy to see that literally billions of surgical instruments are processed in the U.S. annually. Each of these devices has the potential to cause harm to a patient.

Central Service (CS) technicians are responsible for helping ensure that instruments needed for each procedure are safe, functional and available when needed. To reach this critical goal, it is essential that CS professionals can properly clean, decontaminate, package and sterilize instruments. It is also critical they understand how to identify, inspect and test these devices.

Beyond that, CS professionals must ensure that instrument sets and trays are complete and neatly organized to enable the end user to find instruments easily.

It is impossible for any technician to be able to identify every instrument in existence; however, skilled technicians can identify the vast majority of instruments in their facility's inventory. This chapter provides some background information about common instruments and instrumentation-related processes applicable to most facilities.

THE IMPORTANT ROLE OF INSTRUMENT SELECTION AND INSPECTION

Although many instruments may appear similar, they may have very different functions. Each one is designed to perform in a specific situation. Placing the wrong instrument into a set can cause serious problems during a surgical procedure. Many instruments come in various sizes. Placing the wrong size instrument in a set may have the same effect as placing the wrong instrument in the set.

While identifying and selecting the correct instrument for each set is crucial, knowing how to inspect the instrument is just as important. Placing dull scissors or forceps with a missing tooth into a set for example, can cause delays in the procedure and may also harm the patient. Loose or damaged parts can fall off into a patient during a procedure, potentially causing injury to the patient.

Inspecting devices for cleanliness is also important. Instruments may appear clean on the outside, but careful inspection of the entire instrument may show that it was not properly cleaned. Instrument assembly is another vital role of the CS technician. When an instrument tray or set is completed by the CS technician, it will not be checked again until it reaches the point of use. At that point, errors—such as defective or missing instruments—can cause serious problems. (See **Figure 10.1**)

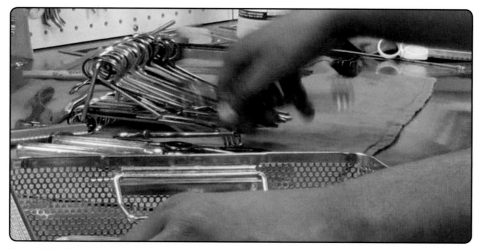

Figure 10.1 Proper instrument set assembly is critical for positive outcomes.

Some Basic Questions

CS technicians usually have some common questions when they begin to learn about surgical instrumentation. Knowing the answers to those questions can help establish a good starting point for instrument care and handling. Some key questions may include the following:

Where do instruments come from?

Physicians identify the specific instruments needed to perform various procedures. Most instruments are purchased by the healthcare facility and maintained by CS. Some instruments are sent to the facility on loan for a specific surgery and must be returned to the vendor after use. *Note: Loaner instrumentation will be discussed in Chapter 11.*

Why must all instrument requirements be so exacting?

The human body is very complex. Surgeons need exactly the right instrument in order to perform specific functions. Devices that appear similar can be used for very different procedures/purposes.

Where do the instruments get their names?

As discussed in Chapter 3, many instruments get their names from the part of the anatomy where they were designed to be used. Instruments are sometimes named after the surgeon who invented them. The Bookwalter retractor, for example, is named after its inventor, Dr. John Bookwalter. Other common examples of instruments named after surgeons include Debakey and Mayo.

Why are instruments so expensive?

Surgical instruments are precision tools. Manufacturing surgical instruments is very labor-intensive process. Most instruments are made using a combination of machine and hand labor. Fine details, such as sharpening, inspection and other steps, are performed by hand. The combination of materials used and labor costs make instruments expensive.

In this era of high technology, CS technicians may imagine that instruments are stamped out on a high-speed assembly line, packaged and then shipped to the customer; however, this is not the case. The manufacturing process requires time-consuming and hands-on labor from highly-skilled professionals.

INSTRUMENT MANUFACTURING PROCESS

The manufacturing process begins with the selection of the materials used to construct the instruments.

Stainless Steel

The study of the surgical instrument manufacturing process begins by considering the raw materials used to create them. Most are produced from **stainless steel**; however, other materials like materials, such as titanium, copper and silver, are also widely used.

Stainless steel can, in fact, stain, spot and rust; therefore, more appropriate name is "stain-resistant." Proper care will ensure that a stainless instrument performs as it should and lasts a long time.

Several types of stainless steel are used to produce surgical instruments. One type (400 series stainless steel) is hard, and used when sharp cutting edges are needed. Instruments produced with 400 series steel include **scissors, osteotomes, chisels, rongeurs, forceps, hemostatic forceps** and **needle holders**. This hardened steel is known as **martensitic** stainless steel.

The second most popular steel used to manufacture surgical instruments is 300 series stainless steel. While it offers high corrosion resistance, this material doesn't provide the hardness properties of its 400 series counterpart; therefore, it is more workable and malleable. Instruments produced with 300 series stainless steel include **retractors, cannulas, rib spreaders** and **suction devices**. This softer type of steel is called **austenitic** stainless steel.

Stainless steel An alloy of steel with chromium and sometimes another element, such as nickel or molybdenum, that is highly resistant to rusting and ordinary corrosion.

Scissors Surgical instruments used to cut, incise and/or dissect tissue.

Osteotomes Chisel-like instruments used to cut or shave bone.

Chisels Wedge-shaped instruments used to cut or shape bone.

Rongeurs Surgical instruments used to cut or bite away at bone and tissue.

Forceps Instruments used for grasping, holding firmly or exerting traction upon objects.

Hemostatic forceps Surgical instruments used to control the flow of blood.

Needle holders Surgical instruments designed to drive suture needles to close or rejoin a wound or surgical site. Also known as needle drivers.

Martensitic (stainless steel) This metal is also known as 400 series stainless steel. It is magnetic and may be heat-hardened.

Retractors Surgical instruments primarily used to move tissues and organs to keep the surgical site exposed throughout surgery.

Cannulas Surgical instruments with a hollow barrel (or lumen) through their center. Cannulas are often inserted for drainage.

Rib spreaders A retractor used to expose the chest.

Suction devices Surgical instruments used to extract blood and other fluids from a surgical site.

Austenitic (stainless steel) This metal is also known as 300 series stainless steel. It is non-magnetic, cannot be heat-hardened and is more corrosion-resistant than martensitic stainless steel.

Manufacturing Steps

The next step in manufacturing a surgical instrument is forging the material to create a stamp of its rough outline from a heated bar of stainless steel. (See **Figure 10.2**) The heating and cooling process used to create an instrument is very important because good forging produces good instruments. Most high-quality forgings come from mills in Germany, but forgings also come from Japan, Pakistan, Malaysia, France and Sweden. After the forging is completed, the instrument must be ground and milled first, and have the excess steel removed. Some instruments require more than 20 milling operations to create the male and female halves and the cutting of **serrations** and **ratchets**.

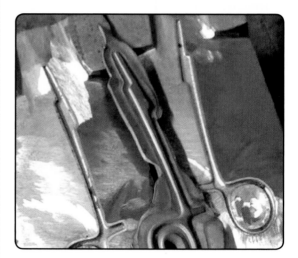

Figure 10.2

In today's instrument manufacturing environment, there is more reliance on machines than in years past. Despite technical advances, however, there is still a significant amount of the milling process that must be done by hand. Instrument manufacturers perform hundreds of quality checks and finishing applications to every instrument during the manufacturing process to ensure quality.

Upon completion of the assembly process, instruments undergo a final heating procedure, called tempering.

After tempering, the instruments are polished. Polishing is necessary to achieve a smooth finish, which ultimately determines the final appearance or finish of the instrument. Surgical instruments can be shiny (mirror finish), or they can have a matte or satin finish (gray-colored surface that does not reflect light). (See **Figure 10.3**) Both finishes are widely accepted and create a smooth surface; however, the mirror finish is smoother, it tends to stain less frequently.

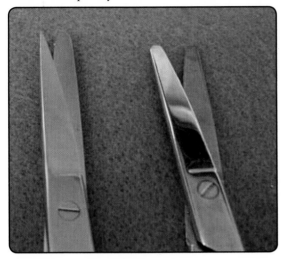

Figure 10.3

Next, the passivation layer is applied. **Passivation** uses nitric acid (HNO_3) to remove all the iron content still found on the outside layer of the instrument. The removal of this iron helps build a protective outside layer of chromium oxide (Cr_2O_3). This layer is highly resistant to corrosion and continues to build up throughout the instrument's life. The passivation layer may become damaged when the instrument is abused by using abrasive cleaners, saline and chemicals not approved for use by the manufacturer.

> **Serrations** Parallel grooves in the jaws of surgical instruments.
>
> **Ratchet** The part of a surgical instrument that "locks" the handles in place.

The instrument is now ready for final inspection and it will be carefully examined. Ratchets, tips, scissor blades, serrations, **box locks** and spot welds will be tested. Finally, the instrument is ready to be etched with the company name and catalog number. Acid chemical, stamping and lasers are some methods used for this process.

> **Box locks** Point where the two jaws or blades of an instrument connect and pivot.
>
> **Passivation** A chemical process applied during the instrument manufacturing process that provides a corrosion-resistant finish by forming a thin, transparent oxide film.

As you have read, the surgical instrument manufacturing process is lengthy and detailed, and requires a significant amount of experience, skill and craftsmanship. A typical manufacturing cycle—from forging to finished instrument—usually takes up to six weeks.

CLASSIFICATION AND OVERVIEW OF SURGICAL INSTRUMENTS

Surgical instruments are designed for a specific surgical purpose. Injury to the patient and destruction of or damage to the instrument can occur when the incorrect instrument is used. For example, one might incorrectly pull a pin using a needle holder instead of a pin puller or a pair of pliers, and this can damage the needle holder.

To properly inspect and test surgical instruments, CS technicians must know the anatomy and points of inspection of the devices, and how to measure them. This will enable them to properly and efficiently assemble instrument sets.

Many of the most common categories of surgical instruments will be discussed in this section.

Hemostatic Forceps

The primary function of hemostatic forceps is to control the flow of blood. **Figure 10.4** identifies the anatomy and points of inspection of a hemostatic forceps. **Figure 10.5** shows the correct way to measure this instrument.

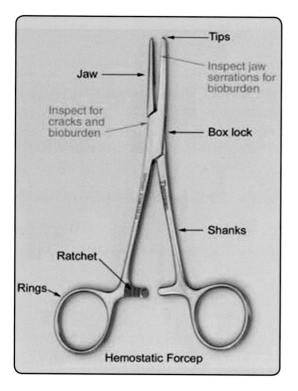

Figure 10.4

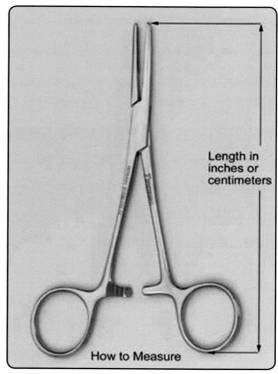

Figure 10.5

Identification of Hemostatic Forceps

Length		Jaw Pattern	Name
3½ inches	8.9cm	Full serrations	Hartman Mosquito (see Figure 10.7)
5 inches	12.7cm	Full serrations	Halstead Mosquito (see Figure 10.7)
5½ inches	14.0cm	Full serrations	Crile Hemostat (see Figure 10.8)
5½ inches	14.0cm	Partial serrations	Kelly Hemostat (see Figure 10.8)
6¼ inches	15.8cm	Full serrations	Rochester Pean
6¼ inches	15.8cm	Full serrations with 1x2 teeth	Rochester Ochsner or Kocher
6¼ inches	15.8cm	Longitudinal serrations and cross-serrated tip	Rochester Carmalt

Figure 10.6

Figure 10.6 provides basic information that can help CS technicians identify several types of hemostatic forceps.

Figure 10.7 identifies two common hemostatic forceps: the Hartman Mosquito 3½" and the Halsted Mosquito 5".

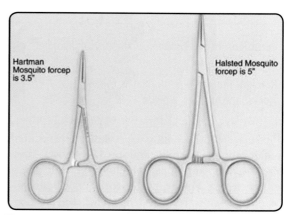

Figure 10.7

Jaw features can consist of full serrations (Crile hemostat) or partial serrations (Kelly hemostat). *Note: These two types of forceps are shown in* **Figure 10.8**. Hemostatic forceps can also have longitudinal serrations (Rochester Carmalt) and serrations with 1x2 teeth (Kocher forceps).

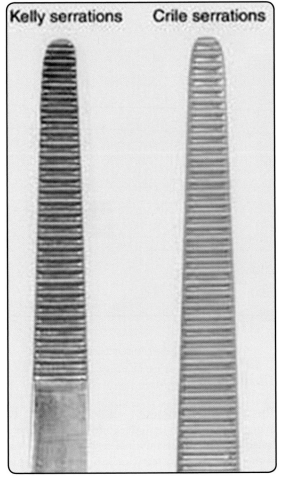

Figure 10.8

Needle holders

These instruments are designed to drive suture needles to close surgical sites. **Figure 10.9** identifies the anatomy and points of inspection of a needle holder, and **Figure 10.10** shows the correct way to measure this instrument.

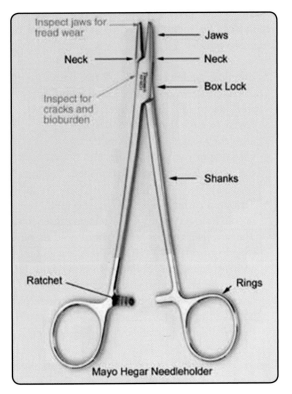

Figure 10.9

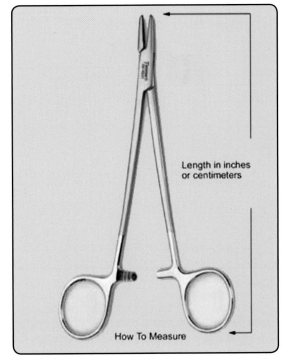

Figure 10.10

Needle holder **jaws** (the portion that holds the needle) can be manufactured of stainless steel or tungsten carbide:

- Stainless steel jaws. There are two patterns of jaw tread: smooth or serrated. Stainless steel jaw treads cannot be repaired, re-jawed, or have the serrations replaced after they wear out. This can occur with one or two years of use, and then the needle holder must be replaced.

- Tungsten carbide jaws. The most popular needle holders in surgical use have these jaws. The key visual factor is the bright gold rings. (See **Figure 10.11**) When gold is placed on an instrument, this indicates that the working portion (jaws) is made of tungsten carbide. Jaws made of this metal are typically preferred because they are harder and last longer, grip the needle more firmly and can be replaced.

Figure 10.11 shows needle holders with stainless steel and tungsten carbon jaws.

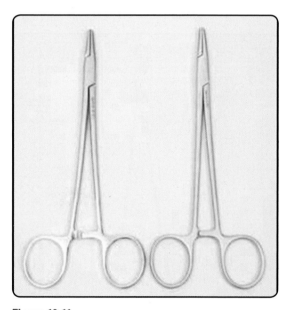

Figure 10.11

> **Jaws** Two or more opposable parts that open and close; used for holding or crushing something between them.

Other names for needle holders are needledrivers, diamond jaws and gold handles. The two most common needle holder designs are Mayo-Hegar and Crile-Wood, and they are shown in **Figure 10.12** *Note: The Crile-Wood is narrower than the Mayo-Hegar design.*

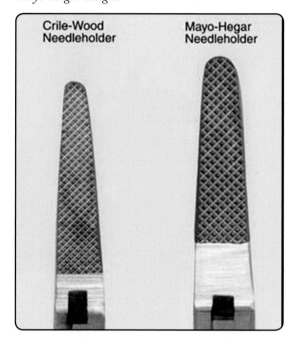

Figure 10.12

Tissue Forceps

The primary function of tissue forceps is to manipulate tissue. A design feature of this tweezer-styled forceps is the multiple-teeth configuration at the distal tips. The teeth assist in grasping tissue and provide a more secure grip. **Figure 10.13** identifies the anatomy and points of inspection of a tissue forceps. **Figure 10.14** shows the correct way to measure this instrument.

The most common teeth configurations for tissue forceps are one tooth on one side and two teeth on the other. With this design the teeth interlock one another, and the teeth configuration is indicated by 1x2. Other common teeth configurations are 2x3, 3x4, 5x6, 9x9, and 1x2 with serrations. Other names for tissue forceps are rat tooth, brown forceps and pickups.

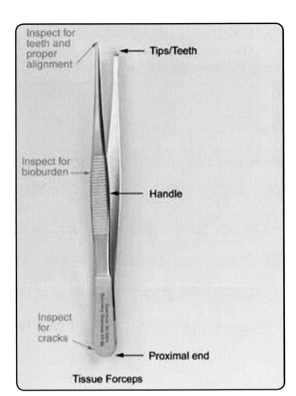

Tissue Forceps

Figures 10.13

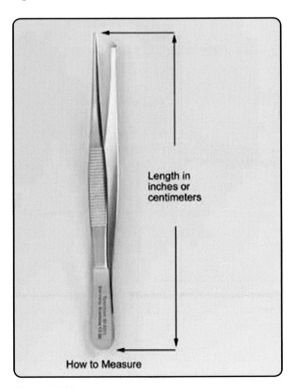

Length in inches or centimeters

How to Measure

Figure 10.14

Dressing Forceps

Dressing forceps are similar to tissue forceps, except they have serrations instead of teeth at the distal end. The primary function of this instrument is to manipulate tissue and pack surgical sites. **Figure 10.15** shows the anatomy of a dressing forceps and points of inspection. **Figure 10.16** shows the correct way to measure this instrument. Other names for dressing forceps are smooth forceps and plain forceps.

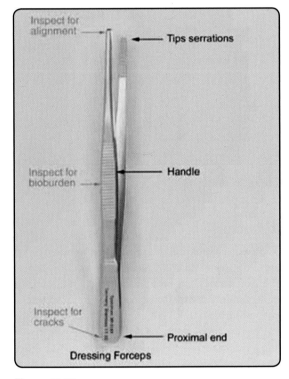

Dressing Forceps

Figure 10.15

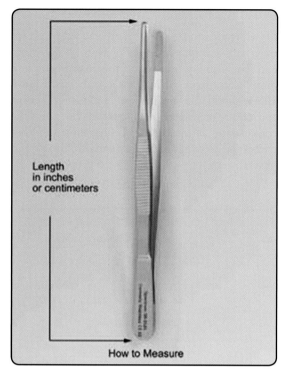

Figure 10.16

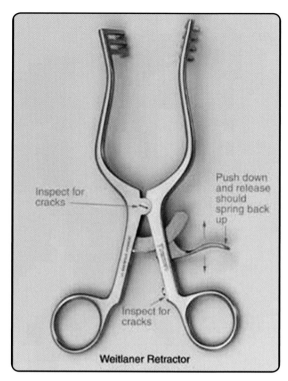

Figure 10.17

Retractors

The primary function of a retractor is to move tissue aside for exposure and visualization of the surgical site. Retractors can be handheld, self retaining or table mounted. Small finger-held retractors move and hold skin and subcutaneous tissues, while larger retractors are used to retract muscle tissue and organs. Self-retaining retractors (**Figure 10.17**) are designed with a mechanical action that keeps them open to retract. To test a self-retaining retractor, simply push down on retractor lever and let it go. If the lever springs up, the instrument is working properly. If the lever remains in the down position, remove it from the instrument set and send the instrument to the repair vendor. Some common self retaining retractors are Weitlaner, Gelpi and Beckman-Adson.

Figure 10.18 shows the points of inspection of a loop handle retractor. **Figure 10.19** shows the correct way to measure a hollow handle retractor.

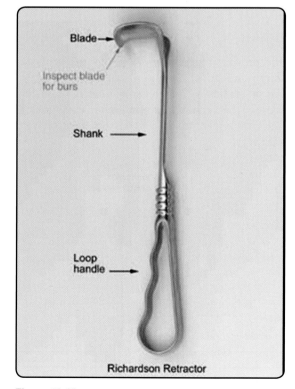

Figure 10.18

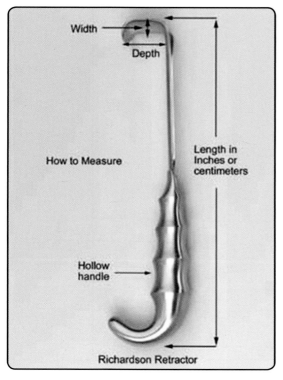

Figure 10.19

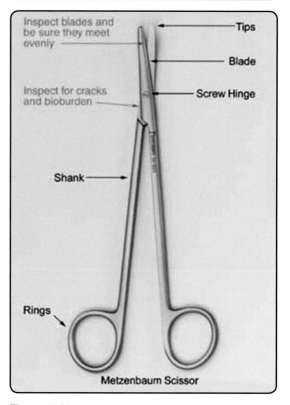

Figure 10.20

Scissors

The primary function of scissors is to cut tissue, suture and other material in the surgical field. For **dissection**, curved scissors are primarily used because their curve allows for better visualization. The opening action of the scissors also helps to dissect and spread tissue. **Figure 10.20** shows the anatomy and points of inspection for scissors. **Figure 10.21** shows the correct way to measure this instrument.

Dissection The process of cutting apart or separating tissue.

Mayo scissors are one of the most popular scissors used and are identified by beveled blades. The second most popular Mayo design is the Mayo Noble. As seen in **Figure 10.22**, it does not have a beveled blade.

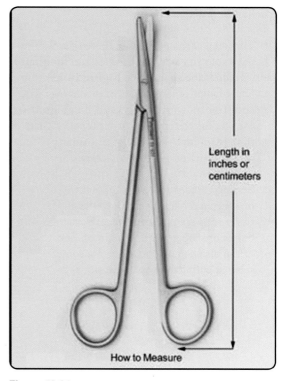

Figure 10.21

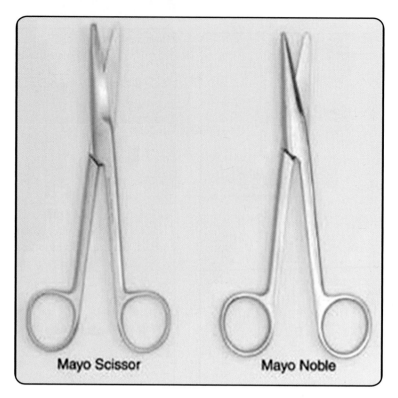

Figure 10.22

Surgical scissors have various blade features for specific surgical applications:

- Tungsten carbide blades – These scissors have gold rings on the handles and tungsten carbide blade edges. (See **Figure 10.23**) Scissors with these blades have a harder and stronger cutting edge, and they allow the scissors to remain sharper for a longer time than other scissors. Their primary design function is tissue dissection.

- Serrated blades – The design feature of a serrated blade is the prevention of tissue slippage or escape during cutting. Serrations are generally found on one of the blades; however, there are some scissors with dual-blade serrations.

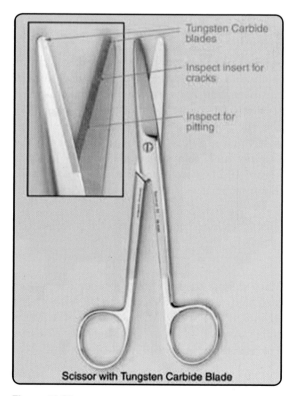

Figure 10.23

• Microgrind or supercut blades – Black rings visually identify these scissors from standard or gold-handled tungsten carbide scissors. The design of a black-handled scissors is to simulate a tissue lancing/slicing action. While all other scissors cut tissue with a crushing action, a black-handled scissors has one blade sharpened like a knife to slice tissue. The other blade is a standard design that causes a guillotine effect. (See **Figure 10.24**) Black-handled scissors must be specially sharpened.

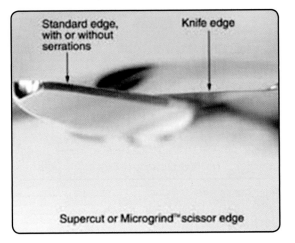

Figure 10.24

Suction Devices

The primary function of suction devices is to extract (suction) blood and fluids from the surgical site. **Figure 10.25** shows the anatomy and points of inspection for a suction device. **Figure 10.26** shows the correct way to measure this instrument. The two most common suction devices are Baron and Frazier suction tubes. These suction devices include a metal stylet that is used during the surgical procedure to unclog the suction channel. *Note: This stylet is not to be used to clean the device. The only cleaning tool for a suction device is the proper cleaning brush.*

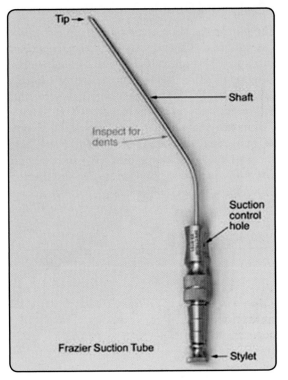

Figure 10.25

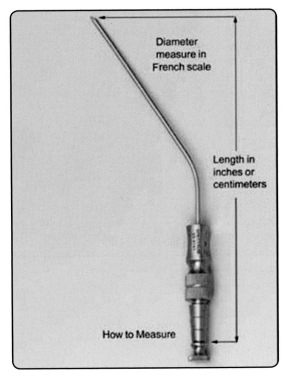

Figure 10.26

Single- and Double-Action Rongeurs

The primary function of a rongeur is to cut or bite away at bone and tissue. The difference between a single-action (**Figure 10.27**) and a double-action (**Figure 10.28**) rongeur is the design of how the jaws close. With a double-action instrument, the surgeon squeezes the handle, which creates two movements for the jaw to close. This double movement reduces the amount of hand strength, so the instrument bites more with less hand strength. The main inspection point on single- and double-action rongeurs is the jaws. Any dents or gouges of the jaws prevent the instrument from working properly.

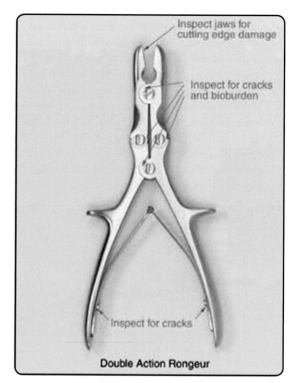

Double Action Rongeur

Figure 10.28

Kerrison/Laminectomy Rongeurs

The primary function of this style of rongeur is to remove the disc or lamina during spine surgery. The distal portion must be inspected after each use to look for bioburden and cutting edge damage. (See **Figure 10.29**) When Kerrison rongeurs are being assembled in trays, it is important to identify the different bite designs (e.g., the 90-degree up bite, as shown in **Figure 10.30**). If a Kerrison rongeur is sticking in a closed position, a repair vendor will need to disassemble, polish, sharpen and re-assemble the instrument.

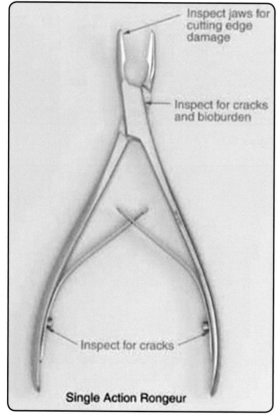

Single Action Rongeur

Figure 10.27

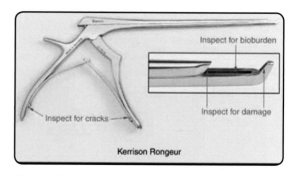

Kerrison Rongeur

Figure 10.29

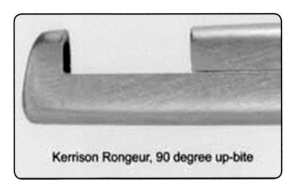

Figure 10.30

Nail Nippers

The primary function of nail nippers (see **Figure 10.31**) is to cut toenails and fingernails and, occasionally, to trim small bone fragments. The cutting surface and edge should be inspected along with the hinge area and spring.

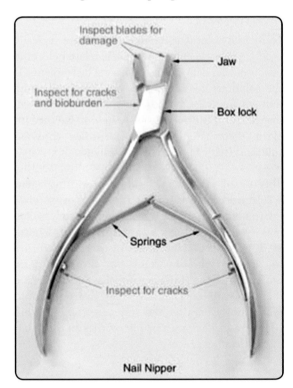

Figure 10.31

Graves and Pederson Vaginal Speculums

The primary use of these medical instruments is to expose the vaginal cavity. **Figure 10.32** shows the anatomy the of a vaginal speculum. One important inspection point is to ensure that the thumb screws are present and functioning. It is also important to inspect all sides of the blades for damage. As noted in **Figure 10.33**, a Pederson blade is narrower than that on a Graves speculum.

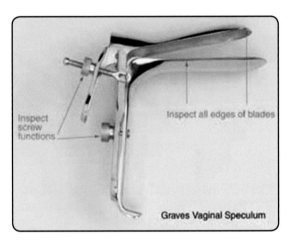

Figure 10.32

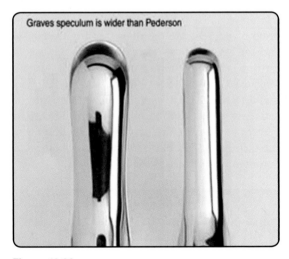

Figure 10.33

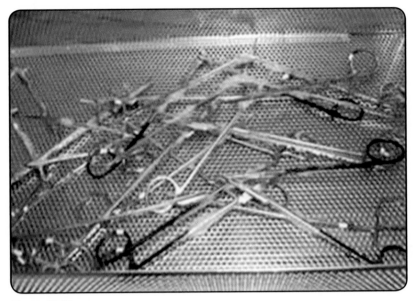

Figure 10.34

POST-OPERATIVE CARE OF SURGICAL INSTRUMENTS

Within minutes, blood can begin to dry on surgical instruments. Users should take precautions to ensure that blood and soil is not allowed to dry on instruments. To prevent damage associated with dried blood, separate the rings (see **Figure 10.34**) and ratchets for box-lock exposure on applicable instruments and cover them with a water-moistened towel. (See **Figure 10.35**) Another useful technique is to spray an enzymatic foam or detergent-based solution onto the instruments to prevent blood from drying. With either approach, the instruments should be transported to the CS decontamination area as soon as possible.

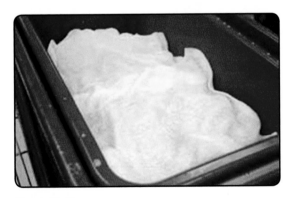

Figure 10.35

SOLUTIONS THAT DAMAGE INSTRUMENTS

Numerous solutions, ranging from those typically used for housekeeping to kitchen-related cleaning purposes, can damage stainless steel instruments. If the solution's container does not specifically note that its intended purpose is for use on surgical instruments, the product should not be used to clean them. **Figure 10.36** identifies common solutions that can damage instruments.

The use of saline as a soaking or rinsing agent accelerates the rusting and pitting of surgical instruments. In many cases, the use of saline may void instrument warranties (See **Figure 10.37**); therefore, controlling instrument exposure to saline is very important. For clinical reasons, Operating Room (OR) personnel cannot eliminate the exposure of stainless steel instruments to saline; however, after the surgical procedures are completed, saline must be removed as an early step in the cleaning process.

Solutions That Damage Surgical Instruments
Betadine
Peroxide
Dish soaps
Soaking in water
Soaking in saline
Bleach
Iodine
Hand soaps
Saline
Long term soaking in rust remover
Long term soaking in stain remover
Porcelain cleaners
Household lubricants
Household powder cleansers
Surgeons' hand scrubs
Laundry detergents

Figure 10.36

Rusts and Stains

Stainless steel is composed of rust-resistant alloys. No steel is truly "stainless," although rusting is relatively rare. Proper processing helps control both staining and rusting.

"Rust" that appears on an instrument is often a stain. A pencil eraser can be used for an "eraser test" to help determine the difference between staining and rusting. After a stain is discovered, use the eraser to remove the discoloration. Then, look at the metal below the discoloration to determine if there are any tiny pit marks. If pit marks are discovered, this is corrosion: the origin of the rusting. If the metal is smooth and clean below the stain, the source of discoloration is a stain; there is no rust.

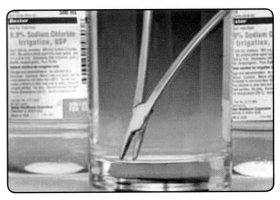

Figure 10.37

INSTRUMENT SHARPNESS TESTING AND IDENTIFICATION

Instrument sharpness testing is essential to monitor the sharpness of surgical instruments. **Figures 10.38** through **10.45** illustrate proper sharpness testing procedures for common surgical instruments.

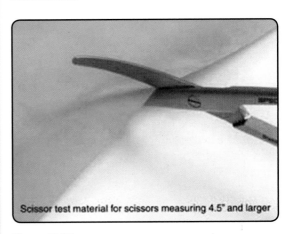

Scissor test material for scissors measuring 4.5" and larger

Figure 10.38

Instrument: Scissors 4.5" and larger.

Test material: Red test material (latex); orange material (latex free).

Test: Scissors must be able to cut through to the tip two to three times. The distal tips of scissors are the most crucial portion because this is where they first become dull. They must cut cleanly through the tips of the instrument.

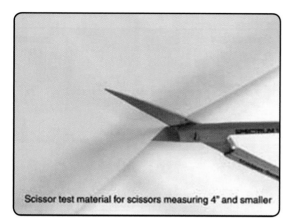

Figure 10.39

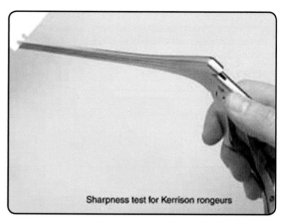

Figure 10.41

Instrument: Scissors 4" or smaller.

Test material: Yellow test material (latex or latex free).

Test: Scissors must be able to cut through the tips two to three times. The distal tips of scissors are the most crucial portion; they must cut cleanly through the tips of the instrument.

Instrument: Kerrison rongeur.

Test material: Index card.

Test: Punch a clean hole through the card.

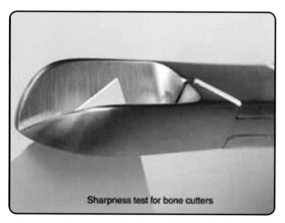

Figure 10.40

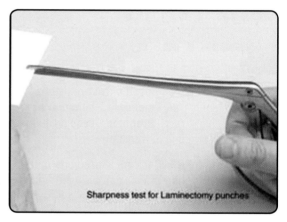

Figure 10.42

Instrument: Bone cutter.

Test material: Index card.

Test: Cut off a piece of the index card.

Instrument: Laminectomy rongeur.

Test material: Index card.

Test: The rongeur should make a clean bite using half the jaw.

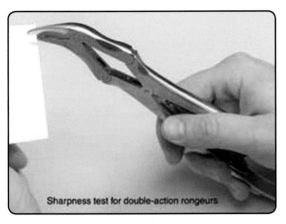

Sharpness test for double-action rongeurs

Figure 10.43

Instrument: Double-action rongeur.

Test material: Index card.

Test: The rongeur should make a clean bite through the card.

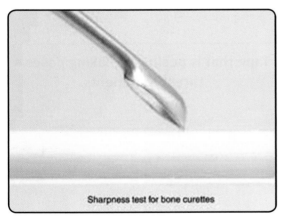

Sharpness test for bone curettes

Figure 10.44

Instrument: Bone curette.

Test material: Plastic dowel rod.

Test: Shave off pieces of the dowel rod.

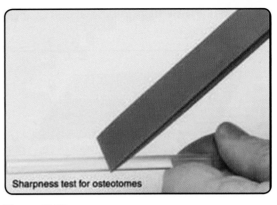

Sharpness test for osteotomes

Figure 10.45

Instrument: Chisels and osteotomes.

Test material: Plastic dowel rod.

Test: Shave off pieces of the dowel rod.

INSTRUMENT IDENTIFICATION METHODS

There are thousands of different surgical instruments and many look quite similar. CS technicians must ensure that the correct instruments are placed into the proper trays. Many healthcare facilities use different instrument marking methods to mark instruments for faster and easier identification.

Marking surgical instruments for identification can be done several ways. The use of tape is one popular method for identifying instruments. Although this is a seemingly simple approach, it is important to follow proper application techniques. What follows are some important steps to ensure proper device taping:

- Clean fingertips with alcohol to remove oils, grease and dirt.

- Wipe alcohol on the site of the instrument where the tape will be placed to remove any lubricant or moisture that might be on the instrument. *Note: Tape should always be placed on the shank of the instrument and never the rings. Tape that is applied to a rounded surface, such as instrument rings, will not adhere to the instrument's surface.*

As shown in **Figure 10.46**, cut the tape on an angle to allow its edge to lay flat.

Figure 10.46

- Wrap the tape one to one and one-half times around the device. Apply the tape with a firm, pulling tension. Be careful not to apply excessive tape. (See **Figure 10.47**)

- After the tape is applied, autoclave the instrument to allow the heat to help bond the tape to the instrument. **Figure 10.48** provides an example of properly applied tape.

Note: Please refer to the tape manufacturer's IFU for special instructions.

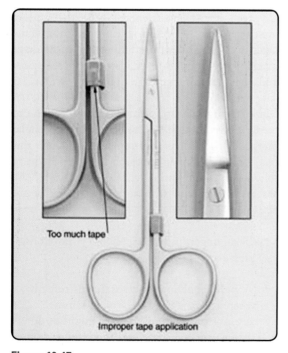

Figure 10.47

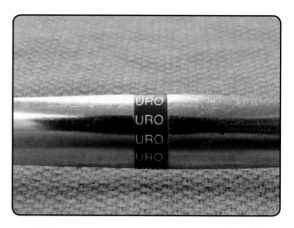

Figure 10.48

When using tape to identify instruments, inspection of the tape each time the device is processed is very important. Tape that is loose, damaged or peeling must be removed and replaced as microorganisms under the loose or damaged tape are very difficult to clean. Peeling and damaged tape can inadvertently fall into the patient potentially causing an infection. (See **Figure 10.49**)

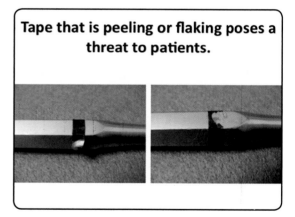

Figure 10.49

Other methods of marking instruments include:

- Acid-base etching – This process can be done by the instrument repair vendor, or a kit may be purchased, so the etching process can be done at the facility. Acid base etching uses a stencil, solutions and electricity to mark stainless steel. This process is semi-permanent, and it can be buffed off during the instrument repair process. (See **Figure 10.50**)

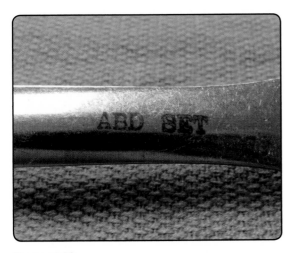

Figure 10.50

- Heat-fused nylon – This color coding is often referred to as "dipping," and is typically done in a repair facility. Heat-fused nylon is a powder-coating process that leaves a thin layer of colored nylon on the instrument. Nylon coating can last years; however, once it begins to chip, all nylon must be removed from the instrument. (See **Figure 10.51**)

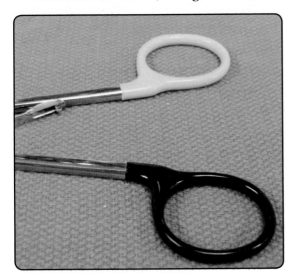

Figure 10.51

- Laser etching – This durable process is usually done by the manufacturer or an outside vendor. (See **Figure 10.52**)

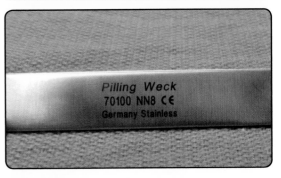

Figure 10.52

- Dot matrix - These systems are relatively inexpensive and can be applied by CS technicians. (See **Figure 10.53**) The two most popular types of dot systems are:

  - The dot marking system, where a small barcode containing the instrument information is applied with pressure-sensitive tape.

  - The dot peen system is done by using a laser or tungsten stylet to implant the information onto an instrument.

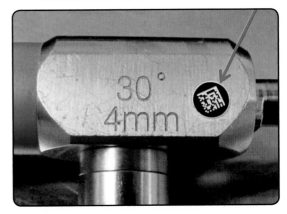

Figure 10.53

INSTRUMENT LUBRICATION

Many surgical instruments with moving parts must be lubricated after each use or in accordance with manufacturer's recommendations. The use of a neutral-pH lubricant extends the life of the instrument, and makes the device easier for the surgeon to use. While most washer-disinfectors will lubricate instruments, some instruments may need to be lubricated again during assembly. Each CS workstation should have lubrication available for this purpose. Lubricants are available in spray bottle formulas. All lubricants must be approved for use as a surgical instrument lubricant and for the type of sterilization method that will be used on the instrument. The point of application should be the instrument's hinged area or any working component, such as a moving/sliding area. (See **Figure 10.54**)

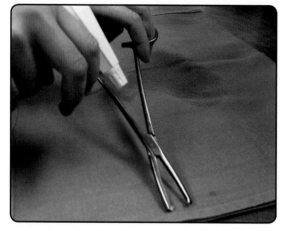

Figure 10.54

TIPS TO PROTECT INSTRUMENTS FROM DAMAGE

Instruments are an expensive asset for any facility. Protecting the instruments is a part of every CS technician's job. When treated properly, many instruments can remain in active service for many years. The following are some helpful tips:

- Always follow the manufacturer's instructions for cleaning, lubrication and sterilization. These instructions were developed by the instrument manufacturer to help ensure the instrument's longevity.

- Place heavy instruments on the bottom or side of the tray. This will help protect the smaller, more delicate instruments.

- Select an instrument tray that allows adequate space for weight distribution. Overcrowding instruments can cause damage.

- All curved instruments should be curved in the same direction to protect tips from being damaged.

- Tissue and dressing forceps should be softly nested together or placed close to each other in the tray or peel pack. Do not push the forceps together. Leave some space between each forceps so the sterilant can reach all surfaces.

- Delicate instruments should be kept in approved micro cases or small protective cases within the surgical tray.

- The use of metal instrument holders, called stringers, can assist in faster sterile field assembly and safer handling of the instruments, especially sharps. Stringers also hold the instruments in the open position during sterilization. (See **Figure 10.55**)

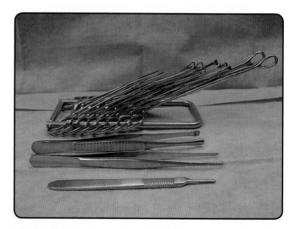

Figure 10.55

- Laser-finished instruments should never have metal-to-metal contact that can damage, chip and scratch the finish during decontamination, tray assembly and transport. A silicon nipple mat can prevent metal-to-metal contact, as can foam or a lint-free towel.

CONCLUSION

Properly identifying instruments and following the proper inspection protocols help ensure instrument trays are assembled correctly and all the instruments are clean and functional. Carefully following the manufacturer's IFU and paying meticulous attention to detail will help keep the instruments in good repair and extend the life of these expensive items.

Central Service technicians are the last to touch instruments before they are received in a procedure area; therefore, their quality of work is critical to successful patient outcomes.

RESOURCES

Centers for Disease Control and Prevention. *FastStats.* http://www.cdc.gov/nchs/fastats/insurg.htm. Accessed March 2014.

Schultz R. *Inspecting Surgical Instruments: An Illustrated Guide.* 2005.

Gregory B. *Orthopedic Surgery.* 1994.

Tighe S. *Instrumentation for the Operating Room.* 1994.

Glaser Z. *Surgical Instrument Quality. Infection Control and Sterilization Technology.* 1997.

Storz Instruments. *The Care and Handling of Surgical Instruments.* 1991.

Reichert M. *Sterilization Technology for the Health Care Facility, Second Edition.* 1997.

CENTRAL SERVICE TERMS

Stainless steel

Scissors

Osteotomes

Chisel

Rongeurs

Forceps

Hemostatic forceps

Needle holders

Martensitic (stainless steel)

Retractors

Cannulas

Rib spreaders

Suction devices

Austenitic (stainless steel)

Serrations

Passivation

Box lock

Jaws

Dissection

Chapter 11

Complex Surgical Instruments

Learning Objectives

As a result of successfully completing this chapter, readers will be able to:

1. Provide an overview of and discuss procedures to care for and effectively process powered surgical instruments

2. Explain important basic concerns when handling and processing endoscopic instruments

3. Discuss detailed information about rigid and flexible endoscopes and their accessories

4. Review general processing and inspection requirements for endoscopes and accessories

5. Identify infection prevention concerns regarding endoscopes and loaner instrumentation

6. Identify basic protocols important for each step in the loaner instrumentation process

INTRODUCTION

Advances in many types of surgical procedures have improved patient outcomes and shortened both hospital stays and recovery time. At the same time, the instruments used in these procedures have become more complex and difficult to process.

From their origin in early times, surgical instruments have evolved from simple devices to the complex surgical instruments used today. Forceps, scissors, needle holders and retractors, along with numerous other simple instruments, are still commonly used, but they are joined by powered surgical instruments, endoscopes and other highly sophisticated and delicate devices with complex components, such as circuit boards and computer chips.

Many of these complex instruments that Central Service (CS) technicians process require special handling and care. This instrumentation may range from a single instrument or a few sophisticated devices in a small tray to those that comprise many trays and consist of hundreds of devices.

Whatever the specialty, the requirements for processing complex instruments remain the same: thorough cleaning, detailed inspection, proper packaging, and sterilization. One of the greatest challenges that CS technicians face is keeping abreast of new and evolving instruments and their specific processing requirements. Complex instruments are costly to purchase and repair and, therefore, represent a large financial investment to the hospital. Due to the associated expense, many facilities may not have back-up instrumentation available, so careful handling of these instruments is essential.

This chapter addresses basic information about some of the complex instruments that may cause processing concerns for CS technicians.

POWERED SURGICAL INSTRUMENTS

The use of drills and saws by physicians dates as far back as 5,000 to 7,000 years ago. In the mid-1800s, the dental industry took the lead in powered instrumentation by developing powered dental drills.

The fields of neurosurgery, orthopedics, otology and dentistry have also played key roles in the development of high-powered surgical instruments now used in every surgical and dental subspecialty. These developments have revolutionized surgery, making procedures both safer and faster.

The size, compactness and design complexity of powered surgical devices range from drills used on the tiniest ear bones to drills and saws used on the largest leg bones. Powered surgical instruments have greatly reduced the brute force historically required for orthopedic surgeries and they have also decreased the time required to perform them. This, in turn, has allowed surgeons to complete surgeries quicker and with more precision.

Materials used to construct powered surgical instruments are varied, so careful selection of cleaning and disinfection products is critical. Products chosen must be compatible with materials used and they must yield successful processing results. Equipment manufacturer's processing instructions must be followed to prevent damage to instruments containing lumens, channels, attachments and

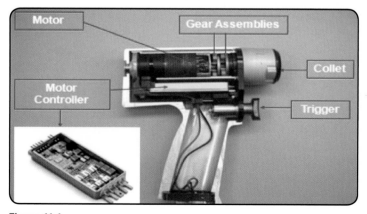

Figure 11.1

multiple moving parts. **Figure 11.1** shows some internal components of a motorized handpiece and demonstrates the complexity of powered surgical instrumentation.

Powered surgical instruments contain several working components that will be damaged if fluid (such as water or a cleaning solution) is allowed to penetrate into the device's interior. **Figures 11.2** and **11.3** illustrate the type of damage that occurs when powered surgical instruments and their accessories are invaded by fluid. CS professionals should be specifically trained to clean, process and handle powered surgical devices and equipment, and ensure that fluid invasion doesn't occur.

Fluid Invasion Damage on a Powered Surgical Instrument

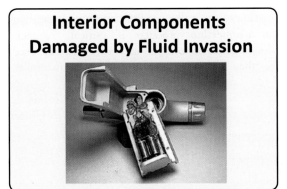

Figure 11.2

Interior Components Damaged by Fluid Invasion

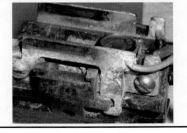

Figure 11.3

Power Sources

There are three main sources of power used for powered surgical instruments: electric, compressed gas (pneumatic) and battery.

Electric-Powered Surgical Instruments

Electric-powered instruments are used when physicians need a lightweight instrument for procedures where access is limited, such as in maxiofacial, dental and small bone (e.g., hand) procedures.

Instruments powered by electricity require a power cable that can be sterilized. One end of the cable attaches to the motorized handpiece on the surgical field; the other end attaches to a power unit (motor/electrical adapter) that plugs into an outlet. These cables require routine maintenance that involves disassembly, cleaning, lubrication, and inspection to look for cuts, nicks and/or other damage. During cleaning, fluid must not enter the cable or handpiece. Many manufacturers recommend connecting the cable to the handpiece during processing to help prevent fluid invasion. Care must also be taken not to bend the connector pins on the cable.

An arthroscopy shaver is an example of an electric-powered instrument. (See **Figure 11.4**)

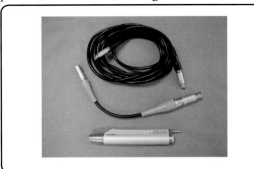

Figure 11.4

The most common problems associated with electric-powered equipment are:

- Damage to electrical parts during cleaning and sterilization.

- Condensation that enters the equipment when seals wear out.

- Electrical contacts that become worn and affect equipment handling.

The following are general guidelines for proper care and handling of electric-powered instruments and accessories:

- Do not immerse the equipment in any solution, including water, unless the manufacturer's Instructions for Use (IFU) specifically state that the device can be submerged.

- Do not use solvents or lubricants, unless specified by the equipment manufacturer.

- Use a brush to clean the distal tip and lumens. Follow the IFU for the correct size and type of brush to use for each area.

- Dry the equipment with a clean, lint-free cloth.

Electric-powered equipment can be operated with a foot switch (foot-controlled pedal). (**Figure 11.5** shows an operational foot pedal and **Figure 11.6** shows a foot pedal damaged by fluid invasion.) Foot switches may have a cable to attach the instrument console, or they may be wireless. To clean foot switches, follow the manufacturer's instructions and avoid pulling on or stressing the power cord or damaging the sensors.

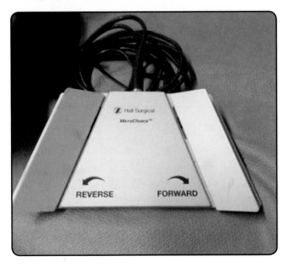

Figure 11.5

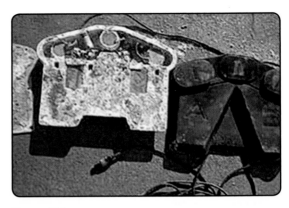

Figure 11.6

Pneumatic-Powered (Air-Powered)

Pneumatic-powered (air-powered) instruments come in various sizes and allow the surgeon to work on small, medium and larger bones. Sternum saws, sagittal saws and drills are popular pneumatic-powered instruments.

Pneumatic-powered instruments require a hose that can be sterilized. (See **Figure 11.7**) One end of the hose attaches to the motorized handpiece on the surgical field; the other end attaches to the source of compressed gas, which can come from a stand-alone cylinder (tank) with a pressure regulator (See **Figures 11.8** and **11.9**), or be "piped in" through a wall or column-mounted regulator panel. (See **Figure 11.10**)

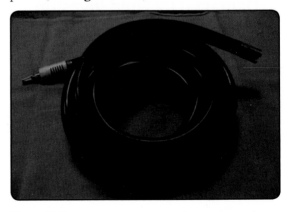

Figure 11.7

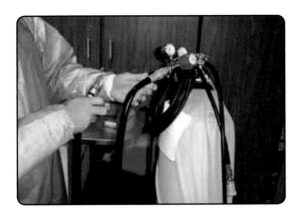

Figure 11.8

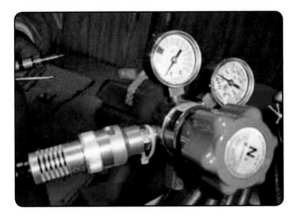

Figure 11.9

Instrument hoses must be carefully inspected for cleanliness. *Note: These hoses are usually black, so it is often difficult to see blood and debris.* Hoses must also be inspected for nicks and other possible damage. They must be pressurized for proper inspection; therefore, an air source is required in the processing area.

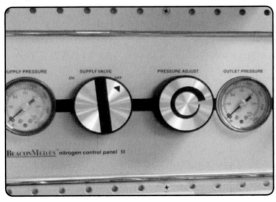

Figure 11.10

If the hose casing becomes damaged (or "bubbled") it must be removed from service. Fluid must not enter the hose or handpiece during processing. Many manufacturers recommend connecting the hose to the handpiece during cleaning to help prevent fluid invasion and related damage.

Different types of powered instruments require different operating pressures, and a chart of these pressures should be available where the instruments are processed. CS technicians must be certain to follow the manufacturer's instructions and test instruments using the appropriate gas. Extreme care is required because testing instruments at an improper pressure can injure the operator and/or severely damage the instrument. **Figures 11.11** and **11.12** provide examples of air-powered instruments.

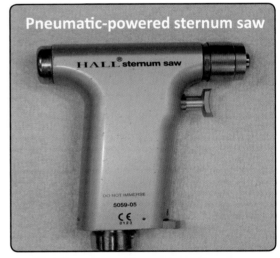

Figure 11.11

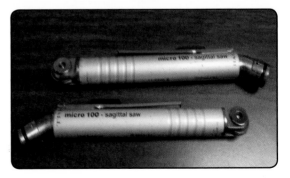

Figure 11.12

To properly care for and handle pneumatic equipment:

- Never immerse in any solution (including water) unless the manufacturer's IFU specifically states the device can be submerged.

- To clean, insert the appropriate manufacturer-recommended cleaning brush into attachments and burr guards. (See **Figure 11.13**)

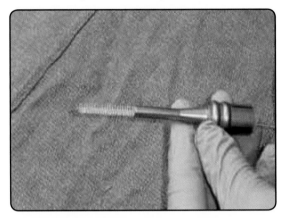

Figure 11.13

- Carefully wipe and rinse the outer casing. (See **Figure 11.14**)

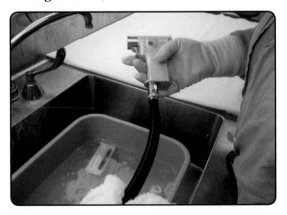

Figure 11.14

- Use a decontamination hose to protect inner components. (See **Figure 11.15**)

How to Create a Decontamination Hose

Decontamination hoses are made by cutting small pieces of damaged pneumatic hoses, placing both regulator ends on the hose, and marking the hose in some way to identify it as nonfunctional. A popular way of marking the hose is with red tape.

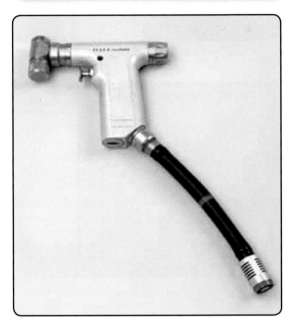

Figure 11.15

- Burr guards must be lubricated according to manufacturer instructions.

Care of Air Hoses

All pneumatic (air-powered) equipment must be attached to an air hose to operate. Sterilization issues are the primary reason air hoses fail because heat from sterilization breaks down the rubber components and O-rings, and causes air leakage. To clean the hose, use a mild detergent. Don't allow fluids to enter hose and never use abrasives to wash the hose liner. Take care when coiling the hose during handling. Proper coil size for sterilization should be nine to 12 inches. Hoses should not be coiled tightly.

Battery-Powered Instruments

Battery-powered surgical instruments are high powered and work well with the procedures performed on larger, denser bones. Total hip and knee replacement surgeries are examples of such procedures. (See **Figure 11.16**)

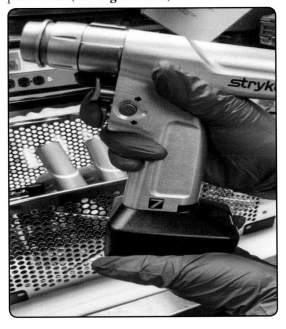

Figure 11.16

Batteries and chargers are specific to each system, and are not interchangeable. Additional space must be provided to accommodate the chargers. (See **Figure 11.17**)

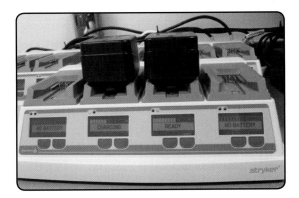

Figure 11.17

Figure 11.18 provides examples of battery-powered instruments.

Examples of Battery-Powered Surgical Instruments

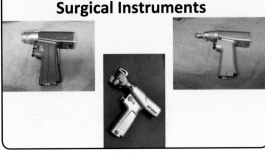

Figure 11.18

Common Powered Surgical Instruments

- Dermatome/dermabraders for harvesting skin grafts or reshaping skin surfaces.

- Cebatomes for removing bone cement.

- Sternal saws to split the sternum and allow access for open-heart surgery.

- Dental drills for repair/reconstructive work on teeth and jawbones.

- Micro drills for reshaping middle ear bones or driving very small wires through bones.

- Wire drivers, drills and saws in the appropriate size and shape to work on the smallest facial bones to the largest bones (such as those in the leg).

- Saws designed to perform specific cutting actions, such as reciprocating or oscillating.

To properly care for and handle battery-powered instruments:

- Never immerse handpieces, attachments or batteries in any solution, including water, unless approved by the manufacturer.

- Clean surgical debris from attachments and handpieces using brushes and a manufacturer-recommended mild detergent.

- Rinse with water, while assuring that the water does not enter the battery contact area.

- Use a decontamination battery to protect electrical components from moisture. (See **Figure 11.19**)

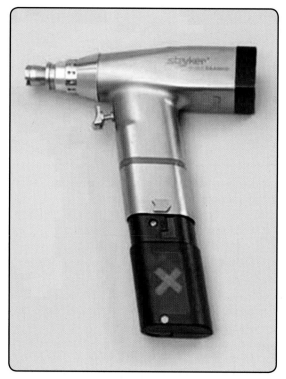

Figure 11.19

How to Create a Decontamination Battery

Locate a dead, unrepairable battery for each style of powered surgical instrument. Use instrument marking tape to make a red "X" on the battery packs and keep these batteries in the decontamination area. When battery-powered equipment enters the Central Service decontamination area, select and insert the appropriate battery pack to protect the electrical components from moisture. *Note: While this does help prevent moisture from entering the unit, care should still be taken to avoid contact with excess moisture.*

- Check all moving parts for cleanliness and function. (See **Figure 11.20**)

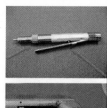
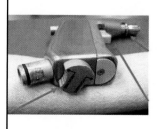
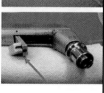

Check Moving Parts of Powered Surgical Instruments

Figure 11.20

- Lubricate the handpiece with the type and amount of lubricant recommended by the equipment manufacturer. *Note: Not all powered instrumentation or accessories are lubricated. Refer to the device's IFU.*

- Some manufacturers recommend operating handpieces to ensure proper functioning, and dispersing lubrication (if added) prior to packaging for sterilization. (See **Figure 11.21**)

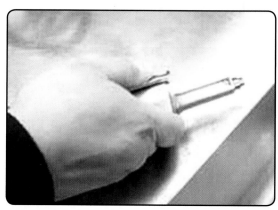

Figure 11.21

• Attach accessories, including batteries, to the handpieces to ensure they fit properly. (See **Figure 11.22**)

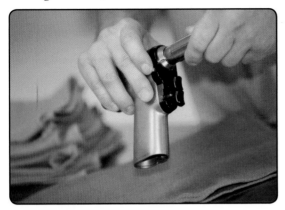

Figure 11.22

• Package and sterilize the device, per manufacturer recommendations. Special racks or positioning devices may be needed to ensure that all device surfaces are properly exposed to the sterilant and to ensure that condensation does not collect. Some types of packaging, such as peel packs, are not suitable for all types of powered instruments and accessories. Check manufacturers' packaging recommendations.

Common Reasons for Powered Equipment Repairs

Powered surgical equipment is expensive to purchase and repair. Everyone who handles this equipment should use caution to prevent damage. Common causes of damage include:

• Corrosion of internal components from condensation, steam, fluid invasion or improper cleaning.

• Physical damage due to mishandling. (See **Figure 11.23**)

• Lack of or improper preventive maintenance.

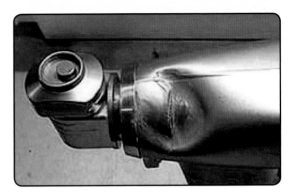

Figure 11.23

Motorized handpieces are very delicate and expensive and require special care. Proper use and handling, along with regular preventive maintenance and service, will help ensure that the devices are available for safe, effective use.

ENDOSCOPES

The term "endoscopy" means "looking inside." Endoscopic procedures allow a physician to look inside the body through the use of an **endoscope**. Endoscopic procedures are considered minimally-invasive because they do not involve a large incision. This minimally-invasive instrumentation allows the physician to perform procedures either through natural body openings like the mouth, nose or anus, or through small incisions that provide access for endoscopic instrumentation. This instrumentation may be used to view a specific area of the body or, with the addition of other instruments, perform multiple types of surgeries.

> **Endoscope** An instrument used to examine the interior of a hollow organ or body cavity.

All endoscopes allow for light and image transmission. Some endoscopes also provide a working channel, allowing the surgeon to perform surgical procedures.

The first endoscopes were developed in Germany in the 1800s; however, the use and development of endoscopes became more popular after World War II. In the 1950s, the flexible endoscope was introduced. Today, fiber optics [a technology that uses glass (or plastic) threads (fibers) to transmit data] and **light-emitting diodes (LED)** are the primary carriers/sources of light for endoscopic surgery.

> **Light-emitting diode (LED)** Semiconductor diode that emits light when voltage is applied.

LED act as tiny light bulbs. Fiber optics do not produce light; instead, they act as wires to carry light generated from an external source. (See **Figure 11.24**)

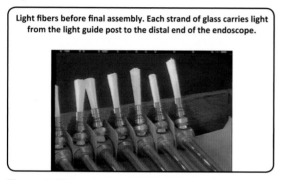

Light fibers before final assembly. Each strand of glass carries light from the light guide post to the distal end of the endoscope.

Figure 11.24

Proper light is a critical factor in endoscopic procedures, as the quality of the image or pictures is largely dependent on light quality and quantity. It is important to check the endoscope, the light source and the carrier (fiber optic cord) to ensure they are in working order each time the endoscope is processed. The dark areas in **Figure 11.25** indicate damaged light fibers.

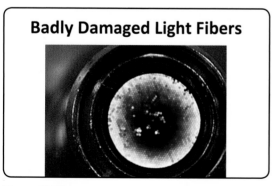

Badly Damaged Light Fibers

Figure 11.25

The second function of endoscopes is to transmit the reflected image back to the surgeon's eye or to a video system. **Figure 11.26** shows endoscopy with the use of a video system. This can be accomplished through the use of fiber optic bundles or computer chips inside the scope.

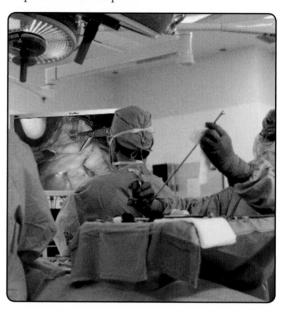

Figure 11.26

Endoscope Classification

The term "endoscope" describes all devices that are used to view inside a body cavity. **Figure 11.27** shows the different classifications of endoscopes.

It is important when discussing endoscopes to properly classify the type of endoscope in use because function, care and handling processes are different for each classification. This section will focus on rigid, semi-rigid and flexible endoscopes.

The classification of rigid, semi-rigid and flexible relates to an endoscope's ability to bend without damaging the device. Rigid and flexible endoscopes can be further classified according to how the image is captured. This divides rigid and flexible endoscopes into two broad categories: video and non-video.

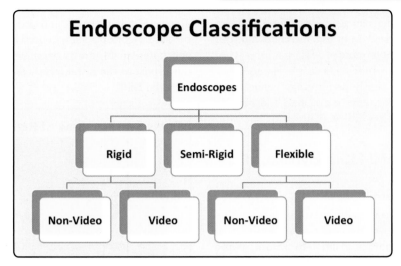

Figure 11.27

Operative and Non-Operative Endoscopes

The first endoscopes were non-operative; meaning the surgeon could view anatomy through the device, but could not perform a surgical procedure, such as a biopsy. Operative endoscope technology permitted surgeons to do much more than diagnose a condition; they could perform corrective surgeries with these new minimally-invasive instruments. Surgical procedures, such as laparoscopy and arthroscopy, came into demand as physicians and patients realized the benefit of shorter hospitalizations, less painful surgical procedures, lower healthcare-associated infection (HAI) risks, and faster recovery times.

An operative endoscope has a working channel (lumen) through which instruments or accessories can be passed to perform surgical procedures. (See **Figure 11.28**)

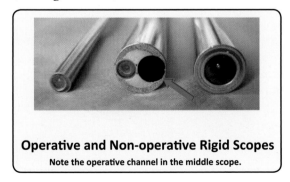

Operative and Non-operative Rigid Scopes
Note the operative channel in the middle scope.

Figure 11.28

Technological advancements continue today across surgical specialties, much of which has been fueled by smaller instruments and endoscopes. For example, surgeons can perform endoscopic abdominal, arthroscopic, urological, otolaryngeal, cardiac and neurosurgical procedures. Recent endoscopic developments permit heart conditions to be treated without opening the chest or cutting the ribs; pituitary surgery can now be performed through the sinus cavity, and salivary gland stones can be removed endoscopically. Further, lesions in the gastrointestinal tract and lungs can be directly visualized, and diagnostic biopsies and therapeutic procedures can be performed without surgery or general anesthesia.

Endoscope Use and Selection

Endoscopes are chosen by the physician based on the type of procedure they are performing. Rigid endoscopes are appropriate for viewing anatomy where there is straight-line access to the site. Semi-rigid endoscopes are useful where the line to the surgical site is relatively straight; however, some slight bending of the scope shaft may be needed to access the site, such as in bladder surgery. Flexible endoscopes are used where straight line access is not possible, such as when viewing the esophagus, lung, kidney or large intestine. Whether a rigid, semi-rigid or flexible endoscope is used, the device acts as the eye of the surgeon. Due to their delicate construction, as well as their size and frequent handling, endoscopes are at risk of being damaged every time they are handled. In a single cycle of use, the endoscope can be handled by eight or more people.

Damaged or poorly-performing endoscopes result in costly procedure delays, staff and surgeon dissatisfaction and, possibly, patient harm.

RIGID AND SEMI-RIGID ENDOSCOPES

Rigid Endoscopes

Rigid endoscopes range in size from the very tiny 1.9mm scopes used for sialendoscopy (internal viewing of the salivary glands) to 15mm scopes used for robotic surgical procedures. Rigid endoscopes can be constructed using rigid rod lenses (non video) or with a video chip mounted in the distal end (video). (See **Figure 11.29**)

All rigid endoscopes are generally manufactured using tubes of stainless steel. Rigid endoscopes are designed to allow for some minimal flexing of the shaft, but damage will occur beyond the flex limits.

A general rule is that a rigid endoscope should not be bent. Fiber optics are housed between the inner and outer tubes and transmit light from the light guide post to the distal end of the endoscope. (See **Figure 11.30**)

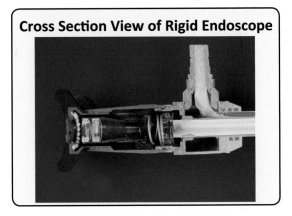

Cross Section View of Rigid Endoscope

Figure 11.30

Operative rigid endoscopes have a working channel that allows the surgeon to pass instruments to perform surgery.

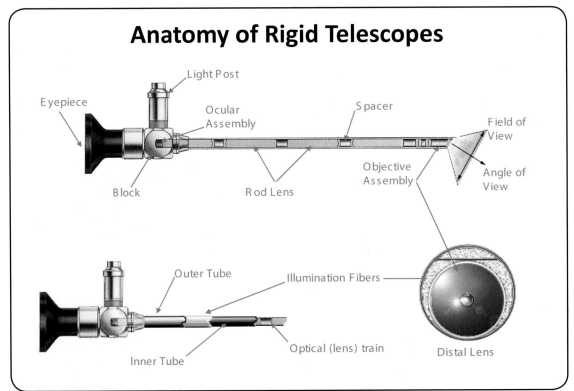

Anatomy of Rigid Telescopes

Light Post
Eyepiece
Ocular Assembly
Spacer
Field of View
Block
Rod Lens
Objective Assembly
Angle of View
Outer Tube
Illumination Fibers
Inner Tube
Optical (lens) train
Distal Lens

Figure 11.29

Specialty rigid scopes provide the ability to change the direction of view. The endoscope pictured in **Figure 11.31** allows the surgeon to change the direction of view by rotating a knob near the eyepiece.

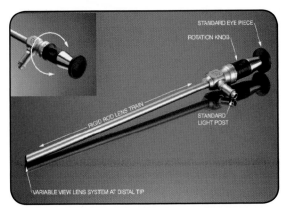

Figure 11.31 Variable Direction of View Rigid Scope

Other specialty endoscopes contain filters that help the surgeon identify diseased tissue when used in combination with pharmaceuticals and/or different spectrum light sources.

Semi-Rigid Endoscopes

Semi-rigid endoscopes are termed as such because the shaft is made of a very thin stainless steel, thus allowing it to bend slightly, without kinking the metal.

Semi-rigid endoscopes are primarily used in urology to view the bladder and the distal portion of the ureter. (See **Figure 11.32**) While they have the ability to bend slightly more than a rigid scope, they will be damaged if too much pressure is applied, or if they are bent beyond their intended limits.

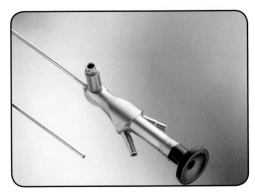

Figure 11.32

RIGID AND SEMI-RIGID ENDOSCOPE GENERAL GUIDELINES FOR DECONTAMINATION

The following are some general guidelines for cleaning rigid and semi-rigid scopes. Check with the individual scope manufacturer for specific instructions.

1. Remove the light source adaptors from the light post. (See **Figure 11.33**)

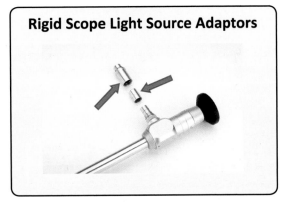

Figure 11.33

2. Use a neutral-pH enzymatic cleaning solution properly diluted per manufacturer's instructions, unless otherwise stated in the scope manufacturer's IFU.

3. Hand wash the endoscope using a soft cloth. Pay particular attention to the distal window, as this is where debris collects and is most difficult to remove.

4. If the endoscope has a working channel, thoroughly brush the channel using only the manufacturer's recommended brush size.

5. Thoroughly rinse the endoscope with treated water and flush the working channel (also with treated water) to remove all traces of enzymatic solution.

6. Dry the outside of the scope with a clean, lint-free cloth. Dry the working channel the per manufacturer's IFU.

New technology allows for the automated washing of non-operative rigid endoscopes. Check the manufacturer's IFU to verify that the tray and scope are approved for automated washing of rigid endoscopes. (See **Figure 11.34**) Automated washing provides multiple benefits:

- Consistent quality of wash.

- Reduced time spent on decontamination by staff.

- Safer devices for handling.

Note: Ultrasonic cleaning cycles must not be part of the automated washing, as damage will occur to the rigid endoscope.

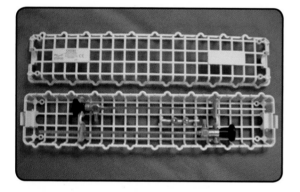

Figure 11.34 Basket and rigidscope approved for (non-sonic) automated cleaning.

RIGID ENDOSCOPIC INSTRUMENTS

Rigid endoscopic instruments come in hundreds of shapes and sizes. Many of them contain lumens that require special care to ensure that they are properly cleaned. Many instruments come with multiple parts, such as a laparoscope with a handle, working insert and outer shaft. (See **Figure 11.35**)

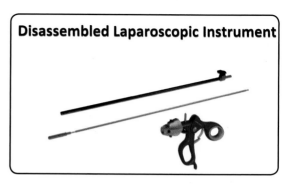

Disassembled Laparoscopic Instrument

Figure 11.35

Care and handling is often complicated due to some instrument designs. If the instrument cannot be easily disassembled into component parts, it may be virtually impossible for a technician to determine that the lumens are clean. This applies to single-piece instruments with flush ports, since the technician cannot visualize the inner lumen to verify that it is thoroughly cleaned. For instruments with flush ports, if the instrument is not flushed properly after every use, there is an opportunity for debris to remain within the lumen after cleaning.

Hidden areas and moving parts can protect soil during the cleaning process. (See **Figure 11.36**)

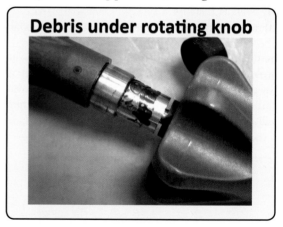

Debris under rotating knob

Figure 11.36

Complex designs, such as resectoscopes, require special attention be paid to all of the areas where debris could remain. Examples include lumens, hinges and covered spaces. (See **Figure 11.37**)

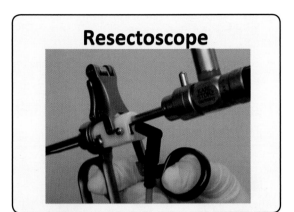

Figure 11.37

ENDOSCOPIC AND ROBOTIC INSTRUMENTATION

Operative endoscopes require special instrumentation. The following section addresses common instruments used with rigid and semi-rigid operative scopes.

Laparoscopic Instruments

Most laparoscopic instrumentation can be easily identified because they are very slender (3mm to 10mm in width) and longer than other instruments. The shafts look like the shaft of pencils or small rods, while the tips have the same design as general instruments with the same name. The distal tip of a laparoscopic Allis forceps, for example, is the same design as the distal tip of a general surgery Allis forceps. (See **Figure 11.38**)

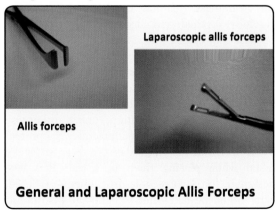

General and Laparoscopic Allis Forceps

Figure 11.38

Some endoscopic instruments are used to cut or cauterize during surgery. These instruments will have insulation covering the shaft. This covering protects the patient from electrical current that flows through the instruments.

Laparoscopic insulation is susceptible to pin holes, cracks, tears and overall loosening. These defects must be identified as the instruments are tested and assembled. Failure to discover pin holes or other damage to the insulation can result in leaked electricity that can damage nearby tissue and organs. These burns can cause infection, extended patient recovery times and other complications.

To inspect the insulation, locate the metal collar at distal tip. (See **Figure 11.39**) The insulation should fit tightly against the collar, and this union should be snug, with no spaces visible. Next, grip the insulation and try to slide it back. If the insulation slides (moves), the instrument needs repair. Finally, visually check the instrument shaft, looking for cuts, cracks and nicks to the insulation, and inspect the insulated handle for chips or cracks.

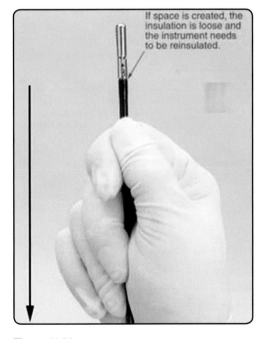

Figure 11.39

Electronic testing devices (See **Figure 11.40**) can detect microscopic holes in the shaft of a laparoscopic instrument. Electronic testing with an approved testing device should be done prior to set assembly on the clean side of the CS department.

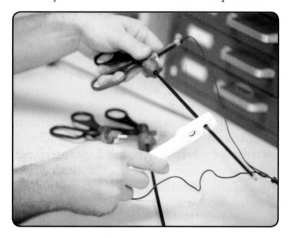

Figure 11.40

Laparoscopic hooks and spatulas are used to cut and/or cauterize. They must be inspected for insulation failure in the shaft and at the distal tip. (See **Figure 11.41**) Cannulated instruments will require a brush for proper cleaning. Always use the brush size and length recommended by the manufacturer.

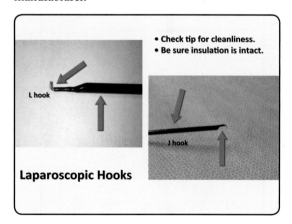

Figure 11.41

Laparoscopic ring handles are available in several styles (See **Figure 11.42**), such as:

- Free handle – No ratchet or spring finger, with an open and close action.

- Spring handle – Opens under slight tension and closes by spring action.

- Ratchet handle – Similar to hemostats with various locking points on the ratchet.

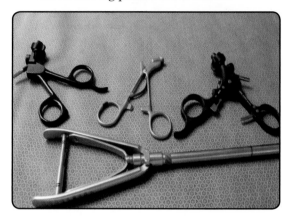

Figure 11.42

While most laparoscopic instrumentation can be mechanically cleaned, careful manual cleaning must take place first. Some laparoscopic instruments, such as scissors, use disposable tips. Disposable tips should be removed and discarded prior to instrument cleaning. Manufacturer cleaning instructions should be meticulously followed. All ports should be flushed and lumens should be brushed. Instruments that come apart should be disassembled. Due to the dark-colored surface, insulated instruments must be carefully inspected for cleanliness. Spatulas and hook tips must be carefully cleaned and inspected for cleanliness because they can be very difficult to get clean.

During assembly, multi-part instruments should be assembled to ensure they are in working condition. Multi-part items should then be disassembled for sterilization, unless otherwise stated by the instrument manufacturer. To protect these instruments from damage, care must be taken when placing them in a tray. If a tray designed for laparoscopic instruments is used, care should be taken not to bend the instrument shafts when placing or removing the instrument. Most laparoscopic instrumentation can be steam sterilized; however, refer to the manufacturer's instructions to ensure the proper method of sterilization is used.

Robotic Instruments

In the past several years, robotic surgery has become very popular in many surgical specialties. While both laparoscopic and robotic surgery use small incisions to insert instruments and perform surgery, robotic surgery allows the surgeon to be remote from the patient (either across the room or across a continent). As with laparoscopic surgery, the instruments are complex and require careful attention to ensure they are clean, sterile and functional when needed. (See **Figure 11.43**)

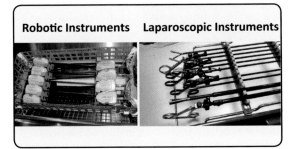

Robotic Instruments   **Laparoscopic Instruments**

Figure 11.43

Robotic instruments are heavier than laparoscopic instruments. Mechanical and electrical components are located in the proximal end of the instrument. Robotic instruments are more difficult to clean than standard laparoscopic instruments because:

- They do not come apart for cleaning.

- The distal end of the instrument rotates.

- There may be multiple channels to flush in each instrument.

Like laparoscopic instrumentation, many of the working tips of robotic instruments look like their general surgery counterparts.

Carefully follow the manufacturer's cleaning instructions. When cleaning the distal tips of the instruments, brush as stated in the IFU, rotating the distal end to ensure the tip is clean. Flush the lumens as instructed by the manufacturer. When

connecting to an irrigating sonic, ensure the sonic is approved for cleaning robotic instruments and the correct connectors are utilized. (See **Figure 11.44**)

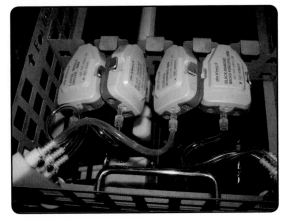

Figure 11.44

Robotic instrumentation is very delicate and complex. Careful attention to the manufacturer's IFU throughout the entire processing process is essential.

Arthroscopy Instruments

Arthroscopic surgery is a type of endoscopic procedure performed on joints. (See **Figure 11.45**)

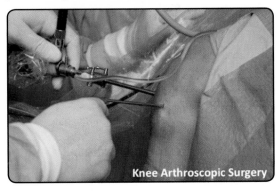

Knee Arthroscopic Surgery

Figure 11.45

Because joints are small, enclosed areas, the instruments used for arthroscopic surgery are smaller than those used on other endoscopic procedures. Unlike laparoscopic instruments, most arthroscopy instrumentation does not look similar to general surgery instrumentation. (See **Figure 11.46**)

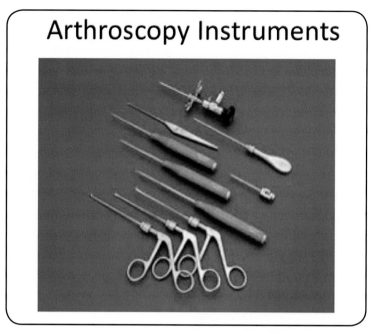

Figure 11.46

Arthroscopy shavers are complex instruments. Shavers can become clogged with debris during surgery, which can make them very difficult to clean. (See **Figure 11.47**)

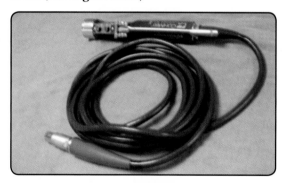

Figure 11.47

Due to the size and design of arthroscopic instrumentation, the manufacturer's IFU must be carefully followed during the entire processing cycle.

FLEXIBLE ENDOSCOPES

The term, "flexible," means capable of bending, thereby allowing the physician to gain easier access to internal body organs. Flexible endoscopes are complex instruments used to visualize inside the body, perform diagnostic tests, surgical procedures and/or to obtain tissue specimens for biopsy.

Flexible endoscopes revolutionized minimally-invasive surgical procedures because they gave surgeons access to parts of the body without performing an open procedure, thus minimizing patient discomfort and length of stay in the hospital.

Like many sophisticated medical devices, the flexible endoscope is a complex, reusable instrument that requires processing between patients.

Flexible Endoscope Components

Flexible endoscopes are comprised of a handle assembly, light source connector and a flexible shaft. The handle features control knobs that, when actuated, cause the distal end of the endoscope shaft to move. Small-diameter flexible endoscopes generally allow movement in two directions: up and down. Large-diameter flexible endoscopes allow movement in four directions: up, down, left and right. Flexible endoscopes can be classified as either fiber optic or video. The difference between the two is how the image is captured and transmitted by the endoscope.

A fiber optic flexible endoscope gathers the image via a series of lenses at the distal end of the endoscope. (See **Figure 11.49**) The image is transmitted to the eyepiece via a fiber optic bundle. Video flexible endoscopes require a power source and a video system to view the image. The image is captured and transmitted as an electrical signal to the viewing monitor.

Distal End of a Flexible Scope

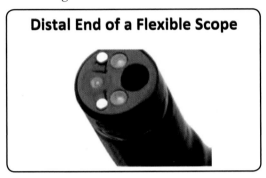

Figure 11.49

The internal components are contained and protected by an external sheath. The sheath is made of materials that can withstand exposure to bodily fluids, and they allow easy insertion and withdrawal. *Note: Care must always be taken when handling flexible endoscopes as sharp bends of the shaft or umbilical cable can cause damage.* Flexible endoscope lengths range from a typical esophagogastroduodenoscope (about 36" long) to colonoscopes (usually 60" or longer). Like rigid endoscopes, flexible endoscopes can also be described as either diagnostic or operative. Operative flexible endoscopes have a working channel that allows passage of a surgical instrument (i.e., Biopsy forceps or diagnostic brushes for scrapings). These scopes may also have channel(s) for suction, irrigation and insufflation to stretch the organ for better viewing.

Different caps are used to protect the scope from damage during various phases of reprocessing. If protective water caps are supplied, these must be in place whenever the scope is at risk of having water enter the scope. Flexible endoscopes may also come with a venting cap that opens the scope to the outside environment. The venting cap is used to allow sterilants, such as ethylene oxide (EtO), ozone or hydrogen peroxide, to enter and exit the scope channels. It is also used for shipping (particularly via air freight) to equalize pressure within and outside the scope. *Note: A venting cap must never be used when the scope will be exposed to fluids, as it will allow the fluid invasion and will likely result in damage.*

Types of Flexible Endoscopes

There are a variety of flexible endoscopes in use today.

Bronchoscope

Bronchoscopy uses a bronchoscope to directly visualize the tracheobronchial tree (bronchus) and allows:

- Diagnosis to secure uncontaminated secretion for culture, to take a biopsy, or to find the cause of a cough or hemoptysis (spitting up blood).

- Treatment to remove a foreign body, excise a small tumor, apply a medication, aspirate the bronchi or provide an airway during a tracheotomy.

Flexible intubation scopes are used to check the placement of endotracheal tubes during intubation.

Gastroscope/Esophoscope

Gastroscopy uses a gastroscope to visually inspect the upper digestive tract (including esophagus, stomach and duodenum), with aspiration of contents and biopsy, if necessary. Esophagoscopy is the direct visualization of the esophagus using a grastroscope.

Colonoscope/Sigmoidoscope

Colonoscopy involves the visual inspection of the entire large intestine with a colonoscope.

Sigmoidoscopy involves the visual inspection of the lower part of the large intestine with a sigmoidoscope.

These are important diagnostic tools, and may be used for biopsy and removal of polyps and to control bleeding ulcers.

Cystoscope/Ureteroscope

A flexible cystoscope is used to visualize the urethra and bladder. Ureteroscopes are used to visualize the ureter and kidney. It is passed through the urethra and bladder to the ureter/kidney to look for obstructions, such as strictures or kidney stones and tumors.

Rhino-Laryngoscopes

Rhino-laryngoscopes are used to visualize and perform procedures within the nose, sinus cavity or upper gastrointestinal (GI) tract.

CLEANING AND PROCESSING FLEXIBLE ENDOSCOPES

Manufacturer IFU, Centers for Disease Control and Prevention (CDC) guidelines, Society of Gastroenterology Nurses and Associates Inc. (SGNA) guidelines (for GI endoscopes) Association for the Advancement of Medical Instrumentation (AAMI) ST91 and hospital protocols must be followed regarding the care, handling and processing of all endoscopes and accessory devices.

Technicians who process endoscopes should also follow standard precautions. They must wear personal protective equipment (PPE), including gloves, gown, face masks and shields (or goggles), and shoe and hair coverings. (See **Figure 11.50)**

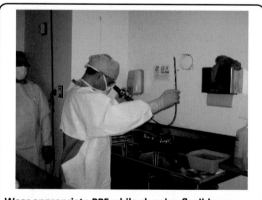

Wear appropriate PPE while cleaning flexible scopes.

Figure 11.50

Endoscopes should be processed in an area large enough to allow for the safe handling of the instruments.

Be sure to follow the scope manufacturer's IFU to ensure that only approved cleaning chemicals are used. Cleaning should be performed with soft, lint-free cloths or sponges and brushes specifically designed for use with the endoscope. Effective cleaning reduces disinfection failures by reducing the presence of organic soil that harbors microorganisms and prevents the penetration of germicides.

When selecting endoscope processing chemicals, one should consider whether:

- The chemical is approved by the specific scope manufacturer.

- The chemical is effective for the intended purpose.

Not All Scopes Are Alike

Due to the significant difference in the processes required for video and non-video flexible endoscopes, it is important to follow the manufacturer's IFU for the model and brand of flexible endoscopes being cleaned. Refer to each manufacturer's scope brand and model IFU.

Basic steps required to reprocess flexible endoscopes

1. Precleaning

2. Leak testing

3. Cleaning

4. High-level disinfecting (HLD)/sterilizing

5. Drying

6. Storing

Precleaning

Precleaning is the removal of gross debris from the endoscope's external surfaces and internal channels. Cleaning begins at the point of use to prevent blood or protein material, including patient debris, from drying on the instrument. Suction channels should be rinsed with clean water to remove as much blood and tissue debris as possible.

The insertion tube or shaft should be wiped with an enzymatic detergent solution approved by the endoscope manufacturer.

Leak Testing

The majority of flexible endoscopes require a leak test be performed prior to submerging the device during cleaning, and prior to HLD or sterilization. A leak test is necessary to ensure that the endoscope is watertight. A leaking endoscope should not be used on any patient, as the endoscope cannot be properly disinfected or sterilized. Depending upon the manufacturer's IFU, leak testing may involve dry leak testing or leak testing the endoscope while it is under water. In either case, the endoscope is pressurized via a hand pump or automated system. Damage from use, incorrect care and handling practices, or improper chemical exposure can lead to leaks in the covering or seals. Leak testing is, therefore, required before further cleaning can occur. It is necessary to consult the manufacturer's instructions for the proper leak testing procedures for the specific endoscope. *Note: Most scope manufacturers require the use of specific leak testers. Ensure the test is performed using the correct tool.*

Dry Leak Testing

Some manufacturers recommend only a dry leak test be performed. To perform this test:

- Attach the leak tester and pressurize the scope. Do not place the scope in water. (See **Figure 11.51**)

- Follow the IFU for pressure testing the endoscope to the prescribed pressure, then manipulate the movable parts of the endoscope by holding the parts in each direction for a minimum of 15 seconds. Watch the leak tester gauge; if the pressure drops, the scope has a leak and should be sent for repair.

Wet Leak Testing

Some manufacturers recommend a wet leak test. To perform this test:

- First, pressurize the scope and check the distal end by submerging only the distal end of the insertion tube into water. The water bath should be clear water (with no chemicals), so air bubbles will be easily seen.

- Rotate the distal end of the endoscope. If no bubbles are observed exiting the bending section then the endoscope is totally submerged.

- After submerging the scope, use a syringe to flush water through all channels to remove any air that remains trapped within the channel; observe the exit area to see if air bubbles appear. (See **Figure 11.52**) Because air rises in water, bubbles can be trapped within the channel and may not emerge unless water is used to flush it out. If air bubbles are observed exiting the endoscope after previously flushing all air out of the channel, a leak has occurred. *Note: The most common areas for leaks is the bending rubber at the distal tip of the insertion tube [from within the working channel(s) or at the control knobs].* **Figure 11.53** shows leak damage to a scope.

- Remove the endoscope from the water and drain. Release pressure. Verify deflation of the endoscope.

- Disconnect the leak tester from the endoscope. *Note: Never disconnect the leak tester while it is submerged; water could enter the leak tester connector, and invade the endoscope's interior.*

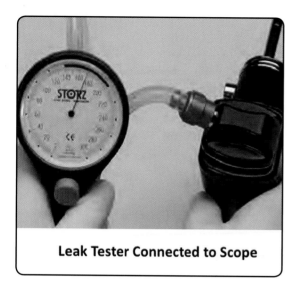

Leak Tester Connected to Scope

Figure 11.51

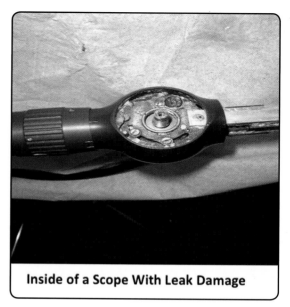

Inside of a Scope With Leak Damage

Figure 11.53

If the endoscope passed the leak test, it is watertight and reprocessing may proceed.

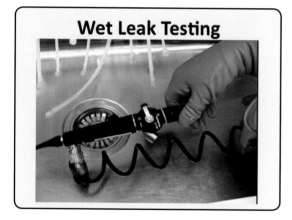

Figure 11.52

Any endoscope that fails a leak test should be immediately shipped to the manufacturer or an authorized repair company for repair. The Occupational Safety and Health Administration (OSHA) requires that medical equipment be decontaminated to the maximum extent possible before transport.

Cleaning Steps for Flexible Endoscopes

The following are general recommendations for cleaning a flexible endoscope. Always consult the scope manufacturer's IFU for specific cleaning information.

1. Thoroughly rinse the endoscope with water to remove all gross debris.

    Detach all removable parts (valves) and completely immerse the endoscope and valves in a mild/neutral-pH enzymatic cleaning solution. (See **Figure 11.54**)

2. Using a syringe or the manufacturer's supplied irrigation tubes and fill channels with cleaning solution.

3. Keep the scope immersed for the time recommended by the manufacturer.

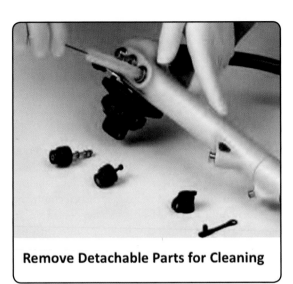

Remove Detachable Parts for Cleaning

Figure 11.54

4. While immersed, use a soft, lint-free cloth or sponge to wipe the exterior of the endoscope. Use a soft-bristle brush to clean the valves and any crevices of the videoscope. Be sure to use the correct size brush for the lumen's opening.

5. Insert a long, flexible brush into the channel at the proximal end of the endoscope. Be sure the brush is the correct diameter to clean the channel, and the correct length to reach the entire length of the channel(s). (See **Figure 11.55**)

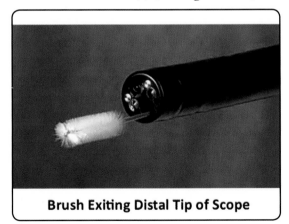

Brush Exiting Distal Tip of Scope

Figure 11.55

6. Carefully push the brush through until the brush exits the distal end. Rinse the bristle of the brush to remove debris and fully pull the brush back through the channel. (See **Figure 11.56**)

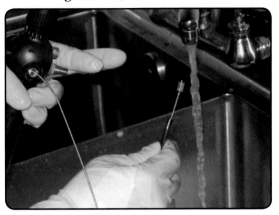

Figure 11.56

7. Rinse the brush again and repeat until the brush remains clean after passing through the channel. Consult the IFU for any special brushing instructions.

8. After the immersion period, remove the endoscope and valves from the cleaning solution and completely immerse them in treated water (water that has been processed to reduce impurities). Be sure to flush all the channels with water to remove the cleaning solution. Discard the water and repeat with fresh water, as recommended by the device manufacturer.

Scopes must be dried thoroughly to prevent the growth of microorganisms. External components can be dried with a soft, lint-free cloth. Internal channels are often dried with an alcohol flush or particle-free, low-pressure (less than five psi) compressed air. Consult the device IFU for specific internal drying instructions.

Quality Programs for Monitoring the Flexible Endoscope Cleaning Process

There is growing concern about the effectiveness of decontamination techniques for flexible endoscopes. Residual organic debris on processed scopes is a concern, and visual inspection is not 100% accurate. Scopes with lumens or channels pose one of the most difficult challenges in cleaning and inspection.

Testing any channel/lumen instrument, especially flexible endoscopes, is important because one cannot see down the channel/lumen.

AAMI TIR 12: 2010, Designing, Testing and Labeling Reusable Medical Devices for Reprocessing in Health Care Facilities: A Guide for Medical Device Manufacturers, recommends that users be able to test and verify their cleaning process.

Cleaning verification of flexible endoscopes should include:

- Visually inspecting both external surfaces and inner housing/channels of the flexible endoscope.

- Testing the cleaning efficacy of mechanical equipment, if used.

- Monitoring key cleaning parameters (e.g., temperature and dilution of chemicals) of both the manual and automatic cleaning process.

- Monitoring the results.

Published studies support testing flexible endoscopes for cleaning effectiveness. Users now have available various technologies that allow the inside of flexible endoscopes to be tested for organic soil residue or microbial contamination. Testing internal and external cleaning effectiveness on a routine basis will help ensure scopes are properly cleaned prior to disinfection or sterilization.

High-Level Disinfection

The minimum recommended practice for endoscope disinfection is HLD with an approved disinfectant.

High-Level Disinfection or Sterilization?

The decision to sterilize or high-level disinfect a surgical device is based upon its use according to the Spaulding Classification System.

To achieve adequate HLD, all internal and external surfaces must be in contact with the disinfectant, according to the disinfectant manufacturer's labeling instructions. Prior to selecting a disinfectant, the scope manufacturer's IFU must be consulted to ensure that the disinfectant is compatible with the instrument. In addition, if an automatic endoscope reprocessor (AER) is used, that manufacturer's IFU must also be consulted.

Several HLD solutions, including glutaraldehyde, ortho-phthalaldehyde (OPA), and peracetic acid solutions, are approved for endoscope disinfection. Testing of the dilution of each of these chemicals is required prior to each use. Ensure that the monitoring processes and strips are correct for the brand and concentration of disinfectant selected.

What about Other Disinfectants?

Some disinfecting agents are not recommended for use on endoscopes and endoscopic equipment. Reasons include incomplete antimicrobial coverage (failure to meet the definition of a high-level disinfectant), toxic exposure to personnel, or physical damage to equipment.

The disinfection process used (manual or automatic) is selected based on the type of scope and equipment available.

Manual Disinfection

Many departments do not have automated equipment readily available to high-level disinfect flexible endoscopes.

General Guidelines For Manual High-Level Disinfection

1. Prepare the disinfectant solution for use, per the manufacturer's IFU.

2. Place the clean scope into the appropriate container containing the HLD solution. Ensure that the scope is fully immersed and remove any air bubbles adhering to the surface of the scope.

3. Use a syringe, the cleaning adaptors, or the supplied irrigation tubes to fill all channels (including air, water, suction/biopsy, elevator and auxiliary water) with disinfectant solution until no bubbles are seen exiting the channels.

4. Place all valves and removable parts in the disinfectant.

5. Set the timer for the correct exposure time.

6. After disinfection is complete, remove the endoscope, valves and removable parts from the disinfectant solution, and rinse the instruments by completely immersing them in treated water. Flush lumens carefully according to the device manufacturer's IFU.

7. Dry the endoscope according to the device IFU.

8. Document all processing information, as discussed in Chapter 9.

9. Label the scope with the date processed or date to process, depending on the facility's scope storage policy. (See **Figure 11.57**)

General Guideline for Automatic Endoscope Reprocessors

AER are machines that clean, disinfect and rinse flexible endoscopes. (See **Figure 11.58**) Their design permits the exterior of the scope and all lumens to be exposed to cleaning, disinfecting and rinsing solutions. To facilitate the flushing of the lumens, specific tubing connections must be connected. Endoscopes are then are placed in the AER after initial cleaning and brushing. The labels of some disinfectants require elevating their temperature above room temperature to achieve HLD. Most AER feature a heater that conveniently and rapidly elevates the temperature to a pre-determined setting. Because they are typically enclosed systems, most AER limit staff exposure to liquid chemical disinfectants and their vapors.

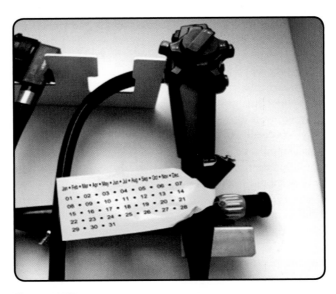

Figure 11.57

When Can An Automatic Endoscope Reprocessor Be Used?

Not all endoscopes and their accessories can be reliably processed in an AER. If not specifically indicated in the AER labeling, ask the scope manufacturer whether the endoscope being used has been tested in the AER.

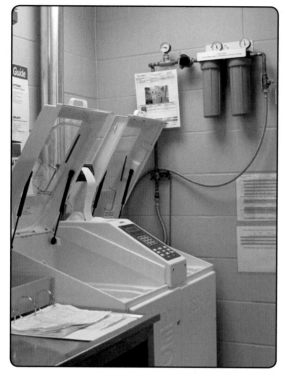

Figure 11.58

Storing

Storage is the final step in flexible endoscope processing. If flexible endoscopes are not stored properly, bacteria could grow, even though the endoscope has previously received HLD or sterilization. Dry endoscopes should be stored in a manner to prevent recontamination or damage from sharp, jagged edges. They should be stored:

- With the insertion tube hanging vertically (not coiled). (See **Figure 11.59**)

- With the weight of the control body supported, and angulation locks off.

- In a dry, dust-free cabinet with good ventilation.

- Without removable parts, such as control valves, distal hoods and caps, in place, to reduce the risk of trapping moisture inside the instrument. These items should be stored with the scope. The water-resistant cap should be removed from the video scopes while they are in storage.

- If multiple scopes are stored in the same cabinet, they should not touch other scopes.

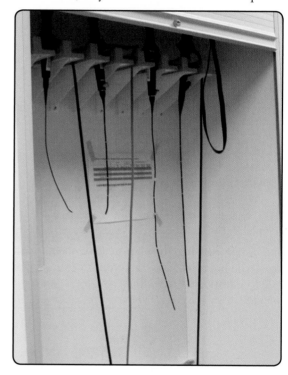

Figure 11.59

Scope Transport

Flexible endoscopes must always be carefully transported because they can be easily broken. If not properly contained, they can become damaged when struck against walls, doorways, carts and other fixtures. To prevent this, endoscopes should always be transported loosely coiled and with their distal tip protected.

Sterilization of Flexible Endoscopes

Package and sterilize the endoscope following the manufacturer's IFU. Some flexible scopes sterilized using low-temperature sterilants may require a venting cap during sterilization. (See **Figure 11.60**)

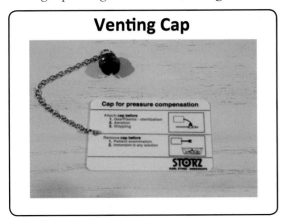

Venting Cap

Figure 11.60

Carrying Cases

The carrying case used to transport endoscopes outside the healthcare environment should not be used to store an endoscope or transport the instrument within the facility. Contaminated endoscopes should be bagged prior to placing them in the carrying case because the case can also become contaminated. A contaminated case could recontaminate endoscopes since the inside of the case has not been decontaminated. Most cases are lined with foam that cannot be properly cleaned and disinfected.

FLEXIBLE ENDOSCOPE ACCESSORIES

With the exception of the water bottle, endoscope accessories consist of two types: diagnostic and therapeutic. Depending upon the type of procedure, various and different diagnostic and/or therapeutic accessories are used with the endoscope.

Water Bottle Precautions

The water in an endoscope's water bottle (See **Figure 11.61**) is sprayed through the water channel to the patient's internal organs. For this reason, the bottle must be cared for properly. The water bottle should be sterilized at least once a day (ideally, after each use). Only sterile water should be used to fill it,

and water should never be stored in the water bottle overnight. Clean and sterilize the water bottle per the manufacturer's IFU.

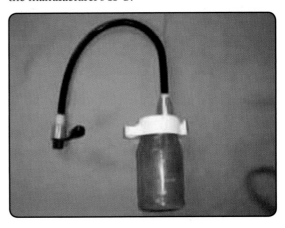

Figure 11.61

Flexible Endoscope Instruments

All reusable flexible endoscope instruments should be carefully cleaned following the manufacturer's IFU. These items usually come in contact with sterile membranes; therefore, they must be sterilized prior to use.

The following are examples of flexible endoscope instruments:

Biopsy forceps. Two distally-located cups or jaws that open or close when a control located at the proximal end is manipulated. Jaws can have smooth or serrated edges. When the edges are open, they expose a sharp spike that grasps the tissue. The tissue is seized between the jaws when they close to prevent tissue slippage. (See **Figure 11.62**)

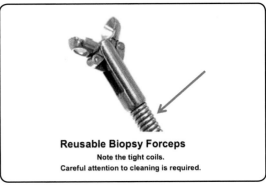

Reusable Biopsy Forceps
Note the tight coils.
Careful attention to cleaning is required.

Figure 11.62

Brush for cytology. A plastic tube that encloses a wire and contains a short brush at its distal end. The brush is inserted through the endoscope's biopsy channel.

Cannulas for opacification. These small plastic (silicone) catheter-type devices have markings for visualization, located at the tip.

Measuring device. This flexible, rod-like accessory is marked at its distal end with a series of spaced bands.

Electro-coagulating ("hot biopsy") forceps. Similar to a biopsy forceps, but has a mechanism to direct electrosurgical current to lesions, so small polyps can be transected and cauterized to prevent bleeding.

Polypectomy snares. Consists of a pre-formed, oval or hexagonal wire loop (when opened) inside a plastic tubular sheath. The loop can be rotatable or nonrotatable, and is manipulated over the polyp and closed around its base like a noose. Electrosurgical current then burns the polyp free.

Polyp retriever. Features finger-like metal prongs inside a tubular plastic sheath. The prongs spread apart spontaneously when they are extruded from the sheath's distal end. The polyp retriever grasps tissue specimens for retrieval after they have been transected or cut free.

Foreign body forceps. Secures and extracts foreign bodies from the respiratory or digestive tracts. It is a modified version of biopsy forceps; the jaws are spoon, claw or serrated.

Stone management instruments. Used for the retrieval of stones from glands (such as salivary), and for retrieval from organs, such as the kidney or ureter. (see **Figure 11.63**)

Electrodes for electrocoagulation. A ball-tipped electrode is located at the distal end of a plastic cannula and is used for electrocoagulation of bleeding points and electrodesiccation of polypoid growths.

Injection needle. Used to inject sclerosis of esophageal varices (stretched veins), and for injection of marking dyes in the layer of loose connective tissue under a mucous membrane to designate the site from which a suspicious lesion was removed. It is a small (25-gauge), specially designed and retractable injection needle attached to flexible tubing.

Laser probe. Made of specially-constructed fiber optic quartz glass bundles, which transmit a laser beam that is passed through an endoscope. When connected to a laser unit, these fiber optic bundles help control bleeding from gastrointestinal lesions and can be used for stone vaporization.

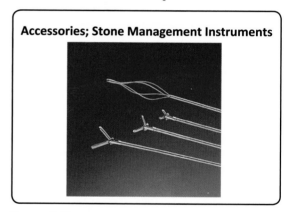

Accessories; Stone Management Instruments

Figure 11.63

FLEXIBLE ENDOSCOPE REGULATIONS AND GUIDELINES

Federal regulations enable endoscope users to maximize safe care for the patient, while also protecting the equipment, users and the environment. In addition to federal laws, state and local governments may have stringent requirements. The following government agencies have rules or laws that impact the use of flexible endoscopes, and their requirements must be reflected in policy development and practice:

- OSHA: Provides broad guidelines and specific requirements to protect employees from workplace infections. www.osha.gov

- Department of Transportation (DOT): Ensures a safe, efficient, accessible and convenient transportation system. Its laws include those relating to the transport of biohazardous materials, such as minimally-processed endoscopes in need of repair. www.dot.gov

- CDC: Publishes disinfection and sterilization guidelines. www.cdc.gov

- U.S. Food and Drug Administration (FDA): Regulates and monitors multiple standards regarding IFU, disinfectants, sterilants and the manufacture of medical devices. www.fda.gov

- U.S. Environmental Protection Agency (EPA): Has issued regulations applicable to endoscope processing. www.epa.gov

- Numerous professional organizations have also developed professional guidelines and standards that impact endoscopy and endoscope processing. The Association for the Advancement of Medical Instrumentation (AAMI; www.aami.org); the Society of Gastroenterology Nurses & Associates Inc. (SGNA; www.sgna.org); the Association for Professionals in Infection Control and Epidemiology (APIC; www.apic.org); the Association of periOperative Registered Nurses (AORN; www.aorn.org); and others have written standards or guidelines for the safe use, reprocessing and care of endoscopes. (See **Figure 11.64**)

ENDOSCOPE-RELATED INFECTION PREVENTION

Effective infection prevention policies and practices are critical for minimizing or eliminating endoscope-related cross contamination. The flexible endoscope is particularly challenging for infection control. Its long, dark and narrow lumens

Sources for Endoscope Guidelines

Association	General Topic
The Society of Gastroenterology Nurses and Associates (SGNA) - (www.sgna.org).	• Guidelines for use of high-level disinfectants and sterilants • Safe and effective handling of glutaraldehyde solutions • Reprocessing flexible gastrointestinal endoscopes
The American Society of Gastrointestinal Endoscopy (ASGE) (www.asge.org).	• Infection control during gastrointestinal endoscopy. • Reprocessing of flexible gastrointestinal endoscopes.
The Association of Professionals in Infection Control and Epidemiology (APIC) (www.apic.org).	• Guidelines for infection prevention and control in flexible endoscopy.
The Association of PeriOperative Registered Nurses (AORN) (www.aorn.org)	• Guidelines for cleaning and processing of flexible endoscopes and accessories.
Association for the Advancement of Medical Instrumentation (AAMI) (www.aami.org)	• Guidelines for chemical disinfection. • ST91: Comprehensive guide to flexible and semi-rigid endoscope processing in health care facilities
American Society for Testing and Materials (ASTM) (www.astm.org)	• Standard practice for effectiveness of cleaning processes for reusable endoscopes

Figure 11.64

pose a fundamental processing concern because they are not directly accessible and are extremely difficult to clean. In addition, if channels are not thoroughly dried after processing and are stored wet, they become a dark and damp environment that is suitable for bacterial growth. Most flexible endoscopes cannot be sterilized by high-temperature, and are functionally and cosmetically sensitive to the chemicals needed for cleaning, disinfecting and/or sterilizing.

Other issues that can negatively impact infection prevention efforts include:

- Failure to leak test or to test correctly. An unidentified hole in the endoscope permits contaminants to grow exponentially with each use, and cleaning chemicals can damage internal components.

- Poor manual cleaning that does not effectively remove bioburden from the endoscope. This reduces the effectiveness of disinfection or sterilization chemicals.

- Failure to follow the original equipment manufacturer's instructions.

- Failure to follow directions on the labels of processing chemicals.

- Failure to use the proper brush size.

- Failure to adequately flush all channels with disinfectant solution.

- Failure to fully immerse the scope in the approved disinfectant.

- Failure to adequately time the length of disinfectant contact.

- Use of disinfectant solutions after their expiration date.

- Failure to sterilize scope instruments.

- Improper scope repair.

- Variations in staff training.

- Improper processing of reusable cleaning accessories.

- Improper storage and transport.

- Processing endoscopes more quickly than is prudent in order to perform more procedures.

- Processing scopes in inadequate space.

- Poor water quality.

- Improper drying and/or storage.

FLEXIBLE AND RIGID ENDOSCOPE CARE AND HANDLING

Due to their sophisticated and complex design, endoscopes are costly devices. On average, a rigid rod-lens endoscope will have a list price from $3,000 to $6,000.

Flexible fiber optic endoscopes have a list price between $8,000 and $25,000, and a flexible video scope can have a price ranging from $12,000 to over $100,000 for some of the advanced video scopes that contain microscopes and ultrasound units. In particular, the cost of repair and replacement of endoscopes is a major expense item, costing many large hospitals over approximately $750,000 or more per year. An average community hospital will spend over $200,000 per year on endoscope repair. It is estimated that 60-75% of scope damage is caused by improper care and handling practices; therefore, the majority of this expense is preventable.

Device damage not only impacts the healthcare organization's bottom line, it also increases stress levels and user frustration as these damaged items are often discovered during use. Damaged equipment delays cases and potentially exposes patients to longer anesthesia times, missed diagnoses and potential harm.

For these reasons, good care and handling practices for endoscopes, endoscope accessories and instruments must be used at all times by all staff members.

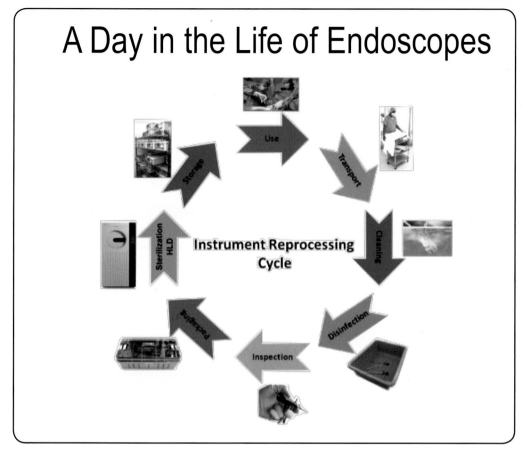

A Day in the Life of Endoscopes

Instrument Reprocessing Cycle

Use • *Transport* • *Cleaning* • *Disinfection* • *Inspection* • *Packaging* • *Sterilization HLD* • *Storage*

Figure 11.65

Endoscope Daily Use Cycle

Care and handling for endoscopes can be examined in each of the various stages of their daily cycle: (See **Figure 11.65**)

- Storage

- Transport

- Use in procedures

- Decontamination

- Preparation and packaging (prep and pack)

- Disinfection or sterilization

Storage

Storage should be broadly considered as any location of an endoscope when it is not in use. By this definition, lying on the back table in the Operating Room (OR) or hanging on the side of a video cart are all forms of storage. Viewing storage in this way enables one to see that storage is much more than just the container or cabinet that houses the endoscope.

If endoscope containers or trays are used, they must be of appropriate size to ensure that the endoscope is fully and properly encased. (See **Figure 11.66**) Bending or kinking a flexible scope can cause damage to the device.

If a tray is used, it should be protective and secure the endoscope so damage will not occur if the tray is tipped or dropped.

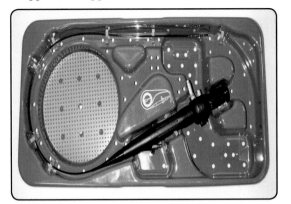

Figure 11.66

Flexible and rigid scopes should not be left in basins because the basin will not protect the scope. If left in a basin, flexible scopes will be too tightly coiled, which could result in potential damage; rigid scopes may fall out of the basin. (See **Figure 11.67**)

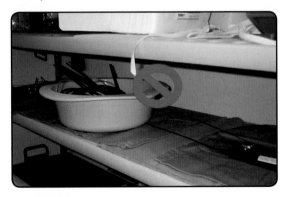

Figure 11.67

Transport

Transporting should be broadly defined as any time the endoscope is moved. By this definition, carrying either by hand, within a tray, or in/on a cart are all forms of transport. In each transport situation, the endoscope must be secured and protected. (See **Figure 11.68**) When carrying by hand, rigid endoscopes should be held by the housing body and not the shaft. Flexible endoscopes should be carried by the handle, while holding onto the distal end of the shaft and umbilical cable (if

present). Endoscopes, even in trays, should not be transported unless safely secured. This will help ensure that they will not fall and become damaged. (See **Figure 11.69**)

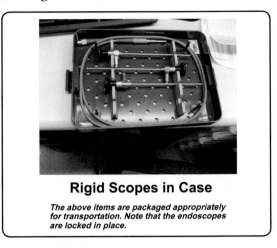

Rigid Scopes in Case

The above items are packaged appropriately for transportation. Note that the endoscopes are locked in place.

Figure 11.68

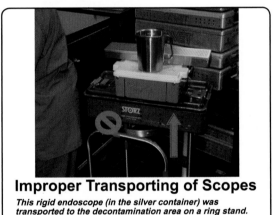

Improper Transporting of Scopes

This rigid endoscope (in the silver container) was transported to the decontamination area on a ring stand. This stand was later moved and the rigid endoscope tray fell, damaging the endoscope.

Figure 11.69

Procedural Use

An estimated 50% of damage to endoscopes and their accessories occurs during procedures. This can be caused by allowing the endoscope to come in contact with something that can cut, burn or otherwise damage the endoscope. Dropping accessory devices, using excessive force during the procedure and improperly storing endoscopes can also result in damage.

Other examples of damage caused by improper use include:

- Cuts in a flexible endoscope shaft caused by placing sharp objects on it.

- Damage caused by shaver blades contacting a rigid endoscope during arthroscopy.

- Laser damage.

- Scopes being dropped.

- Inserting the endoscope through a sheath or bridge where the sheath or bridge are bent, thus bending the endoscope as it passes.

- Inserting an instrument improperly through a working channel.

- Excessive force used by the physician, which can lead to excessive bending.

- Stacking instruments or other scopes on top of scopes. (See **Figure 11.70**)

- Allowing gross soil to dry on the scopes.

- Not securing the scopes prior to transporting.

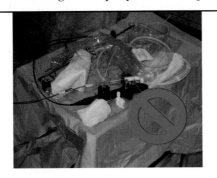

Items Stacked on Scopes
This practice can cause scope damage.

Figure 11.70

Decontamination

Decontamination should begin in the OR/procedure room, with the department staff wiping

off gross contamination and applying enzymatic spray to prevent drying. As directed by the manufacturer, suction channels should be cleared of gross debris by suctioning water or enzymatic solution through the channel. Prompt transport to the decontamination area is very important to prevent soils from drying on the endoscopes, instruments and accessories.

A significant amount of damage occurs to endoscopes in the decontamination area. Reasons may include:

- Improper placement of items in transport containers. (See **Figure 11.71**)

- Improper handling.

- Improper use of cleaning accessories, such as brushes and forced air.

- Improper chemical use.

- Failure to protect instruments and devices from damage.

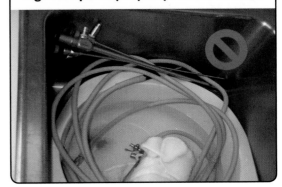

Rigid Scope Improperly Placed in Basin

Figure 11.71

Preparation and Packaging

During the preparation and packaging process, the endoscope and accessories are examined and packaged properly for sterilization.

The inspection process is very important to ensure the proper function of the endoscope. The technician must understand the proper procedures for inspection, and the manufacturer's IFU should be followed. The following are basic guidelines for addressing scope inspection:

- Closely inspect for damage and cleanliness.

- Functions such as light output, image quality and angulations should be examined, if applicable or possible.

- For rigid endoscopes used with bridges/sheaths, fit should be checked to ensure that the two devices go together with little to no force being applied.

- For all endoscopes, the distal and proximal windows should be inspected for cleanliness, and wiped off with 70% isopropyl alcohol and a soft cloth, if necessary.

- For non-video rigid scopes, the image quality should be tested by viewing typewritten print through the scope from a distance of about one inch. (See **Figure 11.73**) The image should be closely examined in the center and for 360 degrees around the outside edge to ensure that there are no blurry or dark areas. *Note: Most flexible fiber optic endoscopes have a focus adjusting mechanism near the eyepiece.*

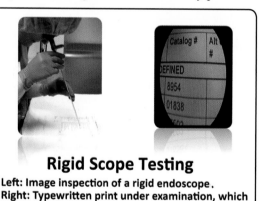

Rigid Scope Testing
Left: Image inspection of a rigid endoscope.
Right: Typewritten print under examination, which should be round, bright and clear.

Figure 11.73

Looking through an endoscope while viewing objects across the room is not an appropriate way to inspect image quality. Distance, color and patterns can obscure imperfections in the image.

- For non-video rigid endoscopes, the light fibers should be checked by pointing the distal end of the endoscope toward a light source and inspecting the light fibers to ensure that the color is white and that there are no (or minimal) broken light fibers.

Prep and pack is complete when the inspected endoscope is securely placed in the tray and properly prepared for sterilization.

Sterilization

Due to the variations in sterilization requirements for endoscopes, it is recommend that the manufacturer's IFU be carefully followed.

ENDOSCOPE CAMERA CARE AND HANDLING

Endoscope cameras are complex devices that typically range from \$5,000 to over \$25,000 each. **Figure 11.79** shows one type of endoscopic camera. An average repair cost is \$3,500 and camera damage resulting in major repairs can cost over \$9,000. The most common damage to cameras includes:

- Cuts in the cable.

- Cable/button damage due to improper chemical exposure.

- Damage to the coupler due to dropping or misuse.

Major damage occurs when components within the camera are affected, such as the imaging chip and/or circuitry boards. Dropping the camera can shift the prism or sensors. Fluid invasion through a button, cable or breach in the housing will also cause significant damage.

Endoscopic Camera

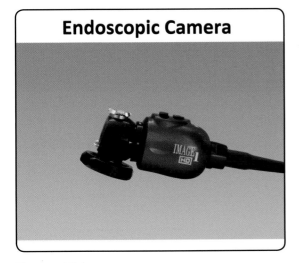

Figure 11.74

Camera Cleaning

The manufacturer's IFU should be followed to help ensure proper care and handling of the camera, including cleaning. The use of improper chemicals is a major contributor to premature failure of external components. In general, cameras should be precleaned in the operating/procedure room to remove gross debris and then transported to the decontamination area as quickly as possible to prevent drying of debris. An inspection of the camera should be performed, closely examining the camera cable for any cuts, nicks or other damage. *Note: Any damaged camera, including those with holes in the cable, must be sent for repair and should not be used in any procedure.*

Cleaning is performed using a soft cloth and a neutral pH enzymatic solution. Particular attention must be paid to the camera window. This window must be perfectly clean. If the camera has a water cap for the cable, this must be applied prior to submerging the camera. Disinfection and/or sterilization processes must be performed according to the manufacturer's IFU.

Camera Inspection

Inspection of the camera consists of checking the camera coupler by inserting a rigid endoscope onto a coupler. Most couplers open by turning in a counter-clockwise direction, and close by turning in a clockwise direction. The coupler tightens on the endoscope eyepiece, and should hold the endoscope so that the endoscope does not rotate within the coupler. If the endoscope rotates, try to tighten the coupler again. If the endoscope continues to rotate, the camera should be sent for repair. The cable and buttons should be inspected for any signs of cuts or other damage. Electrical connections should be inspected for any signs of damage or corrosion.

Image quality cannot be checked without the use of a complete video system and an endoscope.

ENDOSCOPE REPAIR

The best way to control repair costs of endoscopes and endoscope accessories is to manage and monitor care and handling practices to reduce damage.

When repairs are needed for any scope or accessory instrument, only qualified repair sources should be used.

Before any repaired or exchanged endoscope is placed back into service, a qualified staff member should inspect, clean and disinfect (or sterilize) the device prior to use.

STAFF EDUCATION

CS technicians working with complex medical instrumentation, such as endoscopes, must be thoroughly trained in proper processing protocols. Competency should be reviewed annually using a competency checklist. See the sample checklist illustrated in **Figure 11.75**.

Department-wide education is key to effective infection prevention in endoscopy and should be updated with any adopted change to chemicals or processes.

Sample Competency Checklist

Level:
0 - Cannot perform skill independently
1 - Requires assistance to perform skill
2 - Performs skill independently
N/A - Not Applicable

Method:
D - Demonstration
V - Verbal

Skill	Level/Method
Transports items according to departmental procedure	
Organizes and prioritizes work load appropriately	
Performs leak testing according to manufacturer's IFU	
Knows what product to use on each item for cleaning and disinfecting	
Understands the purpose of using alcohol to facilitate drying	
Knows how to and what to check for after cleaning the scope	
Knows how to and what to check for after cleaning the camera	
Knows how to and what to check for after cleaning the light cord	
Understands and can identify the different sizes and degree angles in scopes	
Can identify the different cameras	
Performs appropriate inspection and testing, according to manufacturer's IFU	
Knows how to correctly package all items for sterilization	
Handles all items with appropriate care	
Is familiar with and follows manufacturer instructions for handling and processing	

Figure 11.75

Other Specialty Instruments Create Processing Challenges

Each specialty service within the Operating Room and other areas within the facility and associated clinics typically have instrumentation that requires special care and handling. Examples include:

- Neurology – Stereotactic biopsy systems, aneurysm clip systems and testing electrodes
- Cardiology – Cardiac endoscopes
- Electro Physiology – Cables and cords

Each instrument must also be processed following the manufacturer's recommendations.

LOANER INSTRUMENTATION

Loaner instrumentation gets its name because the instrumentation is loaned from a vendor for a special case or procedure. Loaner instrumentation comes in many sizes and variations, and represents different challenges pertaining to ordering, receiving, decontamination, assembly, sterilization, storage and return of the borrowed items. Loaner instrumentation, once primarily used in orthopedic and neuro-surgical specialties, is now used in almost all surgical and procedural specialties. Facilities borrow instrumentation from manufacturers and distributing vendors because:

- The technology behind the instruments may change rapidly, causing instruments to be outdated rapidly.

- The cost of the instrumentation to perform relatively few procedures is prohibitive.

- More specialty cases are being performed than what the facility's instrument inventory can support.

- A physician or surgical specialty wants to trial the new instrument(s) or technology.

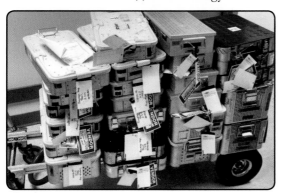

Figure 11.76

Loaner instrumentation may be received as one instrument or as numerous trays for a specific procedure. (See **Figure 11.76**) Each instrument requires special attention during processing. As the concept of borrowing instruments continues to grow, departments may receive several hundred trays in one day. Many of these instruments require special disassembly, cleaning and assembly protocols

making them a challenge in most CS departments. It is important to have these loaned instruments delivered with enough time to properly process them for the scheduled procedures. After the procedure, enough time should be allowed to properly clean and disinfect these instruments prior to returning them to the loaning vendor.

> **Loaner instrumentation** Instruments or sets borrowed from a vendor for emergency or scheduled surgical procedures that will be returned to the vendor following use.

Loaner Receipt and Inventory Procedures

Loaner instruments may be received at the facility in several different ways. Company representatives may personally deliver the instruments, or they may also arrive by next day carriers, U.S. mail and local courier services. This makes managing the process difficult. Policies and procedures need to be in place so standard practices are followed when receiving, handling and returning these expensive instruments.

The CS technician should log receipt of loaner instrumentation and implants with information including:

- Date

- Time

- Signature of delivery person

- Initials of receiving person

- Surgeon's name

- Patient's name or identifier

- Number of trays

- Number of implants

As soon as possible after receipt, loaner instruments should be inspected. This process should be done with the vendor representative, whenever possible.

The following steps should be taken when loaner instruments are received:

- Check each instrument to ensure proper function.

- Verify that the manufacturer's IFU are received (and up to date), and kept in the department's files.

- Complete inventory control check to verify the types and numbers of instruments and implants.

- Perform a quality assurance check by visually inspecting instruments and implants for damage.

Because the quality of the previous cleaning is unknown, it is advisable to wear gloves during the inspection process.

When completed properly, an inventory control sheet provides valuable information to protect the facility and the vendor. (See **Figure 11.77**)

Responsibility for the instruments should not be taken until the above procedures are completed, as the facility will be responsible for lost or damaged instruments.

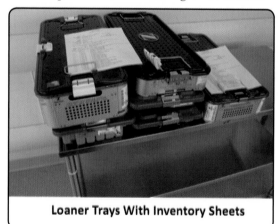

Loaner Trays With Inventory Sheets

Figure 11.77

Decontamination of Loaner Instrumentation

All loaner instruments should be cleaned and decontaminated upon receipt and after use. Instruments that appear clean (even those received in sterilized containers or wrap) should be considered contaminated and must be properly cleaned. Loaner instruments can be difficult to clean and debris can be hidden in lumens, hinges and crevices. Each manufacturer has specific instructions about the type of enzymatic detergent, temperature and mechanical cleaning method to be used.

Loaner Instrument Inspection and Assembly

After cleaning and decontamination, CS technicians must inspect each device for cleanliness and functionality, and then assemble and prepare the loaner instrumentation for sterilization. Each instrument should be examined for residual bioburden and for any defects that might cause it to malfunction. (See **Figure 11.78**) Defective instruments should be documented and reported to the appropriate supervisor to prevent delays in scheduled procedures.

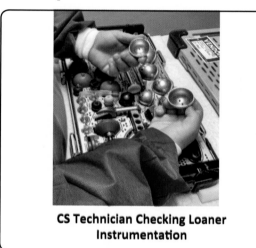

CS Technician Checking Loaner Instrumentation

Figure 11.78

Loaner instruments should be packaged according to the manufacturer's IFU.

Trays placed in another container system must be validated by the instrument manufacturer for use in that specific container. It is important to note that manufacturer-configured trays should not be reconfigured unless sterilization parameters for the new configuration has been validated by the manufacturer.

Each manufacturer establishes instructions for the sterilization of their instruments and sets. These instructions are based, in part, on the tray configuration and the complexity of the instrumentation. Facilities must follow the sterilization times and temperatures established by the manufacturer to help ensure sterilization of the loaner instruments.

Loaner Instrument Handling and Storage

After the loaner instruments have been sterilized, they should be moved to a department area with low traffic and allowed to cool away from the direct airflow of cooling vents. Trays should not be handled until properly cooled, which could take several hours. After cooling, trays should be handled as little as possible to prevent contamination or damage to the wrap. Care should be used when handling and moving the trays after the cooling process has taken place. These trays are often heavy and their packaging may be easily compromised (torn) if not handled properly. Loaner trays should be handled as little as possible and should never be slid across a surface. They should always be lifted and set on storage shelves or case carts for use in the OR. Use of transport trays is recommended to avoid damaging the processed trays. (See **Figure 11.79**)

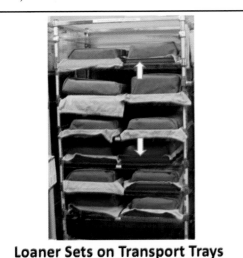

Loaner Sets on Transport Trays

Figure 11.79

After the loaner trays have been used in the procedure suite, they must be processed. Each instrument should be carefully cleaned and decontaminated according to manufacturer instructions prior to releasing them to the vendor representative, or before sending the trays back via courier or shipping company. Vendor representatives may be in a hurry to take the instruments to another facility. Regardless, all instruments must be thoroughly cleaned and decontaminated prior to release.

Sometimes, loaner instruments are loaned to a facility for an extended time. These instruments should be stored in a protected area to decrease the potential of instrument loss or damage.

An exit inventory of all loaner instruments is recommended to help ensure that any missing or damaged instrumentation is identified in a timely fashion.

CONCLUSION

As technology advances, surgical instruments and equipment will become more complex, and this has been evident with endoscopic equipment and accessories. Central Service technicians will continue to be challenged with keeping current with new technologies and standards impacting endoscopic equipment, instrumentation and accessories to ensure that patients are provided with safe and functional devices for their treatment and care.

RESOURCES

International Association for Healthcare Central Service Materiel Management. *IAHCSMM Position Paper on the Management of Loaner Instrumentation.* 2011.

Centers for Disease Control and Prevention. *Guideline for Disinfection and Sterilization in Healthcare Facilities.* 2008.

Association for the Advancement of Medical Instrumentation. *ANSI/AAMI ST58: 2015, Chemical Sterilization and High-level Disinfection in Health Care Facilities.*

Association for the Advancement of Medical Instrumentation. *ANSI/AAMI ST79, A3 2012, A4 2013, section 6, Comprehensive Guide to Steam Sterilization and Sterility Assurance in Health Care Facilities.* 2012.

American Society of Gastrointestinal Endoscopy. *Multisociety Guideline on Reprocessing Flexible Gastrointestinal Endoscopes.* 2011.

Association for the Advancement of Medical Instrumentation. *AAMI TIR12, Designing, Testing and Labeling Reusable Medical Devices for Reprocessing in Health Care Facilities: A Guide for Device Manufacturers.* 2010.

The Society of Gastroenterology Nurses and Associates. *Guideline for Use of High-Level Disinfectants & Sterilants for Reprocessing Flexible Gatrointestinal Endoscopes.* 2013.

Olympus America Inc. Two Corporate Center Dr., Melville, N.Y. 11747-3157; 800.548.5515.

Circon Corp. 6500 Hollister Ave., Santa Barbara, Calif. 93117-3019; 888.524.7266.

Karl Storz Endoscopy-America Inc. 600 Corporate Pointe, Culver City, Calif. 90203-7600; 800.421.0837.

CENTRAL SERVICE TERMS

Endoscope

Light-emitting diode (LED)

Loaner instrumentation

Chapter 12

Assembly and Packaging

Learning Objectives

As a result of successfully completing this chapter, readers will be able to:

1. Explain the set up and function of the assembly area

2. Review basic procedures to prepare pack contents for packaging

3. Explain the basic objectives of the packaging process and review basic selection factors for materials to be used with specific sterilization methods

4. Provide an overview of reusable packaging materials

5. Provide an overview of disposable packaging materials

6. Discuss basic package closure methods

7. Review general packaging concepts:
    • Package labeling
    • Special concerns
    • Sterility maintenance

INTRODUCTION

When instruments have been cleaned, they are transferred to the **assembly area** of the Central Service (CS) department. This area is also known as the preparation and packaging (prep and pack) area, and its here where instruments are inspected to ensure that they are clean and in good working order before they are packaged for sterilization. This is a critical step because it is the last time the instruments will be handled before being dispensed to the Operating Room (OR) or other user area. Potentially serious problems can arise if a defective or unclean instrument arrives in the user department. When these incidents are detected, delays occur. When they are not detected, risks to the patient increase; therefore, it is imperative that protocols for inspection, assembly and packaging are followed at all times. Like other areas of the CS department, attention to detail is critical in the assembly area. CS professionals working in this area of the department must understand the configuration of their work area and the specific requirements that must be followed to work safely and effectively in that area.

> **Assembly area** A clean area of the Central Service department where instrument inspection, assembly and packaging are performed. The assembly area is sometimes called the Preparation and Packaging (prep and pack) area.

ASSEMBLY AND PACKAGING AREA

The Physical Environment

The assembly/pack and prep area is a designated clean area; therefore, meticulous care must be taken to maintain that cleanliness. Airflow plays a critical role in keeping the assembly area clean and free of contaminants. Air pressure in the clean assembly area should be positive in relation to outside hallways, the decontamination area, break rooms, and other adjacent areas, with the exception of the sterile storage area. The purpose of this positive airflow is to ensure that when the doors to the assembly area are opened, air flows outward instead

of into the work area. Positive airflow reduces the risk of airborne bacteria being introduced into the area.

Maintaining proper temperature is also critical. Temperature in the assembly area should be between 68° and 73°F (20° to 23°C). Relative humidity should be maintained between 30% and 60%.

Housekeeping standards for the assembly area should be the same as those for delivery rooms and the OR. To reduce the amount of bacteria in the area, fixtures, work tables and all other furniture in the area should be constructed of non-porous easy to clean materials. In addition to routinely cleaning surfaces, care must be taken to minimize dust and lint in the area. Dust and lint may settle on pack contents and be introduced into the patient's body during a procedure.

> ## The Danger of Lint
>
> Lint is composed of fine fibers that separate from items, such as wraps, towels and other textiles, paper and more. Lint can be carried on air currents and deposited anywhere. Microorganisms often adhere to lint. When lint is introduced into the sterile field, it can settle into a wound and cause infection.
>
> CS departments should make every effort to minimize lint. Good cleaning practices and compliance with attire and housekeeping protocols can reduce lint and the chance of it entering the OR or inside of packs.

To further maintain environmental cleanliness, hand hygiene stations (handwashing sinks and waterless, alcohol-based hand rubs) should be conveniently located and readily accessible to all CS staff.

Proper lighting in the assembly area is essential. Work performed in this area is very detailed and inadequate lighting can lead to errors and eye strain.

Dress Code and Personal Behaviors

Personal cleanliness and adherence to dress code is essential for preventing microorganisms and contaminants from entering the work area. The cleaner the environment, the less chance there is of contaminants entering a pack.

Nail polish and artificial nails should not be worn in the prep and pack area because there is a potential for nail polish to chip and artificial nails to fall off. Natural fingernails should be clean and be kept at a length that does not extend beyond the fingertips. Long nails harbor bacteria that may hinder effective handwashing. **Figure 12.1** shows a technician in proper attire for the preparation and packaging area.

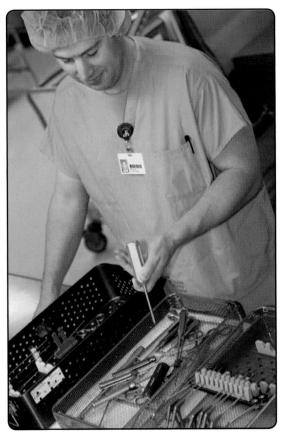

Figure 12.1

According to ANSI/AAMI ST79:2010/A4:2013, *Comprehensive guide to steam sterilization and*

sterility assurance in health care facilities, all head and facial hair (except for eyebrows and eyelashes) should be completely covered with a surgical-type hair covering. Jewelry and wristwatches should not be worn in the area because they can harbor microorganisms.

All staff members in the area must monitor their cleanliness and change scrub attire if it becomes soiled. They must also perform hand hygiene, as necessary. CS professionals should not bring items into the area that may contaminate hands (e.g., money, personal items and personal electronics). *Note: CS personnel should consult their facility's policy about the use of personal electronics and how it relates to infection prevention.*

Traffic Control and Environmental Management

Everyone assigned to the prep and pack area should be mindful and protective of that clean environment. Traffic should be restricted and traffic control requirements must be followed. Care must be taken to ensure that items that may serve as vehicles for microorganisms are not allowed into the area. (See **Figure 12.2**)

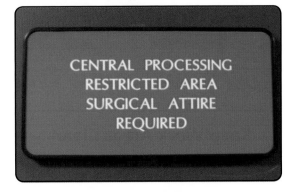

Figure 12.2

Food and beverages are not allowed in the prep and pack area. Food and drinks may attract insects and rodents, and residues left on hands after eating may transfer to instruments and impede the sterilization process.

CS technicians assigned to the prep and pack area should always be mindful of potential contaminants that could have a negative impact on the packs they are assembling. Personal behaviors, such as following dress code, performing proper hand hygiene and avoiding situations that pose a threat of contamination, all help protect the patient.

Work Area Requirements

The work area in prep and pack should be adequately sized to perform inspection, testing and assembly duties. Supplies needed for those processes should be readily available. Equipment, such as computers, printers and specialized instrument testing devices, should also be readily available. (See **Figure 12.3**) The work area should be routinely cleaned to reduce bacteria and lint. (See **Figure 12.4**)

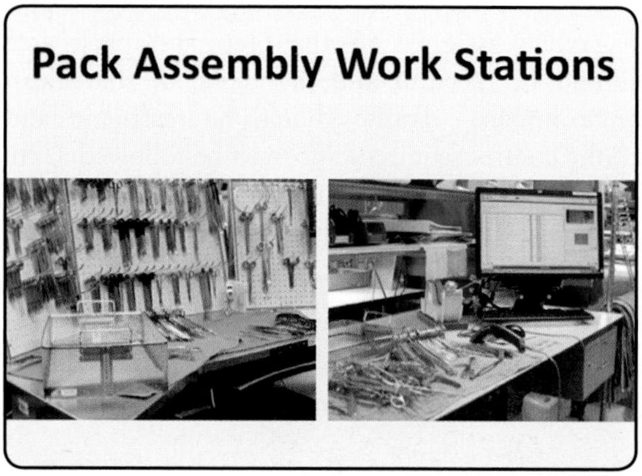

Pack Assembly Work Stations

Figure 12.3

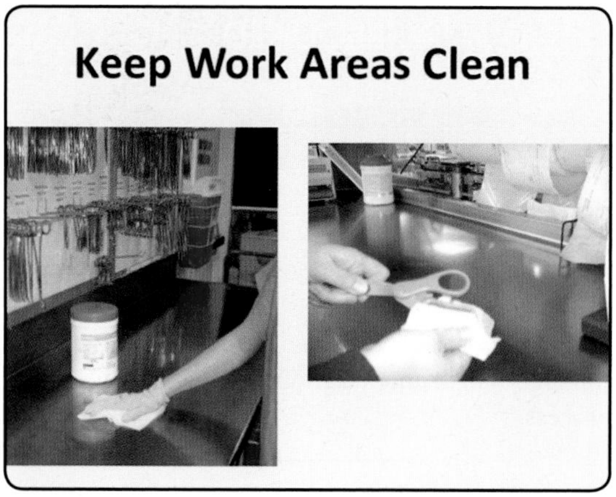

Keep Work Areas Clean

Figure 12.4

PRIMARY GOALS OF PACK PREPARATION

CS professionals assigned to the prep and pack area must understand the primary goals of creating an instrument pack. The first goal is to create a pack that meets the users' needs. The acronym"FAN," which stands for Functional, Accurate and Neat, can help reinforce that goal.

- Function. Each item in the pack must function as it was designed. This means that scissors must be sharp, clamps must hold securely, and multi-part items must be complete and functional when assembled. Technicians reach that goal by understanding how instruments operate and by relying on specific test methods to ensure that they work properly.

- Accurate. Instruments must be correct and quantities must be exact. Technicians meet this goal by learning to identify specific instruments, working from an up-to-date pack content list and verifying that all specifications for the pack — including quantities and configuration — are correct.

- Neat. Pack contents must be organized, and instruments must be easy to locate. Disorganized packs may waste time or delay treatment and care.

> When assembling any pack for sterilization, remember the "**FAN**" principle.
>
> All items must be **F**unctional, **A**ccurate and **N**eat.

In addition to creating organized packs that contain correct and functional instruments, CS technicians must also arrange pack contents in a manner that facilitates the appropriate sterilization process. As technicians arrange pack contents, they must also take precautions to protect instruments from possible damage or content shifting that may occur during handling and transport.

Technicians must then adhere to the packaging method recommended by the instrument manufacturers — one that is appropriate for the sterilization method that will be used for the items being packaged. Finally, technicians must use the proper packaging technique, as instructed by the manufacturer.

GENERAL GUIDELINES FOR PREPARATION OF PACK CONTENTS

Most instruments are prepared in groups called packs, sets, trays or kits. *Note: The specific name (kit, tray, set or pack) is determined by the healthcare facility.* Smaller groups of instruments used for smaller procedures in areas outside of the OR, such as suturing, wound irrigation or cutdowns (accessing deep veins for intravenous fluid delivery), are often called procedure trays (also known as floor trays). No matter what type of tray is being assembled and regardless of its size, preparation of pack contents begins with planning.

Clearly-written and illustrated procedures for preparation of items to be packaged (usually called count sheets) should be readily available and used by all personnel each time pack preparation procedures are performed. Many packs have unique characteristics that may require special configurations and preparations. Count sheets provide specific information that helps ensure all packs are assembled, packaged and sterilized according to exact specifications.

Item requirements for tray contents are usually identified by users. For example, a surgeon and OR staff would determine the contents of specific surgical trays. Pack content information may be collected and maintained in a manual (paper) system, or the information may be gathered and maintained with a computerized system (See **Figure 12.5**). Whichever method is used, the same basic information is provided to the assembler:

- Correct and complete name of the tray.

- A detailed list of tray contents, including item quantities, sizes and catalog or reference numbers.

- Essential steps for preparation and inspection, and for assembly and disassembly of device(s) according to the manufacturer's written directions and/or specifications.

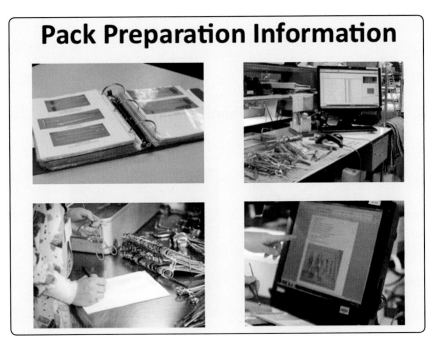

Pack Preparation Information

Figure 12.5

- Specific instructions for correct placement of items in the tray.

- Sterilization method and required cycle used for processing tray.

- Type(s) and size(s) of packaging to be used.

- Type and placement of internal and/or external chemical process indicator(s), in accordance with the facility's policies.

- Destination or storage location of the tray (i.e., Emergency Department or OR Cabinet 32, Shelf 4).

Once the information needed for assembly has been obtained, the pack contents can be assembled. All items to be sterilized must be completely dried prior to assembly and packaging, as water left on instruments can interfere with the sterilization cycle. Moisture issues affect different sterilization processes in multiple ways:

- Steam cycles – Moisture will change the wet/dry steam ratio.

- Ethylene oxide (EtO) cycles – Moisture will form ethylene glycol, which is harmful to staff and patients.

- Hydrogen peroxide and ozone cycles – Moisture will cause the cycle to abort.

Note: Some manufacturers recommend that lumens be moist for steam sterilization. If the manufacturer specifically requires this for steam sterilization, only those lumens should be moistened.

Pack Assembly

Before items can be assembled into trays, sets or packs for sterilization, they must be inspected and in some cases, tested to ensure that they are clean, correct and functional.

Inspection Guidelines

Each instrument should be carefully inspected upon assembly and packaging. Chapters 10 and 11 addressed inspection techniques for several common instruments. What follows are some basic guidelines for instrument inspection during pack preparation. *Note: Be sure to consult the manufacturer's IFU for inspection requirements for specific instruments.*

Inspect for cleanliness. Even though instruments have been cleaned, there may still be instances where some soil was not removed. (See **Figure 12.6**) Organic material, such as blood or other contaminants, will interfere with sterilization and optimal functioning. Inspecting instruments for cleanliness adds a safeguard to the process by reducing the chance that a soiled instrument is delivered to a user area.

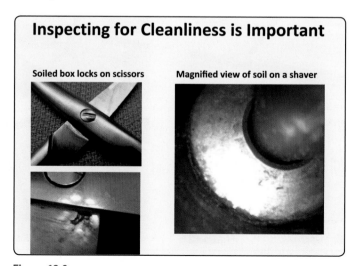

Inspecting for Cleanliness is Important

Soiled box locks on scissors

Magnified view of soil on a shaver

Figure 12.6

If a soiled instrument is detected during the inspection process, it should be sent back to the decontamination area for proper cleaning. The tray that the soiled instrument was in should also be sent back to the decontamination area, as other instruments may have also been contaminated through contact with the unclean instrument. *Note: Do not attempt to clean the instrument in the assembly area. Doing so may contaminate the immediate area and may cross contaminate other areas of the department.*

Inspect for damage. Instruments may become damaged through use, misuse, transport and processing. Look for cracks, breaks, bent tips, misalignment and other signs of damage.

Inspect for signs of wear. Even with the best of care, instruments eventually begin to show signs of wear. Scissors and other sharp instruments become dull, surfaces break down, springs may weaken, screws may loosen and moving parts may begin to stick.

Damaged and worn instruments should be removed and sent for repair or discarded, as necessary. The continued use of broken or excessively worn instruments could put patients and/or facility personnel at risk. (See **Figure 12.7**)

Check multi-part instruments. Instruments that have been disassembled for cleaning should be reassembled and tested for proper function, and then disassembled again for sterilization. (See **Figure 12.8**) *Note: Small parts, such as wing nuts, should be placed in an approved containment device.* (See **Figure 12.9**) When placing disassembled instruments inside the tray, keep all parts close to one another, so they can be readily accessible in the OR.

Examples of Sharpen and Repair Tags

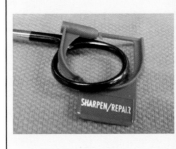
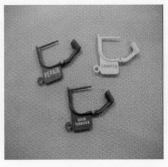

Figure 12.7

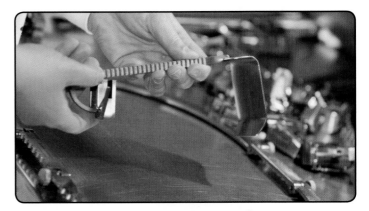

Figure 12.8

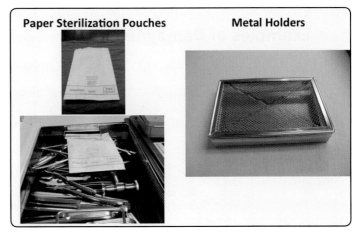

Figure 12.9

Scissors Sharpness Testing

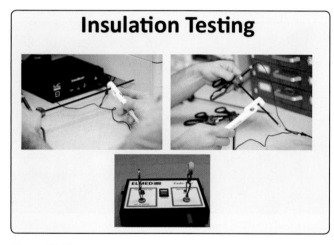

Figure 12.10

Insulation Testing

Figure 12.11

Examples of Demagnetizers

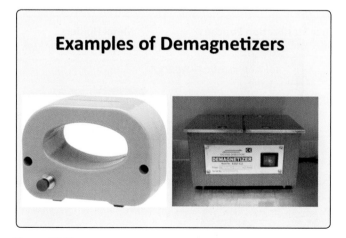

Figure 12.12

Testing

All instruments must be inspected before assembly. Some instruments must also be tested. For example, scissors should be tested for sharpness (See **Figure 12.10**) and the insulation of electrosurgical instruments must be tested between uses. (See **Figure 12.11**)

Demagnetizers. Occasionally, instruments may become magnetized. This is a source of frustration for the surgeon, especially with needle holders, as magnetization may make working with suture needles very difficult. Demagnetizers work by reversing the magnetic field away from the instrument. **Figure 12.12** provides examples of demagnetizers.

Tools for inspection. There are many tools available to help with instrument inspection. Magnifying lamps and computer magnifiers can enlarge areas to help detect residual soil, wear and damage. (See **Figure 12.13**)

Photos of instruments and instrument configurations (either hard copy or computerized) can also help ensure that items are assembled correctly.

Instrument scanning systems, instrument etching and instrument tape can help CS technicians identify devices and assist with pack assembly. (See **Figure 12.14**)

Instrument holding trays. Groups of instruments for a specific procedure or specialty are contained together in trays specifically designed to protect the devices and facilitate the sterilization process. (See **Figure 12.15**) Other instrument groups are contained in trays that can be adapted to several configurations. (See **Figure 12.16**) In most cases, the container is selected when the instrument tray is put into the surgical instrument system.

Magnification Devices

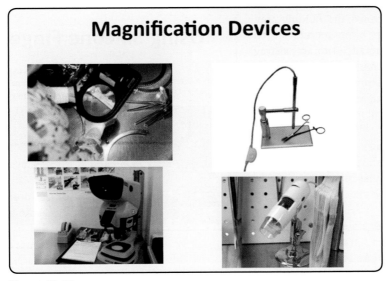

Figure 12.13

Instrument Identification

Scan Readable Codes   **Etching and Tape**

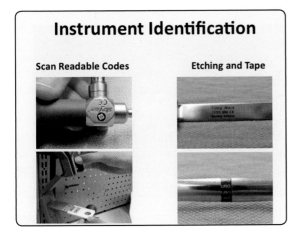

Figure 12.14

Trays That Can Hold Multiple Configurations of Instruments

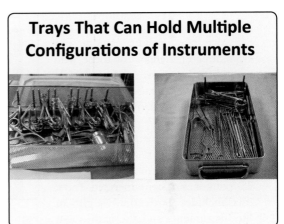

Figure 12.16

Examples of Trays Designed for Specific Instruments

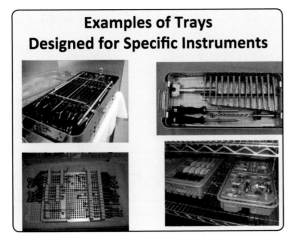

Figure 12.15

The following are points to consider when using instrument holding trays:

- Use the holding tray correctly.

- Read the manufacturer's IFU and use the tray as instructed. Failure to do so can damage instruments or cause the sterilization process to fail. For example, trays with silicone finger mats must be aligned with drainage holes to help ensure air and water removal during steam sterilization. (See **Figure 12.17**)

- Do not overcrowd the holding tray. Overcrowding often occurs when instruments are added to an existing tray. Over time, physicians' needs may change and instruments may be added to trays, creating a situation where the tray is too small for its contents. (See **Figure 12.18**) When this happens, there is a greater risk of instruments being damaged. In some cases, severe overcrowding may impact sterilization and drying.

- Don't create overweight trays. Be aware of tray weight and density recommendations from the manufacturers of sterilizers, instruments and packaging systems. In addition to possible issues associated with heat-up and drying, excessive tray weight can present ergonomic challenges for those who must lift the trays. ANSI/AAMI ST77, *Containment devices for reusable medical device sterilization* and ANSI/AAMI ST79, *Comprehensive guide to steam sterilization and sterility assurance in health care facilities*, recommend a maximum weight of 25 pounds for containerized trays; this includes both the weight of the instruments and the instrument container. (See **Figure 12.19**)

- Protect instruments from damage. As discussed in Chapters 10 and 11, all instruments should be protected from damage when handled. Delicate and sharp instruments are of special concern. Sharp points may be protected with special holders, commercially-available tip guards, silicone mats, holding brackets, posts or foam sleeves. **Figures 12.20** and **12.21** provide examples of methods to protect instruments. Suppliers of protective devices should be consulted to ensure that the devices are permeable to the sterilant being used.

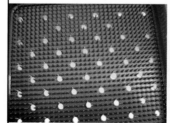
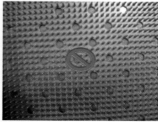

Using Silicone Finger Mats

Correct – Openings aligned

Incorrect – Openings offset and closed. No path for air removal and water drainage.

Figure 12.17

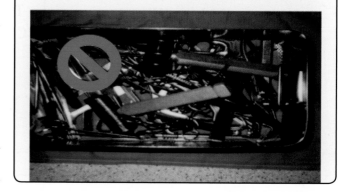

Do Not Overload Trays

Figure 12.18

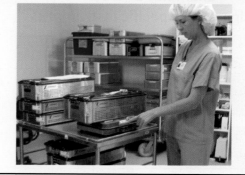

Technician Weighing Loaner Trays in the CS Instrument Receiving Area

Figure 12.19

For example, latex tubing should not be used to protect instrument tips, as it may prevent the sterilant from making direct contact with the instruments.

Examples of Tip Protectors

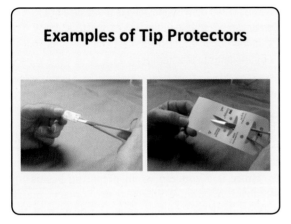

Figure 12.20

Examples of Instrument Protectors

Silicone finger mats   Foam protectors

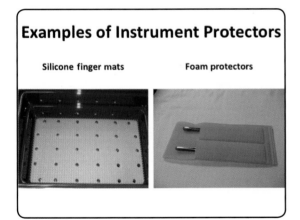

Figure 12.21

Instruments that open, such as scissors and hemostats, should be kept in unlocked, open positions to enable the sterilant to reach all parts. Devices such as instrument stringers and racks can be purchased to keep hinged instruments open. (See **Figure 12.22**) Always follow the manufacturer's IFU for specific requirements.

Protect the alignment of forceps tips by placing all tips in the same direction. (See **Figure 12.23**) Forceps tips can also be protected by using an approved containment device.

Examples of Devices Used to Keep Hinged Instruments Open

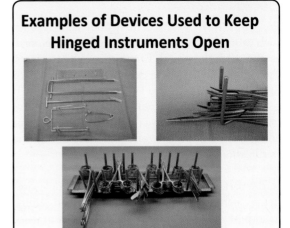

Figure 12.22

Protect Forceps Tips

Correct   Incorrect

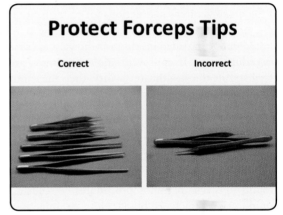

Figure 12.23

The most important thing to remember with all pack preparation is that all items must be functional, accurate and neat/organized because the next time the pack is accessed, it will be used for patient care.

Assembly Procedures

Pack contents and pack configurations are unique. CS technicians must apply basic principles to pack assembly to create packs that can be successfully sterilized and meet the users' needs. The following section provides an overview of general assembly guidelines.

Procedure Trays

Procedure trays are used in patient care settings such as nursing units and in procedure areas, such as the Radiology and Emergency Departments. Procedure trays are often designed to include all or most of the items needed for a minor procedure. It is important to disassemble multi-part items and place all items in trays in a manner that prevents air entrapment and pooling of condensate during the sterilization process.

In the past, the inclusion of disposable (single-use) items, such as needles, scalpel blades and suture, in trays was common; however, today, this practice is uncommon. To sterilize single-use items, the manufacturer's IFU (including resterilization instructions) must be on file and carefully followed. If the manufacturer's instructions for resterilization of a single-use item cannot be obtained, the item should not be included inside an in-house sterilized procedure tray. If approved single-use items are sterilized in the healthcare facility, they must not be resterilized if they are returned unused.

Gauze sponges and surgical (huck) towels were also commonly used in procedure trays in the past; however, many studies now show that lint from these items can be transferred to a patient wound — even in minor procedures — causing complications, such as blood clots or infection. Prepackaged sterile towels purchased from an outside vendor or processed in house should not be opened and used on trays because they may **super heat** within the sterilization cycle. If super-heating occurs, the tray they are in (and other trays within the load) will potentially be unsterile. Towels should be laundered after sterilization to rehydrate the fibers prior to sterilization. Prepackaged, sterile towels from an outside vendor should not be laundered unless the IFU have been obtained from the towel manufacturer because these towels are usually made of lower-quality material to allow for single use and no relaundering.

Super heating   Super heating steam occurs when dry steam becomes too hot compared to saturated steam. Dry steam rises to a temperature higher than the boiling point of saturated steam. This commonly occurs when dehydrated linen is processed in a steam sterilizer. Due to the lack of moisture, dry steam is not an effective sterilant and will often char or burn items in the sterilizer.

Basin Sets

Basin sets should be assembled in a way that allows moisture to drain from them during sterilization. Moisture is a concern when preparing basins for sterilization because when steam contacts metal, it is immediately cooled when the heat from the steam transfers to the metal. As this occurs, the steam condenses and forms water droplets on the metal. When multiple basins are sterilized together, **wicking material**, such as a surgical towel (See **Figure 12.24**) or specially-designed wicking materials, can be used to facilitate drying.

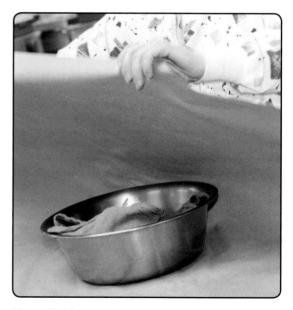

Figure 12.24

If basin sets are too dense, the excess amount of metal may cause condensation, thereby creating a wet pack. To avoid this problem, additional absorbent materials may be added. Very dense sets should be divided into two separate sets.

All items that will collect water must be placed in the same direction to facilitate drainage. When multiple basins are sterilized, there should be at least a one-inch size difference in basins that will be placed together to allow for condensate drainage and drying.

> **Wicking material**   An approved absorbent material that allows for air removal and steam penetration, and facilitates drying.

Instrument Trays

As with procedure trays, each instrument tray should have a detailed count sheet available during instrument assembly. Technicians should never try to assemble an instrument tray from memory, as the contents change, or items could easily be forgotten. Technicians should avoid counting total tray contents as a method of assembling instrument trays (e.g., counting a total of 100 instruments instead of verifying each type of instrument needed). Each instrument should be identified, inspected, verified against the count sheet and placed properly in the tray.

Standardization of the instrument arrangement within each tray is important. Instrument trays should look the same, regardless of which technician assembled them. This saves time and reduces stress for the user. The order or arrangement in the tray should be determined by the CS manager and user department personnel.

It is important to note that CS technicians must place the required number of instruments in the tray. Placing too few or too many will disrupt the instrument count and may delay a surgical procedure while the needed instruments are located. Instrument substitutions should not occur, unless approved by the user department. If packaging an incomplete instrument tray is

unavoidable, the users should be notified and the tray should be clearly marked to indicate what is missing. (See **Figure 12.25**)

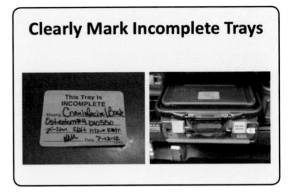

Clearly Mark Incomplete Trays

Figure 12.25

Instruments of the same type should be arranged together to facilitate their location during an emergency. Hinged instruments may be grouped together on racks, tray pins or stringers to ensure that instruments with locks are maintained in the open position. Heavier items must be placed at the bottom of the tray to avoid damage to more delicate instruments. Delicate instruments should be protected using items such as approved foam pouches, tip protectors, silicon mats, holding brackets or posts. Instrument protectors should be approved by the manufacturer for the type of sterilization method to be used.

The use of towels or tray liners for cushioning instruments or wicking should be determined based on the metal mass in the tray and the external package manufacturer's IFU.

Gauze sponges should never be used as additional packaging (wicking) material in trays or packs. Surgery staff count gauze sponges during procedures, and their counts must be exact. The introduction of additional sponges into the OR as packaging material may cause confusion and affect sponge counts.

There may be sterilant penetration or weight distribution concerns that prevent the "perfect tray" arrangement requested by the user department. CS managers should inform user department personnel about sterilization limitations. The ultimate goal must always be to create a tray that can be successfully sterilized.

Powered Surgical Instruments

Manufacturer instructions should always be followed when preparing powered surgical instruments for sterilization. This includes the use of the correct disassembly and lubrication procedures. Trigger handles should be placed in the safety position, and power switches should be turned off before placing the instruments in the tray.

Powered surgical instruments often use a sterilization container supplied by the manufacturer. (See **Figure 12.26**) Extended or special sterilization conditions may be required and details about these procedures should be supplied by the instrument's manufacturer. After items are inspected, disassembled (if necessary) and placed in a container according to the manufacturer's instructions, the tray is ready to be packaged for sterilization.

Powered Surgical Instrument in Manufacturer's Tray

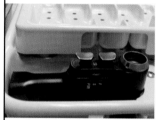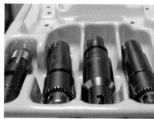

Figure 12.26

Specialty Instruments

Specialty instruments, such as laparoscopic instruments, robotics, endoscopes, cameras and others, are of special concern for CS technicians. Manufacturer IFU must be carefully followed to ensure that proper disassembly, assembly and

sterilization procedures are completed. Many of these specialty instruments are contained in specialty containers to prevent damage during handling.

Single Instruments

The term "single instrument" is used to describe instruments that are to be packaged alone and it can also refer to like instruments packaged together (e.g., a single Mayo scissors or a package of six Kelly clamps). These instruments should be assembled according to the department's established protocols for size and number of instruments.

Surgical Supplies

Numerous non-instrument surgical supplies, such as cotton balls and dressings, may be required by users. Most of these items are available as commercially-sterilized products and it is often more cost effective to purchase them presterilized. If the facility chooses to process them internally, however, these and similar items should be wrapped individually or in usable quantities, based on the product manufacturer's IFU and the user's need. These items should not be sterilized without the manufacturer's IFU on file within the department. Due to the linting factor, most surgical supplies should not be sterilized inside trays or packs.

QUALITY ASSURANCE MEASURES - INTERNAL CHEMICAL INDICATORS

Part of the assembly process for every pack includes a quality assurance test designed to measure sterilant penetration. Incorrect placement of pack contents, incorrect packaging methods or incorrect loading can impede the sterilization process by creating air pockets or barriers that can prevent the sterilant from penetrating the pack and making direct contact with the items inside. Internal **chemical indicators (CIs)** are designed to identify those issues before a pack is used. *Note: Sterilization process monitoring methods are covered in detail in Chapter 17.*

Examples of
Internal Chemical Indicators

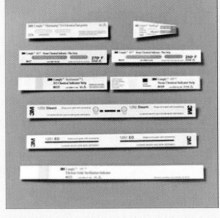 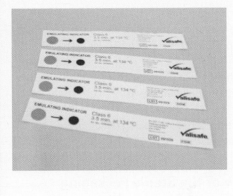

Figure 12.27

> **Chemical indicators (CIs)** Devices used to monitor the presence or attainment of one or more of the parameters required for a satisfactory sterilization process.

A CI is a small, disposable test that helps the user verify that the pack contents were exposed to a sterilant. (See **Figure 12.27**) When exposed to the specific sterilant they are designed to detect, their color changes, providing a visual indication of the presence of sterilant in the pack. When the pack is opened at point of use, it is checked by the user. Users will not use a pack that has a failed internal CI. They will also not use a pack that does not contain a CI.

When used properly, the CI becomes a very important early warning that something may be wrong with some aspect of the sterilization process. CIs should be placed inside each pack in the area considered the least accessible by the sterilant being used. That may or may not be in the center of the pack's contents. In some cases, multiple CIs may need to be used if there are multiple areas that could pose a challenge for sterilant penetration. Multi-level trays should have a CI placed in the most difficult area for sterilant penetration on each level of the tray.

Commonly-used internal CIs include:

- Class 5 integrating indicators are designed to react to all critical parameters and to be equivalent to or exceed performance requirements, over a specified range of sterilization cycles. When used inside a **process challenge device (PCD)**, non-implant loads may be released with the appropriate results indicated on the CI.

- Class 6 emulating indicators, also called verification indicators or cycle specific indicators, are designed to react to all critical parameter of a sterilization cycle. Class 6 indicators are designed to be run within one specific cycle (e.g., 270°F, four-minute exposure). This is the only cycle this specific indicator may be used. If a 275°F, three-minute exposure cycle is to be run, an emulator specifically made for that cycle must be used.

Note: It is important to use the appropriate indicator for the intended method of sterilization and cycle.

> **Process challenge device (PCD)**   Object that simulates a predetermined set of conditions when used to test sterilizing agent(s).

BASIC PACKAGING PROCEDURES

Once items have been cleaned, inspected and assembled, they are ready to be sterilized. In order to maintain their sterility, items must be packaged before they are sterilized. That packaging helps maintain the integrity (sterility) of the sterile items until they are opened and used.

The following sections discuss packaging selection and application.

Overview of the Sterile Packaging Process

CS technicians must select the appropriate packaging material and apply it correctly to create a pack that can be sterilized successfully and maintain sterility until it is opened.

One can draw some comparisons between food packaging and sterile packaging. Both types of packaging must protect items and keep them from becoming contaminated before they are used. Both can be compromised in a way that affects the package's contents and makes them unsafe for use.

Sterile packaging is designed with **tamper-evident seals,** so users can tell if the package has been opened. (See **Figure 12.28**) Many food products use these tamper-evident seals on their packaging for the same reason. There are several packaging options for food products and sterile items, and not all types of packaging are appropriate for all items and processes. For example, soup could not be packaged in aluminum foil, carried to work and heated in a microwave oven. Sterile item packaging must also consider the sterilization process that will be used.

CS technicians must be familiar with the various packaging materials available for sterilization and they must be able to select the packaging, which is most appropriate for the item to be packaged and the sterilization process to be used. CS technicians must also be able to apply the selected packaging in a manner that facilitates the sterilization process and protects the package contents during the storage and handling that follows sterilization.

> **Tamper-evident seals** Sealing methods for sterile packaging that allow users to determine if the packaging has been opened. Tamper-evident seals allow users to determine if packages have been opened (contaminated) and help users identify packages that are not safe for patient use.

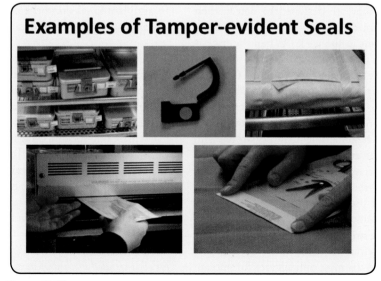

Examples of Tamper-evident Seals

Figure 12.28

Objectives of the Packaging Process

There are three primary objectives for any sterilization packaging system. It must:

- Allow penetration of the chosen sterilant and be compatible with any other requirements of the specific sterilization process, such as drying.

- Maintain the sterility of the package contents until the package is opened.

- Create a package that can be opened aseptically (without contaminating the contents) by the user.

Packaging systems must also:

- Have a sealing method that is tamper evident

- Be nontoxic

- Be nonlinting

- Be easy to use

- Be cost effective

The FDA classifies sterilization packaging as a Class II medical device (a device that presents a potential risk). The consequences of using a nonsterile item during a surgical procedure can be life-threatening. In addition to selecting and applying the appropriate packaging material, CS technicians must also be able to construct packages that allow the sterilization process to be successful and protect the package contents from contamination.

Selecting the Appropriate Packaging Material

The first step in the packaging process is to select the appropriate type of packaging material and method. Different types of packaging are needed for alternative sterilization methods, and styles of packaging may vary based on package contents.

CS technicians must make good packaging choices. Since there is no single packaging material for all situations, CS technicians must select the material that is best suited for the sterilization process to be used. Only materials specifically designed for sterilization packaging and approved by the FDA are acceptable. In addition, there are other special concerns based on the sterilization method that will be used:

- Packaging used for steam sterilization must be capable of withstanding high-temperatures of 250°F to 275°F (121°C to 135°C). The packaging must allow air removal and steam penetration to the contents, and permit drying of the contents and packaging material.

- Packaging choices for ethylene oxide (EtO) sterilization must allow adequate penetration of the gas sterilant and removal of the residual gas (aeration).

- Packaging choices for hydrogen peroxide sterilization must tolerate a deep vacuum draw without absorbing the sterilant, interrupting the cycle or damaging the contents. Packaging must also be cellulose free.

- Packaging choices for ozone sterilization should be cellulose free, such as spunbond-meltblown-spunbond and spunbond polyolefin (both of these products are discussed later in this chapter).

In addition to selecting the appropriate packaging material, CS technicians must understand how to use sterilization packaging appropriately to achieve the desired results, sterilant penetration, barrier effectiveness and aseptic opening.

Packaging systems used in healthcare facility-based sterilization are generally classified into reusable packaging and disposable (single use) packaging materials. Each packaging system has advantages and limitations. The following sections provide some basic information about common packaging systems and their application.

REUSABLE PACKAGING MATERIALS

There are two basic types of reusable packaging material: woven fabric and rigid containers.

Woven Fabric Materials

Before the early 1980s, woven textiles were the reusable packaging material of choice; however, new technologies have increased the choices for sterilization packaging. The standards for manufacturing today's packaging materials have been based on penetration and microbial barrier capability measurements for a minimum of 140-thread count (threads per square inch) **muslin**.

Muslin, Type 140 cotton, calico, and barrier cloth are common names for fabrics made of 100% unbleached, loosely-woven cotton fibers. Muslin wrappers are generally made of two-ply (double thickness) fabric fastened together as one wrap. (See **Figure 12.29**).

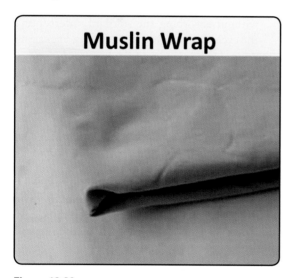

Figure 12.29

Other woven fabrics used in sterilization are:

- Duck cloth

- Twill

- Treated barrier fabrics

Note: Canvas is not recommended as a packaging material because its tight weave impedes steam penetration and drying.

> **Muslin** Broad term describing a wide variety of plain-weave cotton or cotton/polyester fabrics with approximately 140 threads per square inch.

Textile packaging is still the packaging method of choice for some healthcare facilities. The selection of reusable textiles is often impacted by costs and/or environment sustainability concerns (the desire to reduce the waste generated by disposable packaging materials). Some facilities contract with off-site companies to pick up used textile wraps and then launder, inspect and return them to the facility for reuse.

Textile packaging requires more labor because it must be laundered and inspected to ensure that there are no tears, punctures, worn spots or stains from previous use. That inspection is performed using a light table that has a light source built into the tabletop to help spot small holes and punctures. As the wrap is passed over the lighted table top, light shines through small holes and punctures making them easier to identify.

If holes, punctures or worn spots are discovered, the linen wrap must be repaired using a heat-sealed patch designed to cover the hole. The size of the surface area covered by heat-sealed patches on reusable fabrics should be considered before the fabric is reused. (See **Figure 12.30**)

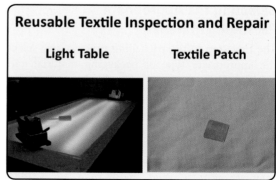

Figure 12.30

Reusable materials with approved heat-sealed patches can be effectively sterilized; however, the limit (the percentage of exposed area that can be patched) depends on the method of sterilization, positioning in the sterilizer, number of layers of patched fabric and type of fabric patch. Some patching materials are not fully steam penetrable, but are surface sterilized only. Although the sterilant entering through unpatched areas may be sufficient to sterilize the pack contents, excessive use of non- or semi-permeable patches may hinder the sterilization process. A facility's Infection Prevention and Control Committee should investigate the use of patched wraps to establish an "accept/reject" standard for the total surface area of patch that is permitted for use within the facility.

If stains are discovered, the wrap should be re-laundered. If stains cannot be removed, the wrap should be removed from service.

Textiles must also be de-linted as needed to minimize the risk of lint entering the sterile pack and, ultimately, the sterile field. (See **Figure 12.31**) Reusable textiles can be a significant source of lint. If lint enters a patient's incision, it may cause negative effects.

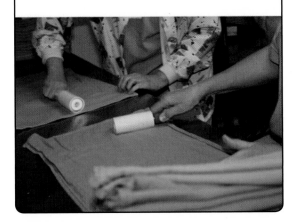

De-linting Reusable Textiles

Figure 12.31

When assembling linen packs, their size is limited to 12" (height) x 12" (width) x 20" (length), and they are not to weigh more than 12 pounds. Maximum density must not exceed 7.2 pounds

per cubic foot because higher densities may reduce sterilant access to all contents.

Linen wrappers should be securely applied without compressing package contents. Contents must be packaged with sufficient spacing to enable the sterilant to reach all surfaces.

Tight packaging will not allow for fiber swelling (expansion); when expansion occurs the sterilant will not penetrate the material. It is possible to wrap even a small pack so tightly that its density will be too great for adequate sterilant penetration. Muslin-type wrappers must always use a sequential type wrapping process. *Note: This topic is discussed later in this chapter.*

Rigid Container Systems

Rigid container systems are box-like structures with sealable and removable lids. They are made of anodized aluminum, stainless steel, plastic or a combination of these materials. Rigid containers have lids and filters that allow sterilant penetration while providing a microbial barrier. Filters may be disposable (a synthetic spunbond product) or reusable (with ceramic filters or a valve system). Rigid containers consist of an inner basket to hold the instruments and an outer container that acts as a protective barrier. Both the inner basket and outer container have handles for ease of carrying.

Figure 12.32 identifies the common components of a rigid sterilization container system's outer container.

Some manufacturers of rigid container systems recommend that times for instrument sterilization, drying and aeration be extended when using their containers. It is important to consult the specific container manufacturer's IFU before using a rigid container system. Rigid containers are regulated by the FDA, and containers are required to have a 510(k) premarket submission certifying they will perform as an effective packaging material.

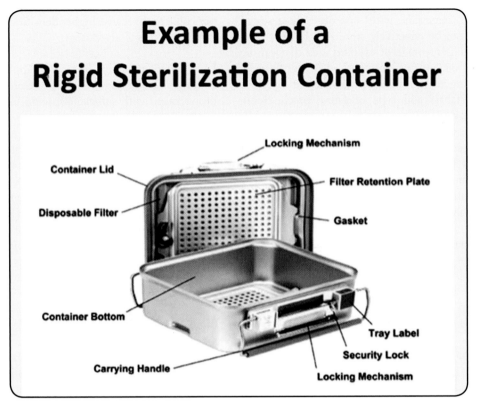

Example of a Rigid Sterilization Container

- Locking Mechanism
- Container Lid
- Filter Retention Plate
- Disposable Filter
- Gasket
- Container Bottom
- Tray Label
- Security Lock
- Carrying Handle
- Locking Mechanism

Figure 12.32

Advantages and Disadvantages

There are several advantages of rigid sterilization containers. They:

- Provide an excellent barrier to microorganisms.

- Are easy to use.

- Eliminate torn wrappers.

- Help protect instruments from damage during processing, storage and transport.

> **Rigid container system** Instrument containers that hold medical devices during sterilization and also protect devices from contamination during storage and transport.

There are also potential disadvantages to the use of these systems, including:

- Safety concerns linked to ergonomics. Some large (12"x23"x6") empty containers weigh approximately seven to nine pounds. This requires CS technicians to use good body mechanics when lifting and moving containers. *Note: Loaded instrument baskets must be added to this base weight, and employees should be able to comfortably carry a container or instrument set at waist height.*

- Additional cycle time may be required to thoroughly dry the container. Sterilization efficacy is also impacted as a container's weight increases because of excess condensation. **Wet packs** have been noted and discussed for many years. While it is difficult to generalize about specific causes of wet packs, it is known that heavier sets and those with greater metal mass are more likely to experience this problem, especially when instruments are not properly disbursed in the container.

Wet pack   Package or container with moisture after the sterilization process is completed.

- Plastic containers may require longer dry times because they lack metal, which produces heat by conduction to help drying.

- Additional space may be needed to store those containers that are larger than traditional wrapped containers. (See **Figure 12.33**)

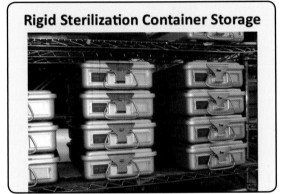

Rigid Sterilization Container Storage

Figure 12.33

- Additional labor may be required since the containers must be cleaned between uses. This may also affect washer loads if a mechanical washer is used. (See **Figure 12.34**)

- Latching mechanisms on containers create potential problems. When latches and welds break, the containers cannot be used. Also, sharp edges can injure employees.

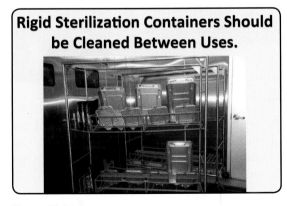

Rigid Sterilization Containers Should be Cleaned Between Uses.

Figure 12.34

- Filter retention plates may become dislodged and contaminate instruments. *Note: Some manufacturers have addressed this potential problem by modifying or changing the design of the container's filter retention plate.*

Cleaning and Inspection Procedures for Rigid Containers

To clean a rigid sterilization container, first remove its disposable filters or release its filter protector/holder. Valve-type closures must be cleaned according to the manufacturer's written instructions. Interior baskets must be removed and cleaned. Dividers/pins may need to be removed if they interfere with the cleaning process.

Cleaning and rinsing instructions provided by the container manufacturer should be followed. Particular attention should be given to the type of detergent used. For example, some containers cannot be exposed to certain chemicals, such as high alkaline solutions.

Inspection should also focus on the top and bottom valve or filter mechanism and the latching mechanism. For example:

- The filter retention plate should be intact and not bent; the retention plate should seat over the filter and securely lock into place.

- The retention post should be secure and not move.

- If using disposable filters, they should be checked for holes prior to placing in the container. (See **Figure 12.35**) Filters should fit the space allotted, with no folding or crimping of edges. Filter material must be approved for the type of sterilization to be used.

Check Filters Before Use

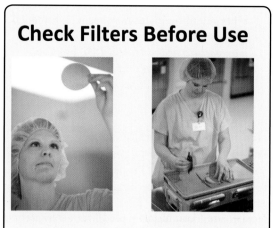

Figure 12.35

- If using reusable valves, they should be clean and debris free, with no breaks or chips in the valve mechanism. (See **Figure 12.36**) Valves should fit securely and not move once seated.

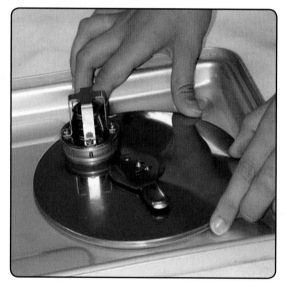

Figure 12.36

- The lid gasket should be clean and free of cracks and nicks. There should be no ridges on the gasket. *Note: Ridges are caused by a tight fit between the top and bottom of the container.* (See **Figure 12.37**)

Check Gaskets for Cleanliness, Damage and Signs of Wear

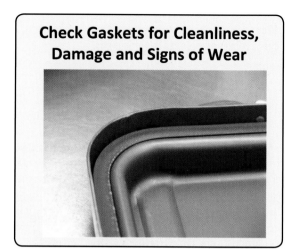

Figure 12.37

- Rivets in the handle area should be checked to ensure that they are secured and not separating from the container. If loosened, they can become a safety hazard and a pathway for entry of bacteria.

- Handles should move up and down easily. Ensure the latch springs are in place. (See **Figure 12.38**)

Check Handles for Function and Cleanliness

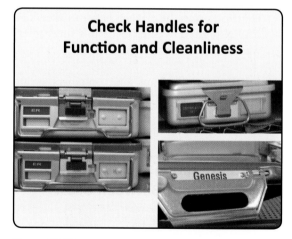

Figure 12.38

As noted earlier, the weight of instruments placed in the container is an important concern. The number of instruments placed in the tray must not exceed the quantity that can be effectively sterilized and dried.

Rigid containers should be carried by both of their handles (not by the lid) to avoid breaking the container's seal or damaging the instruments inside.

DISPOSABLE PACKAGING MATERIALS

Disposable (nonwoven) materials were introduced as "engineered fabrics" in the 1940s, and have made their way into everyday life. Coffee filters, teabags, vacuum cleaner bags and disposable diapers are all examples of "engineered fabrics" (also referred to as disposable nonwoven materials). These materials are used in both disposable flat wraps and rigid container filters. (See **Figure 12.39**) Before using, both disposable flat wraps and rigid container filters should be inspected for tears or holes that may have occurred during transport and handling. These materials are a popular choice for sterilization packaging because they have excellent barrier effectiveness and can be discarded after use. There are three types of disposable packaging materials in common use: paper, polyolefin plastic and disposable nonwoven wraps.

> ### Important Note: Be Aware of Packaging Expiration Dates
>
> Some disposable packaging materials contain expiration dates from the manufacturer. It is important to check for an expiration date prior to using any disposable packaging material. Since the expiration date usually indicates a decrease in the packaging's ability to perform at optimal standards, including microbial barrier properties.

Papers are commonly used as sterilization packaging materials. It is important to ensure that the paper packaging is intended for use as sterilization packaging, and that it has been approved by the FDA. *Note: Papers containing cellulose cannot be used in hydrogen peroxide or ozone sterilizers because cellulose absorbs the sterilant and reduces penetration. As this occurs, the contents being sterilized may not be exposed to the proper amount of sterilant.*

Disposable, nonwoven materials play a significant role in sterilization packaging.

Flat Wrap

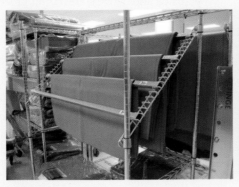

Rigid Container Filters

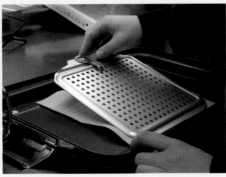

Figure 12.39

Kraft-type papers (medical grade) are generally smooth surfaced, and they are available in sizes to accommodate many medical devices, and porous or soft-good items. Pouches of medical-grade papers specially formulated for sterilization are also available. Pouches with both sides consisting of Kraft-type paper can be used to hold small parts and instruments inside the instrument sets. (See **Figure 12.40**)

Example of Kraft-type Paper Pouches

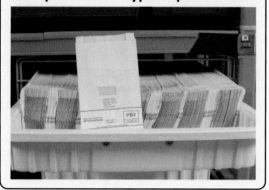

Figure 12.40

Kraft-type papers (also known as crepe paper) can also be purchased as flat wraps. These products may be utilized in steam and EtO sterilization but cannot be used with hydrogen peroxide or ozone sterilization.

Paper/plastic and spunbond polyolefin-plastic combinations (called peel packs or peel pouches) are the most commonly-used packaging materials for small instruments and lightweight items. (See **Figure 12.41**) They are called peel-pouches because after they are sealed, they must be peeled open for aseptic opening.

There are two basic types of combination peel pouches:

- Paper/plastic combinations – These are typically acceptable for use with steam and EtO sterilization processes.

Example of a Peel Pouch

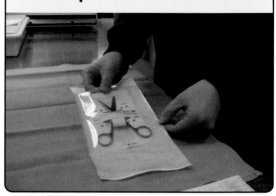

Figure 12.41

They are not compatible with hydrogen peroxide or ozone sterilization. As suggested by their name, they have a paper side and a plastic side. The plastic side allows visibility of the package contents, and the paper side allows sterilant penetration. *Note: Sterilant cannot enter through the plastic side, so proper positioning is important to achieve sterilization.*

- Spunbond polyolefin-plastic combinations (Sometimes referred to as Tyvek® pouches) - These are used for hydrogen peroxide and ozone sterilization. Like paper/plastic combinations, they have a plastic side, so package contents are visible. The other side is composed of polyolefin that contains no cellulosic materials and is, therefore, compatible with hydrogen peroxide and ozone sterilization processes.

Important Note: Use Caution When Selecting Peel Pouches.

Paper/plastic and spunbond-polyolefin packages look alike. Paper/plastic combinations are not compatible with hydrogen peroxide and ozone sterilization and spunbond-polyolefin combinations will melt in high-temperature processes, such as steam sterilization.

Flat wraps are another commonly-used packaging material. Instead of inserting objects into a ready-made pouch and sealing it, flat wrap requires the user to "create" a barrier package using specific folding techniques. (See **Figure 12.42**)

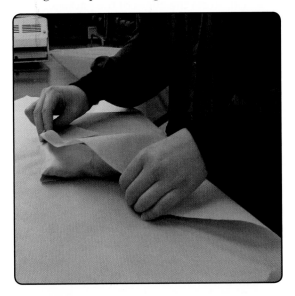

Figure 12.42

One nonwoven packaging material, spunbond-meltblown-spunbond (SMS), is a popular flat wrap. It is made by a process in which polyolefin layers (synthetic materials softened by heat and hardened by cooling) are exposed to high heat and are pressure-bonded together to form sheets. Flat wrapping products constructed of nonwoven SMS fabrics for sterilization wrapping are designed as single-use disposable products, and must never be reused. These materials are available in a range of weights and a wide variety of sizes. Flat wraps are also available as single- or double-sheet wraps that are bonded together.

The use of each packaging material has advantages and disadvantages. CS technicians must ensure that they select the type of packaging most suitable for the item(s) being packaged and the type of sterilization selected. CS technicians can then begin preparing the package contents for packaging and the sterilization process to follow.

WRAPPING TECHNIQUES

Peel Pouching Techniques

Peel pouches are usually used for smaller, lightweight items. They are also useful when it is important to see the contents of the package, such as when a description of the contents is difficult to view on the label. Peel pouches are available on rolls that allow CS technicians to cut off the length desired for each package, and they are also available in precut sizes. Inserts or tip protectors help to protect a pouch's contents from damage and prevent the tips from penetrating the package. If inserts or tip protectors are used, ensure that the material is appropriate for the type of sterilization method to be used, and that it is nontoxic and free of non-fast dyes. (See **Figure 12.43**)

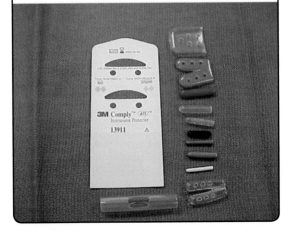

Figure 12.43

Before placing items in the peel pouch, carefully inspect the pouch to ensure there are no tears or holes. Items should be placed in the pouch, so the end of the item to be grasped during presentation (i.e., Finger rings of an instrument) will be presented first when the package is opened at the point of use. *Note: This is the chevron end for pre-made pouches.* **Figure 12.44** illustrates the chevron end of a pre-made pouch. It is designed in a manner that makes it easier to open. This reduces the risk of product contamination during aseptic opening.

Instrument tips should always face the plastic side of the package to avoid penetrating the paper side and contaminating the contents.

Hinged instruments must be packaged in a manner to keep the instrument open for sterilization. This can be accomplished by using commercially-purchased products.

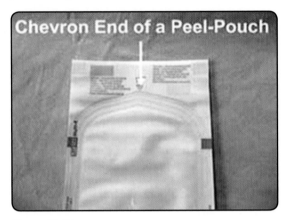

Figure 12.44

Pouches must be sized and applied properly to allow for adequate air removal, sterilant penetration and drying.

To allow space for package contraction and proper circulation, leave about one inch ($^{1}/_{4}$" per side of the package) of space between the items in the pouch and the sealed edges. When packaging is too small, the packaged instruments cause stress on the sides of the pouch. (See **Figure 12.45**) Stress compromises the package's barrier and will likely rupture the side seams of the package during the harsh air removal and heat-up phases of the steam sterilization process, or the high vacuum phase of the hydrogen peroxide sterilization process. Items placed in packages that are too small can also rupture the seams during normal handling and transportation. Pouches should not be too large because movement of the items inside the pouch may result in the contents sliding from end to end or side to side. The excessive movement of the contents could break seals or puncture the pouch's paper. (See **Figure 12.46**) Pouches should not be over-filled because this can cause the paper to

tear, or the seals to rupture during sterilization or handling. (See **Figure 12.47**)

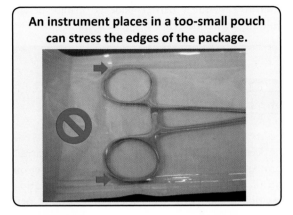

Figure 12.45

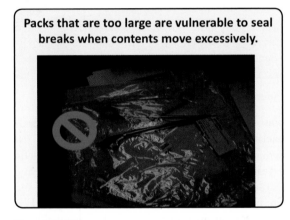

Figure 12.46

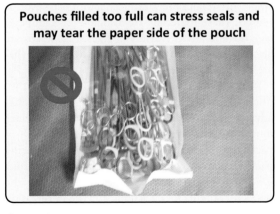

Figure 12.47

Trapped air acts as a barrier to heat, moisture and sterilant penetration, so it is important to remove as much air as possible before sealing. To remove trapped air, gently push the pouch's top and bottom layers together just prior to sealing. *Note: Applying too much pressure can damage the pouch.*

Paper/plastic pouches must only be labeled on the plastic side or on areas specifically provided by the manufacturer (e.g., on fold-over paper flap seals). Writing on the paper side of the pouch will cause damage to the package, which may not be noticeable, but which may compromise the barrier protection. Use only pens approved for writing on the plastic surface and approved for the sterilization method to be used. Using the wrong type of pen such as a ballpoint pen can damage the packaging.

Pouches must be closed using a tamper-evident seal, so there is no danger of packages being opened and resealed for later use. After a sterile package is opened, it is contaminated, and may not be resealed and reused.

Common ways that paper/plastic and polyolefin-plastic packages can be used to meet specific packaging needs include:

• Wrap within a pouch – Sometimes (usually to accommodate unique sterile presentation issues) it is desirable to place a single wrapped package into pouch. The initial wrap is done using the flat wrap packaging and wrapping method. It is not necessary to seal the wrapped item. The wrapped item is then inserted into the appropriately sized pouch. The pouch should be sealed and labeled. *Note: The manufacturer's IFU for both the peel pouch and the flat wrap must be reviewed to see if this process*

is approved. Using this method if not approved by both manufacturers could result in an unsterile product.

• Double pouches – While double pouching is not necessary for sterility maintenance, it may be required for aseptic presentation of multiple items or for instruments having more than one part. Double pouches are prepared by placing the item(s) into one paper/plastic pouch and sealing it. This pouch is then placed inside another slightly larger pouch and sealed. (See **Figure 12.48**) Care is needed when selecting the appropriate sequential sizing. The same rules apply for the inside peel pouch as for pouching instruments (leave about one inch—$^1/_4$" per side of the package). Never fold the inner pouch because this can interfere with air removal and sterilant penetration. (See **Figure 12.49**) Place the smaller inner package paper side to paper side and plastic side to plastic side to help ensure sterilant penetration, drying and content visibility.

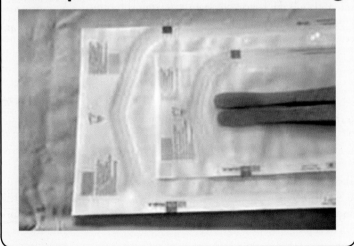

Example of Double Peel Pouching

Figure 12.48

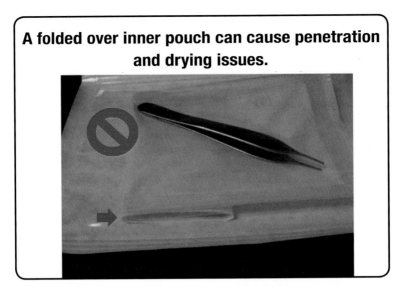

A folded over inner pouch can cause penetration and drying issues.

Figure 12.49

Flat Wrapping Techniques

Flat wrapping procedures are primarily used for large packages, but they may also be used for smaller items. They involve use of either reusable woven textiles (linens) or disposable nonwoven wraps.

There are two methods of using flat wrapper packs:

- Sequential – The package is wrapped twice and is "a package within a package." The term "sequential" indicates that the contents have been wrapped in sequence (one after the other). This method is used for muslin, Kraft-type paper and single layers of SMS wraps.

- Simultaneous – The package is only wrapped once, but it requires a special double-layered synthetic nonwoven material bound on two or four sides.

The advantage of sequential wrap is that it affords a "second chance" for sterile presentation. The disadvantages: sequential wrap requires more time for wrapping and unwrapping.

The advantage of simultaneous wrap is reduced labor costs and increased output in the CS and OR. The disadvantage is that the absence of the second

layer removes the "second chance" aspect during aseptic opening/presentation.

There are also two techniques for wrapping packages and both are used with the sequential and simultaneous wrap methods:

- Square fold – This is also called the in-line or parallel fold; it is most frequently used for larger packs and instrument trays.

- Envelope fold – This is more commonly used for individual items, small packs and most instrument sets.

Regardless of the packaging system used, flat wrappers should be inspected for holes and tears prior to use. Wraps must be free from holes, tears, abrasions or any other deviations that could allow bacteria to enter the package.

CS technicians are responsible for creating a package that will protect the contents, allow for sterilization and allow for aseptic opening from flat sheets of wrapping material. This requires that every package be created according to specific protocols. The following photos illustrate the proper techniques for sequential and simultaneous wrapping in both the envelope and square styles.

Figures 12.50 through **12.60** illustrate sequential wrapping techniques using the envelope style. In this method, flat wraps are applied one after the other (in sequence).

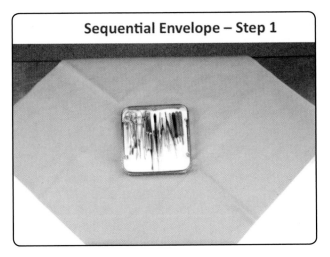

Sequential Envelope – Step 1

Figure 12.50

With the sequential envelope technique, the wrap is placed on the table to form a diamond shape. The item to be wrapped is placed in the center of the wrap, parallel with the edge of the table.

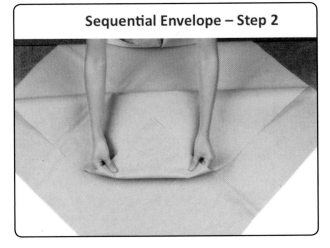

Sequential Envelope – Step 2

Figure 12.51

The lower corner is brought up to completely cover the contents and the tip is folded back on itself to form a flap. This flap may be used later to assist with opening the pack aseptically.

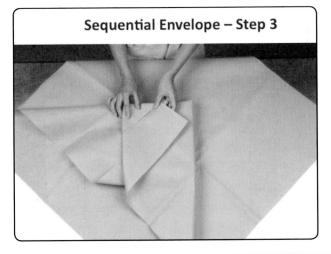

Sequential Envelope – Step 3

Figure 12.52

Fold the left corner over the contents and fold the tip back to form a flap. Ensure the entire tray/pack is covered with this fold.

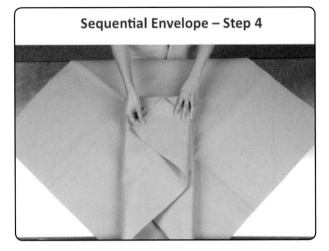

Figure 12.53

Fold the right corner over the left fold and fold the tip back on itself to form a flap. Ensure the entire tray/pack is covered with this fold.

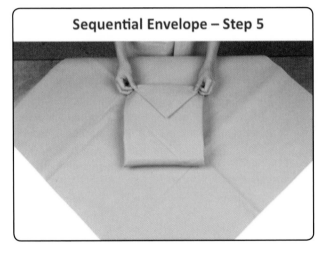

Insert Figure 12.54

Bring the top corner down over the contents and tuck the corner under the right and left folds, leaving a small tab visible for easy opening.

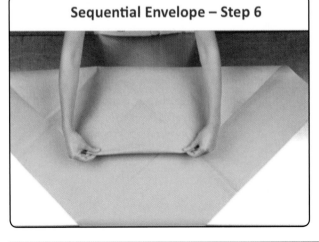

Figure 12.55

The second wrap is applied by placing the single wrapped item into the center of the remaining wrap and then repeating the wrap sequence to form a package within a package.

The lower corner is brought up to cover the single wrapped item and the tip is folded back on itself to form a flap.

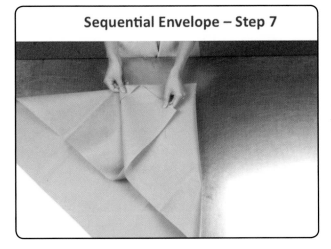

Sequential Envelope – Step 7

Figure 12.56

Fold the left corner over the single wrapped item and fold the tip back to form a flap. Ensure the entire tray/pack is covered with this fold.

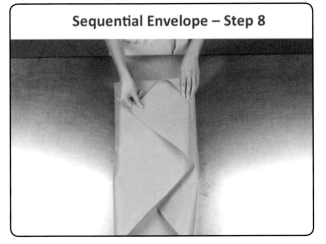

Sequential Envelope – Step 8

Figure 12.57

Fold the right corner over the left fold and fold the tip back on itself to form a flap. Ensure the entire tray/pack is covered with this fold.

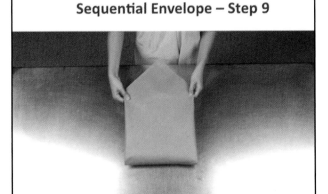

Sequential Envelope – Step 9

Figure 12.58

Bring the top corner down over the single wrapped item.

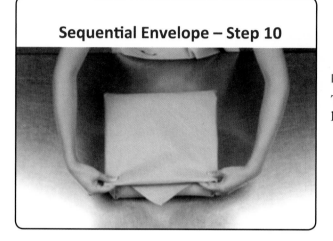

Figure 12.59

Tuck the corner under the right and left folds, leaving a small tab visible for easy opening.

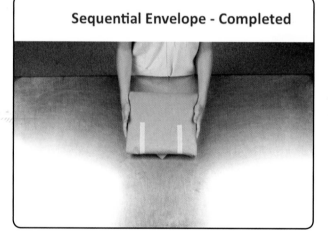

Figure 12.60

The package is then secured with indicator tape to complete the wrap process.

Figures 12.61 through **12.70** illustrate sequential wrapping techniques using the square style. This method is primarily used for large packs.

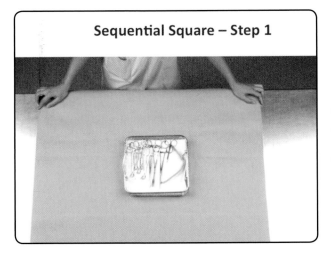

Sequential Square – Step 1

Figure 12.61

The edge of the wrapper is placed parallel with the table.

The instrument tray is placed square in the center of the wrapper parallel with the edge of the wrapper.

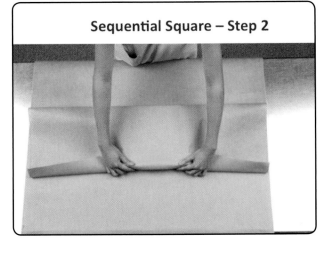

Sequential Square – Step 2

Figure 12.62

The edge of the wrapper is folded over the top of the contents. The edge is then folded over itself to form a cuff. This cuff will facilitate aseptic opening of the pack when used. Ensure the entire tray/pack is covered with this fold.

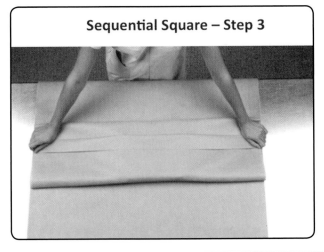

Sequential Square – Step 3

Figure 12.63

The upper edge of the wrap is brought down over the contents and folded back on itself to form another cuff overlapping the original cuff. Ensure the entire tray/pack is covered with this fold.

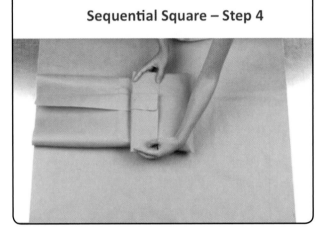

Figure 12.64

The left edge of the wrapper is folded over the pack and back onto itself to form a cuff. Ensure the entire tray/pack is covered with this fold.

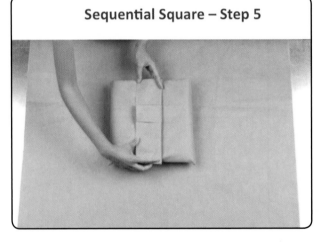

Figure 12.65

The right side of the wrapper is folded over the pack, overlapping the previous fold and folded back to form a cuff. Ensure the entire tray/pack is covered with this fold.

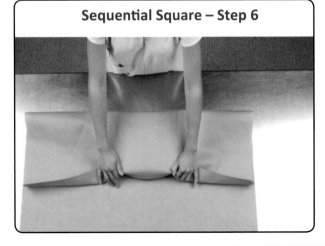

Figure 12.66

The second wrap is applied by placing the single wrapped item into the center of the wrap and repeating the steps performed for the first wrap to create a package within a package.

The edge of the second wrapper is folded over the single wrapped item. The edge is then folded back over itself to form a cuff. Ensure the entire tray/pack is covered with this fold.

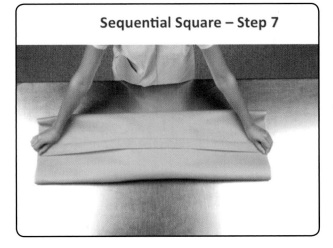

Sequential Square – Step 7

Figure 12.67

The upper edge of the wrap is brought down over the single wrapped item and folded back onto itself to form another cuff overlapping the original cuff. Ensure the entire tray/pack is covered with this fold.

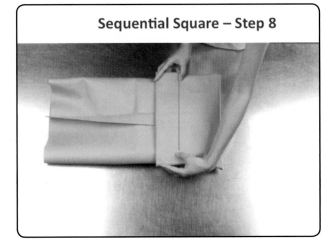

Sequential Square – Step 8

Figure 12.68

The left edge of the wrapper is folded over the pack and back onto itself to form a cuff. Ensure the entire tray/pack is covered with this fold.

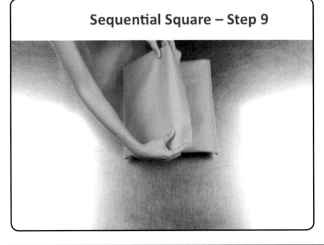

Sequential Square – Step 9

Figure 12.69

The right side of the wrapper is folded over the pack overlapping the previous fold and folded under. Ensure the entire tray/pack is covered with this fold.

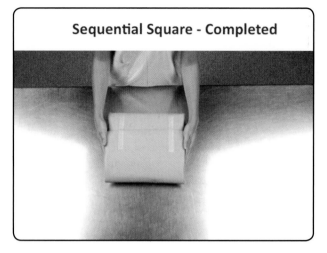

Figure 12.70

The package is secured with indicator tape.

Simultaneous wrapping uses two layers of synthetic nonwoven material, such as SMS bound on two or four edges. Since the material is already double layered, the contents are only wrapped once. Both methods are acceptable, although one may be more appropriate for specific situations.

Figures 12.71 through **12.77** illustrate simultaneous wrapping techniques using the envelope style. In this method, flat wraps are applied together.

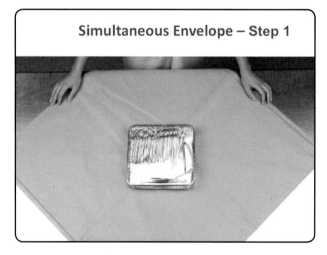

Figure 12.71

With the envelope simultaneous technique, one application of simultaneous wrap is placed on the table surface in diagonal or diamond format. Simultaneous wrap is two sheets of wrap bonded together.

Center the instrument tray between the right and left edges of the wrap.

Simultaneous Envelope – Step 2

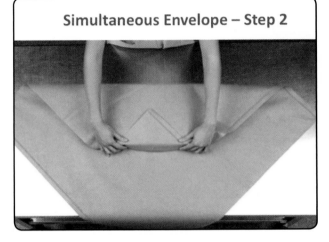

Figure 12.72

Bring the bottom corner of the wrap up and over to completely cover the instrument tray.

Fold the tip back onto itself to form a flap. This flap is used later to assist in opening the pack aseptically.

Simultaneous Envelope – Step 3

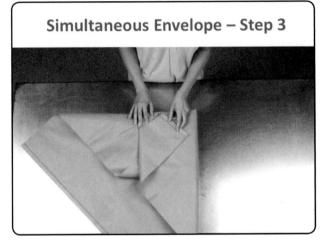

Figure 12.73

Fold the left corner over the contents and fold the tip back to form a tab. Ensure the entire tray/pack is covered with this fold.

Simultaneous Envelope – Step 4

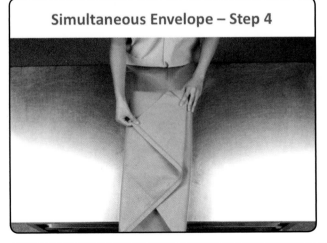

Figure 12.74

Fold the right corner over the left fold and fold the tip back onto itself to form a tab. Ensure the entire tray/pack is covered with this fold.

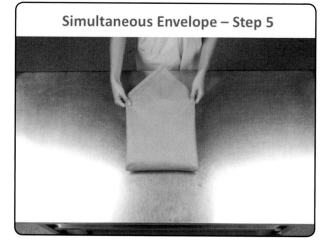

Simultaneous Envelope – Step 5

Figure 12.75

Bring the top corner down over the contents and fold it toward the body.

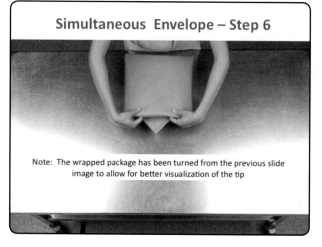

Simultaneous Envelope – Step 6

Note: The wrapped package has been turned from the previous slide image to allow for better visualization of the tip

Insert Figure 12.76

Tuck the corner under the right and left folds. A small tab may be incorporated for easy opening.

Ensure the wrap is not too tight or too loose; either way compromises the effective sterilization of the package contents.

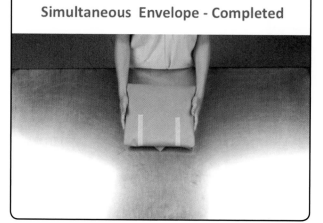

Simultaneous Envelope - Completed

Figure 12.77

The package is then secured with indicator tape to complete the wrap process.

Figures **12.78** through **12.83** illustrate simultaneous wrapping techniques using the square style. This method is primarily used for large packs.

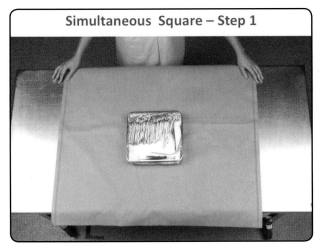

Simultaneous Square – Step 1

Figure 12.78

With the simultaneous square technique, place one application of simultaneous wrap—that is, two sheets of wrap specially bonded together —on the table surface in a rectangular- or square-shaped format.

Center the instrument tray between the left and right edges of the wrap.

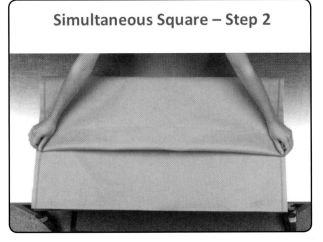

Simultaneous Square – Step 2

Figure 12.79

The edge of the wrapper is folded over the top of the contents covering the entire item. The edge is then folded back over itself to form a cuff. This will facilitate aseptic opening of the pack when used.

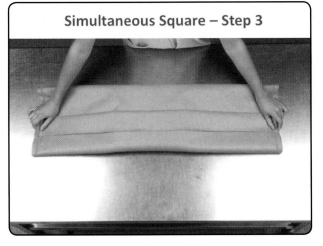

Simultaneous Square – Step 3

Figure 12.80

The upper edge of the wrap is brought down over the contents and folded back onto itself to form another cuff over lapping the original. Ensure the entire tray/pack is covered with this fold.

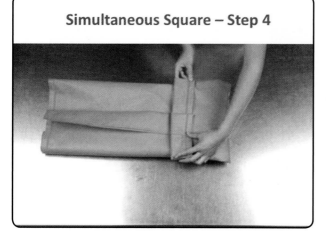

Simultaneous Square – Step 4

Figure 12.81

The left edge of the wrapper is folded over the pack and folded over itself to form a cuff. Ensure the entire tray/pack is covered with this fold.

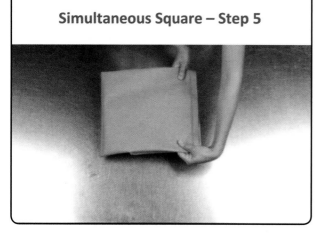

Simultaneous Square – Step 5

Figure 12.82

The right side of the wrapper is folded over the pack overlapping the previous fold. Ensure the entire tray/pack is covered with this fold.

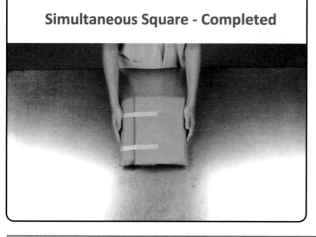

Simultaneous Square - Completed

Figure 12.83

To complete the wrap process, the final fold is tucked under and secured with indicator tape.

Choose the properly-sized wrap for either method. The wrapper must be large enough to completely contain the contents without leaving excess material that could inhibit sterilant penetration and release. Wrappers must be snug, but not so tight as to impede sterilant entry or exit. If the wrapper will also be used to create a sterile field, it must be of sufficient size to extend at least six inches below the edge of the surface being covered.

METHODS OF PACKAGE CLOSURE

Overview

The purpose of a package closure is to seal the package securely, maintain the sterile integrity of the contact area during transport and storage, and prevent resealing if the package is opened or the seal is compromised.

Only approved closure methods should be used to seal a sterile package. There are several types of package closures and CS technicians must ensure they use the appropriate packaging method.

Acceptable Closure Methods

Several methods of package closure are acceptable for use:

- Tapes designated as "indicator tapes" are considered best practice because they are

made specifically to withstand sterilization, and change color after being exposed to the sterilization process. They do not, however, provide proof that adequate sterilization of package contents has occurred. Indicator tapes or indicator stickers that change color after exposure should be used on every package to avoid mixing processed and unprocessed packages. (See **Figure 12.84**)

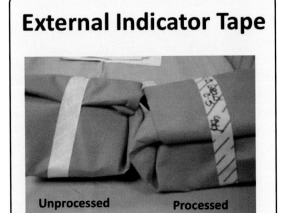

External Indicator Tape

Unprocessed   Processed

Figure 12.84

- Specially manufactured elastomer bands or similar closures are only acceptable if the manufacturer of the wrap material explicitly recommends their use. If recommended, care

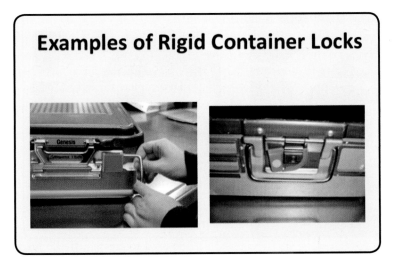

Examples of Rigid Container Locks

Figure 12.85

is needed to select the properly-sized bands that allow a snug fit, without creating excessive wrinkles or folds in the fabric that may reduce the effectiveness of sterilant penetration. If bands are used, the label or indicator stickers should be placed in a way that any attempt to remove the band will damage the band and reveal the compromised status of the pack. *Note: Band applications are designed for specific packaging methods and should only be used as recommended by the specific manufacturer.*

- Rigid container systems have tamper-evident seals, which are secured to the outside of the container and lock the top and bottom of the container together. (See **Figure 12.85**) Ensure the locks are securely in place prior to sterilization. Rigid container seals are designed to break when the seal on the container has been broken. The most common types are plastic components that lock in place and must be broken to open the container. Small bands that tighten as they react to heat during sterilization can also be placed on certain types of rigid containers and these will break when the seal of the container is broken.

- Heat sealing is a peel pouch closure method. There are several varieties of heat sealers available. (See **Figure 12.86**) The manufacturer of the sealer and/or pouch material must verify that the two are compatible. If they are not, the seal may not bond, or there may be burn-through; both actions will compromise the seal. Multiple-band or wide-band heat sealers should be used to reduce the possibility of an incomplete seal. The manufacturer's instructions for temperature settings, applied pressure and contact times should be written into procedures and always be followed.

The package is placed inside the jaws of the heat sealer, and the two sides are fused together. Be sure to follow the heat sealer and packaging manufacturers' instructions to ensure appropriate exposure times and temperatures. Inadequate exposure times or temperatures may cause inadequate seals and those that exceed recommendations may cause package damage. CS technicians should use extra caution when operating heat sealers to avoid burns.

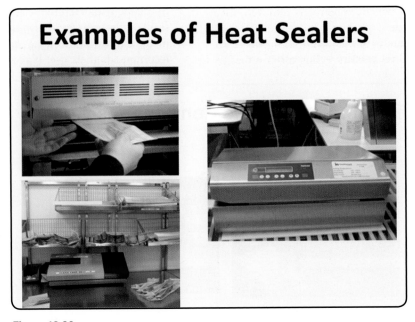

Examples of Heat Sealers

Figure 12.86

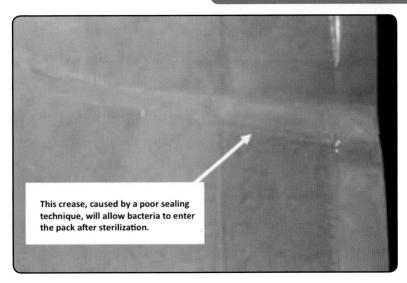

This crease, caused by a poor sealing technique, will allow bacteria to enter the pack after sterilization.

Figure 12.87

Heat seals must be observed for bubbles and creases. (See **Figure 12.87**)   Seals that are not smooth and complete will allow bacterial contamination after sterilization.

- Self-adhesive seals. Some paper/plastic and polyolefin-plastic packages contain self-adhesive seals that do not require heat. An adhesive portion is covered with a removable strip at one end of the self-adhesive sterilization pouch. When it is removed, that portion of the seal should be carefully folded over the opening of the package. **Figure 12.88** shows a CS technician sealing a self-adhesive sterilization pouch. Care must be taken to avoid gaps, wrinkles or creases which compromise the seal integrity for both heat-seal and self-seal closure systems.

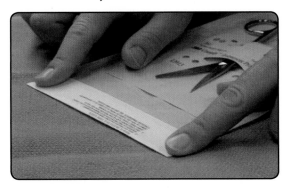

Figure 12.88

- Sealing tape is sometimes used to secure pouch openings. Care is needed to ensure that the seal is secure, without compromising gaps. Proper taping technique includes the folding of corners, so the side edges of the top corners are parallel to the bottom edge of the pouch. Ensure that the plastic is folded onto the plastic (not paper-to-paper), so sterilant access is not impeded. Then fold the open bottom edge over the folded corners. Seal with tape overlapping the edge of the pouch by about $1/4$ inch. Observe carefully to ensure that there are no gaps, creases or wrinkles, and that the tape has completely covered the pouch's open edge and is securely attached to the plastic.

Do Not Use!

Several package closure methods are never appropriate:

- Do not use safety pins, staples or other sharp objects to seal packages. Punctures create holes that allow contamination. Even the smallest space (hole) is large enough to allow bacteria to pass.

- Do not use paper clips or binding clips. They can be removed and replaced without evidence of barrier compromise.

- Avoid using tapes that are not designed specifically to withstand the rigors of sterilization.

CS technicians must use closure methods specifically designed for the packaging material that is chosen. They must also check the seals on all packages before dispensing them to user units. Any seals that appear to have been broken or opened should not be issued or used. (See **Figure 12.89**)

PACKAGE LABELING

It is essential that all packages be labeled before sterilization. The label must be complete and accurate to ensure that the correct packs are selected and opened.

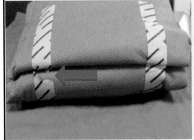
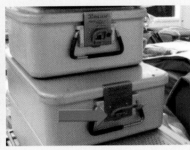

Examples of Broken Seals

Figure 12.89

Label information should include the following:

- Description of package contents.

- Initials of package assembler/packager.

- Lot control number.

- Identification of sterilizer and cycle to be used.

- Date of sterilization (unless contained in the lot control number).

- Assigned storage location.

- The requesting department or the surgeon's name may also be included on the label for special request items.

Standardized abbreviations and terms help avoid confusion. Slang terms and nicknames should not be used. Labeling is necessary for the end user and also for sterilization processing, quality assurance, stock rotation and inventory control purposes. Correct labeling is also critical in the event of a sterilization load recall.

CS technicians with the responsibility for labeling packages must use clear, legible handwriting and accurate descriptions. Confusion caused by an illegible or inaccurate package label can compromise patient safety because items may be misplaced, or the label may be misread and incorrectly dispensed. Either situation can cause a delay in patient care and treatment.

Labeling should be documented on label-sensitive tape; flat wraps and peel pouches; commercially-available, pre-printed, adhesive labels; in-house computer-generated labels (See **Figure 12.90**); or on the plastic side of a peel pouch.

Note: Do not write directly on flat wrap packaging material.

For pouches, the labels or written information should not be placed on the paper or spunbond polyolefin side, as they may inhibit the microbial barrier properties.

Approved felt tip pens are generally used for marking, but they should be indelible, non-bleeding, nonfading and nontoxic, and able to withstand the sterilization method used.

Printed Pack Labels

Computerized instrument systems generate labels that are easy to read and contain barcodes for tracking.

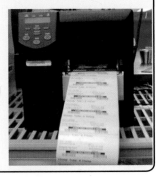

Figure 12.90

Examples of Peel Pouch Loading Racks

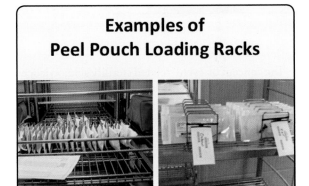

Figure 12.91

Special Packaging Concerns

Several basic packaging concerns require special mention:

- All packaging materials should be held at a temperature between 68°F to 73°F (20°C to 23°C), and at a relative humidity ranging from 30% to 60% for a minimum of two hours prior to sterilization. This will permit adequate sterilant penetration and prevent super heating of the product during sterilization.

- Packaging procedures should be performed only by the department responsible for sterilization. Other departments (e.g., OR, Delivery Room, Emergency Department, and X-ray) whose personnel might prepare and package their own instruments and supplies before sending them to CS for sterilization should be discouraged from this practice. Often, CS technicians do not know about all items in the package, and it could be processed inappropriately. Also, supplying packaging materials to each of these departments is not cost effective. If a facility does allow instrument preparation outside the CS department, personnel must receive training on the proper methods of processing those devices.

- Paper/plastic pouches should be positioned in the sterilizer standing on edge in loading racks, or they should be placed in baskets specifically designed for these packages. They can also be held on edge by an alternate means (e.g., a peel pouch rack or tray pins), (See **Figure 12.91**) and they must be properly spaced. Pouches should be loosely spaced in the basket to ensure the sterilant can reach the breathable paper side of each pouch, as the plastic side is not penetrated by air, steam or other sterilants. Arrange the pouches paper-to-plastic in a perforated or mesh bottom tray.

- Paper/plastic pouches should not be placed inside wrapped trays or containers.

- All packaging systems must be handled with care. Although they provide protection and a barrier for medical devices, they are not impenetrable and can be compromised by rough handling and contact with sharp surfaces. There are several devices on the market to help protect larger trays from damage, such as tears in wrap. Facilities may choose to use those devices if they are experiencing issues with wrap integrity. (See **Figure 12.92**)

- Observe pouch contents and outside packaging of flat wrap or containerized instruments for moisture after sterilization and again prior to storage. Remember: Steam condenses on a metal's surface when heat is transferred to the metal. This condensation can allow contamination of the contents. Prevention of

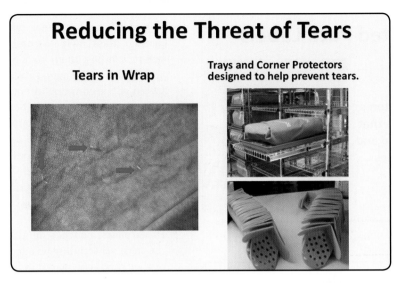

Reducing the Threat of Tears

Tears in Wrap

Trays and Corner Protectors designed to help prevent tears.

Figure 12.92

condensation is only possible when sterilizers with heated dry cycle capabilities are used; however, limiting sterilizer contents and following good loading practices can usually prevent the problem.

- All sterilized packages, whether sterilized by the facility or purchased as sterile, ready-to-use products, should be inspected to ensure the packaging material and/or the seals have not been compromised prior to placing into sterile storage, prior to dispensing and prior to opening the package.

Sterility Maintenance

Sterilized packages must maintain their content sterility until opened.

Traditionally, the sterility of a package has been thought of as "**time-related**." That is, the package was considered sterile until a specific expiration date was reached. Then the package was taken out of inventory and processed. The Joint Commission (TJC) and the Association of periOperative Registered Nurses (AORN) now recognize sterility as "**event-related**."

The concept of event-related sterility acknowledges that microbial contamination of a sterile package is caused by an event, such as improper handling or transport, rather than by time alone. For example, one may purchase a carton of milk at the grocery store with an expiration date that is several days away; however, if he/she forgets to put the carton of milk in the refrigerator, it will become warm and sour. Even though the milk had an expected shelf-life, an "event" happened that caused its shelf life to be shortened.

Event-related sterility depends on the quality of the wrapper material, handling procedures, storage and transport conditions, and the number of times the package is handled before use.

By closely controlling the environment and events to which a sterile package is exposed, rather than just the time the package is in storage, the probability of package contamination can be minimized.

Note: Expiration dates on commercial products must be adhered to as they reflect product usability or stability, rather than sterility of the contents. Packages that contain dated products must be labeled with the earliest expiration date.

Event-related sterility will be fully discussed in Chapter 16.

> **Sterility (time-related)** A package is considered sterile until a specific expiration date is reached.
>
> **Sterility (event-related)** Items are considered sterile unless the integrity of the packaging is compromised (damaged) or suspected of being compromised (damaged), regardless of the sterilization date. This is sometimes referred to as ERS.

Sterility Maintenance Covers

Protective plastic overwraps (called dust covers or sterility maintenance covers) can be applied to packages after sterilization to protect the package from dust, moisture and other contaminates. (See **Figure 12.93**) The plastic material should be at least 2 to 3 mil thick. Steam-sterilized items must be thoroughly cooled and dried, and EtO-sterilized items must be aerated before they are overwrapped in plastic. The seal of the dust cover should be secured with either a heat seal or security-tape sealing process. The overwrap should be clearly marked as a "dust cover" or "protective overwrap" to prevent its use as part of the sterile field. Protective overwraps are not to be placed in the sterilizer; they should be placed over properly cooled, presterilized items only.

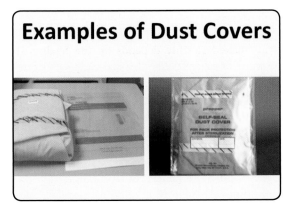

Examples of Dust Covers

Figure 12.93

There are basic protocols for applying a dust covercover; however, specific manufacturer instructions should always be followed:

- Perform hand hygiene prior to handling the sterile package.

- Dust covers must be applied as soon as the package is cool enough to do so. Placing items in dust covers after an extended period of time may place potential contaminates in a perfect environment for microbial growth.

- Select a dust cover slightly larger than the item to be packaged.

- Carefully place the sterile item inside the dust cover; ensure the sterile package label is visible. Gently compress the package to remove air and seal the dust cover.

Note: The expiration date of any item in a dust cover is not extended by placing the item in a dust cover.

CONCLUSION

Medical devices and supplies used in patient treatment and care are made of various materials and configurations. No single assembly method or packaging system meets all requirements for packaging and sterilization of all devices. Central Service technicians must understand assembly and packaging concepts, and follow best work practices for preparing packages to help ensure that devices dispensed for patients are functional and safe.

RESOURCES

Association for the Advancement of Medical Instrumentation. *ANSI/AAMI ST79:2013. Comprehensive guide to steam sterilization and sterility assurance in healthcare facilities.* Sections 8, 10.5 and 10.6.

Association of periOperative Registered Nurses. *Recommended Practices for Cleaning and Caring for Surgical Instruments and Powered Equipment.* Standards, Recommended Practices, and Guidelines. 2014.

Association of periOperative Registered Nurses. *Guidelines for PeriOperative Practice: Packaging Systems.* Guidelines for PeriOperative Practice. 2015

Truscott W. *SSI Prevention Pointers from Industry.* Infection Control Today. 2010.

CENTRAL SERVICE TERMS

Assembly area

Super heating

Wicking materials

Chemical indicators (CIs)

Process challenge device (PCD)

Tamper-evident seals

Muslin

Rigid container system

Wet pack

Sterility (time-related)

Sterility (event-related)

Chapter 13
Point-of-Use Processing

Learning Objectives

As a result of successfully completing this chapter, readers will be able to:

1. Define the term Immediate Use Steam Sterilization and review the industry standards

2. Describe point-of-use processing and examine its requirements

3. Explain the basic procedures necessary to safely perform Immediate Use Steam Sterilization

4. Address point-of-use processing for heat-sensitive medical devices

INTRODUCTION

The majority of processing takes place in the Central Service (CS) department; however, there are times when processing is performed at the point of use. There are two basic types of **point-of-use processing**. The first is **Immediate Use Steam Sterilization (IUSS)**, which consists of cleaning, steam sterilization and immediate delivery of heat-resistant items to the procedure room. This process is designed for instances when there is no time to send the item(s) to the CS department for processing. The second type of point-of-use processing is designed for heat-sensitive items. Regardless of the process used, the goal is to provide an item that is safe for patient use. This chapter will examine methods of point-of-use processing.

> **Point-of-use processing** That which occurs when a medical device is processed immediately before use, and/or close to the patient care area.
>
> **Immediate Use Steam Sterilization (IUSS)** Process designed for the cleaning, steam sterilization and delivery of patient care items for immediate use; formerly known as flash sterilization.

IMMEDIATE USE STEAM STERILIZATION

A Brief History

In patient care, there are always unexpected events that require quick action. Instrument demands become urgent when there is an immediate patient need and no instruments are ready for use. In previous years, "flash" sterilization was designed for use in the Operating Room (OR) for emergencies and immediate use. Flash sterilization was a process where unwrapped instruments were steam-sterilized using an abbreviated cycle (a cycle with no dry time) in order to ready the instruments for patient use.

In 2009, the name flash sterilization was replaced with a new term (and process): Immediate Use Steam Sterilization (IUSS). Items processed using IUSS are cleaned according to their manufacturers' Instructions for Use (IFU), placed in containers specifically designated for IUSS sterilization and

sterilized according to manufacturer instructions. (See **Figure 13.1**)

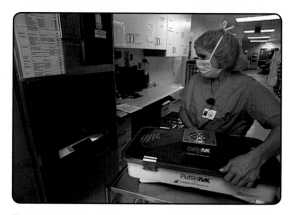

Figure 13.1

> ### What Happened to "Flash"?
>
> Many Central Service professionals will remember the term "flash" sterilization and may ask what happened to that term. "Flash" referred to the abbreviated steam sterilization cycle of an unwrapped device. With the move to Immediate Use Steam Sterilization (IUSS), the process shifted from an unwrapped container to a sealed containment device that provides greater protection from contamination during transport.

Processing devices for immediate use can be safe and effective, but only if all steps recommended by the device manufacturer are followed. This includes proper cleaning, decontamination, sterilization using the correct cycle and aseptic transfer to the point of use. Those performing IUSS are responsible for processing every item in a way that best ensures it is safe for reuse. Shortcuts, such as improper cleaning in the interest of saving time, can jeopardize patient safety. Following validated manufacturer's IFU and controlling process quality helps protect patients from infections and prolongs the life of instrumentation.

A multi-society IUSS Position Paper providing information about the change to IUSS was developed in 2011 by the Association for the Advancement of Medical Instrumentation

(AAMI), the Association of periOperative Registered Nurses (AORN), the International Association of Healthcare Central Service Materiel Management (IAHCSMM), the Accreditation Association for Ambulatory Health Care, ASC Quality Initiative and the Association of Surgical Technologists (AST). The paper provided support for the change to IUSS and offered additional information about the process.

Standards and Recommended Practices

Several associations have developed standards to help ensure IUSS procedures are performed properly.

Association for the Advancement of Medical Instrumentation

AAMI standards are not law; however, they are the recognized industry standards for sterilization and may be relevant in any legal proceeding. AAMI standards represent a national consensus and many have been approved by the American National Standards Institute (ANSI).

ANSI/AAMI ST79, *Comprehensive guide to steam sterilization and sterility assurance in health care facilities,* is a broad document covering recommended practices for steam sterilization. The document states that IUSS can be performed when deemed appropriate, and when all of the following conditions are met:

- Items are needed for immediate use.

- Items are dissembled and thoroughly cleaned according to the manufacturer's IFU, with approved detergents and water to remove soil, blood, body fats and other substances.

- Lumens are brushed and flushed under the water with appropriate cleaning solutions, and items are thoroughly rinsed.

- The device manufacturer's written instructions on sterilization cycle and exposure times, temperature settings and dry times are followed.

- Processed items are transported in a manner to prevent contamination.

The Association of peri-Operative Registered Nurses

AORN publishes its Guidelines for Perioperative Practices, formally titled Perioperative Standards and Recommended Practices. Surveying agencies refer to the AORN guidelines, as well as the AAMI standards. AORN guidelines state that:

- IUSS should be kept to a minimum and should only be used in selected clinical situations and in a controlled manner.

- IUSS should only be used when there is no time to process the items using the preferred (wrapped) method.

- Devices undergoing IUSS should be subjected to the same decontamination processes as in AORN's *Guidelines for PeriOperative Practice: Sterilization and Disinfection.* Guidelines for PeriOperative Practice. 2015.

- The items must have manufacturer's instructions for IUSS.

- Manufacturer's recommendations for cleaning, exposure times, temperatures and drying times are followed.

- Processed items are transferred to point of use aseptically.

- Staff is educated on the IUSS process.

- Recordkeeping allows for the tracking of the device after use.

Surveying Agencies

IUSS is designed for urgent situations when there is not sufficient time to send an item through the normal **terminal sterilization** process. Surveying agencies are closely monitoring IUSS to ensure everything is being done by the healthcare facility to decrease this practice and ensure that where and when IUSS is practiced, the processes are done correctly.

> **Terminal sterilization** The process by which surgical instruments and medical devices are sterilized in their final containers, allowing them to be stored until needed.

The Joint Commission

In 2009, The Joint Commission (TJC) revised its position statement on IUSS and emphasized that three critical steps of processing must be followed to ensure sterility. TJC requires that complete documentation must be available for each IUSS cycle, so the device is traceable to the patient if a problem should arise. In the recent past, TJC focused on how many IUSS cycles were run and how to reduce the amount of IUSS sterilization in any facility. Now, in addition to focusing on IUSS reduction, TJC surveyors are focusing on the IUSS process to ensure all processes are completed properly. They expect the same safeguards and quality controls to be in place, regardless of who operates a sterilizer or where the sterilizer is located. The following are the four key areas TJC surveyors will focus their attention:

- Cleaning and decontamination. Before an item can be sterilized, it must be properly cleaned and decontaminated according to the manufacturer's recommendations.

- Sterilization. The manufacturer's instructions must specify the type of cycle (e.g., gravity displacement and dynamic air removal) and length of time needed for sterilization. Some instruments may require an extended cycle or a specified dry time; some instruments cannot undergo IUSS at all. The manufacturer's IFU must specify that the item can undergo IUSS cycles.

- Transfer to the sterile field. Aseptic transfer from the sterilizer to the sterile field is required to prevent recontamination of the sterilized item.

- Frequency of IUSS use. Lack of instrumentation is not an excuse for IUSS. A plan should be in place to reduce IUSS cycles.

Examples of TJC findings could include failure to adequately clean the instruments before IUSS, inappropriate use of chemical indicators and unsafe transporting of instruments back to the procedure room after they have been sterilized.

Centers for Medicare and Medicaid Services

The Social Security Act mandated the establishment of minimum health and safety standards that must be met by providers and suppliers participating in Medicare and Medicaid programs. These standards are found in the 42 Code of Federal Regulations. The Secretary of the Department of Health and Human Services has designated the Centers for Medicare and Medicaid Services (CMS) to administer the standards compliance aspects of these programs.

Like TJC, CMS has established requirements regarding the use of IUSS:

- The same multi-step process used to prepare instruments for terminal sterilization must be completed for IUSS.

- Parameters for all phases of the sterilization cycle must be determined by consulting the IFU for the instrument(s), sterilizer and containment device.

- Each IUSS cycle must use physical monitors and chemical indicators. At least weekly, the sterilizer must be tested with a biological test for each IUSS cycle.

- If IUSS must be used for an implant, a tracking system should be in place to trace the IUSS load to the patient.

- Medical instruments and devices processed using IUSS must be contained in a packaging system labeled for the IUSS cycle(s) used.

- Items sterilized by IUSS must be used immediately.

CMS also indicates that IUSS is not acceptable in the following circumstances:

- When sterilizing implants, except in documented emergency situations.

- For post-procedure decontamination of instruments used on patients with possible Creutzfeldt-Jakob Disease (CJD) or other prion diseases.

- When devices or loads have not been validated for the specific cycle used.

- On single-use devices.

PROCEDURES FOR IMMEDIATE USE STEAM STERILIZATION

Safe and effective IUSS requires that all steps in the process be done properly each and every time to achieve sterilization and maintain sterility of instruments and instrument sets all the way to the point of use. Improperly sterilized or contaminated instruments used in a surgical procedure can result in serious concerns, from surgical site infections to increased costs and legal liability.

Precleaning

Precleaning of instrumentation is a necessary step to help promote effective, thorough decontamination and sterilization. AORN guidelines state that items should be kept free of gross soil during surgery. These standards are critical factors when items are to be prepared for IUSS. Soil is easier to remove when items are properly pre-treated in the OR.

Point-of-Use Decontamination

Thorough decontamination of medical devices is required for IUSS to be safe and effective. Manufacturers of sterilizers and medical devices assume that the level of contamination has been adequately reduced on the surfaces of instruments before they are placed in the sterilizer. **If items are not properly cleaned, they cannot be sterilized.**

Standard precautions require that staff handling contaminated devices wear the appropriate personal protective equipment (PPE). This includes gloves, hair covering, eye protection, masks, fluid-impervious gown or jumpsuit, and shoe covers. PPE should be removed and discarded, and not worn outside of the cleaning/decontamination area.

Manufacturer instructions for instrument processing should be available and consulted to ensure proper cleaning and decontamination before IUSS. These may contain special cleaning instructions, such as the disassembly process and the recommended use of cleaning solutions and mechanical cleaners. Instruments must be cleaned as thoroughly at the point of use as they would in the CS decontamination area. Items must be decontaminated in an area designed to clean instruments, and never in a scrub or handwashing sink. Surveying agencies will check to ensure that the staff is trained in proper cleaning methods.

Prior to placing instruments in the sterilizer, instruments must be carefully inspected to ensure they are clean and functional. Instruments must be placed in the sterilizer in a manner that facilitates full steam contact.

Immediate Use Steam Sterilization Cycles

Steam sterilizers used for IUSS are usually placed in close proximity to user areas. (See **Figure 13.2**) There are two types of steam cycles commonly used: gravity displacement and dynamic air removal, which includes the prevacuum and steam flush pressure pulse (SFPP) cycles. The type of cycle to be used depends on the manufacturer's IFU. **Figure 13.3** shows minimum IUSS cycles as identified by AAMI. *Note: Steam sterilization processes are discussed in detail in Chapter 14.*

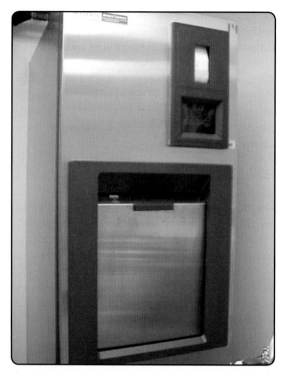

Figure 13.2

Consult the manufacturer's IFU for exposure times and cycles when using containment devices or packaging systems.

Safe Transport after Immediate Use Steam Sterilization

Instruments subjected to IUSS should be transported to the point of use in a manner that reduces the potential for contamination. Failure to take appropriate measures to protect IUSS processed instruments after their removal from the sterilizer and during transport to the point of use will increase the potential for contamination and the patient's risk for acquiring a surgical site infection. *Note: Use of the single wrapped method helps protect sterile instruments; however, this method cannot be used unless the sterilizer has the "single wrapped" function built into the system.* Utilizing sealed rigid containers approved for IUSS offers the best protection for the sterile instruments. Instruments processed in these rigid containers still cannot be stored for later use, unless approved by the U.S. Food and Drug Administration (FDA); therefore, the items must be used as soon as possible after the sterilization cycle is complete.

Staff Education

Educating staff members who perform IUSS is important to decrease the possibility of errors that could occur during the process. Staff members should receive initial training and competency assessment, followed by continuing education at regular intervals to review and update their knowledge.

QUALITY CONTROL MONITORS FOR IMMEDIATE USE STEAM STERILIZATION

The efficacy of every sterilization cycle must be monitored. The quality assurance of each process includes physical, chemical and biological monitors. All of these monitors should be carefully watched and reviewed to identify potential issues.

AAMI Minimum Recommended IUSS cycles			
Type of sterilizer	**Load configuration**	**Temperature**	**Time**
Gravity displacement	Nonporous items only (e.g., routine metal instruments, no lumens)	270°F (132°C)	3 minutes
	Nonporous and porous items (e.g., rubber or plastic items, items with lumens) sterilized together	270°F (132°C)	10 minutes
Prevacuum	Nonporous items only (e.g., routine metal instruments, no lumens)	270°F (132°C)	3 minutes
	Nonporous and porous items (e.g., rubber or plastic items, items with lumens) sterilized together	270°F (132°C)	4 minutes
Steam-flush pressure-pulse	Nonporous or mixed nonporous/porous items Manufacturers' instructions	270°F (132°C)	4 minutes

Figure 13.3

Note: Sterilization monitoring processes are discussed in Chapter 17.

A dynamic air removal test, as the name implies, is only done in dynamic air removal sterilizers. This test should be run each day the sterilizer is used.

Recordkeeping

IUSS records allow for traceability of every item sterilized to the patient. It is important to keep accurate and complete records that include evidence of cycle performance, such as sterilization cycle printouts and biological and chemical indicator results. Sterilizer cycle records should include:

- Patient identification. There must be a way to identify the patient on whom the items were used in the event of a problem, such as sterilization cycle failure or the patient acquiring a healthcare-associated infection.

- The sterilizer and sterilizer cycle identification.

- The instrument(s) sterilized in the cycle.

- The cycle parameters.

- The reason the IUSS cycle was run (e.g., instrument dropped on floor).

- Operator's signature or other identification.

No national standard exists for how long sterilization records should be kept. Local statute requirements and individual facility policies should be followed.

POINT-OF-USE PROCESSING FOR HEAT-SENSITIVE DEVICES

Low-Temperature Disinfection and Sterilization Processes

Advancing sterilization technologies have changed the way procedures are performed. The medical devices used in many procedures have changed, as well. Many of the medical devices used today are heat sensitive. In other words, processing them in

a heated process, such as with steam, will lead to damage. Facilities must look to low-temperature methods to safely process those heat-sensitive items.

There are several types of low-temperature options for point-of-use processing. Selection is determined by the types of items that will be processed and their compatibility with that low-temperature process.

In some cases, the decision to process heat-sensitive items at point of use is made in an effort to reduce instrument turnaround time. In others, it is made to reduce the distance that unwrapped processed items must be transported before use.

The choices for point-of-use processing for heat-sensitive medical devices include high-level disinfection (HLD) or sterilization. The level of biocidal process required is based on the intended use of the item. Options include wrapped processes (e.g., vaporized hydrogen peroxide or hydrogen peroxide gas plasma) where the device is packaged and processed through a type of chemical sterilization cycle, or an unwrapped process where the device is processed using a liquid chemical. (See **Figure 13.4**)

Note: The wrapped sterilization processes mentioned above are discussed in detail in Chapter 15.

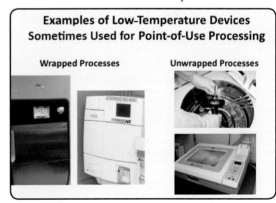

Examples of Low-Temperature Devices Sometimes Used for Point-of-Use Processing

Wrapped Processes   Unwrapped Processes

Figure 13.4

All low-temperature processes utilize a chemical process. CS technicians must understand the specific type of process used in their facility and must be educated on proper handling and operational procedures, as well as safety protocols for the specific process.

Preparation of Devices for Low-Temperature Processes

As with IUSS processes, proper preparation is critical to the success of the low-temperature point-of-use process. Items must be cleaned thoroughly. Any soil remaining on the device will result in a failed process and will pose a danger to the patient. Items must be prepared for the low-temperature process according to the manufacturer's IFU.

If using a wrapped process, items must be wrapped using packaging that is compatible with the process to be used. Those packages must be positioned correctly within the sterilizer.

When using an unwrapped process, technicians must also be certain to position the device correctly. Any connections between the device and the processor must be appropriately connected to ensure the proper flow of liquid through the device.

As with all HLD and sterilization processes, the medical device manufacturer must have approved the device for the specific biocidal process to be performed.

Quality Control Monitors for Point-of-Use Low-Temperature Processes

Quality control monitors will vary depending on the process used; however, there are some commonalities:

- The process must be monitored

- Items processed must be logged

Monitoring will be unique to each low-temperature process. For manual HLD using a soak process, the solution must be checked for Minimum Effective Concentration (MEC).

For mechanical processes, testing should be performed according to the equipment and chemical manufacturer's IFU. That testing may include chemical, biological or diagnostic tests.

All items processed at point of use must be logged and those records, along with documentation of quality testing, should be kept on file.

CONCLUSION

Point-of-use processing meets a specific need in procedural areas. Although it is performed away from the Central Service department, the basic principles of reprocessing and the need to accurately follow the device manufacturers' instructions remain the same. When performed appropriately, point-of-use processing can provide items that are safe for patient use.

RESOURCES

Association of periOperative Registered Nurses. *Guidelines for PeriOperative Practice: Sterilization and Disinfection*. Guidelines for PeriOperative Practice. 2015.

The Joint Commission. The Joint Commission Accreditation Manual. 2013.

Centers for Disease Control and Prevention. *Guidelines for Disinfection and Sterilization in Healthcare Facilities*. 2008.

AAMI, AAHSP, AORN, APIC, ASCQC, AST, IAHCSMM. Statement on Immediate Use Steam Sterilization. 2011.

Association for the Advancement of Medical Instrumentation. ANSI/AAMI ST79: *Comprehensive Guide to Steam Sterilization and Sterility Assurance in Healthcare Facilities*. 2013.

PeriOperative Practice: Sterilization and Disinfection. Guidelines for PeriOperative Practice. 2015

Gillespie S. Flash Sterilization: Many Users, Many Questions About This Technique. Biomedical Instrumentation & Technology. Vol. 44, No. 1. (p 62). 2010.

Nania P. Immediate Use Steam Sterilization: It's All About the Process. AORN Journal. Vol. 98, No. 1. 2013. (pp. 32-38).

Rutala W, Weber D. Guideline for Disinfection and Sterilization in Healthcare Facilities. Centers for Disease Control and Prevention. 2008.

U.S. Department of Health and Human Services, Centers for Medicare and Medicaid Services. Ref: S&C:14-44-Hospital/ CAH/ASC. 2014. http://www.cms.gov/Medicare/Provider-Enrollment-and-Certification/SurveyCertificationGenInfo/ Downloads/Survey-and-Cert-Letter-14-44.pdf (Accessed 10-1-14).

Conner R. Sterile Processing in the Surgical Suite, 2014 FGI Guidelines Series, Update #4, September 2014.

CENTRAL SERVICE TERMS

Point-of-use processing

Immediate Use Steam Sterilization (IUSS)

Terminal sterilization

Chapter 14

High-Temperature Sterilization

Learning Objectives

As a result of successfully completing this chapter, readers will be able to:

1. Discuss factors that impact the effectiveness of sterilization

2. Discuss the advantages of steam sterilization

3. Explain the anatomy of a steam sterilizer and identify the function of each major component

4. Provide basic information about the types of steam sterilizers

5. Explain basic information about steam sterilizer cycles

6 Describe the conditions necessary for an effective steam sterilization process

7. Explain basic work practices for steam sterilization

8. Review sterilization process indicators and explain the need for quality control

INTRODUCTION

High-temperature sterilization is the process of choice in many healthcare facilities. It is achieved by subjecting items being processed to thermal energy from moist heat (steam) or dry heat. High-temperature sterilization has long been recognized as an effective way to kill microorganisms. Steam is the most frequently-used sterilant for devices not adversely affected by moisture or heat because of its successful record of safety, efficacy, reliability and low cost. In fact, other methods are only used when the object being processed cannot withstand the heat and/or moisture required for steam sterilization. By contrast, dry heat sterilization is seldom used because of the required lengthy exposure times.

As with all sterilization methods, devices to be processed must first be thoroughly cleaned, decontaminated and properly prepared. Cleaning involves the removal of all visible soil and decontamination kills most, but not all, microorganisms. Sterilization is required to kill any remaining microorganisms, including spores.

Sterilization failure could result in serious, even life-threatening, patient outcomes. A Central Service (CS) technician must understand the anatomy of a steam sterilizer to better understand how it operates, and how it impacts quality outcomes and patient safety.

FACTORS THAT IMPACT STERILIZATION

The success of every sterilization process is not guaranteed. Several factors and conditions impact the effectiveness of all sterilization methods, including those using high temperature. These factors include:

- The type of microorganisms present; some microorganisms are more resistant to the sterilization process than others.

- The design of the medical device; complex devices present a challenge to the sterilization process.

- The number of microorganisms (**bioburden**) present; when there are more microorganisms on a medical device, the sterilization process becomes more difficult.

- The amount and type of soil present; soil acts as a shield to protect microorganisms.

Note: The cleaning process is absolutely essential as a first step in processing. A device can be cleaned without sterilizing, but sterilization cannot be achieved if a device hasn't been thoroughly cleaned.

> **Bioburden** The number of microorganisms on a contaminated object; also called "bioload" or "microbial load."

ADVANTAGES OF STEAM STERILIZATION

Steam is the sterilant of choice for several reasons:

- Low cost

- Rapid sterilization cycles

- Relatively simple technology

- Leaves no chemical residues or byproducts

Steam sterilizers date back to the early days of formalized healthcare. Prior to steam sterilization, boiling water was commonly used to kill bacteria. Scientists recognized the need to increase temperatures beyond the boiling point to kill greater numbers of heat-resistant bacteria. **Figure 14.1** is an illustration of the first pressure steam sterilizer (autoclave) that was developed in 1880 by Charles Chamberlain, a colleague of Louis Pasteur. The autoclave resembled a pressure cooker and was able to use pressurized steam to reach temperatures of 248°F (120°C) and higher. Although it looks primitive by today's standards, it was the first generation model of the steam sterilizers used today.

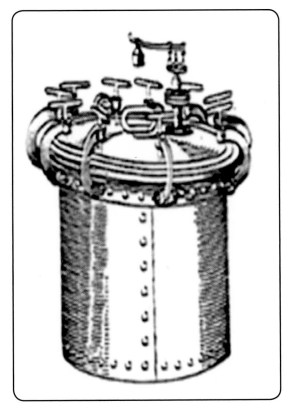

Figure 14.1

ANATOMY OF A STEAM STERILIZER

Steam sterilizers come in many sizes and cycle choices, from small tabletop sterilizers used primarily in clinic and dental settings, to mid-sized and large units designed to sterilize large quantities of items. **Figures 14.2**, **14.3** and **14.4** illustrate various sizes of steam sterilizers.

Tabletop Sterilizers

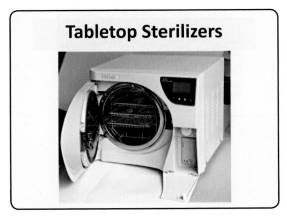

Figure 14.2

Cart and Carriage Loading Sterilizers

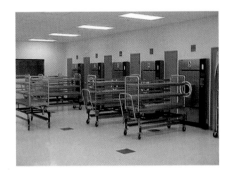

Figure 14.3

Floor Loading Sterilizer

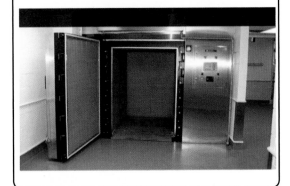

Figure 14.4

A CS technician must know the anatomy of a sterilizer to better understand how it operates.

Components of Steam Sterilizers

Jacket

CS departments typically use jacketed sterilizers. The illustration in **Figure 14.5** shows a cutaway diagram of a steam sterilizer and illustrates how steam from an external source enters the jacket. In most hospitals, steam is supplied to the sterilizers from a main steam line; these units themselves do not generate the steam. Smaller sterilizers in clinics and dental practices usually manufacture their own steam or get their steam from an independent generator. **Figure 14.6** provides an example of a steam generator.

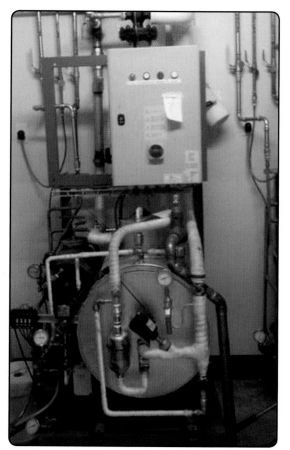

Figure 14.6

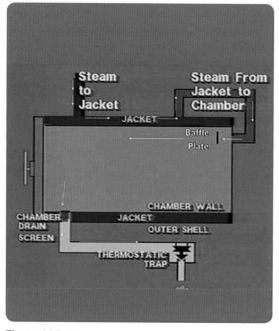

Figure 14.5

The interior chamber walls of the sterilizer are heated by steam in the metal jacket. This helps minimize the amount of condensation (moisture) that forms when hot steam contacts the chamber walls as a cycle begins. **Figure 14.7** shows the condensation that forms during the steam cycle. The jacket surrounds the sides, top and bottom of the vessel, and steam circulates in this space to pre-heat the interior chamber walls.

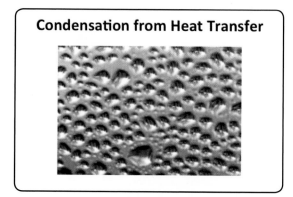

Condensation from Heat Transfer

Figure 14.7

The outside of the jacket is covered with insulation to help prevent condensation from forming on the jacket's outer and inner walls. This insulation also provides a safety feature because it reduces the likelihood that personnel working behind the sterilizer will be burned. The outer shell is typically located behind a wall and is not readily visible to the sterilizer technician. **Figure 14.8** shows the insulation covering the sterilizer jacket.

The door gasket is designed to maintain a tight seal that prevents steam from escaping from the chamber and air from entering the chamber. (See **Figure 14.9**)

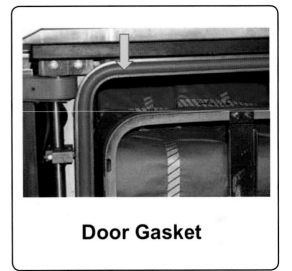

Door Gasket

Figure 14.9

On most steam sterilizers, the chamber drain is located at the front or center of the floor. The drain screen must be cleaned at least daily, and more often, as needed. Debris in the chamber drain screen can impede cycle performance. (See **Figure 14.10**)

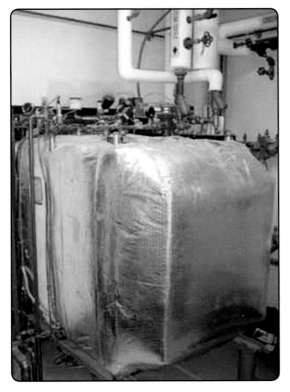

Figure 14 .8

Door, Gasket and Chamber Drain

The door is the weakest part of a steam sterilizer. It has a safety locking mechanism that automatically activates when chamber pressure is applied and it can only be unlocked when pressure is exhausted. Some model sterilizers use radial arm locking doors, which can be tightened, but not loosened, while the chamber is under pressure. Some sterilizers have active gaskets with pressure behind them to seal the chamber.

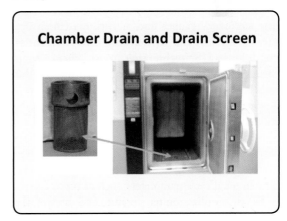

Chamber Drain and Drain Screen

Figure 14.10

Thermostatic Trap

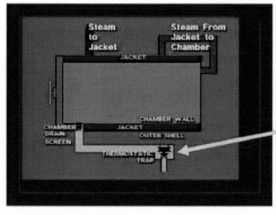
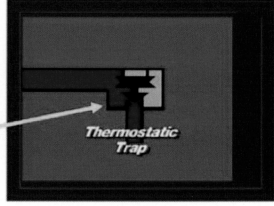

Figure 14.11

Thermostatic Trap

As seen in **Figure 14.11**, the thermostatic trap is located in the drain line. The drain and the area surrounding it are the coolest areas in the sterilizer. A sensor in the chamber drain measures steam temperature and automatically controls the flow of air and condensate from the sterilizing chamber.

Gauges and Controls (Monitors)

The sterilizer's gauges and/or controls (monitors) provide a visual and written record of sterilization conditions. CS technicians must check them throughout the sterilization cycle to ensure that necessary parameters are met. A printout from a steam sterilization cycle usually contains the following information:

- Date and time the cycle began.

- Selected cycle parameters, such as type of cycle, sterilization temperature and dry times.

- A written record of actual cycle activities (e.g., temperatures, exposure times and pressure). Some steam sterilizers can also provide the information in a digital format (see **Figure 14.12**), and some can even be integrated into an instrument tracking system. Older

steam sterilizers have circular patient charts that record sterilization activities. Charts are changed daily and the time listed on the chart is aligned with the recording pen to the correct time of day. The date and sterilizer location are noted on the graph, and the pens are checked daily to ensure they are recording. Charts or printouts are signed by the sterilizer operator, indicating that parameters have been reviewed.

The CS technician is responsible for determining if all sterilization parameters were met and if the load may be released. If any steam sterilization parameter was not met, the supervisor should be notified immediately and the sterilization load should not be released.

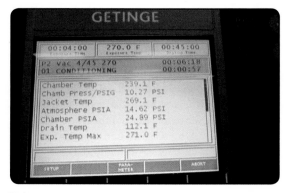

Figure 14.12

TYPES OF STEAM STERILIZERS USED IN CENTRAL SERVICE

Several types of steam sterilizers are available today. Healthcare facilities purchasing sterilizers that will meet their specific needs, including chamber size, style and available cycle options.

Tabletop Sterilizers

Tabletop sterilizers are frequently used in clinics and dental offices. These units operate by having water poured into the sterilizer, either through a port or the bottom of the chamber, and are electrically heated until the water turns to steam. Water quality is an important factor, and is specified in the sterilizer Instructions for Use (IFU). In a tabletop sterilizer cycle steam rises to the chamber's top and as more steam is produced, air is forced out through the drain near the bottom of the chamber. When steam enters the drain, a thermostatic valve closes, which causes the steam to build up pressure until the operating temperature is reached. When the proper temperature is reached, the timer is activated. At the end of the cycle, the relief valve opens to allow the steam to escape. The steam passes through the water reservoir where it condenses back to water. After the pressure has dropped to zero, the door can be opened. As with all sterilizers, CS technicians should carefully review the sterilizer manufacturer's IFU for specific operating instructions.

Gravity Air Displacement Sterilizers

Some small- to medium-sized sterilizers have gravity displacement and dynamic air removal cycles. In a gravity displacement cycles, steam enters the chamber and because air is heavier than steam, the steam forces the cooler air to the bottom of the chamber and out the drain. While their operation appears simple, many mistakes can be made, such as improper loading or unloading; therefore, a thorough knowledge of sterilization theory and practice is essential for those operating these units. Gravity air displacement sterilizers have sophisticated automatic controls, such as temperature-indicating charts and printouts for recordkeeping.

Dynamic Air Removal Sterilizers

Dynamic air removal sterilizers are similar in construction to gravity air displacement sterilizers, except there is a vacuum pump or water ejector. That removes air from the chamber more effectively during the preconditioning phase, prior to reaching the exposure temperature. Dynamic air removal sterilizers usually operate at higher temperatures [270°F to 275°F] (132°C to 135°C) than gravity sterilizers. The preconditioning phase increases the speed of operation and reduces the chance of air pockets in the chamber during the cycle. Dynamic air removal sterilizers use different types of preconditioning methods for air removal. These include variations of prevacuum air removal and above-atmospheric-pressure processes, such as the steam–flush pressure–pulse process (SFPP). The preconditioning cycle removes air from both the sterilizing chamber and the load before the chamber is pressurized with steam to the exposure temperature. Effective air removal is critical for steam penetration.

Prevacuum Steam Sterilizers

In prevacuum steam sterilizers, the dynamic air removal cycle depends on one or more pressure and vacuum sequences at the beginning of the cycle to remove air during the preconditioning phase. Typical operating temperatures are 270°F to 275°F (132°C to 135°C). To ensure air removal in these sterilizers, the integrity of the sterilizers should be checked daily by processing a Bowie Dick (or daily air removal) test. *Note: Bowie Dick air removal tests are outlined in Chapter 17.* Some sterilizers have an automatic cycle (vacuum leak test) to test the vacuum tightness of the chamber.

Steam-Flush Pressure-Pulse Sterilizers

SFPP sterilizers use a repeated sequence of a steam flush and pressure pulse to remove air from the sterilizing chamber and processed materials. Air removal occurs above atmospheric pressure; no vacuum is required. Like a prevacuum sterilizer, this process rapidly removes air from the sterilizer's chamber and wrapped items.

Immediate Use Steam Sterilizers

Immediate use steam sterilizers are located in Operating Rooms (ORs) or surgical suite substerile rooms, Labor & Delivery units and special procedure areas that perform invasive procedures. Their intended use is for the emergency sterilization of instruments when there is not enough time for terminal sterilization. These types of sterilization processes have little to no dry time; therefore, at the end of the sterilization process, instrumentation is expected to be hot and wet. **Figure 14.13** is an example of a sterilizer approved for IUSS cycles.

STEAM STERILIZER CYCLES

Along with understanding the types of steam sterilizers used in the healthcare facility, CS technicians must also understand how these machines function. To begin, CS technicians should be familiar with two basic sterilization cycles: IUSS sterilization and terminal sterilization. Items processed using IUSS must undergo the same cleaning and preparation as items that are terminally sterilized. Time is usually shortened due to the reduced dry cycle. All items do not have IUSS instructions from the device manufacturer; consult the medical device manufacturer's IFU to determine if IUSS is possible and to learn the proper sterilization cycle. Items sterilized using IUSS should be used immediately and cannot be stored for use at a later time, unless such a process has been approved by the U.S. Food and Drug Administration (FDA).

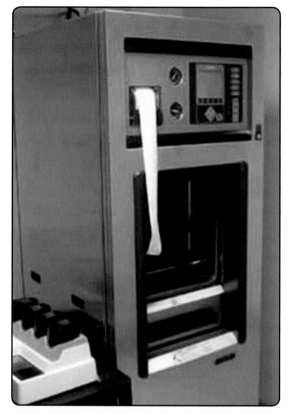

Figure 14.13

By contrast, "terminal sterilization" refers to the sterilization of an item that is expected to be dry upon completion of the sterilization process. Terminal sterilization is most often performed in the CS department, but may be performed in other departments.

A saturated steam sterilization cycle has at least three (and possibly four) phases:

- Conditioning

- Exposure

- Exhaust

- Drying (in most instances)

Conditioning

At the beginning of the sterilization cycle, steam enters at the upper back portion of the sterilizer. As steam enters, air is displaced through the drain. As steam continues to enter the sterilizer's chamber, pressure begins to rise, as does the steam temperature.

Exposure

After the desired temperature is reached, the sterilizer's control system begins timing the cycle's exposure phase. *Note: The instrument manufacturer's IFU should be consulted for the specific time and temperature for each instrument/set sterilized to ensure the cycle is appropriate.*

Exhaust

At the end of the exposure phase, the chamber's drain is opened and the steam is removed through the discharge line. This creates a void in the chamber; filtered air is gradually reintroduced into the chamber and the chamber gradually returns to room pressure.

Figures **14.14** through **14.17** provide illustrations of the conditioning, exposure and exhaust phases in the steam sterilization process.

Figure **14.14** shows (in red) steam entering the chamber, and air being displaced (in green) down the chamber's drain.

Steam Passes through the Thermostatic Trap

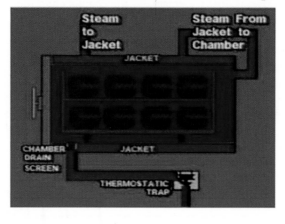

Figure 14.15 shows (in red) steam that has passed the chamber drain screen and travels past the thermostatic trap.

Closed Thermostatic Trap

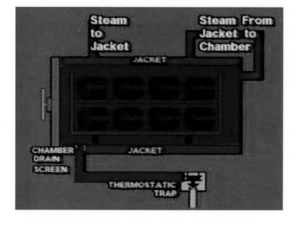

Figure 14.16 shows (in red) the thermostatic trap being closed after the desired temperature is reached.

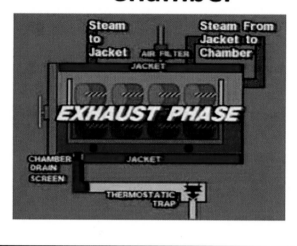

Steam is Exhausted from the Chamber

Figure 14.17 shows (in red) steam being exhausted from the sterilizer.

Drying

Drying begins at the conclusion of the exhaust phase. Dry times are based on the device, packaging and the sterilizer's IFU. At the end of this dry time, the end-of-cycle signal sounds and the door may be opened.

CONDITIONS NECESSARY FOR EFFECTIVE STEAM STERILIZATION

Regardless of the type of steam sterilization method used, the same four conditions (contact, temperature, time and moisture) must be met.

Contact

The most common reason for sterilization failure is the lack of contact between steam and the entire surface of the device being sterilized. This failure may be related to human error or mechanical malfunction. Frequent causes of steam contact failure include:

- Failure to adequately clean the object being sterilized. Any coating of soil, such as protein or oils, can protect the microorganisms from direct steam contact.

- Sets that are too dense or instruments positioned in a way that does not allow steam contact.

- Packages wrapped too tightly. If packs are wrapped too tightly, air becomes trapped and cannot escape.

- Loads that are too crowded. Packs must be arranged with adequate spacing on the cart. If they are packed too tightly, air may be entrapped and steam may not be able to penetrate into all areas.

- Containers that are positioned incorrectly. Basins and other items that can hold water must be positioned, so air can be removed and water (condensed steam) can escape. When sterilizing bottles or other airtight containers, tops must be removed.

- Clogged drain strainer. Most sterilizers have a small drain strainer at the bottom of the chamber to keep lint, tape and other small objects from entering the exhaust line.

- Mechanical malfunctions. Defective steam traps, clogged exhaust lines and similar mechanical malfunctions can occur, and cannot be repaired by a CS technician. A qualified service representative should be called to perform the necessary maintenance.

- Utility malfunctions. Boiler or steam delivery system problems can occur, and a qualified service representative is needed to make repairs, as specified in the sterilizer manufacturer's service manual.

While mechanical malfunctions can occur, many sterilization failures are caused by human error and can be prevented by good work practices.

Temperature

To be effective, steam sterilization must occur at specific temperatures. These temperatures are needed to kill heat-resistant bacteria. The two most commonly-encountered temperatures for steam sterilization are: gravity sterilization 250°F (121°C) and dynamic air removal 270°F to 275°F (132.2°C to 134°C).

Time

The steam sterilization process can only be effective if all items within the load are exposed to the elevated temperatures and steam contact (moisture) for an adequate amount of time. Inadequate sterilization exposure times can lead to failure of the sterilization process.

Figures 14.18 and **14.19** show time and temperature relationships. This data represents the minimum sterilization cycles identified by the Association for the Advancement of Medical Instrumentation (AAMI).

Gravity Air Displacement

Item	Exposure time at 250°F (121°C)	Exposure Time at 270°F (132°C)	Exposure Time at 275°F (135°C)	Drying Time
Wrapped instruments	30 minutes	15 minutes	10 minutes	15-30 minutes 30 minutes
Textile packs	30 minutes	25 minutes	10 minutes	15 minutes 30 minutes
Wrapped utensils	30 minutes	15 minutes	10 minutes	15-30 minutes 30 minutes
Unwrapped nonporous items/ instruments (IUSS Cycle)		3 minutes	3 minutes	0-1 minute
Unwrapped nonporous and porous items in a mixed load (IUSS cycle)		10 minutes	10 minutes	0-1 minute

Figure 14.18

Dynamic Air Removal

Item	Exposure Time at 270°F (132°C)	Exposure Time at 275°F (135°C)	Drying Times
Wrapped instruments	4 minutes	3 minutes	20-30 minutes 16 minutes
Textile packs	4 minutes	3 minutes	5-20 minutes 3 minutes
Wrapped utensils	4 minutes	3 minutes	20 minutes 16 minutes
Unwrapped instruments (IUSS cycle)	3 minutes	3 minutes	N/A
Unwrapped nonporous and porous items in a mixed load (IUSS cycle)	3 minutes	3 minutes	N/A

Figure 14.19

Moisture

Dry, **saturated steam** is required for effective steam sterilization. Saturated steam acts similar to fog because it holds many tiny water droplets in suspension. The moisture content of saturated steam should possess a relative humidity (r.h.) of 97% to 100%. In other words, steam ideally should consist (by weight) of two to three parts of saturated water and 97 to 98 parts of dry, saturated steam.

Saturated steam is similar to air with 100% r.h. When saturated steam cools, water condenses as a liquid. The pressure exerted by saturated steam is constant for a given temperature, and the pressure varies in direct proportion to that temperature. In other words, the higher the temperature, the higher the pressure. To increase steam temperature, pressure must be increased; to decrease the steam temperature, pressure must be decreased.

> **Saturated steam**   Steam that contains the maximum amount of water vapor.

The atmospheric room pressure at sea level is 14.7 pounds per square inch (psi) at room temperature. While the pressure gauges on sterilizers at sea level are set at zero, in reality, the pressure is 14.7 pounds psi. After the sterilizer's door is closed and the sterilization cycle begins, steam is injected into the chamber. Then, the temperature rises, as does the pressure in the compartment. **Figure 14.20** shows the temperature and pressure relationship.

One of the concerns with steam sterilization is super-heated (dry) steam. Super-heated steam reaches higher temperatures than saturated steam, and due to the lack of moisture, it is a poor sterilant. If the steam is not saturated (less than 97% to 100% r.h.), the following two problems can develop (either

---

Steam Table

| Temperature | | Absolute Pressure | Gauge Pressure (lbs/In²) | |
F	C	psia	Sea Level	One Mile Altitude
212	100	14.696	0	2.7
220	104	17.186	2.5	5
225	107	18.912	4	7
230	110	20.779	6	9
235	113	22.800	8	11
240	115.5	24.968	10	13
245	118	27.312	13	15
250	121	29.825	15	18
255	125	32.532	18	20.5
260	127	35.427	21	23
265	129	38.537	24	26.5
270	132	41.856	27	30
270	135	45.426	31	33
280	138	49.200	35	37
285	140.5	53.249	39	41

Figure 14.20

or both of which will interfere with the effectiveness of sterilization):

- Items in the sterilizer will remain dry, and microorganisms cannot be killed as readily as under wet conditions.

- Items in the sterilizer will remain "cool" much longer, especially if they are wrapped. To understand this, think about baking a turkey in an oven with dry heat. It may take hours for the center of the turkey to become cooked compared to one placed in a pressure cooker with saturated steam. Saturated steam is a much better "carrier" of thermal energy than dry air.

BASIC WORK PRACTICES FOR STEAM STERILIZATION

Medical devices must be properly prepared before sterilization to ensure steam will come in contact with all surfaces. This section provides sterilization preparation guidance for processing some common medical devices.

Preparing Devices and Packs for Steam Sterilization

As noted earlier, all devices should be thoroughly cleaned before sterilization.

Effective sterilization requires that the sterilizing agent be in contact with all surfaces for the prescribed time. Air removal, steam penetration and condensate drainage are enhanced by proper positioning, and by the use of perforated or mesh-bottomed trays or baskets. **Figure 14.21** illustrates a mesh bottom tray. Instrument sets should be prepared in trays large enough to equally distribute the mass and the configuration of instrument sets should be evaluated to help ensure they remain dry.

Note: Oils, powders, cork and wood cannot be steam-sterilized.

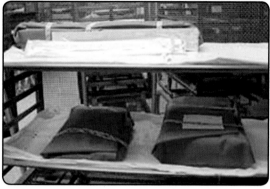

Figure 14.22

* Solid containers must be positioned so air can exit and steam can enter.

* There should be visible space between packs to allow steam circulation and drying.

* When combining loads, place hard goods on the bottom to prevent condensation from dripping onto lower packs.

* Packages must not touch chamber walls.

* Basin sets should stand on edge. They should be tilted for drainage, so if water is present, it will run out. **Figure 14.23** uses an unwrapped basin to illustrate how basins should be positioned for adequate drainage.

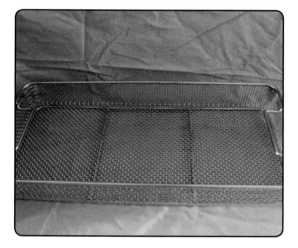

Figure 14.21

Loading a Steam Sterilizer

To ensure full steam contact and removal of air, the sterilizer must be properly loaded to allow adequate air circulation and drainage of the condensate.

Basic procedures for loading a sterilizer include:

* Allow for proper steam penetration and avoid overloading. Packages must be placed for efficient air removal, steam penetration and evacuation.

* If a shelf liner is used, it should only be made of absorbent material. (see **Figure 14.22**)

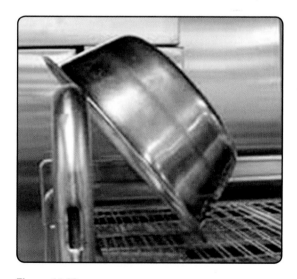

Figure 14.23

• Position textile packs so the layers within them are perpendicular to the shelf. **Figure 14.24** uses two unwrapped towel packs to illustrate how they should be placed on the sterilizer rack to facilitate the sterilization process.

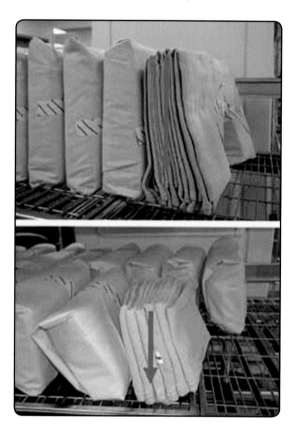

Figure 14.24

• Stand paper/plastic peel pouches on edge using a basket or rack. Placing them plastic side down may cause moisture to remain inside, and placing them plastic side up may cause water to stand on top of the plastic. Place them so the sterilization pouches are placed paper-to-plastic for air and steam circulation.

• When possible, sterilize textiles and hard goods in separate loads. If this is not possible, textiles should be placed on top shelves, with hard goods below to avoid condensation runoff from the hard goods onto the textiles below.

• Surgical instrument trays with perforated bottoms should sit flat on the shelf to maintain even instrument distribution and to facilitate proper drainage. Standing these instrument sets on their edge permits moisture to collect at the standing edge. **Figure 14.25** uses an unwrapped, perforated instrument tray to illustrate how perforated instrument trays should be placed on the sterilizer rack.

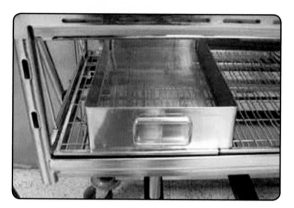

Figure 14.25

Unloading a Steam Sterilizer

When sterilization is complete, follow the sterilizer IFU for opening the door.

When the cart is removed, it should be placed in a low-traffic area where there are no air conditioning or other cold air vents in close proximity. For sterilizers without carts, items should remain in the sterilizer chamber until properly cooled.

The cooling time may be only 30 minutes for small sets or peel pouches, but can take two hours or longer for larger sets. The cooling time must account for critical factors, such as the type of sterilizer used, the design of the device and packaging being sterilized and the temperature and humidity of the room. The packages may still contain some steam vapor. If packages are touched at this point, the vapor present might carry microorganisms from one's hand through the packaging material and contaminate the item.

The load contents should be visibly free of any liquid. Water droplets on the outside of packages or on the rails of carts are signals that every item in the load should be visually inspected. *Caution: Do not touch items during visual inspection.*

Wet items should be considered contaminated, even if they have not been touched.

To unload sterile items:

- Do not unload packages before they are cool. Placing hot or warm packages on cold surfaces will cause condensation to occur beneath and/or between them. If warm packages are placed in plastic dust covers, condensate will be trapped until opened and the moisture may damage items protected by the dust cover.

- Handle the sterile packages as little as possible. Items should not be moved or touched until they have cooled to room temperature.

Controlling Wet Packs

Wet packs may occur when a steam sterilization process is used. Packages are considered wet when moisture in the form of dampness, droplets or puddles of water are found on or within a package after a completed sterilization cycle. Moisture can create a pathway for microorganisms to travel from the outside to the inside of a package. **Figure 14.26** provides an example of condensation (wetness) on the outside of a tray. **Figure 14.27** provides an example of moisture on the inside of a tray. If moisture is present on or in one pack, the problem may be isolated to that one set. To ensure the problem is isolated to only one pack, other packs in the load may be opened to check for moisture. If there are several wet packs from one load, the entire load should be considered "wet." Wet packs cannot be released and should be reported for immediate follow up.

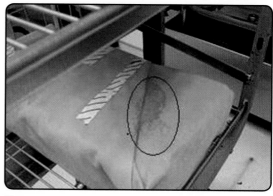

Figure 14.26

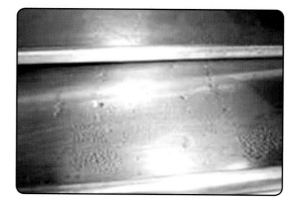

Figure 14.27

A wet pack is considered contaminated and must be completely repackaged and reprocessed. When doing so, all textiles should be relaundered and process indicators in the tray or pack must be replaced.

Wet Pack Documentation

All wet packs should be documented. Because of the complexity of the issue, finding the cause and cure of wet packs and/or wet loads can be difficult as there are many factors to take into consideration. Investigation is a multiple-step process. Documenting wet pack occurrences may identify a pattern that can pinpoint the root cause. For example, documentation may show that only the plastic instrument sets, specialty devices, packages prepared by another department or processed by a specific CS technician are involved. It may also show a pattern of steam usage within the facility or changes in steam quality during a certain time of year. Identifying the root cause of the wet packs is crucial to preventing additional wet packs. External moisture on packs is usually noticed immediately when the packs are removed from the sterilizer. Internal wetness will not be noticed until the packs are opened for use, unless the moisture wicks through the wrap. (See **Figure 14.28**)

Causes of Wet Packs

Primary causes of wet packs arising from CS preparation techniques include:

- Packs that were improperly prepared or loaded incorrectly for sterilization. This is the most frequent cause of wet packs.

- Heavy or dense instrument sets.

- Not using absorbent material to wick moisture between heavy metal, such as basin sets.

- Textile packs wrapped too tightly.

- Improperly prepared items, such as items wrapped while moist.

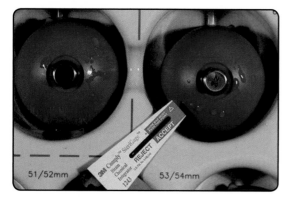

Figure 14.28

- Metal items positioned in a way that allows water to pool or trap steam. Instrument and basin sets that are too dense or overloaded.

- Linen packs wrapped too tightly, causing them to retain moisture.

- Improper placement of concave items, such as medicine cups, in a position that does not allow for drainage.

- Not using the correct filters or incorrect filter placement on a container.

Another reason for wet packs may be the sterilizer itself. Listed below are two of the most common reasons that can be identified by a CS technician:

- Gasket not completely intact.

- Clogged chamber drain strainer.

Other causes of wet packs can only be identified and resolved by a qualified sterilizer service technician. Such causes may include:

- Broken valves.

- Malfunctioning steam traps or drain check valves.

- Faulty sterilizer gauges or controllers.

- Clogged drain line.

- Faulty drain valves.

Wet packs may be caused for reasons occurring outside of CS. As previously stated, these reasons can be attributed to the boiler or stream delivery system. Although CS does not control these factors, it is important to be aware of some of factors from outside CS that can contribute to wet packs, including:

- Steam quality that does not meet the requirements of the sterilizer.

- Blocked steam lines.

- Boiler feed water that contains too many non-condensable gases, including air.

- Boiler not properly maintained.

• Malfunctioning steam traps or check valves.

• Poorly engineered steam piping.

• Increased demands for the steam supply.

Wet packs can also be caused by environmental factors, such as removing a hot load and placing it in an air conditioned area or an area with humidity exceeding 70%.

Extended Sterilization Cycles

Healthcare facilities typically use standard cycles for a majority of items processed; however, medical instrumentation manufacturers are now incorporating complex designs and materials into their devices. They may provide written processing instructions that lengthen the exposure phase of the steam sterilization cycle. This is referred to an "extended cycles."

CS technicians must obtain, review and consistently follow the manufacturer's written recommendations for all of the medical devices they process, including medical devices purchased, consigned or loaned to the facility.

Most medical devices require standard cycle times. Damage to some items can occur if items requiring standard sterilizing times are processed with other devices that require an extended cycle. For that reason, extended cycle items should not be sterilized with items that require a different cycle time. Items should never be sterilized in any cycle that deviates from the specific manufacturer's instructions.

Cleaning and Maintaining Sterilizers

The sterilizer manufacturer's written recommendations for sterilizer maintenance must always be followed. The following general cleaning and maintenance guidelines are illustrative of manufacturer's recommendations:

• Cool the chamber before performing any cleaning or maintenance procedure.

• The chamber drain strainer should be removed at least daily and cleaned thoroughly under running water using a non-abrasive brush and a mild detergent. This procedure may be needed more frequently, depending upon the types of loads processed. If debris is allowed to build up, it may be necessary to soak the strainer before cleaning. **Figure 14.29** shows an improperly-maintained strainer that is clogged and will not allow proper air removal.

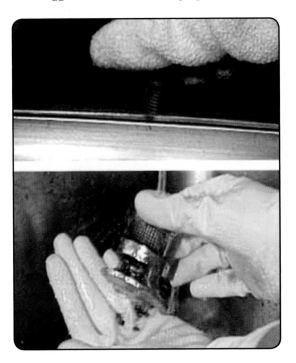

Figure 14.29

• The inside of the chamber should be cleaned according to the manufacturer's instructions. Problems with residue buildup on the chamber's interior can affect the cycle's drying ability. Residues in the chamber can leave deposits on instruments and wrappers. **Figure 14.30** illustrates residue buildup in a sterilizer chamber. Clean with nonabrasive and nonlinting products. Rinse detergent and residue from the chamber thoroughly to avoid deposits on devices during sterilization.

- The door gasket should be inspected and wiped clean daily with a clean, damp, nonlinting cloth. During inspection, look for defects or signs of wear or deterioration, especially if the unit has a vacuum cycle.

- Carriages, carts and loading baskets should be routinely cleaned with a mild solution. Follow the manufacturer's IFU for cleaning and lubrication requirements.

- Carriages, carts and loading baskets should be checked to ensure they are not damaged and can move freely in and out of the sterilizer chamber.

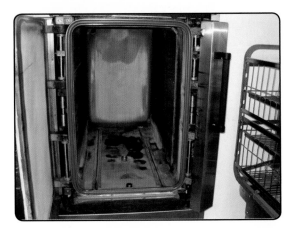

Figure 14.30

- Follow the manufacturer's instructions about the need and method for cleaning and flushing the chamber's drain. Air and steam will not pass efficiently if the drain line is blocked.

- Strong abrasives or steel wool should never be used on the sterilizer because they can scratch the surface and encourage corrosion. While sterilizer chambers are made of corrosion-resistant materials, some steam boiler water treatment chemicals can penetrate the chamber if the surface is damaged. Chambers that have not been properly maintained may require professional cleaning.

- Inspect recording devices daily, including paper charts and printer paper.

STERILIZATION QUALITY CONTROL

Sterilization quality control is an essential part of the sterilization process. Because it is difficult to prove an item's sterility without contaminating it, conditions that indicate sterilization parameters were met must be monitored. Sterilization monitoring is addressed in Chapter 17.

CONCLUSION

Central Service professionals who understand the steam sterilization process reduce the risk of sterilization failure. Knowing when there may be an issue with a steam cycle may allow the load contents to be reviewed and, if necessary, reprocessed before the items are distributed or used on a patient.

RESOURCES

Association for the Advancement of Medical Instrumentation. *ANSI/AAMI ST79:2010 & A1:2010 & A2:2011 & A3:2012 & A4:2013, Comprehensive guide to steam sterilization and sterility assurance in health care facilities.*

Centers for Disease Control and Prevention. *Guideline for Disinfection and Sterilization in Healthcare Facilities.* 2008.

Huys J. *Sterilization of Medical Supplies by Steam, Volume 1, General Theory.* 2010.

CENTRAL SERVICE TERMS

Bioburden

Saturated steam

Chapter 15

Low-Temperature Sterilization

Learning Objectives

As a result of successfully completing this chapter, readers will be able to:

1. Discuss basic requirements important for low-temperature sterilization systems

2. Explain specific requirements for low-temperature sterilization methods commonly used by healthcare facilities:
   - Ethylene oxide
   - Hydrogen peroxide
   - Ozone

3. Review important parameters of the low-temperature sterilization methods

INTRODUCTION

Low-temperature sterilization has become increasingly important due to the development and growing use of delicate, heat- and moisture-sensitive medical devices and surgical instruments. Ethylene oxide (EtO), hydrogen peroxide (H_2O_2) and ozone (O_3) are the low-temperature sterilization methods commonly used in healthcare settings, and each provides terminal sterilization. Chemicals used to sterilize instruments have toxic properties, although levels of toxicity and potential for exposure vary widely, based on the sterilization method and sterilant used. As a result, Central Service (CS) technicians must be trained on how to use them safely and effectively. Each low-temperature sterilization method has advantages and limitations, and it is the responsibility of sterilization professionals to understand when and how to safely use the low-temperature sterilization methods that are available.

LOW-TEMPERATURE BASIC STERILIZATION REQUIREMENTS

Eight basic requirements are important for any type of low-temperature sterilization system:

- Efficacy (effectiveness) - Has the capability of providing the minimum-required **sterility assurance level (SAL)**.

- Safety - There should be no toxic residuals remaining on the packaging or device upon completion of the sterilization cycle.

- Exposure monitoring - Ability to monitor the sterilization process to ensure concentrations of sterilants in the work area remain within any required exposure limits.

- Sterilization performance monitoring - Must be capable of being reliably monitored using physical, chemical and biological indicators.

- Penetration - Quality assurance must be able to penetrate through packaging materials and into lumens and other hard-to-reach areas of the device.

- Material compatibility - There should be no changes in the device's functionality after sterilization.

- Adaptability - Should be compatible with or easily modified to meet existing healthcare practices.

- Approval - Must be cleared by or registered with the appropriate regulatory agencies.

To be effective in the healthcare environment, a sterilization system must satisfy all requirements; failure to meet even one requirement may pose a significant risk to patients and healthcare workers.

Efficacy

To be legally marketed in the U.S., the U.S. Food and Drug Administration (FDA) requires each sterilant and sterilization technology to be rigorously tested against a broad range of microorganisms encountered in today's healthcare environment. The low-temperature sterilization technologies discussed in this chapter use different sterilizing agents and have significantly different processing methods. When used according to the sterilizer's Instructions for Use (IFU), each sterilization method meets the required minimum SAL, as outlined by the FDA, Centers for Disease Control and Prevention (CDC) and other organizations.

> **Sterility assurance level (SAL)** The probability of a viable microorganism being present on a product unit after sterilization.

Safety

Chemicals used as sterilants are designed to destroy a wide range of pathogens; however, the same properties that make them effective sterilants also make them harmful to humans. In particular, in sterilization methods such as EtO, significant toxic residues can build up in medical devices and packaging. To ensure a safe work environment, low-temperature sterilization systems should be

Toxicity Standards for Low-Temperature Sterilants			
Sterilant	OSHA PEL Eight-hour TWA Limit	NIOSH IDLH Limit	Monitoring Required?
Ethylene oxide (EtO)	1.0 ppm	800 ppm	Yes
Hydrogen peroxide (H_2O_2)	1.0 ppm	75 ppm	No
Ozone (O_3)	0.1 ppm	5 ppm	No
PEL—permissible exposure limits; ppm—parts per million; TWA—time weighted average; IDLH—immediately dangerous to life or health			

Figure 15.1

used according to the manufacturers' instructions and appropriate work practices, engineering controls, personal protective equipment (PPE) and monitoring should be employed.

Exposure Monitoring

EtO has been widely used as a low-temperature sterilant since the 1950s. It has potential health risks that require monitoring, long aeration times and other precautions. While safer for healthcare workers, newer low-temperature sterilization technologies also can pose health risks. To ensure the safety of healthcare workers, the Occupational Safety and Health Administration (OSHA) has established **permissible exposure limits (PELs)** for all low-temperature sterilants. These exposure limits are expressed as an eight-hour, **time weighted average (TWA)**: the total allowable worker exposure during an eight-hour period.

> **Permissible exposure limits (PEL)** The maximum amount or concentration of a chemical that a worker may be exposed to under OSHA regulations.
>
> **Time weighted average (TWA)** The amount of a substance employees can be exposed to over an eight-hour day.

The National Institute for Occupational Safety and Health (NIOSH) also has developed standards for Immediately Dangerous to Life or Health (IDLH) concentrations for low-temperature sterilants. **Figure 15.1** lists the standards established by OSHA and the NIOSH for each sterilant.

Sterilizer Performance Monitors

Monitoring sterilizer performance is essential to ensure the successful sterilization of medical instruments and devices and to protect patients. No single monitoring method provides all the information necessary to ensure effective sterilization; therefore, recommended practices state that available information from physical, chemical and biological indictors should be used to assess the effectiveness of a process before releasing a load. It is absolutely essential that CS technicians understand how to read and interpret physical monitoring information and chemical indicator color changes and know how to handle, use and interpret the results of biological indicators.

Penetration

Many modern medical devices and instruments are significantly more complex than their counterparts of just a few years ago. Not only must the sterilant penetrate packaging material (in some cases, multiple layers), it also must reach narrow lumens. If the sterilant cannot reach the most difficult to access site where microorganisms may hide, the sterilization process will not be effective.

The properties of a chemical sterilant impact its ability to penetrate effectively. For example, EtO inactivates microbes by a process called alkylation (seeking out specific proteins in microbes with which to react). This allows EtO to penetrate packaging and materials to reach remote surfaces where microbes may be located. Hydrogen peroxide and O_3 destroy microbes through **oxidation.** Chemicals that are gases at room temperature are more effective penetrants because they will not cause condensation on packaging. In order to monitor the efficacy of all sterilant gases, it is important to place indicators in the most difficult to sterilize area of the load.

> **Oxidation** The process by which several low-temperature sterilization processes, including hydrogen peroxide gas plasma, vaporized hydrogen peroxide and ozone, destroy microorganisms. Oxidation involves the act or process of oxidizing, which is the addition of oxygen to a compound with a loss of electrons.

Materials Compatibility

Medical devices and surgical instruments are composed of a variety of materials that may be affected by ingredients in sterilants; therefore, sterilizers must be tested to establish compatibility with a wide range of materials. Medical device manufacturers typically test the compatibility of their instruments with one or more of the available sterilization technologies; therefore, manufacturer recommendations should be followed to help ensure successful sterilization, instrument integrity, and prevention of damage that may increase costs and limit the availability of instruments for patient procedures.

Adaptability

The low-temperature sterilization process should be compatible with or easily integrated into existing healthcare and instrument processing practices.

Approval

The sterilization system must be cleared and registered with the appropriate regulatory agencies, with a clearly-defined intended use.

ETHYLENE OXIDE

Background

For more than 60 years, EtO gas has been an effective sterilization technology for heat- and moisture-sensitive medical devices and surgical instruments. EtO contributed to the development and increased use of delicate, sophisticated surgical instruments that would be damaged in the intense heat and high moisture required for other sterilization methods. **Figure 15.2** shows an EtO sterilizer.

Efficacy

EtO has excellent microbicidal activity. During the alkylation process, EtO destroys the cell's ability to metabolize or reproduce, which leads to the organism's death.

Penetration

EtO is a small molecule that vaporizes easily and can permeate throughout a wide range of materials, including plastics, to reach recessed areas. It has a high vapor pressure and a low boiling point of 51.3°F (10.7°C). As a result, it is easily maintained in the gas phase.

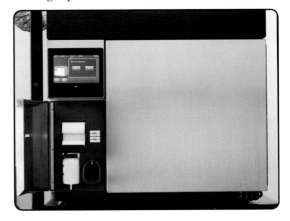

Figure 15.2

Sterilization Cycle and Process Parameters

In healthcare EtO systems, the gas is provided in individual dose cartridges that are placed inside chambers of less than 10 cubic feet. The cartridge is punctured under vacuum. (See **Figure 15.3**) If a leak develops in an EtO system, the vacuum will pull room air into the chamber, rather than allow EtO to be released.

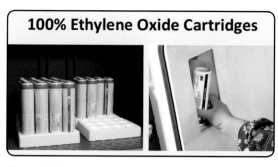

Figure 15.3

The basic EtO sterilization cycle consists of five stages: preconditioning and humidification, gas introduction, exposure, evacuation and air washes. The cycle takes approximately 2 ½ hours, excluding **aeration** time. Upon completion of the sterilization cycle, the items must go through an aeration process to remove all **residual EtO** before the sterilizer chamber can be unlocked and the items removed.

> **Aeration** A process in which sterilized packages are subjected to moving air to facilitate removal of toxic residuals after exposure to a sterilizing agent, such as EtO.
>
> **Residual EtO** Amount of EtO that remains inside materials after they are sterilized.

Operators should demonstrate competency in all parameters of EtO sterilization, as well as possess a comprehensive knowledge of the system. (See **Figure 15.4)**

Safety

EtO is a toxic gas classified by OSHA as a carcinogen and reproductive hazard. To protect CS technicians, EtO sterilizers should be located in a well ventilated area, with a room air exchange rate of at least 10 changes per hour. The sterilizers are usually installed in negative-pressure rooms with contained ventilation systems venting to the outside. (See **Figure 15.5**) Ventilation systems, exhaust lines and floor drains should be periodically checked by qualified personnel to ensure they are working properly.

Today's EtO sterilizers are designed for safety and have many engineering safeguards to prevent personnel from coming in contact with EtO (vapor or liquid). In addition, environmental engineering controls protect CS technicians.

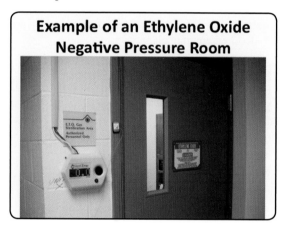

Figure 15.5

To minimize the safety risks associated with the use of EtO, employees should be instructed about:

- Hazards of EtO.

- Sterilizer manufacturer and EtO supplier IFU.

EtO Sterilization Process Parameters	
Gas concentration	450 to 1,200 mg/l
Temperature	98°F to 145°F (37°C to 63°C)
Relative humidity	40% to 80% (critical to the penetration of bacterial cells and successful sterilization)
Exposure time	1 to 6 hours
Aeration time	8 to 12 hours at 122°F to 140°F (50°C to 140°C)

Figure15.4

- Processing procedures.

- Storage and handling of EtO gas cartridges.

- Procedures to reduce employee exposure.

- Use of PPE.

- Principles of EtO monitoring and interpretation of results.

- Handling canceled cycles.

- Applicable OSHA standards.

- **Safety data sheets (SDS)**.

- EtO emergency plans.

Safety data sheet (SDS) A written statement providing detailed information about a chemical or toxic substance, including potential hazards and appropriate handling methods. An SDS is provided by the product manufacturer to the product buyer, and it must be posted and/or made available in a place that is easily accessible to those who will use the product.

Exposure Monitoring

Personal monitoring normally involves the use of devices affixed directly to the employee's clothing in the breathing zone (within one foot of the person's nose) to test airborne EtO concentrations. (See **Figure 15.6**) One limitation of personal monitoring devices is that sampling results are not available until after the actual sampling period has ended. OSHA requires that facilities using EtO sterilization have a system/procedure to immediately alert affected employees in case of an emergency, such as a leak, spill or equipment failure.

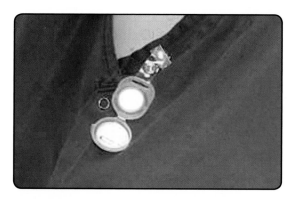

Figure 15.6

Area monitoring is used to measure EtO working area in which EtO sterilizers are used, and the monitoring may identify potential problems. (See **Figure 15.7**) These monitors can potentially detect emergencies and sound an alarm when leaks or spills are detected. Leak detection tests also should be performed.

For specific monitoring requirements refer to federal, state and local regulations.

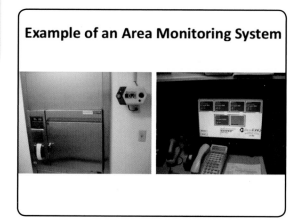

Example of an Area Monitoring System

Figure 15.7

Materials Compatibility

EtO has excellent compatibility with nearly all of the materials used in the construction of both single-use and reusable medical devices; however, as with all sterilization methods, it is imperative that CS technicians follow specific device manufacturer recommendations for the appropriate sterilization process for each specific item.

EtO should not be used to sterilize:

- Liquids. EtO will combine with liquids and may produce harmful chemical byproducts.

- Devices with energy sources. Energy sources could create a spark in the sterilization chamber during the sterilization cycle.

- Leather items. Chemicals used in the tanning process will combine with EtO to form chlorohydrin, which can cause negative health effects.

Packaging

Packaging of instruments should be performed according to standards for packaging products for sterilization. Appropriate packaging materials must be selected based on recommendations of the sterilizer manufacturer. EtO sterilization is compatible with a variety of packaging materials, including paper/plastic or Tyvek peel pouches, approved fabric wrappers, medical crepe paper, polypropylene and most container systems. *Note: Aluminum foil, cellophane, nylon films, polyester, PVC (plastic) films and styrofoam should not be used.*

Loading and Unloading Ethylene Oxide Sterilizers

EtO sterilizers must be properly loaded for effective sterilization. Overloading impedes proper air removal, load humidification, sterilant penetration and aeration. Items should be arranged to avoid contact with chamber walls. Pouches should be placed on edge in wire baskets. Stacking one package on another should be avoided.

Aeration

Because EtO can be absorbed by many materials, aeration is required to remove EtO residual gases before instruments and packaging can be safely handled by healthcare workers, or used for patient procedures.

When the exposure cycle ends, one or more vacuum pulses remove EtO from the chamber. The aeration phase then takes place as warm air circulates through the chamber to remove residuals from instruments. Minimum general recommendations for aeration are eight hours at 140°F (60°C), and 12 hours at 122°F (50°C). The rate of aeration is dependent upon many factors, including the nature of the materials used to construct the device; therefore, the manufacturer of the medical device must provide recommendations for appropriate aeration times and temperatures.

Sterilizer Performance Monitors

An EtO sterilizer should be monitored with physical, chemical and biological indicators. While none of these provide conclusive evidence of device sterility by themselves, they provide a high degree of sterility assurance when used in combination.

- Physical monitors. Include operating pressure gauges, temperature control/measurement devices, timing recorders and humidity sensors. Charts, tapes and graphs detailing the measurements made by physical monitors must be carefully examined before instruments are removed from the sterilizer.

- Chemical monitoring. External chemical indicators (CIs) should be used on the outside of every instrument package to demonstrate that each pack has been processed. Internal CIs should be used inside every package to measure whether the sterilant has penetrated the packaging.

- Biological monitoring. Biological indicators (BIs) are the most accepted means for providing quality assurance for EtO sterilization. (See **Figure 15.8**) The microorganism of choice for EtO is the *Bacillus atrophaeus* spore. Biological monitoring is required for each cycle run in an EtO sterilizer. Follow sterilizer manufacturer's IFU for proper BI placement.

Biological Testing for Ethylene Oxide

Example of a Biological Indicator

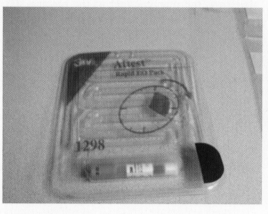

Example of a Biological Incubator

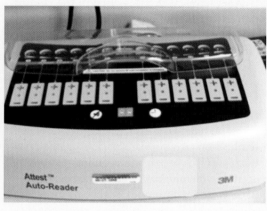

Figure 15.8

HYDROGEN PEROXIDE SYSTEMS

Several types of low-temperature systems use hydrogen peroxide as the sterilant. While the systems operate similarly, there are some key differences in the types of systems.

Hydrogen Peroxide Gas Plasma

Background

The more recent low-temperature sterilization technologies cleared by the FDA are considered oxidative processes. This includes hydrogen peroxide gas plasma. This method is popular due to its safety, relative to EtO, and its rapid cycle times that allow faster turnaround of medical devices. The process uses low-temperature hydrogen peroxide gas plasma for rapid inactivation of microorganisms. The byproducts of the cycle, (water vapor and oxygen) are nontoxic, eliminating the need for a lengthy aeration phase.

Hydrogen peroxide is a highly effective sterilant that sterilizes by oxidation of key cellular components.

Plasma is a state of matter distinguishable from a solid, liquid or gas. Gas plasmas are highly ionized gases.

Efficacy

Hydrogen peroxide gas plasma using a hydrogen peroxide solution ranging from 59% to 95% for the sterilization cycle is proven effective at killing microorganisms. Laboratory tests have demonstrated that the systems destroy a broad spectrum of microorganisms, including Gram negative and Gram positive vegetative bacteria, mycobacteria, yeasts, fungi, lipophilic viruses and hydrophilic viruses, and highly resistant aerobic and anaerobic bacterial spores.

Penetration

Hydrogen peroxide gas plasma sterilizers use deep vacuums, multiple pulse additions of the sterilant, and increased concentrations. These systems can sterilize a wide range of instruments, including some single-channel flexible endoscopes, cameras, rigid endoscopes, light cords, batteries and power drills.

Guidelines have been developed for lumen diameter and length to ensure adequate penetration and efficacy for various cycle parameters. Newer generations of hydrogen peroxide gas plasma sterilizers utilize a higher concentration of hydrogen peroxide (up to 95%) to shorten exposure time and lessen lumen restrictions. There are still some restrictions involving the size, length and number of lumens, and on the type of material and number of instruments per cycle. As always, users should closely follow the instrument and sterilizer manufacturers' instructions and recommendations.

Types of Hydrogen Peroxide Gas Plasma Systems

There are several types of hydrogen peroxide gas plasma sterilizers available, ranging from compact systems with 28- to 38-minute processing times to large-capacity systems with 75-minute cycle times. Different models have different cycle times, load capacities and capabilities for processing instruments. (See **Figure 15.9**)

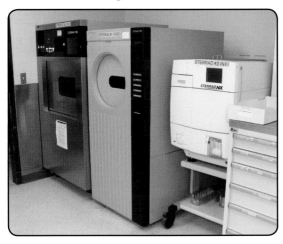

Figure 15.9

Sterilization Cycle and Process Parameters

The phases of hydrogen peroxide gas plasma include:

- Vacuum. The load is heated while the vacuum system removes any remaining water as it evaporates. Air is removed from the chamber and packages until the pressure is reduced to below atmospheric pressure.

- Injection. Once the correct pressure has been reached, a premeasured amount of concentrated hydrogen peroxide is pumped from a cassette into the vaporizer bowl and then vaporized into the chamber.

- Diffusion. The diffusion stage drives hydrogen peroxide vapor into the small crevices and lumens of devices. The chamber returns to atmospheric pressure to accomplish this.

- Plasma. A vacuum decreases the pressure, and radio frequency (RF) energy is radiated within the chamber from an electrode screen. The RF energy ionizes the hydrogen peroxide, creating hydrogen peroxide gas plasma. The injection and plasma phases are repeated a second time.

- Vent. At the end of the second plasma sequence, the RF is turned off. Air is then vented into the chamber through bacterial high-efficiency particulate air (HEPA) filters, returning it to atmospheric pressure. The process byproducts are only water vapor and oxygen. Aeration is not required, and instruments can be used immediately following the 24- to 75-minute sterilization cycle.

Operators should demonstrate competency in all parameters of hydrogen peroxide gas plasma sterilization. (See **Figure 15.10**)

Hydrogen Peroxide Gas Plasma Sterilization Process Parameters	
Time	24 to 75 minutes, depending on the model
Cycle temperature	Less than 131°F (55°C)
Hydrogen peroxide concentration	59% to 95%, depending on the model
Vacuum level	Automatically controlled
Plasma	Automatically controlled

Figure 15.10

Safety

Concentrated hydrogen peroxide liquid can irritate skin and, like other oxidants, is damaging to eyes if direct contact occurs. In the vapor phase, concentrated hydrogen peroxide is irritating to the eyes, nose, throat and lungs; however, a number of safeguards built into hydrogen peroxide sterilizers are designed to minimize the likelihood of personnel contacting hydrogen peroxide in either the liquid or vapor phase.

The hydrogen peroxide is packaged in sealed cassettes (See **Figure 15.11**) containing chemical leak indicators on each side of the package. These change from yellow or white to red when exposed to liquid or vapor hydrogen peroxide. The leak indicator is visible through a clear plastic overwrap to protect personnel handling the cassette. Once the cassette has been placed in the sterilizer, it is automatically advanced by the machine, eliminating any danger of exposure to liquid hydrogen peroxide through handling of the cassette. After five sterilization cycles, the cassette is automatically ejected into a collection box for safe disposal.

To minimize the likelihood of exposure to hydrogen peroxide when removing items from a canceled cycle, CS technicians should **always wear latex, vinyl (PVC) or nitrile gloves**. As with any chemical used for sterilization, healthcare workers should consult the SDS and follow all manufacturer recommendations and departmental procedures.

To minimize hydrogen peroxide risks, employees should be instructed about:

- Hazards of hydrogen peroxide.

- Storage, handling and disposal of hydrogen peroxide cassettes.

- Handling canceled cycles.

- Applicable OSHA standards.

- The use of PPE.

- Applicable SDS.

- Recommendations for routine maintenance of sterilization equipment.

Exposure Monitoring

Monitoring of the area around the system during operation should be conducted according to the manufacturer's IFU and established guidelines.

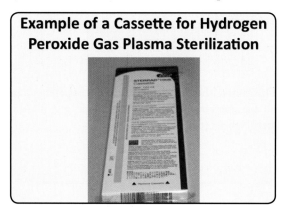

Example of a Cassette for Hydrogen Peroxide Gas Plasma Sterilization

Figure 15.11

Materials Compatibility

Hydrogen peroxide gas plasma sterilization is compatible with a wide variety of materials found in medical devices and surgical instruments, including some flexible endoscopes, semi-rigid ureteroscopes, cameras, light cords, batteries, power drills, rigid scopes and more.

Many items processed in high-temperature sterilization systems, such as stainless steel instruments, are also compatible with hydrogen peroxide gas plasma; however, hydrogen peroxide gas plasma is not compatible with:

- Liquids and powders.

- Any material that absorbs liquids.

- Items that contain cellulose, such as cotton, paper or cardboard, linens, huck towels, gauze sponges or any item containing wood pulp.

Manufacturers of newer low-temperature sterilization technologies, such as hydrogen peroxide, have active device testing programs. These involve cooperative testing with device manufacturers to evaluate sterilization efficacy and materials compatibility. If hospital personnel have a question about the compatibility of a device with a specific sterilization process, the product manufacturer should be contacted.

Packaging

Packaging materials can affect the penetration of hydrogen peroxide. Packaging materials used in the sterilizers should be designed to optimize diffusion of the hydrogen peroxide and not interfere with the RF energy or absorb hydrogen peroxide. Trays and container systems from the sterilizer manufacturer and Tyvek pouches are compatible. Check with tray and sterilizer manufacturers before purchase and use of containers.

Cellulose-containing packaging materials, such as paper/plastic pouches, cellulose-based disposable wrappers and muslin wraps, should not be used with hydrogen peroxide gas plasma sterilizers because they absorb the peroxide and inhibit effective penetration.

Loading Hydrogen Peroxide Gas Plasma Sterilizers

As with other low-temperature sterilization technologies, hydrogen peroxide gas plasma sterilizers must be properly loaded for effective sterilization. If the available amount of hydrogen peroxide is reduced because it reacts or is absorbed before reaching all surfaces, a sterilization failure could occur; therefore, the chamber should not be overloaded. (See **Figure 15.12**)

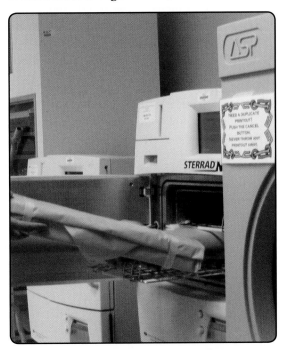

Figure 15.12

Excess moisture remaining on devices can cause the cycle to abort. Consult the manufacturer's IFU for suggested drying methods.

Sterilizer Performance Monitors

Hydrogen peroxide gas plasma sterilizers should be monitored with physical, chemical and biological indicators. Sterilizer performance monitors include:

- Physical monitors. Hydrogen peroxide gas plasma sterilizers operate on a fixed automatic cycle controlled by a microprocessor. All critical parameters are monitored during the operation of the cycle and a printed record documenting the process parameters is provided at the end of each cycle. If any process parameter does not meet established acceptable limits, the cycle will be canceled and the printed record will indicate the reason for the cancellation.

- Chemical monitoring. External CIs should be used on the outside of every instrument package to demonstrate exposure to hydrogen peroxide gas plasma. Internal CIs should also be used to demonstrate exposure to hydrogen peroxide. Internal CIs should be placed at challenging locations inside packs.

- Biological indicators. The microorganism of choice for hydrogen peroxide gas plasma biological indicators is the *Geobacillus stearothermophilus* spore. AORN Guidelines recommend that biological monitoring should be performed at least daily, preferably with each load. (See **Figure 15.13**) Follow the sterilizer manufacturer's IFU for proper BI placement.

Example of Hydrogen Peroxide Gas Plasma Biologicals and an Incubator

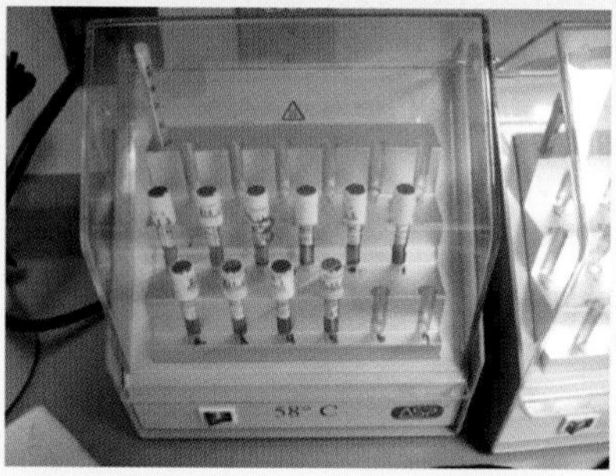

Figure 15.13

Vaporized Hydrogen Peroxide

Background

Low-temperature sterilization technology utilizing vaporized hydrogen peroxide (VHP) has been available to hospitals in the U.S. since 2007. As with hydrogen peroxide gas plasma, VHP systems utilize an oxidative process and provide a rapid cycle time that improves the throughput of medical devices and surgical instruments. (See **Figure 15.14**)

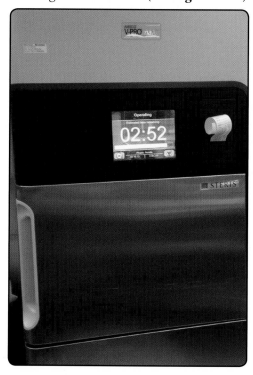

Figure 15.14

Efficacy

Vaporized hydrogen peroxide sterilization uses a 59% hydrogen peroxide solution. It has been shown to be effective against a broad spectrum of pathogens, including spores, bacteria, mycobacteria, nonenveloped viruses, enveloped viruses, cysts, fungi and protozoa.

Penetration

Vaporized hydrogen peroxide is injected four times during each sterilization cycle. Upon completion of the fourth injection hold period, the load is automatically aerated in the sterilizer. The VHP is exhausted from the chamber through a catalytic converter that converts the VHP to water and oxygen.

Types of Vaporized Hydrogen Peroxide Systems

There are two types of VHP sterilizers. One system has a single, preprogrammed, 55-minute sterilization cycle for use with both lumened and nonlumened instruments and devices. The second system offers two preprogrammed cycles: a 28-minute cycle for nonlumened instruments and a 55-minute cycle used to sterilize instruments with lumens and non stainless steel mated surfaces. Review manufacturer's guidelines for details about instrumentation that can be processed in both systems and cycle types.

Sterilization Cycle and Process Parameters

The sterilization cycle of VHP systems operates at low pressure and temperature, and is suitable for processing heat- and moisture-sensitive medical devices. The hydrogen peroxide vapor is generated by injecting aqueous hydrogen peroxide into a vaporization chamber (See **Figure 15.15**) where the solution is heated and converted to a vapor, and then introduced into the sterilizer chamber under negative pressure. The phases of VHP systems include:

- Conditioning. To remove air and excess moisture from the chamber and packaging, the chamber is evacuated and then recharged with dry, sterile air.

- Leak test. Vacuum is held to ensure a leak tight chamber.

- Sterilization. Enhances penetration by injecting hydrogen peroxide vapor into the chamber with a series of four pulses, each followed by a hold period.

- Aeration. Upon completion of the last VHP injection hold period, the load is automatically aerated in the sterilizer. The chamber VHP is exhausted through a catalytic converter that changes the VHP to water and oxygen. No special venting is required.

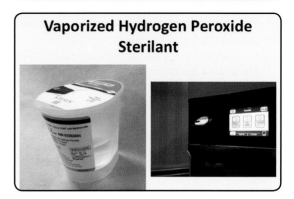

Vaporized Hydrogen Peroxide Sterilant

Figure 15.15

As with all methods of sterilization, operators must demonstrate competency in all parameters of VHP sterilization. (See **Figure 15.16**)

Vaporized Hydrogen Peroxide Sterilization Process Parameters	
Cycle temperature	Less than 122°F (50°C)
Hydrogen peroxide concentration	59%
Time	28 to 55 minutes
Other	Preset cycles

Figure15.16

Safety

Concentrated hydrogen peroxide is corrosive to skin, eyes, nose, throat, lungs and gastrointestinal tract. Under normal conditions of use, the VHP sterilizer operator is not exposed to the contents of the sterilant container. The sterilizer automatically dispenses and injects liquid hydrogen peroxide into the chamber. After each sterilization pulse, hydrogen peroxide vapor is removed from the chamber and converted to water and oxygen. An aeration phase facilitates the removal of hydrogen peroxide residuals from instruments and packaging. To avoid exposure to hydrogen peroxide when removing items from a canceled cycle, CS technicians should always wear latex, vinyl (PVC) or nitrile gloves.

To minimize risks, employees should be instructed about:

- Hazards of hydrogen peroxide.

- Applicable SDS.

- Handling canceled loads.

- Applicable OSHA standards.

- The use of PPE.

- Storage, handling and disposal of hydrogen peroxide cartridges.

Exposure Monitoring

No personal or area monitors are required. Testing to check for hydrogen peroxide vapors in the environment around the sterilizer has shown acceptable VHP levels during typical sterilization cycle conditions.

Materials Compatibility

Vaporized hydrogen peroxide sterilization is compatible with a wide range of medical instruments and materials, including telescopes, cameras, light cables, batteries and many lumened devices. Instrument materials compatibility evaluations have been completed to ensure that VHP sterilization systems are safe for medical instruments; however, the user must select the correct cycle for the instruments being processed. The VHP system is not intended to process liquids, linens, powders or any cellulose materials.

Packaging

Packaging materials can affect the penetrating capability of vaporized hydrogen peroxide. Packaging materials approved for use with VHP sterilization include polywrap, a nonwoven sterilization packaging made of 100% polypropylene. Tyvek also has been validated for use with VHP systems. Trays and organizers are available from the manufacturer that allow gas penetration and are compatible with the VHP process.

Loading Vaporized Hydrogen Peroxide Sterilizers

Vaporized hydrogen peroxide sterilizers must be properly loaded for effective sterilization. Items to be sterilized are placed on a rack system within the aluminum chamber. Organizers are also available that allow for positioning of instruments in the tray. To ensure successful sterilization, the chamber should not be overloaded. **Figure 15.17** shows a properly loaded sterilization chamber.

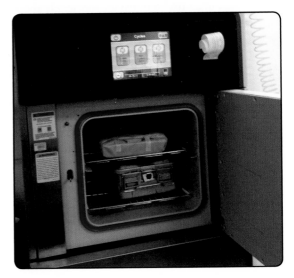

Figure 15.17

Sterilizer Performance Monitors

VHP sterilizers should be monitored with physical, CIs and BIs. As previously mentioned, none of these indicators provide conclusive evidence of device sterility by themselves; however, when used in combination, they provide a high degree of sterility assurance.

Sterilizer performance monitors include:

- Physical monitors. Vaporized hydrogen peroxide sterilizers operate on fixed automatic cycles controlled by a microprocessor and are designed and validated to independently monitor key process cycle parameters.

- Chemical indicators. CI strips for VHP sterilization change color when exposed to the VHP process. They should be used in each pouch, pack or tray as a process indicator to show that items have completed a cycle.

- Biological indicators. BIs are used for periodic biological monitoring of the VHP process. (See **Figure 15.18**) The microorganism of choice for VHP is the *Geobacillus stearothermophilus* spore. Biological monitoring is required each day the the sterilizer is used, but recommended every cycle. Follow sterilizer manufacturer's IFU for proper BI placement.

Example of Vaporized Hydrogen Peroxide Biologicals and an Incubator

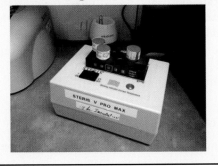

Figure 15.18

OZONE STERILIZATION

Background

O_3 is a low-temperature sterilization method that received FDA clearance in 2003. The system generates O_3 used for sterilization, eliminating the need to purchase or handle a sterilant. The system also does not require aeration and medical devices and surgical instruments can be used as soon as the 4½-hour cycle is complete. (See **Figure 15.19**)

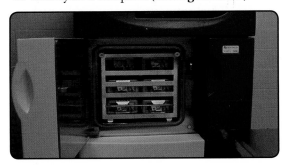

Figure 15.19

Efficacy

O_3 sterilizers generate sterilant using medical-grade oxygen and water. O_3 is highly effective as an oxidizing agent for low-temperature sterilization. O_3 sterilizes by oxidizing proteins and enzymes, causing the death of the organism.

Penetration

O_3 is a contact sterilant, and the process used for O_3 sterilization is similar to that used for other low-temperature sterilization methods. O_3 is highly reactive and has penetration limitations similar to hydrogen peroxide. It has some restrictions relating to the size and length of lumens, and sterilizer and device manufacturer recommendations must be consistently followed.

Sterilization Cycle and Process Parameters

The 4½-hour O_3 sterilization cycle is composed of two identical half cycles. After instruments have been loaded into the chamber, the door is closed and the cycle begins. A vacuum is drawn followed by a humidification phase. O_3 is then injected into the chamber, and the sterilization process begins. When the first half-cycle has been completed, the steps — from the vacuum to the O_3 injection phases — are repeated, followed by a final ventilation phase to remove ozone from the chamber and packaging. At the end of the sterilization cycle, the O_3 is converted to oxygen.

The O_3 sterilizer is controlled by a programmable logic controller. All critical process parameters are monitored during the cycle. At the end of each cycle step, the process parameters are printed. During the sterilization cycle, if one of the critical process parameters is not reached, the cycle will abort, and the reason for the interruption will be displayed on the screen and printout.

OSHA regulations require that operators demonstrate competency in all parameters of O_3 sterilization. (See **Figure 15.20**)

Ozone Sterilization Process Parameters	
Cycle temperature	87.4°F to 97°F (30.8 to 36°C)
Ozone concentration	59%
Relative humidity	85% to 100%
Time	4 hours, 30 minutes

Figure 15.20

Safety

O_3 reacts strongly with other molecules, and high levels of O_3 are toxic to living systems. At low levels, it is a respiratory irritant. OSHA, FDA and NIOSH regulate O_3 as a toxic gas. O_3 is a bluish gas with a very pungent characteristic odor. The odor threshold for humans is from 0.003 to 0.01 ppm. It is possible to detect O_3 at a concentration lower than the exposure limit for an eight-hour period, which is 0.1 ppm, as established by OSHA.

The O_3 sterilizer design limits the risk of exposure of hospital personnel. All O_3 produced passes through a catalyst that converts it back to oxygen before being exhausted into the room. Since the O_3 gas is created in an enclosed O_3 generator within the unit, there is no handling of the sterilant. The O_3 sterilizer possesses built-in safety features that protect the user from exposure to high O_3 concentrations.

To minimize O_3 risks, employees should be instructed about:

- Hazards of O_3.

- Handling canceled loads.

- Applicable SDS.

- Applicable OSHA standards.

Exposure Monitoring

No personal or area monitors are required, although O_3 sterilization requires a well ventilated room with 10 air exchanges per hour.

Materials Compatibility

O_3 sterilization is compatible with most reusable medical devices currently sterilized by EtO, other oxidative methods, peracetic acid or steam. O_3 sterilization is compatible with many heat-sensitive surgical and diagnostic instruments, including those containing polymers. The process is not recommended for sterilizing sealed ampules, liquids, natural rubber, latex and fabrics. O_3 sterilization of implants has not been validated. Medical devices should always be processed by following the device manufacturer's recommendations and instructions provided by the manufacturer of the sterilization system.

Packaging

The manufacturer of the O_3 sterilizer recommends specific wraps, peel pouches and rigid (anodized aluminum) containers for packaging of items to be processed. Other forms of packaging should be verified as acceptable before use.

Packaging made of woven fabric or metal foils are inappropriate for use with the O_3 process, as well as packaging that creates a solid barrier, such as hermetically-sealed (airtight) packs or any other packaging not specifically recommended by the manufacturer.

Loading Ozone Sterilizers

As with all low-temperature sterilization methods, O_3 sterilizers must be properly loaded for effective sterilization. Also, if the available amount of O_3 is reduced because it reacts or is absorbed before reaching all surfaces at remote load locations, a sterilization failure could occur; therefore, the chamber should not be overloaded.

Sterilizer Performance Monitors

Physical, chemical and biological indicators are needed to assess the effectiveness of the O_3 sterilization process:

- Physical monitors. All critical process parameters are monitored during the cycle. At the end of each cycle step, the process parameters are printed. At the end of the cycle, the screen will indicate "cycle completed," and a printout will be produced. During the sterilization cycle, if one of the critical process parameters is not reached, the cycle will abort and the reason of the interruption will be displayed on the screen and printout.

- Chemical indicators. CIs should be placed outside and inside every pack to identify packages that have gone through the process from those that have not, and to demonstrate that the sterilant has penetrated the packaging.

- Biological indicators. A process challenge device has been developed for routine process monitoring of O_3 sterilization. The BI for O_3 sterilization contains *Geobacillus stearothermophilus* spores. Biological monitoring is required each day the sterilizer is used, but recommended every cycle. Follow the sterilizer manufacturer's IFU for proper BI placement.

REVIEW OF LOW-TEMPERATURE STERILIZATION PROCESSES

Figure 15.21 compares the four low-temperature processes discussed in this chapter.

Advantages and Disadvantages of Low-Temperature Sterilization Technologies		
Sterilization Method	**Advantages**	**Limitations**
100% Ethylene Oxide (EtO)	• Penetrates medical packaging, many plastics and device lumens • Compatible with most medical materials • Simple to operate and monitor • Single-dose cartridge and negative-pressure chamber minimizes the potential for gas leak and EtO exposure	• EtO is toxic, flammable, a carcinogen and mutagen • Requires lengthy aeration time to remove EtO residue (eight to 12 hours) • Requires personal and area monitoring • EtO emission regulated by states • EtO cartridges should be stored in flammable liquid storage cabinet
Hydrogen Peroxide (H_2O_2) Gas Plasma	• Safe for the environment • Leaves negligible toxic residuals—no aeration required • Compatible with most medical devices • Fast cycle time of 24 to 75 minutes (varies with model type) • Used for heat- and moisture-sensitive items • Sterilant contained in a multi-use cassette to prevent user contact with hydrogen peroxide • Simple to operate and monitor • Easy installation (requires only an electrical outlet)	• Hydrogen peroxide may be toxic at levels greater than 1 ppm TWA • Avoid prolonged inhalation and contact with skin and eyes • Gloves should be worn when removing items from a canceled load • Cellulose (paper), linens, liquids and powders cannot be processed

Figure 15.21

Sterilization Method	Advantages	Limitations
Vaporized Hydrogen Peroxide	• Safe for the environment • Leaves negligible toxic residuals—no aeration required • Compatible with most medical devices • Used for heat- and moisture-sensitive items • Fast cycle time of 28 to 55 minutes (varies with model type) • Sterilant contained in a multi-use cartridge to prevent user contact with hydrogen peroxide • Simple to operate and monitor • Easy installation (requires only an electrical outlet)	• Hydrogen peroxide may be harmful at levels greater than 1 ppm TWA • Avoid prolonged inhalation and contact with skin and eyes • Gloves should be worn when removing items from a canceled load • Cellulose (paper), linens, liquids and powders cannot be processed
Ozone (O_3)	• Safe for the environment • Compatible with most medical devices • Used for heat- and moisture-sensitive items • Leaves negligible toxic residuals • No sterilants to handle	• Respiratory irritant at low levels • Require a well-ventilated room with 10 air exchanges per hour • Long cycle time (4 hours, 30 minutes) • Natural rubber, latex, textile fabrics, copper, brass, bronze, zinc and nickel cannot be processed

Figure 15.21

CONCLUSION

Today's instrumentation is far more sophisticated and complex than devices of the past, and many of their materials cannot withstand the high-temperatures or moisture required for steam sterilization.

When procedures are carefully followed, these methods are safe for patients, medical devices and Central Service technicians.

RESOURCES

Center for Devices and Radiological Health, U.S. Food and Drug Administration. *Updated 510(k) Sterility Review Guidance K90-1; Guidance for Industry and FDA.* 2011.

Rutala W, Weber D. *Guideline for Disinfection and Steril-ization in Healthcare Facilities.* 2008.

OSHA Fact Sheet: Ethylene Oxide. 2002.

Occupational Safety and Health Administration. *Chemical Sampling Information: Ozone.* 2007.

Centers for Disease Control and Prevention. *Documentation for Immediately Dangerous to Life or Health Concentrations (IDLH): NIOSH Chemical Listing and Documentation of Revised IDLH Values.* 1994.

Occupational Safety and Health Administration. *Understanding OSHA's Exposure Monitoring Requirements.* 2007.

Occupational Safety and Health Administration. *Guideline for Hydrogen Peroxide.*

Chaunet M, Dufresne S, Robitaille S. The Sterilization Technology for the 21st Century. TSO3. 2007.

Carter P, Wright M. *The lowdown on low-temperature steril-ization for packaged devices.* Healthcare Purchasing News. July 2008.

Reichert M, Schultz J. *Is new ozone sterilizer right for your OR?* OR Manager. 2003.

Centers for Disease Control and Prevention. *Guideline for Disinfection and Sterilization in Healthcare Facilities.* 2008.

Scheider MS. *New Technologies for Disinfection and Sterilization. Principles, Practices, Challenges, and New Research.* Association for Professionals in Infection Control and Epidemiology. 2003.

Conway RA, et al. *Environmental Fate and Effects of Ethylene Oxide.* Environmental Science & Technology. 1983.

Kobayashi H, Yoshida R. *Hydrogen Peroxide Varour in the Proximity of Hydrogen Peroxide Sterilisers.* Japanese Journal of Environmental Infection, Vol. 26, No. 4. 2011.

Kobayashi H, Yoshida R. *Hydrogen Peroxide Vapourised from Surface of Fiberscope after Low-Temperature Hydrogen Peroxide Sterilisation.* The Japanese Journal of Medical Instrumentation, Vol. 83, No. 3. 2012.

Robinson NA, Eveland RW. *Using HPG sterilization for heat-sensitive devices.* Healthcare Purchasing News. STERIS Self-Study Series. January 2015.

Association of periOperative Registered Nurses. *AORN Guidelines, Sterilization Monitoring.* 2015.

CENTRAL SERVICE TERMS

Sterility assurance level (SAL)

Permissible exposure level (PEL)

Time weighted average (TWA)

Oxidation

Aeration

Residual EtO

Safety data sheet (SDS)

Chapter 16

Sterile Storage and Transport

Learning Objectives

As a result of successfully completing this chapter, readers will be able to:

1. Review basic sterile storage considerations

2. Describe basic types of sterile storage shelving

3. Identify procedures for moving sterile items into storage

4. Explain the concept of event-related sterility

5. Discuss basic storage guidelines

6. Discuss other sterile storage and transport concerns:

    • Basic procedures for cleaning sterile storage areas

    • Sterile storage personnel

    • Transporting sterile items

    • Transportation guidelines

INTRODUCTION

A great deal of work goes into ensuring items are sterile and ready for patient use. Once items are sterile, they can easily become contaminated. Extreme caution must be exercised to keep each sterile item safe until it is used. While **barrier packaging** protects sterile items from contamination, it is not an impenetrable barrier. Sterile packages must be protected from events that can cause them to become unsterile. This is accomplished by keeping the items in a safe environment and consistently practicing good handling protocols whenever handling a sterile package. This chapter will examine strategies to help keep items sterile until use.

> **Barrier packaging** Packaging that prevents ingress of microorganisms and allows aseptic presentation of the product at the point of use.

STERILE STORAGE CONSIDERATIONS

After sterilization, or after purchased sterile items are received from an outside vendor, the items are stored until needed. The activities of personnel in the storage area and the environment itself impact the maintenance of item sterility.

Just like at home, if items are not properly protected, or something unexpected happens, stored items may become unusable. If there is a flood in the kitchen, for example food items like flour or sugar in their original packaging could be ruined by the water. If there is a flood in sterile storage, some or all of the packaged items may be ruined. Healthcare sterile storage areas need to be well-planned and constantly maintained to keep items sterile until use.

The sterile storage process actually starts as soon as the sterilizer door is opened at the end of a cycle, or when purchased sterile supplies are received into the facility. (See **Figure 16.1**)

Protecting sterile items from contamination begins with considering the environment where the items will be stored. Providing the proper environment is critical to maintaining sterility. The following are all considerations that must be addressed when determining an appropriate sterile storage area.

Location

The sterile storage area should be located next to or near the sterilization cooling area. This area should ideally be an enclosed room easily accessible from the sterilization, **break out** and case cart staging areas, while being out of the facility's main traffic areas. The storage location should be removed from general traffic flow patterns to minimize airborne contaminants and keep items away from untrained personnel. (See **Figure 16.2**)

> **Break out** The process of removing commercially-sterilized items from their outer shipper containers in an area adjacent to the storage area to prevent contamination that is present on the containers from being introduced into the storage area.

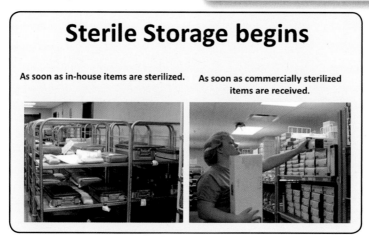

Figure 16.1

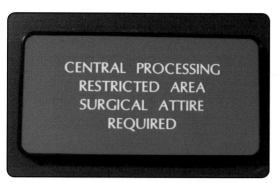

Figure 16.2

This area should be designed and designated for storage of sterile items only. Non-sterile items should not be stored in this area as they could contaminate sterile packaging. While it may be impossible to create a separate sterile storage area, every effort should be made to place items in an area that meets criteria for sterility maintenance. It must be noted that sterile items may be stored in other areas of the healthcare facility, such as nursing units, etc.

Space

When designing or selecting an area for sterile storage, it is important to be sure there is adequate space for storage and cart movement.

When considering floor space needed for proper storage the following must be considered:

- Type and number of instrument trays to be stored. A rigid container usually requires more space than a wrapped tray; however, containers may be stacked on top of each other, while wrapped trays cannot be stacked.

- Adequate space for smaller items and peel packages to allow for appropriate storage techniques.

- Adequate space to store purchased presterilized items, such as surgery procedure packs, gowns and sterile supplies for distribution.

- Adequate room between aisles to allow for cart movement up and down the aisles and to allow for enough space for easy access to all shelves.

- The room set up should allow for thorough cleaning.

- Room for future growth.

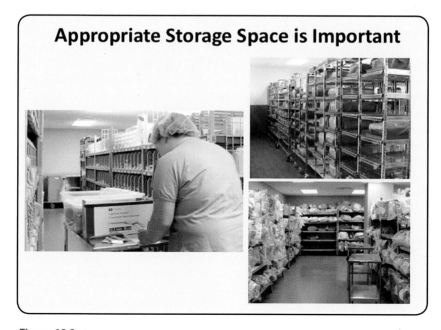

Figure 16.3

Storage Conditions

Sterile storage areas should have no exposed water, sewer or air conditioning lines that could leak and contaminate the items. Work surfaces should be made of easy-to-clean smooth and durable material. There should be no exposed light fixtures, pipes or ducts that can collect and shed dust. The area should be physically separated from other areas of the department. If this is not possible, extra care is required, so air and traffic always flows from sterile to clean to dirty. No pass-through traffic should be permitted.

Air supply to the storage areas should be as clean and dust free as possible, and this usually requires filtration. Because this area will store sterile items, air pressure should be positive in relation to surrounding areas so air flows out of the area when a door is opened, reducing the chance of airborne contamination. The room should also have at least four complete air exchanges per hour.

Temperature in the sterile storage area may be as high as 75°F (24°C), with less than 70% relative humidity. Very dry air can affect seals and cause plastic materials to become brittle. Excessive humidity can cause tapes and labels to lose their adhesion, loosen seals or affect package content identification. Moisture can also condense on the packaging material and seep or "wick" through it while carrying microorganisms to compromise pack sterility leading to wet packs. Moisture also provides an excellent opportunity for fungal growth through the packages. It is important to keep packs at least two inches away from exterior walls, windows and window seals where condensation can form on interior surfaces of exterior walls. Temperature and humidity levels should be checked and recorded at least daily. (See **Figure 16.4**)

This area should have proper lighting so package labels can be easily read. The recommended lighting for this area is 200 to 500 **lux**. There should be no dark corners or blind spots, which could lead to improper product identification and misplaced or forgotten inventory. Adequate lighting is also critical for personnel safety.

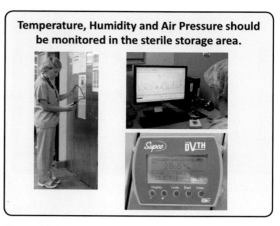

Figure 16.4

> **Lux** A unit of illumination equal to one lumen per square meter.

A hand wash sink or hand sanitizer dispensers should be located in this area. If installing a sink, do not place the sink too close to the shelving units, as water splash could contaminate the sterile packaging.

Storage Shelving

Many companies manufacture shelving that is appropriate for storing sterile supplies. Some facilities have custom-made shelving units to properly fit their allotted space. Regardless of the shelving type, there are several things to consider when choosing or replacing shelving. (See **Figure 16.5**)

* Storage shelving should be designed to protect the sterile product.

* Shelving should be sized to properly fit the stored items without product overhang. Trays that do not properly fit on the shelf pose a safety hazard to all who work in the area. Trays that overhang shelving may also become contaminated by people walking by and brushing against them.

* Shelving must be designed to easily hold the total weight of the trays to be stored.

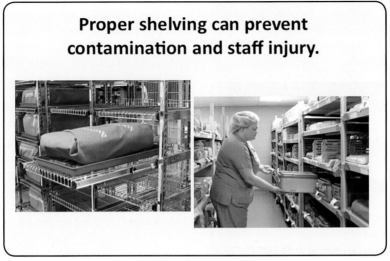

Proper shelving can prevent contamination and staff injury.

Figure 16.5

- Shelving should also be ergonomically friendly for the Central Service (CS) technician.

- Shelving should allow for easy access to the stored product.

- Shelving must be easily cleaned. Metal or plastic shelving is recommended for this reason. Porous materials, such as wood, should not be used as it cannot be properly cleaned and can harbor microorganisms.

Closed Shelving

Closed shelving is the most preferred type of shelving because it protects the sterile packaging from dust, traffic air flow, as well as other environmental and physical challenges within the storage area. (See **Figure 16.6)** Shelves are usually constructed as solid units, allowing for secure storage and easy cleaning. Closed shelving is expensive, so many facilities do not use this system (or it is used only for the most delicate and expensive items.)

Doors should be kept closed at all times, unless items are being accessed. When opening the doors, they should be opened slowly to avoid causing swift air currents that could potentially contaminate the sterile product.

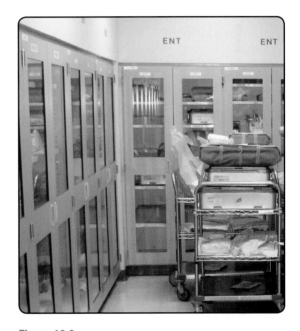

Figure 16.6

Semi-Closed Shelving

Semi-closed shelving is shelving that has at least three solid sides (top and two sides) and forms a closed unit when the shelves are moved together; these units are usually on tracks or have independent wheels. (See **Figure 16.7**) This type of shelving is also expensive; however it is very versatile, user friendly and offers good protection for shelved items. Shelves may be solid or open wire. The bottom shelf must be solid to protect the stored item from contamination. The units should be pushed to the closed position when not accessing sterile product.

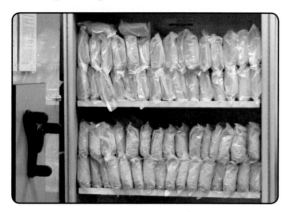

Figure 16.7

Open Shelving

In open shelf storage systems, items are placed on shelves that are not enclosed. Shelves usually have open racks to prevent dust accumulation; however, the bottom shelf must be solid to protect the stored items from contamination. Open shelving is convenient and less expensive than closed shelving; however, packages are more vulnerable to physical hazards (usually accidental) and environmental challenges from cleaning solutions and microorganisms.

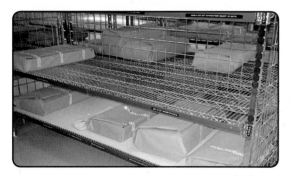

Figure 16.8

Regardless of the system in use, there are a few standards that must be followed.

- The bottom shelf of each unit must be between eight and 10 inches from the floor.

This protects stored items from contamination due to floor cleaning agents and dust.

- The bottom shelf must be solid to protect items from environmental cleaning. If the shelf itself is not solid, commercially-purchased shelf liners may be purchased to line the bottom shelf. (See **Figure 16.8**)

- Although not required, having solid top shelves will help protect sterile items from dust.

- All shelves must be cleaned regularly. Cleaning is discussed later in this chapter.

RECEIPT OF STERILE ITEMS INTO STORAGE

As previously stated, the sterile storage process starts when the sterilizer door is opened after a cycle or upon receipt of purchased presterilized items.

In-House Sterilized Items

Once items are removed from the sterilizer they should be moved to a designated cooling area. (See **Figure 16.9**) This area should be close to the sterilizers because moving the warm cart causes air currents to flow over the warm items. Since the room air is cooler than the sterilized items, this movement can cause condensation making the items unsterile. Air currents can also help microbes penetrate the warm packaging material, again contaminating the sterilized packages.

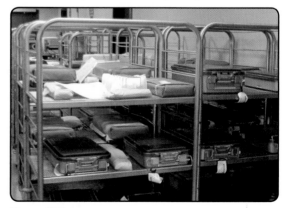

Figure 16.9

Packages should not be touched until they reach ambient (room) temperature. Touching warm packages can cause the packages to become contaminated from microbes on the skin transferring through the warm packaging material.

A temperature meter, such as an infrared meter, is designed to determine the temperature of a package without touching the package. (See **Figure 16.10**)

Once items are properly cooled they may be placed on the storage shelf. Carefully check each item prior to placing it on the shelf. Ensure the indicator tape, peel package seal or container locks are intact. Visible chemical indicators (CIs) should show appropriate color change. There should be no holes or tearing of the package material.

Lift (do not drag) wrapped trays; dragging will cause holes or tears in the packaging material. Wrapped trays should not be stacked on top of each other as stacking causes the lower trays to compress. (See **Figures 16.11** and **16.12**) When the upper trays are removed, air will be pulled into the lower packages, causing contamination. Stacking wrapped trays may also cause holes in the wrapper of the lower trays.

Rigid container systems may be stacked; however, do not stack them too high, as the weight may damage the gaskets of the lower trays. Trays may also be damaged from the weight. Stacking trays too high can also be a safety hazard. Consult the container manufacturer for specific instructions.

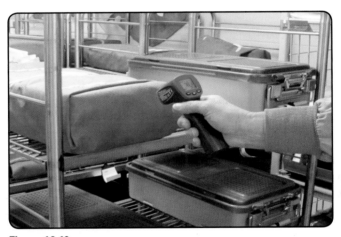

Figure 16.10

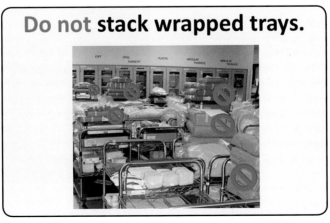

Figure 16.11

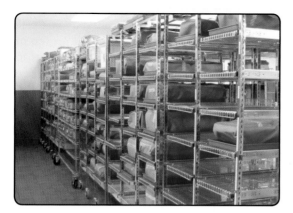

Figure 16.12

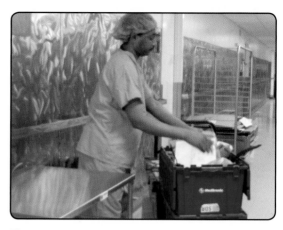

Figure 16.13

Purchased Presterilized Items

Sterile storage areas are also used to store presterilized products from outside vendors. These products are typically received in shipping containers made of corrugated cardboard, although other forms of shipping containers exist. These outer shipping containers should be removed in a controlled break out area as the outside box has been exposed to environmental challenges, including weather, insects, fungus and other microorganisms. (See **Figure 16.13**) Sterile items should not be removed from their outside box on the receiving dock, unless there is an area protected from the outside environment that has been designed for this purpose.

Received items should be delivered to an area close to the sterile storage area where the items can be removed from the outside box. Sterile items should be placed inside a clean enclosed transport cart, tote bin, or container so the items can be delivered to the sterile storage area. Outside shipping cartons should never be allowed in the sterile storage area as they are a major source of contamination. Transfer bins and carts must be cleaned on a regular basis to help keep the sterility of the items intact. Cardboard boxes should be removed from this area as quickly as possible to decrease the chance for cross contamination from the cardboard to the sterile items.

Items should be handled gently during transfer from the box to the transport cart/container. Place items loosely, do not pack items tightly, as it may compromise the items sterility.

Transport items directly to the sterile storage area. Never leave sterile items unattended where others may have access to the items. Curious staff or visitors may handle items and unintentionally damage the packaging causing the items to become unsterile.

Carefully place items on the shelves. (See **Figure 16.14**) Do not pack items tightly, as it will compromise the package sterility and may damage items inside the package. Always follow proper stock rotation procedures.

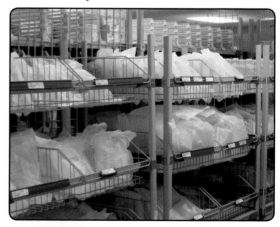

Figure 16.14

EVENT-RELATED STERILITY

Shelf life is related to events that may compromise the pack sterility. Event-related sterility is the concept that sterile products remain sterile until an event occurs to make them unsterile. The following list describes events that may render a package unsterile. This list is not inclusive, as there are many events that can compromise sterility.

Product Life

Some products and packaging material will degrade over time. Using these items once they have expired is unsafe. As items begin to degrade an event has occurred that can affect the items sterility.

Type of Packaging Material Utilized

Many packaging materials have a defined useful life. CS technicians must be sure to follow the manufacturer's recommendations for shelf life before and after sterilization as the products ability to perform appropriately is diminished after the stated expiration date. One of the events that could occur after the expiration date is loss of microbial barrier protection of the packaging. When this happens, items will not remain sterile.

Condition of Package

Package integrity is very important. Rough handling, poor storage practices, moisture, dust and poor transportation procedures are some of the events that can occur to damage a package. Once a package is damaged, the items inside must be considered unsterile. (See **Figure 16.15**)

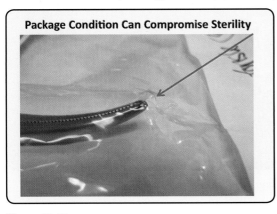

Package Condition Can Compromise Sterility

Figure 16.15

Storage/Transportation Conditions

Clean, dry shelving in the storage area or in the transportation carts is required to keep items sterile. Whether the shelving or carts are opened or closed can affect item sterility. Open shelving allows for greater chance of contamination from the environment or personnel working in the area. Temperature and humidity must be monitored, and ensuring the absence of dust and insects helps maintain package integrity.

Handling

Lack of proper handling can cause items to become unsterile. Handling items while they are still warm, over handling items and the hygiene of the personnel handling the items are all considered events.

All sterile items should be monitored for events that may render them unsterile. If any event occurs to jeopardize an item, the item in question must be removed and processed or disposed of according to the facility's policy. Whenever there is doubt regarding the sterility of a package, the item should be considered unsterile.

BASIC STORAGE GUIDELINES

Once items are delivered to the sterile storage area they need to be carefully placed in their designated storage space. It doesn't matter if the items are processed in house or purchased outside the facility the guidelines for storage of sterile items are the same.

The primary conditions that can adversely affect the ability of a sterile package to maintain its sterility until it is opened by the user at the point of use include:

- Moisture and liquid/fluid contamination.

- Dirt and dust.

- Physical damage to the package, including abrasions, cuts, tears, punctures, broken seals and the breakdown of packaging material (e.g., some plastics become brittle).

Storage environments should be clean, dry and easily accessible by authorized personnel.

Stored items should be arranged so that packages are not crushed, bent or compressed. If the air inside a package is forced out, it can potentially rupture closures and seams. Additionally, by forcing the air out of the pack, a void is created. When the source of compression is released, (i.e., the weight on its top is removed) a slight suction can be created by the void. This can potentially establish conditions for the packs to "suck in" contaminated air.

Per fire codes, stored items should be placed at least 18 inches below sprinkler heads to allow for proper air circulation and allow for water to flow unimpeded during a smoke or fire situation. Spacing must also be planned and maintained to prevent packages from being touched, bumped or leaned upon when the room is cleaned or when personnel are storing or retrieving packs.

Sterile packages should not be stored near or under sinks, exposed water pipes, sewage lines or air conditioning drains.

Always place sterile items on clean surfaces. Do not trust the package barrier to protect contents from soil.

When placing items on shelves or when removing them from the shelf, always check package integrity, including the filter area of rigid containers and ensure all external CIs have turned to the proper color. If sterilized in-house be sure the load (lot) control label is still intact and all seals are securely in place. (See **Figure 16.16**) If the item has an expiration date, ensure the item has not expired. Do not place anything on the shelf until the items have been checked and verified to be intact.

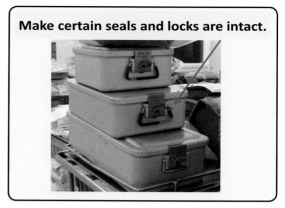

Figure 16.16

Sterile items should fit on the shelf; they should never overhang the edge of the shelf. The shelf edge may cause damage to the item and the overhang can create a safety hazard.

Place heavy items on middle shelves to allow for safe lifting. Light packages should be placed on the higher shelves.

Always lift items, do not drag them across the shelf, as that will damage the packaging and may damage the shelf.

Handle all items gently. Rough handling of sterile packages can cause damage to the packaging, causing the items to become unsterile.

Never place unsterile items on the shelves with sterile items. Unsterile items may contaminate the sterile product. (See **Figure 16.17**)

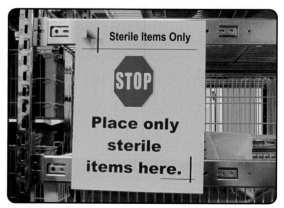

Figure 16.17

Arrangement of Instruments and Supplies

Storage areas for instruments and supplies must be carefully planned. The goal is to help ensure that items are easy to locate and are protected from events that may cause them to become unsterile. Proper use of stock rotation principles is also important to ensure that older items are used first and that supplies with time-sensitive expiration dates are used before they must be discarded.

The logical arrangement of stock improves efficiency, decreases staff injuries and facilitates appropriate stock rotation.

CS professionals should review the manufacturer's IFU to determine if there are any special storage requirements.

Sterile items should be arranged so they are easy to locate. This may best be accomplished by organizing them alphabetically by name, functionality or specialty (related items shelved together) or numerically, based on stock codes. Shelves should be clearly labeled, designating where items should be stored including pertinent ordering information. (See **Figure 16.18**)

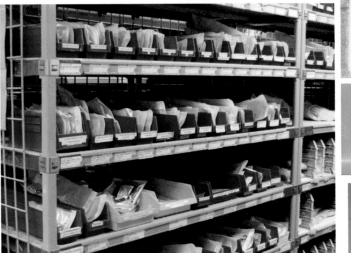
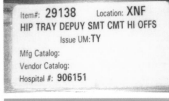

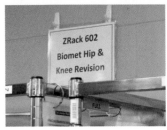

Locator systems help CS manage large numbers of supplies and instruments.

Figure 16.18

Stock Rotation

Sterile packages should be arranged and maintained to allow stock rotation on a **first in, first out (FIFO)** system. This ensures that the oldest items are used first. The longer a sterilized item remains in storage, the greater chance the item can become contaminated, due to handling and environmental issues, such as dust. Even if the item does not become contaminated it may not be able to be opened aseptically. Practicing a FIFO inventory control system prevents a "neglected packs syndrome" where hard-to-reach packs remain in storage much longer than others, and are more likely to be damaged or contaminated. *Note: Items with expiration dates should be used in the order of their expiration dates, with the items that will expire first being used first.*

> **First in, first out (FIFO)** A stock rotation system in which the oldest product (that which has been in storage the longest) is used first.

The goal of a stock arrangement system is to provide minimal pack handling, while allowing FIFO rotation. Many facilities use a left-to-right system: the newest item is placed on the left and the older items move to the right. The pack on the far right is the first to be picked up for use. Other facilities place the new packs in from the back of the shelf, and pick up the oldest from the front of the shelf.

Satellite Sterile Storage

Many facilities store sterile items in user departments. Storage areas for sterile supplies located outside of the CS department, such as in the Operating Room (OR), must follow the same guidelines as stated above and be included in quality assurance and infection prevention audits conducted for the sterile storage area in the department. Regardless of where a sterile item is stored, it must be protected from events that can render it unsterile. If satellite storage sites are used, personnel responsible for the areas should be trained about requirements for sterility maintenance.

CLEANING

To maintain product sterility, it is important to keep the sterile storage area clean and dust and debris free. Standards for environmental cleaning should be the same as those for an OR or Labor & Delivery suite.

The floors should be damp mopped and trash should be emptied at least daily. Walls and vents should also be on a routine schedule for cleaning.

Shelving, racks and other storage devices should also be routinely cleaned. The actual frequency depends on several factors. Closed shelving usually does not need to be cleaned as frequently as opened shelving. The air filtration system in the storage area is also a factor in determining cleaning schedules. The better the filtration system functions, the less frequently the area must be cleaned.

When cleaning the shelves all items should be carefully removed from the shelf. Using a facility-approved solution, wipe the entire shelf, including the sides and top. Alcohol may be used as a drying agent, if approved by the facility's protocols. After the shelves, base and shelf bottom have been cleaned, the wheels should also be cleaned. Be sure the shelves are completely dry before placing items back on the shelf. Also, clean and completely dry all storage bins before placing them back on the clean shelf. Carefully check each item for package integrity and ensure seals are intact. Look for proper external indicator color change and check expiration dates. Ensure the load control number is still on the in-house processed items. As with most processes, sterile storage cleaning should be documented and the documentation maintained for use in the department's quality assurance program. The process for sterile storage shelf cleaning is outlined in **Figure 16.19**.

Shelf Cleaning

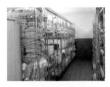
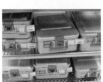
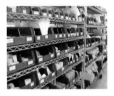

1	Remove all items from the shelves and storage bins.
2	Wipe entire shelf, including sides and top, using a facility-approved solution.
3	Clean all bins and shelf organizers using a facility-approved solution.
4	After cleaning surfaces touched by sterile packages, clean the shelf base, under the bottom shelf, and wheels.
5	Allow to dry thoroughly. *Note: Alcohol may be used as a drying agent, if approved by facility protocols.*
6	Wait until shelves, bins and organizers are completely dry.
7	Place items back in their assigned location. Check items for package integrity, external indicator change, expiration dates and lot control numbers for in-house sterilized items.
8	Document cleaning per the facility's quality assurance requirements.

Figure 16.19

STERILE STORAGE PROFESSIONALS

All CS professionals should maintain a high level of personal hygiene, including clean hair, body, nails (no artificial nails) and clothing at all times. CS technicians should frequently wash their hands or use waterless hand sanitizers according to departmental policy.

Fingernails should be short to reduce the microbial load under the nails, and to minimize the potential for rupturing packages and pouches.

Jewelry is discouraged because it can tear holes in packaging and may harbor microorganisms. Rings, neck and wrist jewelry may become caught in the package, causing damage to the sterilized item and the wearer. If badge lanyards are worn, they should be placed in a pocket or contained in some manner to avoid catching them in the shelving or a package. Lanyards should also be cleaned on a routine basis, so they do not contaminate the sterile items.

Personnel working in the sterile storage area must be properly trained in all aspects of the storage process.

Authorized individuals entering a storage area must follow hand hygiene policies, wear proper attire, be in good health and maintain good personal hygiene.

TRANSPORTING STERILE ITEMS

Transportation of sterile packages should be done in a manner that protects the sterility of the items. It is important to follow the department's established procedures to ensure the items are delivered intact and ready to use. There are several ways to transport sterile items. Regardless of the method used, it is important to protect the items from crushing, bending, falling or other damage. (See **Figure 16.20**)

Hand Carry

It is often faster and easier to hand carry small, lightweight items to the point of use area. Items being delivered should be protected from the environment and air currents from hallway traffic. Carefully place the items to be delivered in a protective cover, such as a dust cover or a clean closed bin. Keep items away from the body to avoid contaminating them. The sterile items should be held with both hands, keeping the items flat so instruments and products do not shift and become damaged.

Cart Transport

Transporting items by cart is easier and safer than hand carrying items. As with shelving, transport carts can be opened or closed. The bottom shelf should be solid to protect the items from dirt and dust contamination. When transporting with open carts, including wheeled tables, items should be covered and protected against the hallway traffic. Items should be placed on the cart flat to protect contents. Trays and packs should not overhang the edges of the cart.

Closed carts are the transportation method of choice, as they provide the best protection for sterile items. (See **Figure 16.21**) Carefully place items inside the cart. Do not overcrowd the cart. The cart doors should close and latch without touching the sterile item.

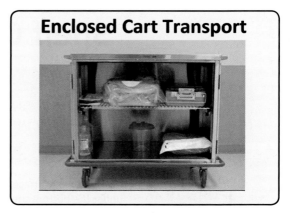

Enclosed Cart Transport

Figure 16.21

All carts should be kept in good repair, and cart doors should be properly attached and dent free. Wheels should be properly maintained so the cart will move easily and quietly.

Elevator/Lifts

Many facilities have dedicated clean elevators for sterile product transportation. These elevators should be used for clean and sterile transportation only. Soiled items should be returned using an elevator designated for soiled items. When using a dedicated lift, items must still be contained because air currents from outside the lift can contaminate the sterile items.

Vehicle

Healthcare facilities today may transport sterile items between sister facilities and to offsite clinics and physician offices. Items should not be transported in the trunk of a car because temperature and humidity levels cannot be properly controlled. There must be clear separation of clean and soiled items within the transport vehicle. The vehicle must be completely enclosed and in good repair, with no holes in the walls that will allow outside contaminates to enter. Sterile items should be placed inside clean, protective bins or carts. Protect the items from movement within the

Sterile Item Transport

Dust Covers   **Open Carts with Bins or Covers**

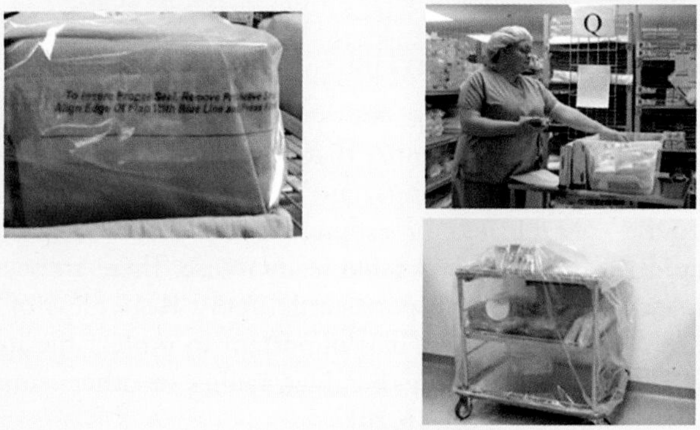

Figure 16.20

enclosed device, as packaging and instruments can be damaged from movement during transport. The cart or bin must be properly secured inside the vehicle to keep it from moving. Temperature and humidity levels should be monitored. When the vehicle is not running, items should not be left inside the vehicle for extended periods of time, as condensation may form inside the sterile packages, making them unsterile. The transport vehicle should be cleaned on a regular basis.

TRANSPORTATION GUIDELINES

Keeping items sterile during transportation is the number one priority. Below are a few basic guidelines to follow when transporting sterile items.

The importance of avoiding contact with sterile packages cannot be overemphasized. This includes bumping into, leaning on, backing into, touching when counting and excessively handling the the packages. When a package is moved or handled, it should not be "cradled." Any sterile items that are dropped to the floor should be considered contaminated and removed, even if no damage is apparent. Jarring and compression upon landing can force dust and airborne microorganisms into the package. The floor could be wet, sharp edges of trays could puncture through the wrap, and dirt could be carried onto the storage shelf to contaminate the next pack placed in that location.

CS technicians and end users must be trained to recognize any signs of sterility compromise. A log of sterile pack contamination events should be maintained and analyzed to implement preventive actions.

When removing the package from the shelf, its front should be lifted from underneath with one hand. The other hand should be placed midway under the package, and the unit should then be lifted off the shelf. Packages should not be dragged or pushed against any surface because this causes friction or abrasion, which can potentially cause a pressure cut or snag and compromise sterility. Shelf liners help create a cushion between the hard surface of the shelf and bottom of the packages. These are recommended if the facility

is experiencing tearing on pack bottoms. This is usually a greater concern with heavy packs, procedure sets and, especially, instrument trays. The edges of the metal trays and weight of the instruments increase the adverse impact of the friction. Burrs or sharp edges on the shelves themselves may also contribute to sterile pack damage.

When packs are removed from storage, they must be carefully inspected for expiration date, tears, abrasion, tracks, worn areas, punctures, compromised seals, dirt and evidence of moisture. The external CI must be checked to ensure that the package was subjected to the sterilization process. If any adverse conditions are noted, the pack should be considered contaminated. The majority of holes in wrap come from mishandling. If the pack contents are reusable, they should be removed from the package for processing. If the contents are disposable, they should be discarded. Single-use wrap should not be reused after it has been sterilized.

All items should be protected from damage, moisture, humidity and dust during transport.

Transport carts and bins should be cleaned before use. Carts and bins should be completely dried before items are placed on or in them.

Carts should be kept in good repair; both for package integrity and staff safety. Doors should be dent free and able to close securely. Wheels must move smoothly and quietly.

Sterile items transported offsite to another facility must be transported in a vehicle specifically designed for sterile transport. The vehicle should have temperature and humidity control, and enough space to completely separate clean from dirty items.

Sterile items should never be left unattended in an unsecured area. Individuals unfamiliar with sterile product handling may inadvertently contaminate them.

Policies and procedures for sterile item transport should always be followed.

CONCLUSION

Maintaining product sterility during storage and transport is one of the most important Central Service job tasks. If unsterile instruments or supplies are used, patients could acquire an infection. Carefully following written storage and transport procedures, and keeping the area clean and maintained will help keep patients safe.

RESOURCES

Association for the Advancement of Medical Instrumentation. *ANSI/AAMI ST79, Comprehensive guide to steam sterilization and sterility assurance in healthcare facilities.* Sections 3.3, 8.9.2-8.11.5. 2013.

Guidelines for PeriOperative Practice: Packaging Systems. Guidelines for PeriOperative Practice. 2015

International Association of Central Service Material Management. *Central Service Leadership Manual,* Chapter 23. 2011.

CENTRAL SERVICE TERMS

Barrier packaging

Break out

Lux

First in, first out (FIFO)

Chapter 17

Monitoring and Recordkeeping for Central Service

Learning Objectives

As a result of successfully completing this chapter, readers will be able to:

1. Discuss the importance of monitoring work areas and processes within the Central Service department

2. Discuss the importance of recordkeeping

3. Explain the types of monitoring needed in each area of the Central Service department

4. Explain the need for monitoring and review of the sterilization process indicators that help assure quality control:
   • Need for monitoring
   • Chemical indicators
   • Sterilization load control information
   • Physical and mechanical monitors
   • Biological indicators
   • Bowie-Dick tests

5. Discuss the importance of employee training and continuing education records

INTRODUCTION

A great deal of planning and effort goes into every aspect of the Central Service (CS) department. From the decontamination area to the storage area, rigid requirements must be met to help ensure the safety of patients and healthcare workers.

Documentation is required to provide a record that those requirements were met; and if requirements were not adequately met, documentation provides a record to assist with performance improvement.

CS technicians are involved in the recordkeeping process across many different functions of their jobs. Records provide evidence that processes were routinely checked, and the information collected provides a quality framework that will be examined by surveying agencies, such as The Joint Commission (TJC), the Centers for Medicare and Medicaid Services (CMS) and state agencies. If the healthcare facility is involved in a legal claim regarding any products that were dispensed from (or processed through) CS, records can help demonstrate that a specific standard of practice was followed.

This chapter provides information about recordkeeping requirements for CS and addresses methods used to **monitor** and document conditions and processes to meet established requirements. Special emphasis will be placed on the methods used to monitor sterilization processes and the recordkeeping required for those processes.

THE IMPORTANCE OF ACCURATE RECORDS

Records are kept to document many processes and conditions in the CS department, including sterilization cycles, preventative maintenance and routine equipment testing and cleaning. It is important to note, however, that records are only as good as the information they contain. Having incomplete records is essentially the same as having no records at all. The following are some facts about CS department records:

- Recordkeeping is mandatory. CS department recordkeeping is not optional. It is as much a part of the job as assembling instruments or operating sterilizers.

- Records must be accurate. Information must be documented as it is, even if the information indicates a process has failed to meet the expected standard.

- Records must be legible and understandable. Handwritten records should be legible to anyone who needs to review them. Slang, unapproved abbreviations and nicknames should not be used, as that terminology may confuse the reader.

- Records must be complete. All information should be documented according to the department's specific requirements.

- Records should be audited routinely. Routine audits ensure that documents contain all necessary information.

Accurate and complete records provide documentation that the CS department is following standards, regulations and its own procedures to help ensure continual adherence to best practices.

> **Monitor** To watch, observe, listen to or check (something) for a special purpose over a period of time.

GENERAL MONITORING

CS technicians should continually monitor their environment to help ensure that the integrity of each work area and the processes performed in those areas are maintained. Some monitoring is informal, such as watching to ensure that everyone who enters the area is dressed appropriately, practices good hand hygiene and follows established traffic control guidelines. This type of informal monitoring is not recorded, but each employee is expected to identify and correct breaches in established protocols. Visual monitoring is especially important when monitoring dress codes in the decontamination area. Visitors, such as loaner instrument vendor personnel or facility employees from other departments (e.g., Maintenance, Biomedical Engineering, Environmental Services, etc.), may not be familiar with or understand the importance of personal protective equipment (PPE) and may endanger themselves if they enter the area without proper attire.

Formal monitoring of the physical environment is also required. For example, room temperature and humidity must be monitored at least daily to ensure they meet the established standard. That data must be recorded. Some departments use electronic devices to collect the data and transfer it to an electronic record, while others collect the data manually. In either case, CS technicians must have that data recorded and accessible. **Figures 17.1** and **17.2** illustrate examples of manual and computerized data collection methods used to monitor temperature and humidity.

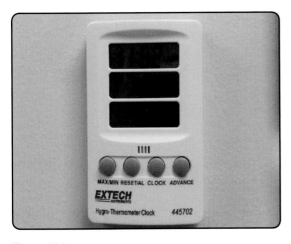

Figure 17.1

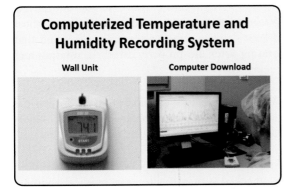

Figure 17.2

CS technicians also monitor their work areas for safety hazards. They learn to keep a watchful eye for unsafe conditions, broken or unsafe equipment, and other issues that may put themselves and others at risk. Once identified, they remedy the situation, if possible (e.g., wiping up a spill) or report it to the appropriate person to initiate a repair or replacement process.

Departmental cleanliness is also monitored by CS technicians. While routine cleaning is performed by the Environmental Services department, there are areas in the CS department that staff are required to maintain (i.e., CS technicians are responsible for keeping their work area clean). This not only means cleaning their work areas at designated times (i.e., at the end of their shift), but also means cleaning the area whenever it becomes contaminated or soiled.

CS technicians are often assigned specific cleaning duties within the CS department. For example, they often are responsible for cleaning cabinets, racks and carts in the sterile storage area. CS staff are assigned to clean those areas because of their understanding of sterile package handling and their ability to handle sterile items, clean storage shelves and return those items to their proper location without compromising the integrity of the sterile packs. The cleaning process in this very important area must be documented to provide a record of routine cleaning.

CS technicians are also responsible for cleaning the transport equipment in their area. Every effort must be made to limit the presence of dust, lint and microbial contamination in the work area. Microbial contamination must be kept to a minimum in all work areas. Excess dust in the work area can easily be transported to items being prepared for sterilization, or onto sterile packages. In either case, that dust may then become airborne and be introduced into an open wound during a procedure.

Figure 17.3 provides an example of a sterilizer loading cart that has not been recently cleaned. The dust and lint pose a significant threat to patient safety.

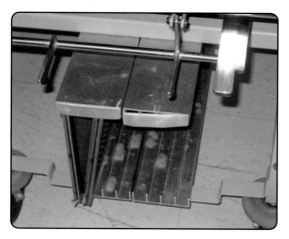

Figure 17.3

CS staff also monitor equipment within their work areas. Some of that monitoring is informal, such as checking the temperature of a heat sealer. Other monitoring is formal. All small electrical equipment has a current preventive maintenance (PM) sticker. Items falling outside of their PM date should be rechecked according to facility policy.

In addition to general guidelines for all work areas, there are unique requirements for each specific work area. The following sections review those requirements.

DECONTAMINATION AREA MONITORING

Monitoring of the decontamination area is important to ensure all cleaning equipment is working properly. If the equipment is not working properly, instruments will not be clean and safe to handle.

Water Quality

Poor water quality will impact every process in the decontamination area. Cleaning chemicals must be used with the recommended water pH and will not function as designed if the water's pH is incompatible with the chemical. Hard water will cause scale to form on equipment, reducing the equipment's cleaning effectiveness. Water quality

should be monitored to ensure that the appropriate dilution of the chemicals utilized is correct.

Commercially-prepared water testing products may be purchased to test water on a weekly or daily basis.

Mechanical Cleaning Equipment

Specific tests are available for each type of equipment. CS technicians must follow the equipment manufacturer's Instructions for Use (IFU) for inspection and testing. If the machine does not meet the inspection requirements outlined by the manufacturer, or if the test fails, the CS manager should be notified immediately. All test results should be documented.

Ultrasonic Cleaners

Ultrasonic cleaners use a process called cavitation to remove soil from instruments. Commercially-prepared tests are available to test the efficacy of the ultrasonic.

Irrigating Ultrasonic Cleaners

Irrigating ultrasonic cleaners are used to help clean lumened instruments. These units also use a cavitation process, but they employ irrigating tubes that flush solution through each lumen. In addition to the cavitation test, the irrigating tubes should be checked to ensure water is flowing freely through the tubes. Test results should be documented.

Washer-Disinfectors

Washer-disinfectors should be visually checked at least daily to ensure screens are clean and that rotating arms are properly attached, rotating and unclogged.

Washer-disinfectors should be tested for proper cleaning ability. Commercially-prepared products are available to assist with the testing process.

At the end of each cycle, physical monitors should be checked. On a washer, the physical monitor is the cycle printout or data log. The printout should be verified by the operator to ensure that the thermal disinfection temperature set by the manufacturer was attained and all other cycle parameters were met.

Cart Washers

Cart washers must be monitored to ensure they are working properly. Floor screens should be checked at least daily to ensure they are free of debris. Check rotating arms or cables to make certain they are operating as intended by the manufacturer.

Cart washers must also be tested to ensure they are cleaning effectively. This can be done using a commercially-prepared test.

HIGH-LEVEL DISINFECTION MONITORING

Many items processed today, such as flexible endoscopes, some respiratory therapy equipment, and other heat-sensitive, Class II semi-critical items, are high-level disinfected. The disinfection process contains many variables that can render it ineffective; therefore, it is important to carefully monitor the process. Surveying agencies review disinfection records as carefully as they review sterilization records.

Chemical Disinfection Monitoring

Test strips are used to ensure the minimum effective concentration (MEC) of the disinfectant solution. (See **Figure 17.4**) When a new bottle of test strips is opened:

- Test the efficacy of the strips, according to the the manufacturer's IFU.

- Document the date the test strips are opened and the final date the strips may be used, per the manufacturer's IFU.

- Document the test results, per facility policy.

Example of Disinfectant Test Strips

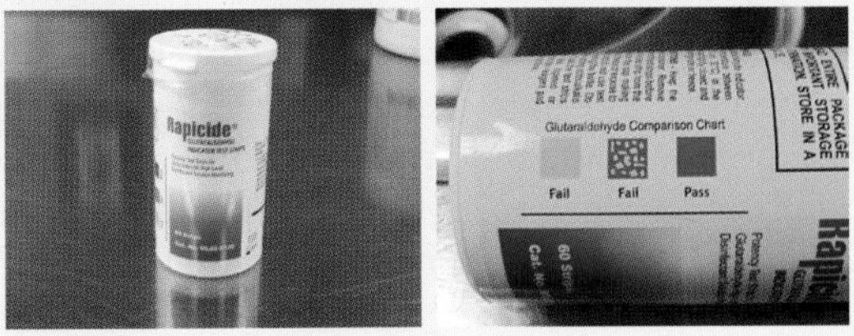

Figure 17.4

Manual Disinfection

Documentation of the manual disinfection process should include the following:

- Date.

- Test strip results (MEC).

- Expiration date of test strips and disinfecting solution.

- Items disinfected.

Note: Some products also require that solution temperature be recorded.

If the disinfected item is a flexible or rigid endoscope, the following must also be documented:

- Name of the technician who cleaned the scope.

- Name of the patient on whom the scope was used (patient ID information, if available).

Automated Endoscope Reprocessor Monitoring

As the name implies, an automated endoscope reprocessor (AER) is used to disinfect endoscopes using an automated process. While this process is less labor intensive than the manual method, monitoring is still just as important.

As with manual disinfection, the disinfecting solution in the AER must be tested for each cycle. The test strips and testing procedure remain the same as with the manual system. The AER manufacturer's IFU must be followed to ensure proper testing of the disinfecting solution.

Most types of AERs have a physical printout of the cycle available after the cycle is complete. This printout should be reviewed to ensure all set parameters were properly met. Technicians should then sign the printout to show the cycle has been reviewed.

Some AERs have a computerized control panel that allows the input of items sterilized in each cycle. If this feature is not available then the items must be manually documented. With the exception of the printout, documentation for AER disinfection is the same as with the manual system.

STERILIZATION AREA

The sterilization process requires a monitoring system to help ensure that sterilization parameters are being met. Because it is difficult to prove an item's sterility without contaminating it through handling, conditions that can indicate that the parameters for sterilization have been met must be monitored.

These sterilization monitoring protocols are an important part of the CS department's monitoring and quality assurance systems. Several control measures must be used to ensure the conditions within the sterilizers are adequate to achieve sterilization.

Process Indicators

Sterilization process indicators help to confirm that packages have been properly exposed to the sterilization process.

ANSI/AAMI ST79:2013, *Comprehensive guide to steam sterilization and sterility assurance in health care facilities* states, "Chemical indicators are designed to respond with a chemical or physical change to one or more of the physical conditions within the sterilizing chamber."

There are two basic types of process indicators: internal chemical indicators (CIs) that are placed inside a package to be sterilized, and external CIs that are placed on the outside of packages.

CIs provide a visual indication to help identify possible sterilization failures. They can detect problems with incorrect packaging, loading or other procedures and can also detect certain equipment malfunctions, such as air leaks, wet steam and inadequate temperature. CIs are an integral part of the sterilization monitoring program and are used in conjunction with physical monitors and biological indicators to demonstrate the efficacy of the sterilization process.

After sterilization, process indicators are examined by the CS technician to ensure complete exposure. If processes such as packaging and loading have been done correctly, the CI will have changed color. By contrast, an incomplete color change may provide the first sign that part or all of a load has not been properly sterilized. While chemical indicators do not verify sterility, they are an important part of the larger sterilization monitoring system.

External Chemical Indicators

External CIs are often the first performance test the user sees upon removing a package from the sterilizer. They provide instant results and visual evidence that the package was exposed to a sterilant. *Note: External CIs do not indicate that the item is sterile.*

External process indicators, including tape, load cards or labels on the outside of the packages, are also examined before the items are dispensed and opened to ensure that proper processing has occurred. (See **Figure 17.5**)

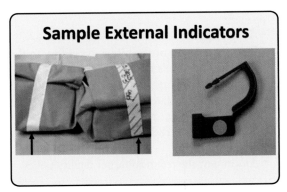

Sample External Indicators

Figure 17.5

Internal Chemical Indicators

Internal CIs are placed inside a package and provide evidence that the sterilant penetrated the package. *Note: Internal CIs do not prove sterility.* **Figure 17.6** provides examples of some CIs.

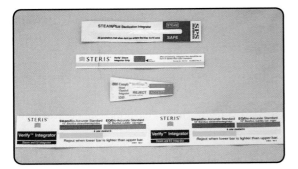

Figure 17.6

CIs should be placed in the area of the package, tray or container considered to be least accessible to sterilant penetration. *Note: This location is not necessarily at the center of the package, tray or container.*

If the interpretation of the CI in a package, tray or container suggests inadequate sterilant penetration, the contents cannot be used and should be returned to the CS department for investigation. *Note: It is possible to have one or more unacceptable indicators in a load because of improper packaging or loading, with the remainder of the load acceptable.*

CIs showing a "fail" result require further investigation to determine the cause. The following could cause a CI test failure:

- Utility or sterilizer malfunction.

- Inappropriate sterilizer loading techniques.

- Not using the correct CI monitor.

- Wrong cycle selected.

- Poor storage of the CI indicator.

- Improper packaging techniques.

- Not following the container IFU.

- Not following the medical device manufacturer's IFU.

Some facilities use CIs that consist of heat-sensitive dye applied to a cardboard strip or a dye that moves along a window. When exposed to a sterilant, these devices gradually change color, thereby integrating a time component to the measurement.

Physical Monitoring

Physical monitors include time, temperature and pressure recorders, displays, digital printouts and gauges. (See **Figure 17.7**) During and at the end of the cycle, and before items are removed from the sterilizer, the operator should review the monitor to ensure all cycle parameters were met.

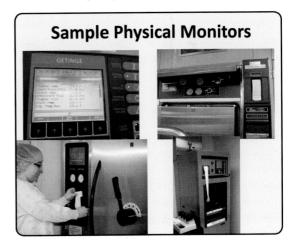

Sample Physical Monitors

Figure 17.7

Upon completion of the cycle, the operator must sign the chart as proof that it was monitored and that all sterilization parameters were met. Physical monitors are needed to detect equipment malfunctions as soon as possible, so appropriate corrective actions can be taken. (See **Figure 17.8**)

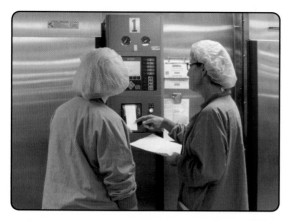

Figure 17.8

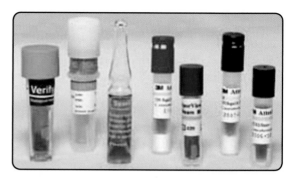

Figure 17.9

If there is any indication of malfunction, the department manager or designee must be notified immediately. The load should be considered unsterile and the sterilizer should be removed from service. It should not be reused until the problem is corrected.

Biological Indicators

Biological indicators (BIs) are one of the most important sterilizer monitors available to the CS technician. BIs are usually ampules that contain a paper strip impregnated with a predetermined amount of live bacterial spores and a solution of growth media. (See **Figure 17.9**) The growth media provides a source for any remaining live bacteria to feed on after sterilization, thus allowing bacteria to grow and be detected. The type of bacteria varies with the method of sterilization, as the spore-producing bacteria most resistant to that sterilization method is used in the test. This test directly determines whether the conditions have been met to kill these resistant organisms. If the most resistant organisms are killed, then less resistant organisms should also be killed. If the proper conditions are not met to kill the spores, then the test organism will grow when incubated after the sterilization cycle.

At the completion of the sterilization cycle, the BI should be incubated according to manufacturer IFU. The load-identifying information must be identified on the BI, in a manner consistent with the IFU. If the bacteria have been killed, there will be no color change or indication of life during incubation. This is known as a negative test result (no growth). If there is a color change in the ampule or there is indication of life through the incubator reading, it is known as a positive test (live bacteria), and items within the load should be recalled and reprocessed.

A test ampule, called a control, should be run at least daily, when a BI is run, and each time a new lot is opened. A control test is the same as the BI, except it has not been put through a sterilization cycle; therefore, the impregnated bacteria will grow when incubated (positive test results). This demonstrates that the ampules in that specific lot are still viable (alive). If the control ampule does not show bacterial growth when incubated (negative test), that means the impregnated bacteria were likely dead before sterilization; therefore, the BI test run with the items being sterilized is inaccurate and will give a false negative reading.

When running a BI and control test, the results CS technicians will look for are a positive reading for the control (growth) and a negative reading for the BI (no growth). All test results and lot numbers must be carefully documented.

A negative BI result does not prove that all items in the load are sterile, or that were all exposed to adequate sterilization conditions. Instead, it shows that all conditions required for sterilization were met. CS technicians must follow proper preparation, packaging and and loading procedures to help ensure proper sterilization parameters will be attained.

BI process challenge devices (PCDs) – addressed further in the next section of this chapter — should be used for routine sterilizer efficacy monitoring (at least weekly, but preferably every day the sterilizer is used). BI PCDs must be used with every implant and they are also required in each load sterilized with ethylene oxide (EtO).

Reasons for Positive Biological Monitors

Positive BI results can be due to an operator error or a sterilizer or utility malfunction. Whenever a positive BI result occurs, its must be investigated to determine its cause.

An operator error can be caused by:

- Using the wrong BI or PCD. Using a BI validated for another mode of sterilization.

- Incorrect placement of the BI in the sterilizer load. BIs placed in the wrong section of the sterilizer, under trays or on their sides may give inaccurate results.

- Not following the BI manufacturer's IFU.

- Incorrect storage of the BI. BIs stored in temperatures that are too cold or too warm can be damaged and lead to incorrect results. Storing BIs where there is inadequate humidity can also impact results.

- Incorrect cycle selection.

- Not loading the sterilizer cart to allow for air removal and sterilant penetration around and through the load. Placing items too closely together (overloading) or placing items on top of the BI can cause an inaccurate test result.

If the cause of the positive BI is not determined, the facility department or outside agency responsible for sterilizer maintenance should be contacted to conduct further investigation. The sterilizer should not be used until the issue is corrected.

Process Challenge Devices

A PCD is designed to challenge a sterilization cycle. These packs may be commercially-prepared or made at the healthcare facility. PCD packs may contain only a CI, but more frequently, they contain a BI and a CI/integrator. For those cycles where a PCD has been developed, the PCD should be used to challenge the sterilization cycle. (See **Figure 17.10**)

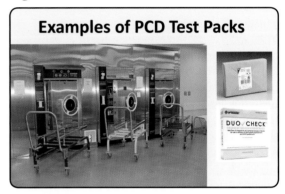

Examples of PCD Test Packs

Figure 17.10

Protocols for using PCDs include:

- The PCD should be labeled with sterilizer load information before being placed into the sterilizer.

- The PCD should be positioned in the chamber according to the sterilizer manufacturer's written recommendations.

- The sterilization cycle should be run. Check the sterilizer and PCD's IFU for specific instructions.

Implants

ANSI/AAMI ST79:2013 recommends that every load containing implantable devices should be monitored with a PCD that contains a BI and a Class 5 integrating CI. An implantable device should not be released before the BI results are known. As with all cycles, the sterilizer operator should review the sterilizer printout and the results of other indicators used to monitor the sterilization process.

Implants should be quarantined until the results of the BI testing are available. In the case of a documented emergency, an implant may be released from the results of the Class 5 CI and physical monitors; however, the BI must continue to be processed to obtain and document a final result. If, due to an emergency, the implantable items must be released before the BI has been read, the release and reason for the release must be documented.

Sterilizer Printouts

Sterilizer printouts should be reviewed and signed by the CS technician responsible for cycle monitoring and if all sterilization parameters were met, the load may be released. It is important for the CS technician to know and understand the parameters that must be met by each type of sterilizer in order to properly monitor the cycles.

Sterilization Load Control Numbers

All items to be sterilized should be labeled with a **load control (lot) number** that identifies:

- Sterilizer identification number.

- Sterilization cycle number.

- Date sterilized – Example: 12-18-2015.

- Some facilities use a **Julian date** on their packages. The Julian date is the number of days that have elapsed since January 1. For example, January 1 is day #001 and December 31 is day #365.

Load control information is usually applied to each package with a labeling applicator gun to place an identification sticker containing the load information. (See **Figure 17.11**)

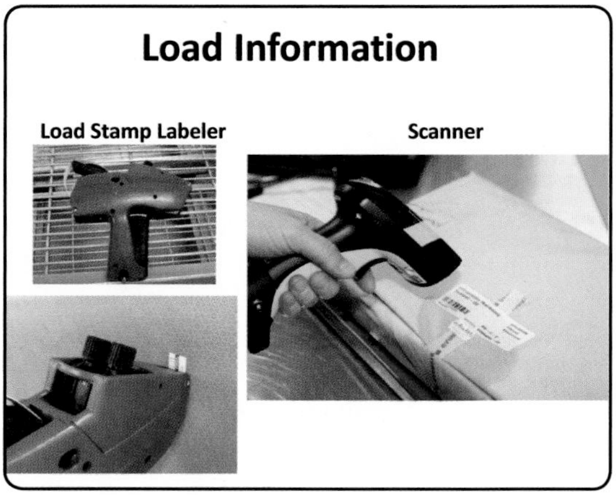

Load Information

Load Stamp Labeler   Scanner

Figure 17.11

Load control (lot) number Label information on sterilization packages, trays or containers that identifies the sterilizer, cycle run and date of sterilization.

Julian date The Julian day or Julian day number (JDN) is the number of days that have elapsed since January 1.

All packages sterilized by the CS department should contain load control (lot) information. Load information helps to retrieve items during recalls and trace problems, such as a positive CI test result.

The following information should be recorded on a load log sheet and maintained for each sterilization cycle:

- Load control number date and time (cycle number) of the sterilizer load.

- Specific items sterilized, including quantity, department and item description (e.g., minor pan 1 OR, towel pack 10 CS, or sternal saw 1 CVOR).

- Exposure time and temperature.

- Sterilizer operator identification.

- Results of biological testing (if applicable).

- Response of the CI placed in the BI test pack, if applicable.

- Results of Bowie-Dick testing, if performed.

This documentation ensures that cycle parameters were monitored and met, and helps personnel determine whether a recall is necessary. *Note: A recall is initiated for a positive BI or nonresponsive CI, wet packs, or other sterility problems. Knowing the contents of the load enables personnel to know where to go to reclaim the packages. This documentation can be compiled manually in a sterilization log book, or there are computer software programs available to compile and maintain these records.*

Validation and Verification

No discussion of sterilization monitoring can be complete without mention of **validation** and **verification** processes. There is a significant difference between "validation" and "verification." Validation is done by the device manufacturer using a documented procedure to obtain, record and interpret the testing results required to determine a process consistently produces a sterile product. Validation requires extensive laboratory testing and retesting of the processes that will be recommended. and the results must be appropriate and reproducible. Testing must also show that the validated sterilization process will not jeopardize the integrity of the product. To validate the sterilization cycle, microbiological challenges are placed in the most difficult to sterilize locations of the device. If it is not possible to reach these areas of the device with a BI, then the device may be inoculated with the specified microbiological challenge via liquid suspension. The medical device is then subjected to three sterilization cycles at one-half the exposure time. In all sterilization qualification runs, the device is packaged (if applicable) in a manner defined by the device manufacturer. The packaging should be appropriate for the device and available to healthcare personnel. The test results must show total microbial kill in the half cycles. Due to the complex requirements, validation cannot be performed in CS.

By contrast, "verification" is performed by the healthcare facility to confirm that the validation undertaken by the manufacturer is applicable to the specific equipment and settings in their facility.

CS technicians perform verification by documenting the procedures to obtain, record and interpret the healthcare facility's test results. The validation provided by the medical device manufacturer provides the framework for these studies.

For information on product verification refer to ANSI/AAMI ST79:2013, Section 10.9.

> **Validation** Procedures used by equipment manufacturers to obtain, record and interpret test results required to establish that a process consistently produces a sterile product.
>
> **Verification** Procedures used by healthcare facilities to confirm that the validation undertaken by the equipment manufacturer is applicable to the specific setting.

Important Note

While product verification can be accomplished in a healthcare facility, the parameters validated by the manufacturer cannot be changed and properly verified. For example, if a manufacturer has validated a device to be steam-sterilized in a 10-minute 270°F cycle, a facility cannot test this item in a five-minute 270°F cycle.

Healthcare facilities do not have the proper products or equipment to properly test and ensure the item is sterile in the shorter cycle. Also, the FDA has approved the manufacturer's cycle, not the healthcare facility's cycle.

Sterilizer Qualification (Verification) Testing

Qualification testing is performed to verify that the sterilizer is in good working condition in the location in which it is being used. This testing also ensures that the sterilizer performs to manufacturer's specifications.

Qualification testing is performed after sterilizer installation, relocation, malfunctions, major repairs, or any time there is a significant change to the utilities connected to the sterilizer. A major repair is considered outside the scope of normal repairs. The replacement of a door gasket is considered a normal repair; however, weld repairs, chamber door replacement, vacuum pump repairs, major piping assembly repairs or rebuilds or control upgrades are considered major repairs.

For more information on sterilizer qualification testing, refer to the sterilizer operation manual and ANSI/AAMI ST79:2013, Section 10.9

STERILIZER-SPECIFIC MONITORING

In addition to the previously discussed monitoring parameters, each sterilization method may have specific parameters that must be monitored to help ensure that it is performing correctly.

Dynamic Air Removal Sterilizers

Dynamic Air Removal Test

This test is also known as a Bowie-Dick test. It is a Class II CI, also known as a specialty indicator. Class II indicators are designed for specific procedures, such as monitoring the effectiveness of the steam sterilizer to remove air from the chamber. (See **Figure 17.12**)

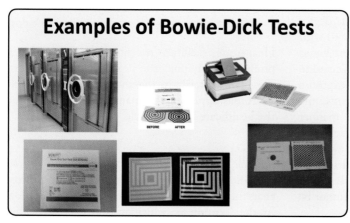

Examples of Bowie-Dick Tests

Figure 17.12

This test should be performed each day the sterilizer is used, at the same time of day and after major repairs. The only items that should be in the chamber during this test are the sterilizer loading carriage (to hold the test), and the test itself. The dynamic air removal test should be placed over the chamber drain and run per the manufacturer's IFU, usually with a reduced sterilization time.

Some sterilizers have a designated air removal test cycle; check to ensure this cycle matches the air removal test manufacturer's instructions. When the cycle is complete, remove the test pack. If the chemically-impregnated sheet has a complete uniform color change, the test is considered negative and the sterilizer is ready to use. If the color change is not uniform and there are blotchy areas of unchanged color, the test is considered positive, and the sterilizer should be taken out of service until the issue can be found and corrected.

Note: Dynamic air removal tests are not run in gravity displacement sterilizers. This is because the air is removed from the chamber using gravity, not a dynamic method.

Leak Testing

Leak testing of dynamic air removal sterilizers is performed to ensure there are no air leaks within the chamber. This test checks the sterilizer's ability to hold a vacuum by testing all the sealed areas and piping to ensure air is not allowed into the chamber during a cycle's vacuum phase. Leak tests should be performed at least weekly in an empty sterilizer chamber. Leak testing is more sensitive than a dynamic air removal test, so it will detect problems before the air removal test might detect the leak. *Note: Refer to the manufacturer's operating manual to determine the acceptable leak test for the sterilizers at the facility.*

Biological Indicators/Process Challenge Devices

The spore-producing microorganism used in steam sterilizer testing is *Geobacillus stearothermophilus*. This bacterium is used because it is a heat-loving bacteria and is, therefore, resistant to the temperatures used for steam sterilization.

It is recommended that commercially-prepared PCDs be used; the materials utilized in the packages remain consistent because they are manufactured for single use, so there is no wear or erosion of the product. If commercially-prepared packs cannot be used, refer to ANSI/AAMI ST79: 2012, Section 10.7.2.1.

Gravity Sterilizers

Biological Indicators/Process Challenge Devices

The spore-producing microorganism used in gravity steam sterilizer testing is *Geobacillus stearothermophilus*.

It is recommended that commercially-prepared PCDs be used; the materials utilized in the packages remain consistent bacause they are manufactured for single use, so there is no wear or erosion of the product. If commercially-prepared packs cannot be used, refer to ANSI/AAMI ST79: 2013, Section10.7.2.1.

Ensure the PCD to be used is designed for gravity sterilizers.

Immediate Use Steam Sterilizers

Biological Indicators/Process Challenge Devices

The spore-producing microorganism used in steam sterilizer testing is *Geobacillus stearothermophilus*.

BIs are processed in Immediate Use Steam Sterilizers (IUSS) without a PCD. This is because items are processed unwrapped or in special containers designed for IUSS. BI ampules should be run in IUSS, according to the manufacturer's IFU. BIs should be run at least weekly, preferably each day the sterilizer is used, and with every load containing an implantable item.

IUSS monitoring includes detailed recordkeeping, so patients can be monitored, if necessary. When an IUSS cycle is run, the following information should be documented.

- Date and time of the sterilization cycle.

- Sterilizer identification (ID).

- Cycle temperature and sterilization time (e.g., 270° F at 10 minutes).

- Item(s) being sterilized.

- Patient identification.

- Reason for sterilizing the item using IUSS.

- CI results.

- BI results, if appropriate.

Multiple Cycle Testing

Some dynamic air removal and immediate use steam sterilizers have the ability to operate in either a dynamic air removal mode or a gravity mode. If a sterilizer is used in both sterilization methods, then BI/PCD testing must be done at least weekly, preferably daily, in both modes. Refer to ANSI/AAMI ST79 and to the sterilizer manufacturer's IFU for specific details.

Tabletop Steam Sterilizers

Biological Indicators/Process Challenge Devices

The spore-producing microorganism used in tabletop steam sterilizer testing is *Geobacillus stearothermophilus*.

Commercially-prepared PCDs are currently not available for tabletop sterilizers. Types of items sterilized varies greatly from facility to facility, so creating a standard PCD would be extremely difficult. To create a PCD for the tabletop sterilizer:

- Select a tray of instruments or package that

represents the most difficult item routinely sterilized in the tabletop sterilizer.

- Once the tray or pack has been identified it should be used for each test performed.

- Place at least one BI and at least one CI in the most challenging area of the tray or pack to sterilize.

After a major repair to a tabletop steam sterilizer, three consecutive test cycles with a PCD should be run and the results should be read before the sterilizer is put back into use.

Ethylene Oxide Sterilizers

Biological Indicators/Process Challenge Devices

BIs are the most acceptable means for providing quality assurance monitoring for EtO sterilization. Like BIs used in steam sterilization, an EtO BI has a carrier that has been inoculated with a known population of a microorganism that is highly-resistant to the sterilant. The microorganism of choice for EtO is the *Bacillus atrophaeus* spore. It is assumed that killing all spores on a standardized BI indicates a successful sterilization cycle; this is because the BI's population and resistance exceeds that of the bioburden on items being sterilized. *Note: This assumption only applies to properly cleaned, prepared, packaged, and loaded supplies. It is recommended that a PCD be run in every EtO load.*

Remember the "4R's"

Process monitoring consists of the "4 R's": Run, Read, Record and Retain. No single monitoring product provides all information necessary to ensure effective sterilization; therefore, recommended practices state that available information from physical, chemical and biological indictors should be used to assess the process before releasing a load.

Note: It is essential that CS technicians are able to read and interpret physical monitoring information and chemical indicator color changes, and know how to handle, use and interpret the results of biological indicators.

Hydrogen Peroxide Sterilizers

There are several different types of hydrogen peroxide (H_2O_2) sterilizers available in today's healthcare market; however, the basic monitoring requirements remain the same for all types of H_2O_2 sterilizers.

Biological Indicators/Process Challenge Devices

BIs are most accepted means for providing quality assurance for hydrogen peroxide (H_2O_2) sterilizers. The microorganism of choice for H_2O_2 is the *Geobacillus stearothermophilus* spore because this bacteria is the most difficult to kill using H_2O_2 methods. As noted earlier, the killing of all the spores on a standardized BI indicates a successful sterilization cycle (assuming supplies have been properly cleaned, prepared, packaged and loaded). A BI PCD should be run at least each day the sterilizer is used, but preferably in every load.

Commercially-prepared PCDs are available; however they are sold to monitor specific sterilizer models. Ensure the correct PCD is being used for the sterilizer.

Ozone Sterilizer

Biological Indicators/Process Challenge Devices

BIs are the most accepted means for providing quality assurance for ozone (O_3) sterilizers. The microorganism of choice for O_3 is the *Geobacillus stearothermophilus* spore because this bacteria is the most difficult to kill using O_3 sterilization. A BI PCD should be run at least daily, each day the sterilizer is used, but, preferably in each load.

PERSONNEL MONITORING

Personnel monitoring can involve several different types of devices. One type of monitoring system uses a badge-type monitor that affixes directly to the employee's clothing in the breathing zone (within one foot of the person's nose). Area monitors are also commonly used. These measure the quality of air in a specific area and alarm if air quality levels are breached.

STAFF EDUCATION

Tasks performed by CS technicians require specific knowledge and skills. The safety of both staff and patients depends on proper execution of specific skills. New instruments, equipment, standards and regulations make ongoing education necessary for even the most experienced CS technicians.

CS departments must provide evidence of the training and education provided for staff. That evidence is usually contained in training documents, competencies and continuing education records.

Training Documents

When a new employee enters the CS department or when an existing employee moves to a new position within the department, the formal process of orienting and training the staff member to their new responsibilities begins. That process should follow a carefully designed training plan that will prepare the employee to correctly perform the required duties. Training and/or orientation documents must be kept on file for each employee as evidence that formal training occurred.

Competencies

Employee competency records are an important monitoring tool for the CS department. Competencies provide evidence that the employee understands specific tasks and is qualified to perform them. Competency records are important for the growth of the department and serve as a basis for a quality improvement (QI) program.

Detailed, step-by-step lists should be developed and utilized for each task performed within the CS department. Competencies should be done during initial orientation, whenever a new device is received, and on a routine basis for daily CS tasks. Some competencies will need to be done annually (i.e., tasks pertaining to sterilizer operation and documentation), while other job duties, such as wrapping techniques, may only need to be done when issues arise or on a rotating basis.

Competency records can be reviewed to determine areas where each employee excels or where more training is needed. They can also be used to show process improvement.

Continuing Education Records

The CS discipline is constantly changing and CS technicians must change with it. Continuing education provides a means of staying abreast of changes in regulations, standards, technology, scientific knowledge and equipment. Continuing education records provide evidence that the employee has kept current and is aware of new best practices. **Figure 17.13** provides an example of an employee inservice, a common method used to help educate CS staff.

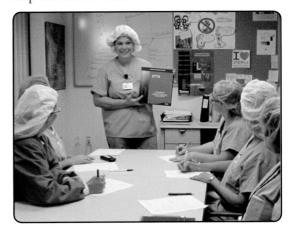

Figure 17.13

Education records should be kept on file for all CS employees and should be monitored to help ensure they are current.

CONCLUSION

Properly and consistently monitoring the Central Service department and processing equipment helps ensure patient and staff safety. It also helps ensure the consistent production of high-quality products.

Every member of the CS department must monitor the environment, work practices, mechanical processes, and training and education to ensure that standards, regulations and best practices are properly and consistently followed.

RESOURCES

Occupational Safety and Health Administration. OSHA Standard 29 CFR 1910.15l(c).

Centers for Disease Control and Prevention. *Guideline for Disinfection and Sterilization in Healthcare Facilities.* 2008.

Association for the Advancement of Medical Instrumentation. ANSI/AAMI ST58, *Chemical sterilization and high-level disinfection in health care facilities,* Section 9.4.4.3.

Association for the Advancement of Medical Instrumentation. ANSI/AAMI ST79:2010 & A1: 2010 & A2: 2011 & A3:2012, Section 10.

CENTRAL SERVICE TERMS

Monitor

Load control number

Julian date

Validation

Verification

Chapter 18

Quality Assurance

Learning Objectives

As a result of successfully completing this chapter, readers will be able to:

1. Define quality in the context of Central Service operations

2. Describe the components of a Central Service quality program

3. Explain the basics of failure mode and effects analysis and root cause analysis

4. Discuss common quality programs:
    • Total quality improvement
    • Continuous quality improvement
    • Total quality management
    • Six Sigma and Lean
    • Other quality programs and standards

5. Review common quality procedures in the Central Service department

INTRODUCTION

Healthcare consumers demand quality in the products and services they receive. They expect nothing less than the best for themselves and their loved ones while using inpatient and outpatient healthcare services. Central Service (CS) professionals must establish appropriate quality levels for the products and services they produce, and ensure that these levels are consistently maintained.

CS technicians directly serve **internal customers** (physicians, nurses and other professionals working in the facility). The success of CS depends upon satisfying the needs of these internal customers, so they can best serve the patients. Quality (or lack of quality) can have dramatic consequences on the health and safety of both patients and facility personnel. Providing quality products and services directly impacts patient outcomes and significantly impacts the department's (and the healthcare facility's) success.

CS technicians are an integral part of quality service throughout the healthcare facility. CS technicians are now processing medical devices for surgery centers, physician's offices, off-site clinics, nursing rehabilitation facilities, dental offices and third-party reprocessors. With emerging antibiotic-resistant bacteria and the ever-increasing complexity of surgical instrumentation, it has never been more challenging or rewarding for CS personnel to consistently provide quality products and services.

This chapter will discuss several established quality indicators to assist in monitoring quality within CS departments. The ultimate goal is high quality patient care. This can best be achieved through comprehensive training programs and ongoing quality monitoring.

> **Customer (internal)** The physicians, nurses and other professional personnel served by Central Service personnel.
>
> **Quality** The consistent delivery of products and services according to established standards. Quality "integrates" the concerns for the customers (including patients and user department personnel) with those of the department and facility.

QUALITY IN CENTRAL SERVICE OPERATIONS

Quality requires CS technicians to look at what they do from their customers' perspectives. In many respects, CS production is only as good as the last device processed or the most recent service provided. One hundred error-free items can be processed, but one imperfect tray or service will be noticed and considered as the department's quality outputs are evaluated. While this may seem unreasonable, it is important to understand that just one error can cause significant harm to patients and employees.

What is Quality?

The concept of **quality** relates to the degree or grade of excellence of a product or service. For example: Emergency Department personnel may believe that an emergency code cart was delivered efficiently (on a timely basis), but the cart might not provide a needed item that was requested on the pick list (supply listing). This indicates poor service quality. By contrast, when a surgical instrument set is needed quickly and the CS department delivers it promptly with all necessary components, poor service quality can still result if the surgical staff was not informed of the set delivery. In short, quality is measured through the eyes of the customers and their concerns relate to both products and service.

The patient must be at the center of every quality concern. CS professionals must provide properly processed products when they are needed. Just being "good" is not good enough. A surgical tray delivered to the Operating Room (OR) on time, but with incomplete or incorrect instruments does not represent quality service and can cause the patient to have a less than desirable outcome due to instrumentation problems. CS technicians accept this responsibility and the challenge to consistently meet requirements.

Looking at functions from customers' perspectives allows the CS team to critically review its processes to determine where improvements can be made. Remember that:

- Increased education should help staff provide a higher quality of service.

- Quality takes time, effort and participation from everyone in the healthcare facility.

- When measuring quality, best practices provide a good starting point.

- CS staff can use their knowledge to increase efficiencies.

How is Quality Identified?

Products and services might be considered "excellent" if they meet one's needs (they do what they are supposed to do). If a new washer-disinfector is properly used, but instruments are still dirty after a complete cycle, the equipment will be judged inferior; however, if the equipment meets expectations (it produces clean decontaminated instruments), it is easier to assume that, "This is a great manufacturer, and I would purchase from this company again."

This feeling provides a subjective view of quality that provides no basis for measurement. What's more, it does not consider the customers' service levels.

Branding is another subjective form of quality identification. If one has a great experience with specific equipment, a future purchase from that manufacturer is more likely than if negative experiences occur.

Products processed by CS professionals should always be complete and properly assembled with no errors. An internal department system should be implemented to identify inferior products before they leave the area. External department information can be obtained from customers by using the count sheets for trays, pick tickets for case carts and requested items, and/or by formal surveys designed to learn about quality dimensions from customers' perspective. (See **Figure 18.1**) Statistics from both internal and external sources should be analyzed, errors should be studied and corrective actions should be implemented to best ensure quality improvement.

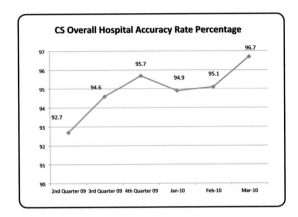

Figure 18.1

COMPONENTS OF QUALITY

Quality is not a quick fix for healthcare facilities. Achieving world class (best in the industry) quality requires a multi-year plan to move a facility from its current quality level to the ideal (highest achievable) quality. For example, the Ritz-Carlton hotel chain, the only U.S. lodging organization to win the prestigious Malcolm Baldrige award for quality, began its quality journey with a benchmark of 60,000 defects per million transactions. It planned a six-year process to move to 0.60 (less than one) defect per million transactions. The Ritz-Carlton's definition of world-class quality also required a 50% reduction in cycle time (the time that passes between an order being placed and being completed). This planned approach to move toward an ideal quality goal is just as relevant to healthcare as it is to hospitality.

Top-level administrators must emphasize quality because their support is critical for success. Most problems affecting the employees' ability to accomplish work are caused by systems and procedures that have, in some way, been required or implemented by top-level leaders.

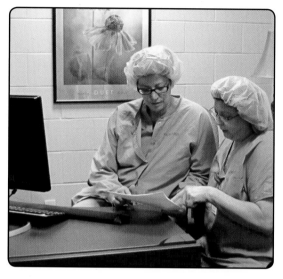

Figure 18.2

Departmental quality should be multidisciplinary, as well as intradepartmental. A true quality program utilizes all CS professionals and a cross-section of its customers. (See **Figure 18.2**)

Empowerment

Empowerment is the action of driving the process of decision-making and implementation down the facility's chain of command. In other words, some decisions that have traditionally been made by managers or higher level departmental staff or administrators are now made by supervisors or front line staff members. Empowerment is typically limited to well defined areas, such as **process improvement** changes within the employee's defined areas of responsibility.

Employees assigned to specific work areas must know how to properly perform all work tasks before they can be empowered. Managers must provide training about the concept of empowerment and they must encourage the sharing of ideas and suggestions that can lead to improvements.

Leadership

Quality requires committed leaders to help manage the data, plan opportunities, establish priorities and empower people to implement process improvements.

Effective leaders define standards to be attained in quality products/services. Those standards will drive the development of strategies that address customer satisfaction and the attainment of the facility's goals.

Departmental leaders, including shift supervisors and lead technicians, should be the first-line "guardians" of the quality program to ensure that all department personnel consistently adhere to the standards and priorities set by senior managers. Employees should help their teammates follow established guidelines. This can be accomplished by interacting with new or less qualified staff members, assisting in ongoing training and participating in daily quality control checks.

> **Empowerment** The act of granting authority (power) to employees so they may make decisions within their areas of responsibility.
>
> **Process improvement** Activity to identify and resolve task-related problems that yield poor quality; the strategy of finding solutions to eliminate the root causes of process performance problems.

Standard Data

Each department must select the data that will be used to monitor its quality processes. **Figure 18.3** provides an example of data that has been collected and compiled for analysis.

Measurement	Goal	Actual	Color
Avg. Trays Backlogged 7am	< 15	42	
Avg. Trays Backlogged 11pm	< 25	76	
# Errors Reported	< 3	2	
% Case Carts Complete Supplies	99%	97%	
% Case Carts Complete Instruments	95%	91%	
% Complete Instrument Trays	98%	94%	
Total Hours per Tray Processed	1.80	2.03	
Staff Productivity	90%	92%	

Figure 18.3

Planning Tools and Procedures

Quality planning can reduce existing problems and prevent potential problems. It involves:

- Studying other facilities. How do other facilities deliver each product and service that their patients/customers want?

- Remembering that the process (not people) is the cause of most problems.

- Thinking about how to improve.

Steps of quality planning include the following:

- Step One: Identify the needs and requests of the department's customers.

- Step Two: Identify an ideal process to consistently address each need/request.

- Step Three: Compare actual steps and outcomes of each process to the ideal outcome (e.g., 100% error-free trays).

- Step Four: Plan process control activities to improve the system.

- Step Five: Measure the errors.

With a good quality system in place, the number of errors should decrease.

Principles of Quality Management

Several principles of quality management form the foundation of a quality process:

- Patient focus – Assuring that patients' needs are the driving force in decision making, problem solving and other activities.

- Process management – Placing the emphasis on managing the process, rather than upon managing the employees.

- Continuous quality improvement – Believing that things can always be done better and then undertaking improvement efforts.

- Fact-based decisions – Basing decisions on facts, rather than assumptions.

Staff Members

To have a successful quality program, all departmental staff members must be fully engaged with the program. While management may set the standards and goals, technicians, for the most part, carry out the processes to achieve success. Providing all staff members with a solid education foundation will help ensure they use critical thinking skills on the job.

Employees must be empowered to address solutions to immediate problems within their realm of expertise. For example, they should be allowed to stop what they are doing to help another employee. They should be able to enlist the assistance of other workers in problem-solving tasks, when necessary. Also, employees who desire additional responsibilities should be allowed to work on longer-term problem-solving projects. This may be done with the use of **cross-functional teams** that select a process problem, analyze it, develop alternatives, offer solutions and make implementation suggestions. It is important for senior leaders to recognize superior staff members and teams.

Cross-functional team Group of employees from different departments within the healthcare facility that works together to resolve operating problems.

Process Management

Studying processes is critical because process problems cause errors. If errors are identified and resolved, patients and customers will experience fewer problems. (See **Figures 18.4** and **18.5**) Also, employees will have greater success in consistently delivering products and services that meet quality standards. Some processes commonly studied for improvement are:

- Instrument set turnaround times.

- Instrument set accuracy.

- Surgical case cart accuracy.

- Inventory fill rates.

The highest levels of quality are difficult to attain and maintain. When quality is not emphasized, inconsistent products, service delays, negative patient outcomes and employee conflicts can arise. These problems contribute to higher costs for the facility and the patient, and lower revenues for the healthcare facility.

Skills Flexibility Matrix Standard				Ratings: 1 = Oriented Only, 2 = Needs		
		# of Skills	Average Skill Rating	J. Abraham	J. Doe	J. Smith
		35	2.6	2.3	2.4	2.5
#	Activity	Skill Trainer	Rating	Rating	Rating	Rating
1	Station Set-Up, Use & Clean Up	JK	3.1	4	4	3
2	Wrapped In-House Items	CN, JK	2.1	1	2	3
3	Container In-House Items	CN, MG	2.9	3	3	3
4	Clean From Hospital Items	JK	2.4	2	3	2
5	Peel Packages	JK	2.2	3	1	1
6	Identification & Use of Indicators	JK	2.4	2	4	3
7	Proper Operation	JK	2.2	1	2	1
8	Troubleshooting	CN, DJ	2.3	1	2	1

Figure 18.4

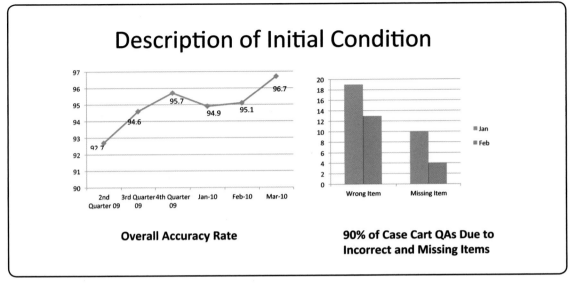

Description of Initial Condition

Overall Accuracy Rate

90% of Case Cart QAs Due to Incorrect and Missing Items

Figure 18.5

QUALITY CONTROL INDICATORS

Purpose of Quality Control Indicators

CS quality control indicators are often used to determine how well the department is meeting its objectives. Several quality indicators should be monitored periodically. (See **Figure 18.6**) Some examples of CS quality indicators are:

- Customer departments receive STAT (urgent) medical supplies within five minutes of request.

- Only sterile supplies with current dates are available on unit supply carts.

- Sterilization processes are acceptable, based upon results of physical, chemical and biological indicators.

- Instrument sets contain clean, functional and correct contents.

- Patient care equipment and supplies are available and in proper working condition.

- Instruments are available for scheduled procedures to avoid the use of Immediate Use Steam Sterilization (IUSS).

- Biological indicators accompany every load requiring biological monitoring.

- Case carts contain correct contents.

ANALYSIS OF QUALITY CONCERNS

Failure mode and effects analysis (FMEA) and root cause analysis (RCA) are two widely used methods to analyze issues discovered within quality systems. Although these methods are not always recognized or practiced in their original form, their popularity has continued to grow. Both concepts are important tools that can be used in a quality program.

Failure Mode and Effects Analysis

FMEA has its origins in the military and industrial fields, and is a method of identifying and preventing problems with products and processes before they occur. The FMEA process seeks to accomplish several things. First, it aims to define the topic that must be addressed (e.g., replacing a hospital boiler), then assemble a group of multidisciplinary staff to identify possible hazards and causes (e.g., poor steam quality, pipe ruptures and service disruption). Finally, the team identifies actions and outcomes for each potential problem. For example, before replacing the boiler, it may be important to rent a temporary steam generator to use if problems arise,

Examples of Technical Quality Control Indicators

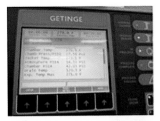
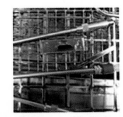
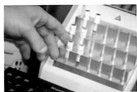
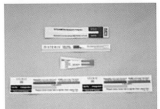
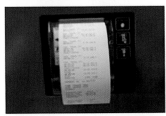
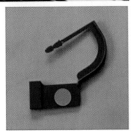
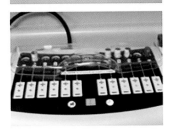
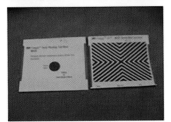
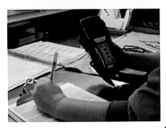

Figure 18.6

so the food service department, OR and CS may remain functional if any of the identified problems occur.

> **Failure mode and effect analysis (FMEA)** A process designed to predict the adverse outcomes of various human and machine failures to prevent future adverse outcomes.
>
> **Root cause analysis (RCA)** A process that "looks backward" at an event to help prevent its future occurrence.

Root Cause Analysis

Root cause analysis (RCA) is a reactive process that uses historical analysis of an adverse outcome to help prevent its recurrence. Assume a washer-disinfector pump malfunctioned and caused instruments to be improperly cleaned. Each event after the pump failure would be examined to determine what could

have occurred and what can be done to prevent this issue in the future. Another example is the tip of a carbide insert on a needle holder breaking during surgery. All members involved with the set will meet to determine what happened and how to prevent this from happening again. Members of this meeting should be:

- The surgeon (How was the instrument used?).

- The scrub technician and circulating nurse (What happened? Was the instrument checked before giving it to the surgeon?).

- The CS manager and the technician who assembled the tray (What are the set policies and procedures for instrument assembly/testing? Was the instrument properly checked?).

- Risk manager (usually serves as meeting facilitator).

- Any other interested parties (instrument repair technician, Infection Prevention personnel).

This group will determine what went wrong at each step of the process and determine how to prevent the problem from happening again.

RCA is widely utilized in the medical field to examine contributing factors to adverse events. Note: *The Joint Commission (TJC) standard LD 5.2 requires facilities to conduct root cause analysis on any* **sentinel event** *that is recurring*.

> **Sentinal event** An unexpected occurrence involving death, serious physical or psychological injury, or the risk thereof.

QUALITY PROGRAM ALTERNATIVES

Many CS departments utilize a quality assurance program because it is comprehensive and requires the gathering of data to ensure that a quality product is regularly produced. The number of items not meeting quality requirements is compared to the total number of items produced. There are many **quality assurance** programs utilized within the healthcare industry. Some of the most popular are:

- **Total quality improvement (TQI)** involves measuring the current output of a process or procedure, and then modifying it to increase the output, increase efficiency, and/or increase effectiveness. TQI recognizes that improvement can occur with an individual, a team, an organizational unit, such as the CS department, or the organization itself.

- **Continuous quality improvement (CQI)** is a statistical method to improve **work processes**. Planning and implementing a CQI program for instrument processing involves the receipt and use of input from decontamination staff, processing employees, clinicians and physician personnel and all others involved in equipment use. This team can assist in identifying where more training is needed (multiple users), where process

changes are needed (multiple departments) and what the expected quality outcomes should be.

- **Total quality management (TQM)** is an organization-wide quality approach based on participation of all members. The aim is long-term success through customer satisfaction and benefit to all members of the organization and society. TQM requires that the facility maintain its quality standards in all aspects of its business. It also ensures work tasks are performed correctly the first time, and that operational defects and waste are eliminated.

The above are just a few of the formal quality programs used in healthcare. Many facilities develop their own quality program utilizing a combination of several of the above programs. As long as the program works for the facility and emphasizes the main focus of quality patient care, it doesn't matter which program or combinations of programs are used.

Figure 18.7 provides an example of a quality report that identifies the types of instrument errors. **Figure 18.8** provides an example of a report indicating progress in efforts to reduce IUSS.

> **Quality assurance** A comprehensive and measured effort to provide total quality. Also, a technical, statistical sampling method that measures production quality.
>
> **Total quality improvement (TQI)** The concept of measuring the current output of a process or procedure and then modifying it to increase the output, increase efficiency, and/or increase effectiveness.
>
> **Continuous quality improvement (CQI)** A scientific approach that applies statistical methods to improve work processes.
>
> **Processes (work)** A series of work activities which produce a product or service.
>
> **Total quality management (TQM)** A quality management approach based on participation of all members aimed at long-term success through customer satisfaction and benefits to all members of the organization and society.

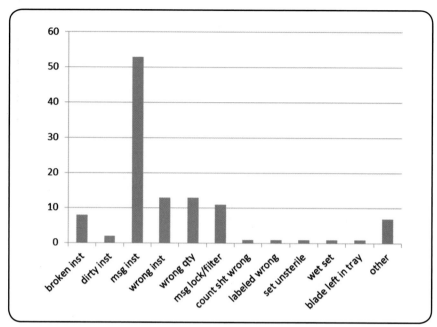

Figure 18.7

CSF - QUALITY
IMMEDIATE USE STEAM STERILIZATION (IUSS)   TOTAL ITEMS

	FY2010	FY 2011	FY 2012	FY 2013	FY 2014
OCTOBER	105	251	27	26	6
NOVEMBER	124	65	42	14	
DECEMBER	134	181	30	14	
JANUARY	80	37	20	4	
FEBRUARY	110	57	31	2	
MARCH	132	203	20	3	
APRIL	140	209	16	4	
MAY	130	90	23	7	
JUNE	195	45	21	3	
JULY	146	33	17	1	
AUGUST	149	69	31	7	
SEPTEMBER	326	79	32	7	
TOTAL	1771	1319	310	92	

This year, our goal for Immediate Use Steam Sterilization (IUSS) is to send *7* or less items out of CSP, unsterile, per month.

We had another great month in reducing immediate sterilization!

This is a great way to increase QUALITY PATIENT CARE!!

Thank you so much!!

Figure 18.8

Six Sigma and Lean Six Sigma

In recent years, healthcare facilities have begun adding **Six Sigma** and Lean Six Sigma programs to their existing quality programs.

Six Sigma

The objective of Six Sigma is to deliver high performance, reliability and value to the end customer. It is a highly disciplined and complex process that focuses on developing and delivering near-perfect products and services in an ongoing quality effort. This process strives to eliminate variations in a product (a tray will look the same each and every time it is assembled, and will look like the same product produced before it), eliminating variations to prevent defects. It focuses on process improvement and variation reduction by use of Six Sigma improvement projects. Two of the processes most used in six sigma are:

- DMADV (define, measure, analyze, design and verify) process is used to develop new processes.

- DMAIC (define, measure, analyze, improve and control) procedures monitor and improve existing processes.

Lean

Lean is a production practice with the key tenet of preserving value with less work (eliminating waste). Eliminating wasteful processes reduces production time and costs.

Lean's strength is its fast implementation. Immediate benefits relate to productivity, error reduction, and customer lead times. Long-term benefits include improvements to financial performance, customer satisfaction and staff morale.

Both Six Sigma and Lean focus on refining the process while reducing defects to an extremely low rate (less than three to four errors per 1,000,000 products produced).

Figure 18.9 provides a comparison of Lean and Six Sigma processes.

> **Six Sigma** A quality process that focuses on developing and delivering near-perfect products and services.
>
> **Lean** A quality process that focuses on eliminating waste in the production of products.

Lean	Six Sigma
Map out the process. In the case of instrument assembly, each step the instruments take from use to reuse is documented.	Map out the process. In the case of instrument assembly, each step the instruments take from use to reuse is documented.
Refine the process. Identify what steps in the mapped process are not necessary.	Identify the defects; where are the mistakes happening?
Developing the new process, based on the information identified during the refining process.	What is causing these mistakes? Correct the actions that are causing the mistakes.
Try the new process.	Try the new process.
Gather, analyze and document data.	Gather, analyze and document data.
Adjust and refine the process, as necessary.	Adjust and refine the process, as necessary.
Monitor and report data.	Monitor and report data.

Figure 18.9

Quality at Work

Being an active participant in any quality process helps ensure the solutions generated are workable for everyone involved. Whether the activity involves the CS workgroup or a broader, cross-functional team, taking the time to examine processes and identify opportunities for improvement is worthwhile.

The following figures provide examples of some common methods to identify issues and improve quality. **Figure 18.10** illustrates a simple process where representatives from two workgroups, the OR and CS, identified issues with trays sent to CS and the OR. Using a simple problem analysis chart fostered better communication, captured issues and gave the group information to make changes to improve their processes.

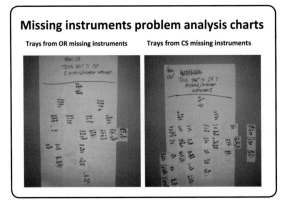

Figure 18.10

Figure 18.11 shows the result of a workgroup's efforts to identify waste in their processes. This information was then used to simplify processes, reduce waste and educate staff.

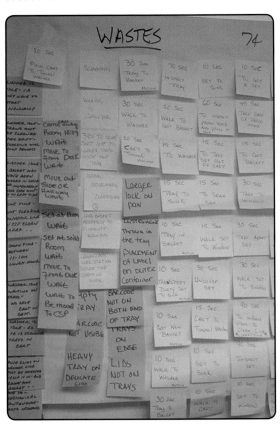

Figure 18.11

| | | SPD Labor Hour Needs | | | | Cycle Starts | |
		Decontam	Assembly	Sterilize	Total	Washer Loads	Sterilizer Loads
1st Shift	7:00	0.3	0.8	0.1	1.2	0.4	0.2
	8:00	0.2	1.0	0.0	1.2	0.3	0.1
	9:00	0.2	0.7	0.0	0.9	0.3	0.2
	10:00	1.8	0.7	0.0	2.5	3.0	0.1
	11:00	3.0	7.4	0.0	10.4	4.9	0.1
	12:00	4.4	12.0	0.3	16.8	7.3	1.2
	13:00	4.2	17.8	0.5	22.4	6.9	2.0
	14:00	4.1	16.7	0.7	21.5	6.7	2.9

Figure 18.12

CENTRAL STERILE PROCESSING

	FY2010			FY2011			FY2012			FY2013			FY2014	
DATE	SETS STERILIZED	EQUIPMENT	DATE	SETS STERILIZED	EQUIPMENT	DATE	SETS STERILIZED	EQUIPMENT	DATE	SETS STERILIZED	EQUIPMENT	DATE	SETS STERILIZED	EQUIPMENT
OCT. 2009	9608	3533	OCT. 2010	9930	4170	OCT. 2011	11883	3873	OCT. 2012	11,775	5,404	OCT. 2013	11,643	6,774
NOV. 2009	8531	3078	NOV. 2010	8941	4003	NOV. 2011	10525	3430	NOV. 2012	10,098	4,813	NOV. 2013		
DEC. 2009	8653	2907	DEC. 2010	8920	4083	DEC. 2011	10947	3388	DEC. 2012	10,242	5,965	DEC. 2013		
JAN. 2010	8480	3374	JAN. 2011	8417	3490	JAN. 2012	10667	2850	JAN. 2013	10,094	6,919	JAN. 2014		
FEB. 2010	8428	2880	FEB. 2011	7820	3255	FEB. 2012	10336	3148	FEB. 2013	9,689	6,157	FEB. 2014		
MAR. 2010	9447	2573	MAR. 2011	9696	3793	MAR. 2012	10999	2813	MAR. 2013	11,066	5,969	MAR. 2014		
APR. 2010	9095	2958	APR. 2011	9712	3297	APR. 2012	9937	2591	APR. 2013	10,517	6,256	APR. 2014		
MAY. 2010	8859	3706	MAY. 2011	9827	2962	MAY. 2012	11153	3163	MAY. 2013	10,088	5,874	MAY. 2014		
JUN. 2010	8890	3609	JUN. 2011	10186	3259	JUN. 2012	10546	4000	JUN. 2013	10,336	6,098	JUN. 2014		
JUL. 2010	8816	3848	JUL. 2011	9991	3674	JUL. 2012	10539	5129	JUL. 2013	9,635	6,635	JUL. 2014		
AUG. 2010	9320	4389	AUG. 2011	11788	3593	AUG. 2012	11783	5287	AUG. 2013	10,339	7,343	AUG. 2014		
SEP. 2010	8869	3960	SEP. 2011	11630	3244	SEP. 2012	10143	4562	SEP. 2013	10,250	7,401	SEP. 2014		
TOTAL	106996	40815		116858	42823		129458	44234		124,129	74,844			

Figure 18.13

Figures 18.12 and **18.13** address labor trends and processing volumes for the CS department. Each provides a tool to address quality issues.

Other Quality Programs and Standards

Quality efforts of healthcare facilities are also impacted by external agencies whose requirements must be addressed. CS technicians should be familiar with the following:

The Joint Commission

TJC is an accreditation organization that ensures quality standards are set, monitored and maintained by member healthcare facilities. It has established many health and safety program requirements for patients and staff using recommended practices and guidelines from agencies and associations, including the Occupational Safety and Health Administration (OSHA) and the Association for the Advancement of Medical Instrumentation (AAMI). Routine and unannounced inspections are used to monitor standards, and each member facility is graded on its performance. TJC requires that any sentinel event be reported and thoroughly investigated to correct the causes.

The Centers for Medicare & Medicaid Services

The Centers for Medicare & Medicaid Services (CMS) is a government agency that focuses on quality in healthcare, as well as patient safety and security. Like TJC, CMS performs announced and unannounced surveys of healthcare facilities to ensure industry standards and regulations are being followed and maintained, and that high quality patient care is the outcome.

National Committee for Quality Assurance

NCQA is a nonprofit organization dedicated to improving healthcare quality. The organization is known for assisting healthcare facilities in identifying how to prioritize quality goals and measure them and promote ongoing improvement.

The Hospital Consumer Assessment of Healthcare Providers and Systems Survey and Value-Based Initiatives

The Hospital Consumer Assessment of Healthcare Providers and Systems (HCAHPS) (pronounced "H-caps") is a standardized survey tool. Hospitals utilize survey results to measure the patient's perception of their experience during their hospital stay. Three broad goals shape HCAHPS:

1. The standardized survey allows meaningful comparisons of hospitals from the patient's perspective.

2. Public reporting of HCAHPS results creates new incentives for hospitals to improve their quality of care

3. Public reporting serves to enhance accountability in healthcare.

The Value-Based Purchasing (VBP) initiatives compare a hospital's HCAHPS scores in a baseline period to those in a later performance period. Healthcare facilities that do not reach HCAHPS goals are penalized through reduced government reimbursement.

Magnet Status

Magnet status is an award given by the American Nurses Credentialing Center to hospitals for quality patient care, nursing excellence and innovations in professional nursing practice.

International Standards Organization

ISO 9000 is an international standard that companies use to ensure their quality system is effective. This process is believed to guarantee that a company consistently delivers quality services and products.

While many healthcare organizations have subscribed to ISO standards, few CS departments have applied or qualified for ISO status.

> **Magnet status** An award given by the American Nurses Credentialing Center to hospitals that satisfy factors that measure the strength and quality of nursing care.
>
> **ISO 9000** An international standard used by participating organizations to help ensure that quality services and products are consistently delivered.

QUALITY CENTRAL SERVICE PROCEDURES

Attaining and maintaining high quality CS standards is everyone's responsibility. Every technician should play an active role in the department's quality program. It is also each technician's responsibility to help or report others who are struggling with a process. Keeping the patient as the focus means helping ensure everyone is properly trained and performing at optimum levels while working in the department. Allowing a known defective product out of the department is inexcusable and can be very dangerous for patients. There are several tools that can be used by technicians to help ensure quality is always addressed:

- Performing departmental audits of each area of the department on a regular basis helps to keep the department and its functions at optimal levels. Audits can be performed by outside departments, such as Safety or Infection Prevention and Control, or they can be done by the CS staff, or a combination of the above. Technicians are a valuable asset to these audits because they know the environment and processes better than anyone else.

- Following the departmental policies, procedures and processing protocols. These documents were developed to help ensure the safety of all CS department members and ensure that all products produced are of the highest quality. Not following policies, procedures and protocols will result in a lower-quality product (i.e., missing, incorrect or soiled instruments) which may harm a patient.

- Keeping current with new technology and appropriately sharing what has been learned with co-workers and supervisors. As technology advances, the ability to check work becomes more effective. New products are always being developed to help check for residual blood and protein.Better products are on the market to check for lumen cleanliness, as well as products that help ensure our processing equipment is working properly. As instrumentation becomes more complex, it becomes more important to utilize technology to help ensure quality products are being delivered.

- Taking an active role in quality improvement processes. CS technicians should take an active role in all process improvement projects. Technicians are very familiar with all department activities and can be a vital asset in helping determine problems and how best to resolve them.

- Assuming responsibility for survey readiness. As part of the CS team, each person is responsible for keeping the department ready for TJC and CMS surveys. Cleanliness, following set practices and knowing the required information on safety, disaster and department processes is a year-round practice.

- Adopting a team mentality. Help co-workers and accept help from them. No one is an expert at all processes within the department. Seek help where skills are not as strong and help those who need assistance.

- Attaining CS certification. Certified technicians know why they perform procedures a specific way. This knowledge of the science behind the practices helps ensure practices will be followed correctly, thus helping ensure a quality product.

CS professionals are expected to consistently attain desired quality standards as they undertake their normal responsibilities. While this is a difficult goal to attain, it is a necessary one. CS technicians have a significant role to play in implementing quality within their facilities. They can, for example, consistently follow all of the instrument procedures discussed throughout this manual. They do not, however, work by themselves. They are an integral part of the entire healthcare team. To ensure the highest quality of patient care, all staff members must work together. The sum of all contributions by all personnel in all departments represents the facility's accomplishments.

QUALITY IN CENTRAL SERVICE PROCESSING AREAS

There are many quality processes that all CS technicians must consistently practice in their daily routine. This section reviews some of these processes on an area-by-area basis within the department.

Decontamination Area

- Always wear personal protective equipment (PPE) when working in this area to protect oneself, other staff, and patients when leaving the area.

- Disassemble all items, where applicable, to ensure all instrument parts are accessible for cleaning.

- Measure chemicals properly. Improperly measured chemicals are not effective cleaners or disinfectants.

- Load and operate equipment properly. Improperly loaded or operated equipment cannot effectively clean instruments.

- Follow all written procedures for cleaning and disinfection. Ensure that items are cleaned and disinfected according to the manufacturer's Instructions for Use (IFU).

- Check processing equipment before use to ensure that it is in proper working order. Improperly working equipment can harm staff and patients.

Preparation and Packing Areas

- Check for holes in all wrappers and disposable filters to ensure that they are intact before sterilization. Even normal handling can sometimes cause a small percentage of wrappers and filters to become damaged prior to use.

- Never use a wrapper, filter or instrument that has fallen on the floor. If this occurs, instruments should be recleaned, and wrappers and filters should be discarded.

- Use only U.S. Food and Drug Administration-approved wrappers and containers approved for the specific method of sterilization utilized.

- Always follow count sheets. Even if one has extensive experience performing the assigned task, changes may have occurred to a case cart or instrument count sheet. Remember that patient care personnel require the correct supplies when they are needed.

- Check instruments for functionality, cleanliness, alignment, proper assembly and sharpness. Failure to do so could result in patient harm.

Sterilization Area

- Always load sterilizer carts as trained. Improperly loaded carts can result in wet or nonsterile loads.

- Ensure the sterilizer parameters are set properly for the load contents. This should include proper temperature, exposure and dry time.

- Always verify physical and chemical indicators after a sterilization cycle to ensure that the process was properly completed.

- Do not touch sterilized items until cool.

- Properly complete all documentation including load, biological and implant logs.

Storage and Distribution Areas

- Always follow established pick sheets to ensure that all items are picked and delivered.

- Ensure transport and case carts are clean and dry before placing items on or inside them.

- Check product packaging for compromised integrity, expiration dating and appropriate color changes of all indicators.

All Central Service/Distribution Areas

- Pay attention to the job at hand: Excessive visiting or other distractions, like a loud radio, can lead to errors.

- CS professionals should not do anything they have not been trained to do. They must always inform someone when they are asked to perform a process/function in which they lack training.

- If a CS professional is unsure about a completed project, they should ask someone to check their work. This is much better than to have an incomplete or wrong item leave the department.

- If distracted, check the entire project to ensure that it is done correctly.

- If a CS professional can't perform to a 100% level, they should not do the project. Also, they should not start a project if they know someone else will need to finish it.

- Recheck all work. The short time required to do so can eliminate an incident in a patient care area.

- Remember that neatness counts.

- Always help other staff members.

- If something appears wrong, speak up.

- Report inoperative or damaged equipment.

- Attend as many educational inservices, seminars, infection prevention, service technician and vendor-sponsored programs as possible. The more education a CS technician can attain, the better they will become on the job.

- Always follow the established departmental policies, procedures and protocols. They are in place for a reason. which usually is to protect staff and the patients.

- Remember that quality is the responsibility of every employee, and every employee must be involved, motivated and knowledgeable if the CS department is to consistently produce and deliver quality products and services. (See **Figure 18.14**)

CONCLUSION

Quality is everyone's responsibility in the healthcare environment and must remain at the core of Central Service operations. Paying careful attention to all policies, procedures and protocols, actively participating in all quality projects, and helping co-workers are all cornerstones to CS quality.

A team-based approach to quality can provide measurable results that improve patient care and on-the-job satisfaction.

Quality Improvement Results

Measure	Before	After	% Improvement	Lean Tools
Daily capacity and demand	378 trays per day	437 trays per day	14% increase	Visual management layout
Rewashes	96 rewashes per day	34 rewashes per day	64% reduction	Standardized work, visual management
Reduction in walking	30 secs per tray	15 secs per tray	100% reduction	Layout
Receiving errors	14 trays per day	9 trays per day	35% reduction	Standardized work, visual management

Figure 18.14

RESOURCES

Key Elements of Quality: Customer, Process and Employee www.ge.com/sixsigma.

Making Customers Feel Six Sigma Quality. www.ge.com/sixsigma.

Six Sigma: What is Six Sigma? http://isixsigma.com.

CENTRAL SERVICE TERMS

Customer (internal)

Quality

Empowerment

Process improvement

Cross-functional teams

Failure mode and effects analysis (FMEA)

Root cause analysis (RCA)

Sentinel event

Quality assurance

Total quality improvement (TQI)

Continuous quality improvement (CQI)

Processes (work)

Total quality management (TQM)

Six Sigma

Lean

Magnet status

ISO 9000

Chapter 19

Managing Inventory within the Central Service Department

Learning Objectives

As a result of successfully completing this chapter, readers will be able to:

1. Explain the importance of inventory management in the healthcare facility

2. Define the role of Central Service technicians as it relates to inventory management

3. Explain basic inventory terms used in healthcare facilities

4. Explain the cycle of consumable items

5. Discuss the partnership between Central Service and Materiels Management

6. Describe guidelines for handling commercially sterilized packages

7. Describe common inventory replenishment systems:

   • Periodic automatic replenishment-level systems

   • Automated supply replenishment systems

   • Exchange cart systems

   • Requisition systems

   • Case cart systems

   • STAT orders

8. Discuss the role of healthcare facilities in sustainability efforts and the reduction of waste

INTRODUCTION

A patient enters the hospital for a surgical procedure. Throughout the admission process, the patient wonders, "Will the procedure go as planned? Will there be much postoperative pain? How long until I can return home? How long before I able to go back to my normal activities?" The patient does not wonder if the healthcare facility has all the supplies needed for the surgery and postoperative care. The patient trusts that these supplies will be available, and trusts in those supplies availability with his/her life.

Providing procedural support requires a vast amount of instrumentation, supplies and equipment. Every surgery requires both reusable items, such as surgical instruments, as well as disposable (consumable) items, such as suture, bandages, syringes, needles, etc. Failure to provide items needed for patient care and treatment directly impacts patient safety; therefore, inventory management in the healthcare facility is critically important.

It takes a tremendous amount of communication, coordination and planning to ensure that every patient has every item needed for every procedure. In most facilities, purchasing, receiving and distribution of supplies is the responsibility of the Materiels Management department. To ensure that needs are met at all times, the overall inventory management and distribution process requires input from users and from dispensing areas like Central Service (CS). CS technicians play an important role in inventory management due to the large number of inventory items that pass through the CS department.

Inventory items that arrive in the CS department can be classified under two basic categories: **operational supplies** and **patient care supplies**. Operational supplies are defined as items needed for the CS department to operate effectively. Examples include detergents, sterilization wrap and sterilization testing products. Patient care supplies are defined as supplies that will be dispensed for patient treatment and care. Examples include: catheters, implants and bandages. **Figure 19.1** provides examples of products in basic CS inventory categories.

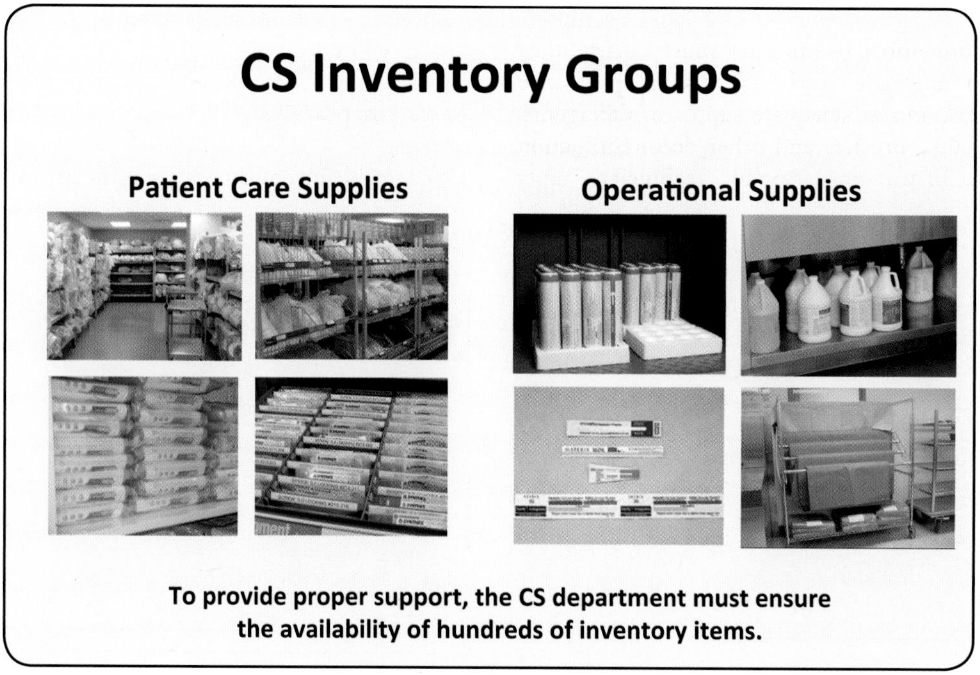

CS Inventory Groups

Patient Care Supplies

Operational Supplies

To provide proper support, the CS department must ensure the availability of hundreds of inventory items.

Figure 19.1

Both supply categories are very important to patient care. It is easy to see how a shortage of patient care supplies would impact patient care; however, it is also important to realize that a shortage of operational supplies would also impact patient care. Imagine trying to provide clean and sterile instruments without detergents or sterilization wrap.

> **Operational supplies** Supplies needed for the operation of the CS department. Examples include detergents, sterilization wrap, sterilization testing products, etc.
>
> **Patient care supplies** Supplies dispensed for patient treatment and care. Examples include catheters, implants, bandages, etc.

As discussed in Chapter 1, the scope of service (responsibilities) of CS departments varies. Some departments provide supplies for the entire facility. Other CS departments may only provide supplies for surgery. Regardless of the department's scope of service, all CS technicians are involved in the inventory management process in some way.

Case cart technicians work with consumable inventory supplies dispensed for each procedure. Decontamination technicians must ensure they have an adequate stock of personal protective equipment and an adequate supply of detergents, disinfectants, brushes and other decontamination supplies. Instrument assembly technicians must ensure that they have an adequate supply of packaging materials, chemical indicators, package closure supplies and other assembly supplies. In some cases, they may need to ensure they have replacement components, such as screws, plates, and pins for implant trays. Sterilizer operators must make certain they have sterility assurance tests, such as biological indicators and Bowie-Dick tests. For some types of sterilizers, they must maintain an adequate supply of the sterilant.

WHAT IS INVENTORY?

The term **inventory** has a broad meaning in healthcare facilities. It refers to both **reusable** and **consumable** items. Before beginning a discussion about inventory, it is important to become familiar with some key terms and concepts.

There are three specific types of inventory in the CS department:

- Consumable inventory items include supplies, such as detergents, disposable wraps and sterility assurance products.

- Reusable inventory items (with a lower cost) include items, such as transport carts, rigid sterilization containers, and many instruments.

- Reusable inventory items (with a higher cost) include items such as mechanical washers and sterilizers. In the healthcare facility, high cost, reusable inventory items are called **capital equipment**.

Consumable items and both higher- and lower-cost reusable items are considered **assets**. They represent a significant financial investment by the healthcare facility and must be managed in a way that enables the facility to get the most benefit from them at the lowest cost possible.

Consumable inventory has a specific life cycle. It is purchased, stored until use, used and replaced. (See **Figure 19.2**)

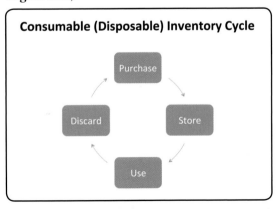

Consumable (Disposable) Inventory Cycle

Figure 19.2

This chapter will focus on the management of consumable assets as they relate to the CS department.

> **Inventory** Reusable equipment and consumable items used to provide healthcare services for patients.
>
> **Reusable (inventory)** Relatively inexpensive assets, such as medical devices and sterilization containers, that can be reused as healthcare services are provided to patients.
>
> **Consumable (inventory)** Assets, such as wrapping supplies, processing chemicals, and other items that are consumed (used up) as healthcare services are provided to patients.
>
> **Capital equipment** Relatively expensive assets, such as sterilizers or washers, that require significant advance planning for their purchase.
>
> **Assets** Something of value that is owned by an organization or person.

WHERE DOES INVENTORY COME FROM?

Every healthcare facility has hundreds and oftentimes thousands of items in its inventory. Each item serves a specific purpose. Some inventory items are used regularly, such as detergents for the decontamination area. Others, like certain specialty catheters, are used less often, but must always be available when needed. Unavailability of certain items may compromise patient safety by delaying treatment or care. All of these items represent a financial investment and must be managed properly to keep costs down. Managing inventory is one of the primary responsibilities of the Materiels Management department.

> ### Material or Materiel?
>
> The words "Material" and "Materiel" are often inter-changed; however, they do have different meanings.
>
> "Material," when used as a noun, refers to the elements, substances or parts that comprise something. (e.g., building materials, such a bricks, lumber and nails.
>
> "Materiel," when used as a noun, refers to supplies or equipment that an organization uses in any operation of business.

The Materiels Management department is responsible for the purchase, receipt and delivery of items to user departments. It oversees the flow of supplies and equipment coming into the healthcare facility. Buyers in the Materiels Management department search for and procure (purchase) items using a variety of tools and strategies to ensure they are able to meet the facility's needs at the lowest possible cost.

Most health systems belong to purchasing groups that enable them to purchase items at pre-negotiated discount pricing. These group purchasing organizations (GPOs) represent many healthcare facilities. GPOs are able to negotiate contracts for products and services that enable facilities (members of the GPO) to receive special, reduced pricing.

Materiels Management plays an important role in the supply chain by helping ensure that everything necessary to support patient care is available when needed.

Once items are received at the healthcare facility, they are checked in to verify that what was ordered was received. From there, items are placed into storage. In most facilities, a large portion of inventory items are stored in the Materiels department. Then, items are delivered to various areas, as needed. **Figure 19.3** reviews the four steps in the flow of materiels through the healthcare facility.

HANDLING COMMERCIALLY-STERILIZED ITEMS

When commercially-sterilized items are brought into a healthcare facility, care must be taken to ensure that those items are not compromised during storage, handling and distribution. That means that those items must be stored in a manner that will protect each package from events that may render it unsterile.

Chapter 16 identified requirements for sterile storage. It is important to note that those same requirements apply to all sterile packages. Although the types of packaging may differ in appearance

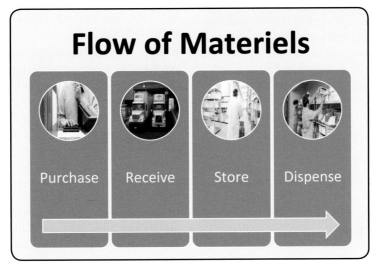

Flow of Materiels

Purchase · Receive · Store · Dispense

Figure 19.3

Important Information Provided on Package Labels

Category	Type of information	Why it is important
Manufacturer information	1. Manufacturer's name 2. Product name and specifics (size, etc.) 3. Product reference number 4. Date of manufacture 5. Batch (or lot) number 6. Product serial number 7. Expiration information	**#1-#3** Important for: • Reordering purposes • Verifying that the correct product is being dispensed **#4-7** Important for: • Tracking product to patient • Product recalls • Stock rotation
Sterility information	1. Sterility statement 2. Expiration date	**#1** Important for: • Determining if a product was supplied sterile **#2** Important for: • Determining the shelf life of the product
Storage information	1. Storage temperature limits 2. Moisture or humidity limits 3. Fragility	**#1-#3** Important for: • Ensuring that items are stored as required by the manufacturer
Safe use instructions	1. Identification of single-use items 2. Notification of latex contents 3. References to product instructions for use	**#1** Important for: • Ensuring single-use items are not processed **#2-#3** Important for: • Providing patient safety information

Figure 19.4

and feel, commercially-sterilized packages are vulnerable to the same potential contaminants as in-house sterilized items. Items should be stored in a clean area — away from moisture, dust and other contaminants that can compromise packaging. Dust on the outside of a package can be easily transferred into the Operating Room (OR) and introduced into that clean environment, possibly contaminating it.

As with every sterile package, care must be taken to ensure that the integrity of the package is maintained until use. CS technicians must understand storage and handling requirements, and they must be able to understand the basic information provided on each commercially-sterilized package.

Commercially-Sterilized Package Information

Unlike in-house sterilized items, commercially-sterilized packages come with printed instructions that contain pertinent information for CS technicians. Most product packaging contains information regarding product manufacturer, sterility, storage, and safe use. **Figure 19.4** reviews the types of information commonly found on commercially-sterilized packages and labels, and explains why that information is important to CS.

Manufacturers employ several symbols to convey information on package labels. Those symbols are designed to provide information that is easily understandable in the usually small space of a product label. **Figure 19.5** provides a review of common commercially-sterilized symbols and their meanings.

Symbol	Meaning	Symbol	Meaning
REF	Reference number (catalog number)	**LOT**	Lot number (batch code)
SN	Product serial number	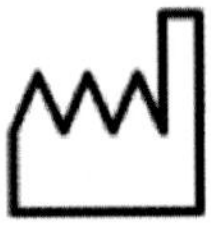 2005-01	Date of manufacture
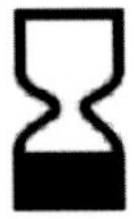 2009-01	Use by date	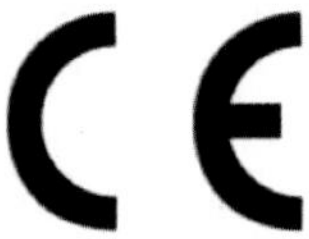 C E	The CE mark is an identification mark that indicates that a product has complied with the health and safety requirements, as published by European directives.
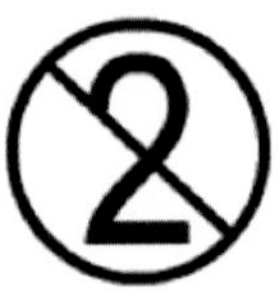 ②	Do not reuse	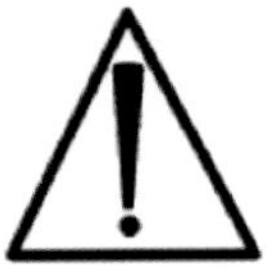 ⚠	Attention; see instructions

Figure 19.5

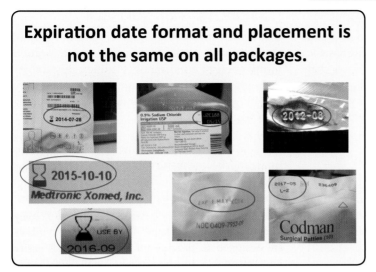

**Expiration date format and placement is
not the same on all packages.**

Figure 19.6

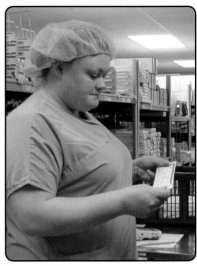

Figure 19.7

Expiration Dates

Many medical products on the market today have expiration dates and these are very important for CS technicians. It is important to note that even if a healthcare facility uses an event-related shelf life policy, expiration dates on medical products must be checked and items that have reached the end of their stated shelf life must not be used.

Identifying expiration dates can be difficult because there is no standard requirement for where they are placed on a package. For that reason, CS technicians must be diligent when checking packages for expiration dates. When new products that have expiration dates are received, all staff handling the packages should be educated on the existence and location of the expiration information. **Figure 19.6** provides examples of locations of expiration date information on commercially-sterilized packages.

Not all packages have an expiration date. Some products use an event-related shelf life system. Those packages will have a statement indicating that the package is sterile, unless opened or damaged. In a storage area filled with commercially-sterilized items, there will most likely be a combination of items with expiration dates and items with event-related sterility statements. It is important to know which items have expiration dates, and to check those dates each time a package is dispensed.

Inspection

Regardless of whether an item uses event-related or date-related shelf life, it must be inspected before being dispensed. That inspection is part of a multi-check safeguard. While it is true that the package will be inspected at the point of use, CS can reduce delays by identifying package integrity issues before they reach the point of use.

Inspections should include a visual check to ensure that the packaging has no holes, tears, signs of moisture or other visible damage. Packages that show excessive handling (wear) should also be identified. Expiration dates (if present) should be checked. **Figure 19.7** shows a CS technician checking a package before dispensing it.

ITEM LOCATOR SYSTEMS

Every healthcare facility has hundreds and, perhaps, thousands of medical supplies. Each one can impact patient safety if it cannot be located when needed. Poorly-organized storage can also lead to loss or damage, which can impact a facility's budget.

Every medical supply storage system must have a system in place that enables all employees who handle supplies to locate a specific product quickly. Systems usually use an alpha, numeric or alpha/numeric system to enable employees to easily locate supplies.

LOSS OF STERILE ITEMS

Ideally, disposable items are purchased, used and replaced; however, there are times when a disposable item may fall out of that sequence. When that happens, the item is lost, which may delay patient care and treatment and cost the facility money for replacement. **Figure 19.8** lists some common causes for the loss of sterile items.

Common Causes of Waste (Loss)

Expiration	The item was not used before the end of its designated shelf life.
Contamination	The item suffered an event that rendered it unusable.
Obsolescence	The item was replaced by a newer, different item.
Loss	The item was lost and cannot be located.
Theft	The item was taken by an unauthorized individual.

Figure 19.8

Each of the above examples represents a financial loss to the healthcare facility.

TRANSPORT OF COMMERCIALLY-STERILIZED PACKAGES

Equipment, such as carts and totes used to transport devices/supplies, must be frequently cleaned. Items that are to be transported outside the facility must be contained in appropriate containment devices, as they are transported. These transport devices must be cleaned routinely to ensure that bioburden is removed.

Care should be taken to protect packages from contamination during transport. Items should not be exposed to conditions that may compromise the sterility of the package, such as excessive temperatures, humidity or moisture.

DISTRIBUTION OF SUPPLIES

Distribution involves moving supplies throughout the facility, generally from their storage location to the point of use. In most facilities, this activity includes distributing consumable supplies from the storeroom or CS to clinical units, including the OR.

The goal of distribution is to move the correct items in appropriate quantities to the right places at the right times and in the most cost effective manner possible. The method of supply distribution used will vary depending on frequency and/or volume of use, peak activity times, the amount of storage space available in the areas to which the supplies are distributed, and other factors. For that reason, it is important to note that no single distribution method is the best choice for all facilities. Each healthcare facility will need to assess its particular needs and develop a system that will best suit those needs. In most cases, many different methods of distribution will be used to meet the needs of different departments.

> **Distribution** The movement of supplies (primarily consumable supplies from the storeroom to clinical units, and processed supplies from Central Service to the Operating Room) throughout the facility.

Carts and Totes used to Transport Sterile Items Must be Kept Clean.

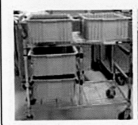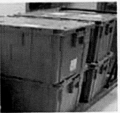

Figure 19.9

Inventory Replenishment and Distribution Systems

The method(s) used to replenish needed consumable supplies throughout the healthcare facility must be carefully considered and planned to best manage costs, to have items available when needed and to minimize the supply efforts of responsible staff members. Effective systems are, to the extent possible, automatic (little or no intervention by the user or user department is necessary to reorder).

The following are examples of inventory replenishment and distribution systems commonly used in healthcare facilities:

Periodic Automated Replenishment Level Systems

Periodic automated replenishment (PAR) systems establish a standard level (PAR) for each supply item stored in a specific department. This level is usually jointly determined by the user department and Materiel Management staff. After these levels are set, there is typically no need for items to be ordered by clinicians. Instead, CS/Materiel Management (CS/MM) personnel inventory (count) each area that houses inventory. They check the current on-hand supply and note the quantity of each item still available. The amount needed to bring the quantity of supplies to the agreed-upon standard (PAR level) is determined and automatically transmitted to the Materiel Management department (or vendor) who will send the required supplies. **Figure 19.10** shows checking and restocking PAR levels on a shelf.

> **Periodic automatic replenishment (often called PAR level or PAR system)** An inventory replenishment system in which the desired amount of products that should be on hand is established, and inventory replenishment returns the quantity of products to this level.

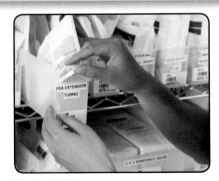

Figure 19.10

Automated Supply Replenishment Systems

Automated supply replenishment systems use a computerized system to gather and track the issuing of patient items. PAR and reorder levels for each item are established. Clinical staff scan or push a button to account for each item removed from the inventory location. An order is generated at a scheduled time for all items that are at or below their reorder point, and the order for the entire location is then placed. The supply pick list is printed and is used to gather replacement products to refill the unit.

Automated systems are generally **interfaced** with the healthcare facility's Materiels Management system for managing inventory. The use of these interfaces reduces the amount of staff required to perform these functions.

> **Automated supply replenishment system** Replenishment system in which items removed from inventory are automatically identified and tracked. When a reorder point is reached, item information is generated on a supply pick list in the central storeroom, or with a contracted vendor. Items are then issued and transferred to the appropriate user area.
>
> **Interfaced** An area or system through which one machine is connected to another machine in order to share information. For example, two computers may be interfaced, or a computer and a sterilizer may be interfaced.

Benefits of automated systems relate to the facility's size and the number of items being monitored. These systems are expensive and may not be cost justified for all or some of the remote storage locations. **Figure 19.11** provides examples of equipment used in an automated system.

Examples of Automated Replenishment Systems

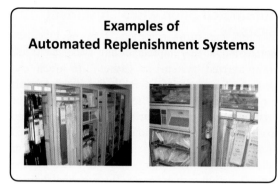

Figure 19.11

Exchange Cart Systems

An **exchange cart system** is an inventory replenishment method that involves the exchange of a freshly-filled supply cart on a user unit. Supply items and quantities on the exchange cart, as well as its location, are determined by user unit staff and CS/MM personnel. At a pre-determined time, a full cart is brought to the unit. The partially-depleted cart is returned to the replenishment area, and remaining items are inventoried to determine the supplies and quantities that were used. The cart is then replenished with the supplies needed to return the cart back to full inventory. As supplies are removed from inventory and added to the cart, they are charged to the budget of the unit that "owns" the cart. At the scheduled time, this full cart is delivered to the unit, the depleted cart is retrieved for restocking, and the cycle repeats. **Figure 19.12** provides an example of exchange carts that are designed to stock anesthesia supplies.

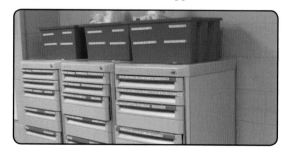

Figure 19.12

An advantage of an exchange cart system is that it is "automatic" unless there is a need to change the cart's items or quantities. Clinical staff do not need

to order these items, and Materiel Management staff does not have to determine which supplies are needed.

Disadvantages associated with exchange carts include the need for duplicate inventory and carts. The system is labor-intensive and requires adequate space to stage the carts. In addition, unless the system is well-managed, numerous unused supplies will be transported back and forth each cycle. This system does work well for emergency medical supply carts (code carts), which are exchanged for a newly-restocked cart each time they are used. (See **Figure 19.13**)

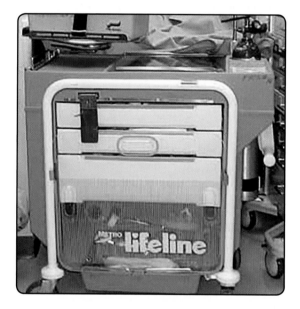

Figure 19.13

Exchange cart system An inventory system where desired inventory items are placed on a cart assigned a specific location and quantity. A second duplicate cart is maintained in another location and exchanged on a scheduled basis to ensure that sufficient supplies are available at all times.

Requisition Systems

Even when PAR level or exchange cart systems exist, it will still be necessary to order additional supplies. That usually happens because of insufficient quantities on hand or because a specific item is not included among those routinely provided. **Requisition systems** exist in every facility.

Requisition systems require users to request (order) needed supplies by completing a requisition. Requisitions may be manual (paper based) or computer generated. Manual systems do not offer the productivity advantages of computerized systems. Requisition systems that electronically requisition supplies typically eliminate the need for Materiels Management personnel to re-enter ordering information from a paper order form. The accuracy and productivity improvements associated with automated data entry are lost when manual requisition systems are used. **Figure 19.14** provides an example of a technician completing a requisition for special order catheters.

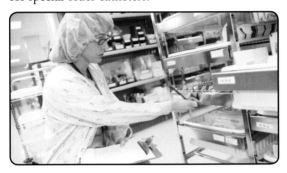

Figure 19.14

Requisition system A method of inventory distribution where items needed are requested (requisitioned) by user department personnel and removed from a central storage location for transport to the user department.

Specialty Items

Every facility has a need for patient-specific and infrequently ordered specialty items that are not maintained in the routine replenishment system. CS technicians must understand the requisition, ordering, tracking and replenishment processes used by their facility for these items. If a patient is scheduled for surgery and a specialty item is needed, it may need to be ordered several days before surgery to ensure that it is available. If an item is not available when needed, patient safety may be compromised.

Case Cart System

Perhaps the most common form of inventory management and distribution in the CS department is the case cart system. In a case cart system, items needed for each specific procedure are assembled in individual carts by CS staff and delivered to the department where the procedure will be performed. There are several benefits to case cart systems, including:

- Reducing the amount of space needed for supply storage in the user department.

- Promoting more standardized infection prevention practices.

- Reducing operational costs associated with supply and instrument management.

- Allowing more efficient equipment and supply tracking.

Case cart systems range from those providing disposable supplies or instruments for each procedure to comprehensive systems, which provide each case's instrument, supply, equipment, and implant needs. While they are most commonly used for the OR, case cart systems can be used anywhere that procedures requiring supplies and instruments are performed, including Cardiac Catheterization labs and Labor & Delivery (L&D) units. When implemented correctly, these systems help to meet the needs of each physician and still maintain an orderly system for tracking and handling supplies, instruments and equipment.

In a case cart system, specific needs for each procedure are identified by users. These needs are compiled on a requisition form called a preference card (or pick list). The preference card usually contains two components: the first is a list of instruments, supplies and implants needed for the specific procedure; the second component contains notes that are helpful to the procedure room staff.

When a procedure is scheduled, a copy of the list of needed items is sent to CS, and the case cart is assembled. (**See Figure 19.15**) That case cart is delivered to the OR (or other user unit) before the procedure. Additional unanticipated needs are communicated to CS, as necessary, and CS responds to those additional requests.

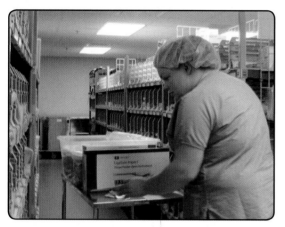

Figure 19.15

Following the procedure unused, unopened (clean and sterile) items are returned to storage; waste is separated, bagged and removed; reusable linens (if used) are bagged; and all opened and soiled instruments are sent to the decontamination area for processing. This process is repeated multiple times throughout the day as additional procedures are performed. (See **Figure 19.16**)

Case cart systems can also provide effective control of supplies and instruments. Because a separate case cart is assembled for each individual procedure, it is easier to track what is actually used, and identify supplies and instruments that are often requested, but seldom used. Quantities of supplies can then be reduced, which can reduce the amount of inventory that must be on hand. Close monitoring of instrument usage allows the facility to shift instruments not being used to other areas where they are needed. Monitoring can also identify instrument shortages, which may be addressed with scheduling changes and/or the purchase of additional instrumentation.

Case cart systems enhance infection prevention practices. Because all instruments are returned to the decontamination area immediately after use, decontamination and sterilization processes can begin immediately. CS technicians assigned to processing in a case cart system devote most of their time and efforts to preparing items for reuse. That is their primary job function, so they become specialists in cleaning, inspecting, assembling and sterilizing complex instruments. This expertise yields better infection prevention practices.

Case cart systems rely on user input to be effective. Physicians and other healthcare personnel utilizing

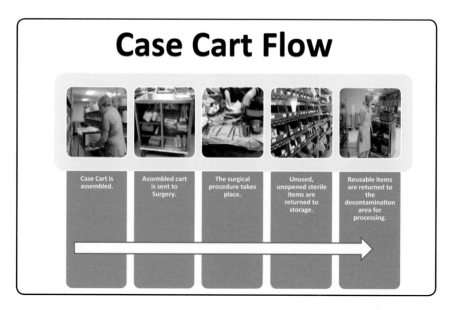

Figure 19.16

the case cart must identify their specific needs in advance. These needs are then transferred to pick lists that CS staff use to assemble each cart. Care should be taken when developing requisitions to ensure that products are standardized, whenever possible. Routine follow up is needed to adjust requisition quantities to actual usage. Properly stocked case carts should be delivered to the user unit. Personnel assigned to the case cart area must maintain direct contact with unit staff, so additional items can be supplied as needed. After the procedure is completed, used and reprocessable items must be returned to the decontamination area. CS technicians should return uncompromised items to stock and then proceed with inventory replenishment and charging activities.

While case cart systems typically use carts assembled as needed for specific procedures, most systems also utilize some form of preassembled carts that remain assembled and "on standby" for emergency situations. These carts are used for STAT situations (for example, emergency cesarean sections) when there is no time for cart assembly.

An effective case cart system requires good communication between OR and CS personnel. As cases are performed, CS and OR staff must be in constant communication to ensure that items are correct and arrive on time. Personnel in each department must be familiar with one another's routine duties and workflow patterns. Frustration can be eliminated if, for example, OR personnel understand the steps involved in processing instruments for another case. Instead of questioning instrument turnaround times, they will understand that this time is required for safe, effective cleaning, inspection, assembly and sterilization.

CS technicians working with case cart systems should have good medical terminology skills and a thorough understanding of surgical instruments, so they can easily communicate with their OR counterparts. They must also remain up to date about new products because they serve as the link between the inventory system and the user department. Along with effective oral communication skills, case cart systems rely heavily on written procedures

and communications. Personnel from all user departments must establish procedures for product handling, outage notification and scheduling. Even the best-planned case cart system will be substandard without good communication.

Case cart systems also require upkeep. As instruments and supplies are added to or removed from the system, physician's preference cards must be updated to reflect changes in the system. (See **Figure 19.17**) Failure to update preference cards to reflect current needs can result in unavailability of supplies and instruments, which can then lead to compromised patient safety and user frustration.

Case cart systems require significant input from CS professionals, and to be efficient, they require a full array of processing skills and inventory management methods.

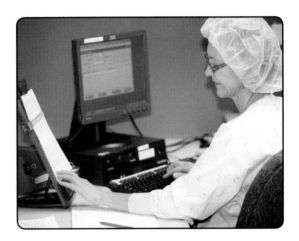

Figure 19.17

STAT Orders

Emergency supply orders requiring immediate action (STAT orders) are a fact of life in every facility. STAT orders can also occur for a procedure scheduled for the next day, if the item is not available. These orders are time consuming and costly to fill, and they usually disrupt routine inventory management activities. Consider, for example, times when additional external resources, such as overnight air shipments or borrowing from another facility may be required. All reasonable efforts to minimize the need for STAT requests should be made; these include reviewing why they occur, and how they can be prevented.

Many STAT requests result from deficiencies in a poorly-managed daily supply and distribution system. STAT requests can become a patient safety issue if the root cause is not addressed, and routine reviews may determine if PAR level adjustments will help ensure appropriate inventory levels. When STAT requests result from improper planning by clinical staff, Materiel Management and CS managers should assist in the planning and education efforts to resolve the issue. While OR staff cannot predict that an emergency patient will require a specific **non-stock item**, they may be able to plan for such a need and ensure that the item is available.

> **Non-stock items** Items that are not carried in the central storeroom or in Central Service storage area but are purchased from an outside vendor, as needed, and then delivered to the requesting department.

SUSTAINABILITY

The Materiels Management department is also often involved in **sustainability** efforts. More and more healthcare facilities are taking sustainability into consideration when selecting supplies. Items that can be recycled or otherwise help reduce waste can benefit patients, healthcare facilities and the environment.

Many facilities are moving toward systems that allow them to reduce the amount of waste being generated. CS departments may be involved in those efforts. (See **Figure 19.18**)

> **Sustainability** Processes designed to reduce harm to the environment or deplete natural resources, thereby supporting long-term ecological balance.

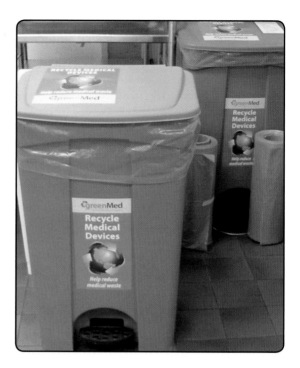

Figure 19.18

THE ROLE OF CENTRAL SERVICE IN INVENTORY MANAGEMENT

Although the primary responsibilities of procurement, receiving, storage and distribution may be performed outside the CS department, CS technicians still play an important role in the healthcare facility's inventory management system. CS technicians are responsible for several key duties, including:

- Learning processes at their specific healthcare facility, such as:

  › How orders are placed.

  › How to identify items.

  › How to locate items.

  › How to properly dispense items.

- Knowing how to stay informed of new products as they enter the system.

- Understanding and following information contained on commercially-sterilized packages.

- Handling sterile products with care.

- Reporting concerns, such as:

  › Excessive, unexpected demand on specific products.

  › Low quantities.

  › Frequent outages.

  › Storage issues.

Each step in the life cycle of a sterile medical supply is an important one. Through keen observation and best work practices, CS technicians can protect the integrity of products until they reach their point of use.

CONCLUSION

Inventory management is an important part of every healthcare facility. Managing inventory effectively and efficiently assists caregivers in providing quality care at lower costs. More importantly, it helps ensure that the items needed to provide patient care and treatment are available when needed.

When Central Service and Materiel Management staff work together to manage and control inventory, they help create a safe environment for the patient, while increasing provider and patient satisfaction.

RESOURCE

International Central Service Materiel Management. *Central Service Leadership Manual*, Chapters 9, 23, 24. 2010.

CENTRAL SERVICE TERMS

Operational supplies

Patient care supplies

Inventory

Reusable inventory

Consumable inventory

Capital equipment

Assets

Distribution

Periodic automatic replenishment (PAR)

Automated supply replenishment system

Interfaced

Exchange cart system

Requisition system

Non-stock items

Sustainability

Chapter 20

The Role of Central Service in Ancillary Department Support

Learning Objectives

As a result of successfully completing this chapter, readers will be able to:

1. Discuss the role of the Central Service department in supporting ancillary departments

2. Discuss strategies for managing patient care equipment

3. Explain the importance of communication and coordination as it relates to ancillary support

INTRODUCTION

While the Operating Room (OR) is the Central Service (CS) department's largest customer, it is by no means its only customer. CS departments provide support for other areas of the healthcare facility by providing instruments, disposable supplies and equipment. Providing service to diverse departments and ensuring they have all the proper items when needed can be challenging. This chapter will focus on common support services provided by CS departments.

IDENTIFYING THE CENTRAL SERVICE DEPARTMENT'S SCOPE OF SERVICE

The level of service provided by the CS department varies by healthcare facility. In some facilities, the services provided by CS are limited to servicing the needs of the OR, and providing reprocessing and sterilization services for instruments used in other departments. In other facilities, the CS department may be responsible for providing sterile instruments, equipment and supplies to healthcare units throughout the facility. CS departments that provide services to areas outside of the OR must ensure that they develop a system that meets the needs of all patients and providers in the safest, most timely and cost-effective manner possible.

PATIENT CARE EQUIPMENT

Along with instruments and supplies, CS departments manage a large portion of the healthcare facility's patient care equipment. Tasks include assembly, delivery, tracking, retrieval, decontamination and storage. Effective handling of this equipment is an important part of the CS department's job. Managing it properly can have a significant impact on patient safety.

Patient care equipment must be readily available when needed. This requires that it be safe, functional, ready to use and free from soil and contaminants. CS technicians are responsible for ensuring that these requirements are met. They must also manage equipment in a manner that minimizes costs to the healthcare facility. An effective patient care equipment management program is essential for managing these costs.

Specific guidelines should be developed for the cleaning, preparation and tracking of patient care equipment. Failure to properly manage equipment can have a dramatic impact on patient and employee safety. Equipment that has not been properly cleaned poses an infection threat to patients and healthcare workers. That threat is magnified because the equipment may be handled by several workers during the course of preparation, storage and distribution. If it is not properly assembled and ready for use, there may be a delay in treatment if staff must obtain necessary components, such as tubing, collection devices and pads. Equipment that is not accurately tracked can be "lost" within the system. This inavailability may cause treatment delay or add unnecessary expense if it becomes necessary to rent additional equipment to replace the missing equipment.

> **Patient care equipment** Portable (mobile) equipment used to assist in the care and treatment of patients. Examples include: suction units, temperature management units, infusion therapy devices, etc.

There are numerous types of patient care equipment in healthcare today. Some general device categories include infusion therapy, temperature management, wound care and suction. Examples of specialized categories include equipment used for maternal and infant care, bariatric care, patient monitoring, specialty surfaces and beds. Many devices are cleaned, tracked and dispensed through CS. Specific types, models and brands will vary from facility to facility.

Basic Types of Patient Care Equipment

Understanding the purpose of basic types of patient care equipment can improve customer service. **Figure 20.1** identifies and defines some of this equipment that is typically handled by CS professionals. CS technicians must also understand requirements for cleaning, inspecting, preparing, storing, dispensing and tracking patient care equipment. Each step in the patient care equipment process is an important component of a comprehensive patient care equipment program.

Equipment	Purpose
Breast pump	Mechanical device that extracts and collects milk from the breast.
Continuous passive motion (CPM) device	Device that treats synovial joints (hip, knee, ankle, shoulder, elbow, wrist) following surgery or trauma. The device moves the affected joint regularly, without patient assistance.
Defibrillator	A device that applies a brief electroshock to restore the rhythm of the heart.
Enteral nutrition (infusion) pump (also called a feeding pump)	A device that provides nutrition to patients who cannot ingest food because of recent surgery, or because digestive organs do not function properly.
Foot pump	A device that artificially stimulates the venous plantar plexus (the large vein located in the foot). It increases blood circulation in bed-ridden patients by simulating the motion produced during walking.
Gastric suction unit	A device that aspirates (withdraws) gastric and intestinal contents.
Hot and cold therapy devices	A device used to reduce swelling, pain and muscle cramps. Also used to treat arthritis, pyrogenic infection and gastrointestinal cramps. Depending on the required therapy, water is cooled or heated and then runs through a disposable pad, which is wrapped around the area being treated. Smaller (heat-only) devices similar to electric heating pads are used on sore muscles.
Hyper/Hypothermia unit	A device that pumps heated or cooled water through a coiled pad to therapeutically raise or lower body temperature. *Note: These pads are much larger than hot or cold therapy device pads.*
Infant incubator	A device that creates and controls the environment (temperature and humidity) of newborns.
IV infusion pump	A device that mechanically controls the administration of intravenous (IV) therapy fluids.
Intermittent suction device	A device that starts and stops suctioning at periodic intervals.
Microdrip pump	Intravenous infusion pump with a drop control that emits a drop that is smaller than a normal drop.
Oral suction device	A device that suctions mucous from oral and nasal cavities.
Patient-controlled analgesia (PCA) pump	A device designed to provide automatic (self) administration of pain medication.
Sequential compression device (SCD)	A device designed to limit the development of deep vein thrombosis (DVT) and peripheral edema in immobile patients.
Suction pump	A device that provides suction by altering the expansion and contraction of air within a cylinder at regular intervals. Also known as aspirators, they use a continuous or intermittent pump and a collection container to aspirate (withdraw fluids or air from a cavity) in patients with lung or throat problems. They can also be used to provide wound drainage, usually from the chest or abdominal areas.
Portable suction unit	A mechanical suction device powered by battery or electrical current, used in various facility locations.
Wall suction unit	A mechanical suction device that must be attached to a wall suction (outlet) for power.
Wound VAC therapy	A device that provides negative pressure wound therapy by using controlled suction to close large wounds and promote faster healing.

Figure 20.1 Patient care equipment

A Close Look at Responsibilities

CS departments maintain the flow of the patient equipment system. They also partner with the **Biomedical/Clinical Engineering department** (Biomed). Technicians in the Biomedical/Clinical Engineering department perform safety inspections and function tests on medical equipment. They are specially trained to inspect, test and repair patient care equipment. CS technicians should not attempt to perform equipment testing and maintenance functions, unless they have received specific training and approval to do so. Biomedical technicians must also not clean used equipment, unless they have been properly trained.

When equipment enters a healthcare facility, it must be safety checked and tested by a Biomedical technician before being cleared for patient use. These items must also receive periodic follow-up inspections, scheduled according to the equipment manufacturer's Instructions for Use (IFU) and the healthcare facility's policies. Biomedical professionals maintain complete records about routine checks, repairs and other important information for all patient care equipment in the facility.

> **Biomedical/Clinical Engineering department**
> The hospital department responsible for performing safety inspections and function tests on medical equipment. It is frequently abbreviated to "Biomed department" and is also known as the Healthcare Technology Management department.

The Joint Commission (TJC) requires that **preventive maintenance** (PM) standards be established for healthcare equipment. The following information should be recorded and maintained for each piece of patient care equipment:

- Assigned equipment location.

- Ownership status (rented, leased, owned, borrowed).

- Schedule for PM.

- PM history.

- Hospital-defined PM standards.

- Repair history.

> **Preventive maintenance (PM)** Service provided to equipment to maintain its proper operating condition by providing planned inspection, and by detecting and correcting failures before they occur.

CS and the Biomedical department partner in several ways. Each time patient care equipment is returned to the CS for cleaning, its preventive maintenance sticker should be checked. Items due for a preventive maintenance inspection should be routed to the Biomedical department, rather than be returned to service. (**Figure 20.2** is an example of a PM sticker.) As part of their routine inspection process, CS technicians should also check for damaged (cracked, torn or frayed) electrical cords, cracked equipment casings, loose knobs and switches, and other signs of damage that should be corrected before the item is reused. All equipment that appears to need repair should also be routed to Biomedical personnel for inspection. Equipment-related issues can be minimized when all staff remain alert to obvious signs of the need for equipment inspection and/or repair. This, in turn, increases the level of patient and employee safety.

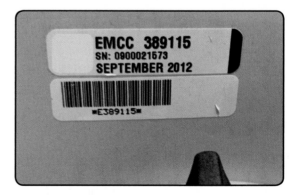

Figure 20.2

Handling Used (Soiled) Patient Care Equipment

All patient care equipment used must be considered contaminated and handled as such, regardless of its appearance. *Note: Patient care equipment may not be visibly soiled and may appear clean; however, it is likely to harbor microorganisms that may pose a threat to patients and staff.* CS technicians make routinely-scheduled rounds to pick up soiled equipment from user units (See **Figure 20.3**) and transport it to the decontamination area for cleaning. In some cases, they may also make special trips to user departments to retrieve specific equipment. In either case, the equipment should be considered contaminated and transported according to soiled item transport guidelines. Disposable components, such as pads, tubing and suction canisters, should be removed from each piece of equipment and discarded at the point of use. Only those items that will be cleaned and reused should be transported to the decontamination area.

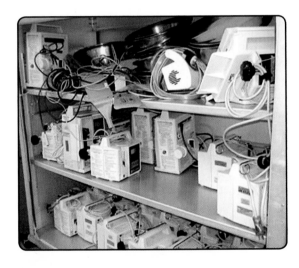

Figure 20.3

Cleaning Patient Care Equipment

Patient care equipment should be cleaned per equipment manufacturer instructions and the healthcare facility's infection prevention protocols. The manufacturer's cleaning instructions are typically found in the operator's manual that accompanies the equipment when it is purchased. Alternatively, the manufacturer can be directly contacted and, in many instances, instructions are available on the manufacturer's website. Whenever a new item of patient care equipment is brought into the facility, CS professionals should receive written instructions about procedures for cleaning and handling. All surfaces, including cords, switches and crevices, must be thoroughly cleaned. **Figure 20.4** illustrates an area that may be missed without using the IFU.

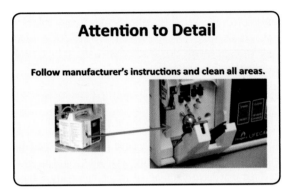

Attention to Detail

Follow manufacturer's instructions and clean all areas.

Figure 20.4

Managing Inoperative Equipment

Equipment that is nonfunctioning should be identified and tagged by the user. (See **Figure 20.5**) CS technicians must ensure that equipment tagged for repair is routed to the Biomedical department after cleaning. If an equipment malfunction causes harm to a patient, it should not be disassembled or have its settings adjusted. It should be removed from service and returned immediately to the Biomedical department for inspection and follow up. Since it will not have been disassembled or adjusted, Biomedical technicians can better establish how the equipment was assembled or used, and they can recognize clues about the cause of the malfunction, such as incorrect assembly or operator error.

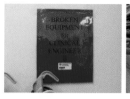

Inoperative equipment should be tagged and routed to Biomedical/Clinical Engineering.

Figure 20.5

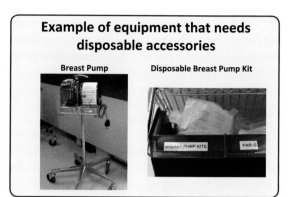

Example of equipment that needs disposable accessories

Breast Pump   Disposable Breast Pump Kit

Figure 20.6

Preparing Equipment for Use

Patient care equipment should be prepared for use and stored in a "ready to dispense" state. Preparation for use may include assembly, the addition of new disposable components, such as tubing and pads and a check and/or replacement of batteries per the equipment manufacturer's assembly instructions. (See **Figure 20.6**)

Some patient care equipment requires water for operation. CS technicians should become familiar with the equipment manufacturer's recommendations for the care of water reservoirs and how to fill them properly. CS technicians should also be aware of any testing that they need to perform prior to dispensing for use.

Storage of Patient Care Equipment

After patient care equipment has been cleaned, inspected and assembled, it should be placed in storage until needed. In most cases, storage is confined to the CS department (See **Figure 20.7**) or a secure location nearby. Sometimes, however, it may be stored in user units. This makes it more accessible for nursing and other patient care staff and reduces waiting time when the equipment is needed immediately.

All equipment should be stored in a clean, secure location, away from high traffic areas, such as visitor hallways.

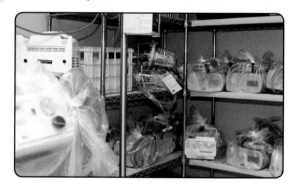

Figure 20.7

Some types of patient care equipment have battery back-up systems that must be recharged. An adequate number of electrical outlets is needed in all applicable storage areas to enable these items to be plugged in at all times for battery recharge. (See **Figure 20.8**). While this equipment is designed to run using electricity, there may be times when patients are moved while still connected to equipment, and during power disruptions, when the equipment must rely on pre-charged batteries to function.

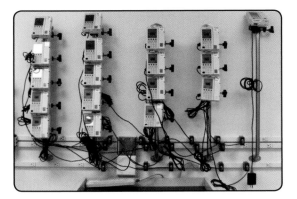

Figure 20.8

Tracking Patient Care Equipment

Tracking patient care equipment is a challenge for any CS department. The equipment is mobile and in many cases, small, and it can easily be placed in an incorrect location, set aside on a user unit or otherwise misplaced. Equipment that is difficult to locate can cause equipment shortages, which may delay treatment, necessitate short-term rental of replacement equipment, and increase the healthcare facility's operating costs.

There are several ways to track patient care equipment. It can be done manually, using a paper system that tracks each equipment item's specific identifying number. Alternatively, it can be done using computerized programs that automate the tracking process by using barcodes that are applied to the device. (See **Figure 20.9**) In some hospitals, equipment is tracked with radio frequency computer chips applied to each device that send signals to a locator system. Regardless of the type of tracking system used, the main goal is to provide information:

• About the current location of the equipment.

• To charge patients for use of the equipment, if applicable.

• On equipment usage and trends.

Tracking patient care equipment allows CS professionals to monitor locations and helps ensure that equipment is available when needed. That information can also be used to justify additional equipment.

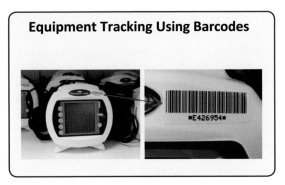

Equipment Tracking Using Barcodes

Figure 20.9

PROCURING NEW AND ADDITIONAL EQUIPMENT

New technologies and increased need (patient volume) often require healthcare facilities to procure additional patient care equipment. New equipment may be purchased, leased or rented, or it can even be loaned to the healthcare facility by a manufacturer. There are advantages and disadvantages to each approach, and the facility should make decisions based upon its specific needs.

Equipment Purchase

This method of equipment acquisition has been used by healthcare facilities for decades. Facility personnel identify the need for specific equipment, determine the type (model, style or brand) that is required, budget for its purchase and incorporate it into the system. The equipment is then owned by the healthcare facility.

Equipment Lease

As with purchasing, healthcare facility personnel must determine equipment needs. From there, they contract with a manufacturer or leasing company to lease (use) the equipment for a specific time period. At the end of the contract, the healthcare facility can usually return the equipment (and acquire a newer technology) or purchase it.

Equipment Rental

Equipment rental differs from leasing because it is usually done on a short-term basis. For example, leasing contracts may be for months or years, but rental contracts may be as short as a single day. When renting, the healthcare facility identifies an immediate need, usually because high patient volume has created a demand for existing equipment that has caused a shortage, or because of the unique needs of a specific patient. In either case, the healthcare facility then contracts for a short-term rental with an equipment rental company.

Manufacturer's Loan

Manufacturers occasionally provide equipment to healthcare facilities as part of an agreement in which the facility will use the manufacturer's disposable products, such as pads, tubing and sleeves.

Decisions about the type of equipment acquisition process that will be most beneficial to the healthcare facility should be made by facility administrators.

Whichever method is used to acquire equipment, the CS technician's responsibilities remain the same: to provide clean, safe and complete equipment and to maintain the availability of that equipment by coordinating workflow.

OTHER PATIENT CARE EQUIPMENT CONCERNS

Equipment Maintenance and Repair

All mechanical equipment must be properly maintained and will sometimes require **repair**. Preventive maintenance will help identify potential problems before they occur. PM is conducted on a routine, scheduled basis, and is designed to ensure that equipment is in proper operating condition. Equipment repair is performed as needed when equipment fails to function properly, and when it appears to be damaged.

Both preventive maintenance and equipment repair should only be performed by trained biomedical equipment technicians or the equipment manufacturer.

> **Repair (equipment)** Procedures used to return equipment to proper operating condition after it has become inoperative.

PROCEDURAL SUPPORT

Procedure Trays and Kits

Many procedures are performed within the healthcare facility and CS departments often provide the sterile instruments necessary to perform those procedures. Procedures that are done outside of the OR can be divided into two categories: those performed in a designated **procedure area**, and those performed at the patient's bedside. In either case, safe and accurate instruments and supplies are critical to patient safety.

> **Procedure area** An area within the healthcare facility that conducts invasive and minimally-invasive procedures requiring instruments, supplies and equipment.

The CS department is the provider of sterile instrumentation and often provides trays and kits for procedure areas located outside the OR. Common procedure areas include:

- Cardiac catheterization lab.

- Emergency department.

- Labor and Delivery.

- Minor procedure rooms.

- Radiology.

- Endoscopy.

Just as each procedure area provides a very different type of treatment, each area will also have different types of trays, instruments and supplies.

Disposable or Reusable?

When a facility determines whether to use disposable or reusable trays and kits, several factors are taken into account, such as physician preference, logistics, storage and replenishment cost.

When reusable trays and kits are used, a process must be adopted to help ensure that instruments are returned to CS for reprocessing. When disposable instruments are used, CS staff must identify and remove disposable instruments that are inadvertently returned to CS, so they are not reprocessed.

Regardless of the type of tray used (disposable or reusable), the user department must identify the tray's contents.

Managing Reusable Instruments

In addition to reprocessing instruments for ancillary departments, many CS departments also perform the function for off-site entities, such as affiliated clinics. (See **Figure 20.10**) Care must be taken to help ensure that the process for transporting soiled instruments meets biohazard transport and infection prevention guidelines, and that the return of clean instruments follows specific protocols for sterile item transport.

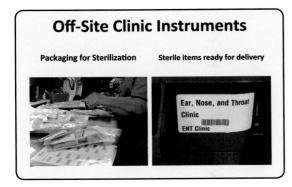

Off-Site Clinic Instruments

Packaging for Sterilization   Sterile items ready for delivery

Ear, Nose, and Throat Clinic

ENT Clinic

Figure 20.10

If instruments are purchased and brought into the ancillary department through a channel other than CS, the user units must also provide written manufacturer IFU to the CS department.

As with the instruments used in the OR, the CS department should develop tray listings and written reprocessing protocols for all items processed for ancillary departments.

UTENSILS AND OTHER MEDICAL EQUIPMENT

CS departments may also be involved in handling utensils, such as wash basins and equipment, as well as transport devices and specialty beds. In many cases, the CS department is the only space in the facility that has the proper equipment and facilities to clean these devices. As with all items reprocessed through CS, manufacturer's reprocessing instructions should be obtained, made readily available to staff, and followed.

COMMUNICATION AND COORDINATION IS KEY

Any discussion of service to ancillary departments must address communication and coordination. Meeting the needs of many departments with various specialties can be challenging. Careful planning and good communication are critical.

Basic questions must be addressed for each item and CS technicians must be aware of the procedures for each unit. Important information includes:

- What is needed? (Which items will be available for the specific unit?)

- When will items be needed? (As requested, on standby in the user unit?)

- How will communication take place? (Phone? Computer-generated message?)

- Where will the items be stored?

- How will the items be delivered? (Stocked on the unit? Delivered upon request? Delivered on courier rounds?)

- How will items be returned? (Picked up by CS? Delivered to CS by the user unit? Delivered by courier?)

For the system to run smoothly, everyone must understand and follow the appropriate process. Inavailability of instruments or equipment could jeopardize patient safety.

CONCLUSION

Modern healthcare relies on equipment, instruments and supplies to provide patient care. Each healthcare department fills a specific need and requires specific items to fulfill its mission. The Central Service department provides the support to enable ancillary departments to provide quality patient care.

RESOURCE

U.S. Food and Drug Administration. *Medical Device Reporting 21 CFR 803.* 2014.

CENTRAL SERVICE TERMS

Patient care equipment

Biomedical/Clinical Engineering department

Preventive maintenance

Repair

Procedure area

Chapter 21

The Role of Information Technology in Central Service

Learning Objectives

As a result of successfully completing this chapter, readers will be able to:

1. Provide an overview of the use of information management systems in Central Service departments

2. Discuss the use of computers and information systems to support activities within the healthcare facility and Central Service department

3. Recognize that tracking systems enhance Central Service operations

4. Explain why tracking systems must address the specific needs of the healthcare facility and Central Service department

5. Review some features of available instrument and equipment tracking systems

INTRODUCTION

Central Service (CS) professionals must responsibly manage the equipment, instruments and supplies in their facility and entrusted to them. These items are in constant movement between departments as they are dispensed, used and replaced or processed. To maintain order and ensure the availability of items for patient care, CS staff must track each item to:

- Ensure that it can be quickly located.

- Determine when consumable supplies should be replaced.

- Monitor item usage.

- Maintain accurate records of processes, such as sterilization and distribution.

- Assist with quality assurance processes and regulatory compliance.

- Capture information for financial analysis.

Historically, all recordkeeping (documentation) performed in the CS department was done manually. Now most departments use some form of automated information management system to track products and document processes. Some departments use a combination of manual and computerized tracking, while others employ a fully integrated information management model throughout the entire facility.

Some common types of computer-based information systems used in the CS department include those for instrument tracking, sterilization logging information, case cart pick lists, patient care equipment tracking, inventory management, staffing analysis and individual productivity data. (See **Figure 21.1**)

ROLE OF COMPUTER-BASED INFORMATION SYSTEMS

CS professionals must maintain and manage a significant amount of data as supplies, instruments and equipment are stocked and issued to the Operating Room (OR) and various other users. Computers can promote basic and numerous advanced capabilities to support operational activities for healthcare Materiel Supply Chain Management and CS processing. CS technicians require a solid understanding of how computers are currently used to serve the department's core mission and functions.

Computers and information systems continue to evolve rapidly. When CS personnel are involved in evaluating and/or selecting a new computer-based application or system, they must be aware of the latest trends and technological advancements that are relevant to their role in the healthcare setting.

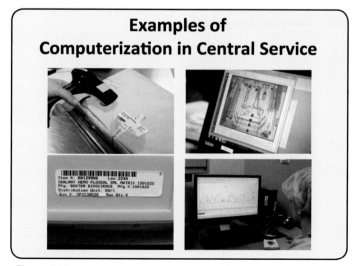

Figure 21.1

Overview of Information Technology in the Healthcare Setting

The modern healthcare environment uses information technology to provide accurate and efficient management of a very complex set of business processes. Ideally, information technology and systems are used to ensure patient safety, demonstrate quality of care, and provide efficient operational and financial management for the healthcare organization.

There are few, if any, aspects of healthcare where information technology or systems are not employed. While an organization may be currently using a mixture of computerized and/or manual processes, it is reasonable to assume that any of the manual processes in use are being routinely evaluated for conversion as resources and budgets allow.

To support the needs of the global patient population today, and in the future, the healthcare industry is intensely focused on continual improvements to the environment of care and our ability to adopt and utilize all of the tools at our disposal to provide high quality healthcare at an optimal cost.

Increasingly, emphasis is on point-of-care and point-of-use computing with mobile solutions suitable for the bedside and use in CS work areas. (See **Figure 21.2**) This has become possible with the development of electronic recordkeeping systems and wireless network capabilities that provide real-time data communication. These systems can be supported with the use of laptop computer-on-wheels (COW) solutions, tablet-based computing, and even smart phones. Computer technology will continue to advance in this manner for the foreseeable future.

Information technology is often the cornerstone of initiatives to transform healthcare. One key reason is that it can be used to clearly demonstrate accountability through the volume of data captured.

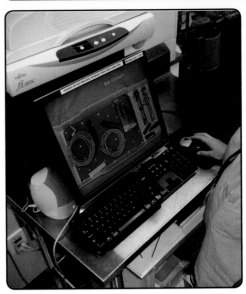

Figure 21.2

A clear understanding of the systems that can be utilized by CS management and staff is important for two critical reasons:

- The core mission is to support patient safety and quality patient care. Information systems can be used to ensure these objectives are accomplished.

- Using available systems appropriately will enhance the ability to provide efficient and cost-effective patient care.

It is also important to understand that many of the systems used in healthcare are integrated (interfaced), meaning they communicate with each other electronically. Integration is essential for eliminating redundant data entry, promoting efficiency and reducing the risk for inaccurate or conflicting data from being entered into the system. While we might receive information needed to perform certain tasks from a particular system, some of the information being used is actually coming from another system. For example, when pick lists are generated for building surgical case carts, they might be printed from the OR scheduling system; however, it is likely that certain information on the pick list, such as the product catalog number and bin locations, is created and managed in the materiels management information system (MMIS).

This is also important to CS because the department sometimes creates and manages information that feeds other systems. For example, if the department uses an electronic sterile processing information system, when inventory information is updated, that may be communicated to the OR scheduling system for use on physician preference cards.

The healthcare facility's information management system utilizes many components to meet a wide variety of needs. **Figure 21.3** provides an example of common components that comprise that system.

- Clinical information systems are at the heart of the core mission of a healthcare provider. They capture data related to direct patient care.

- Admissions and registration, also known as admissions, discharge and transfer (ADT) systems, are used to manage inpatient and outpatient registration. This is important to CS because patient census information is received from the ADT system.

- Electronic medical record or electronic health record (EMR/EHR) is the library of data related to the care provided to a patient by the organization. Healthcare providers must comply with "meaningful use" requirements. This ensures the certified EHR technology is being used to improve quality, safety, efficiency and care coordination, and maintain privacy of patient health information. *Note: The other clinical information systems will transmit relevant information to the EMR/EHR.*

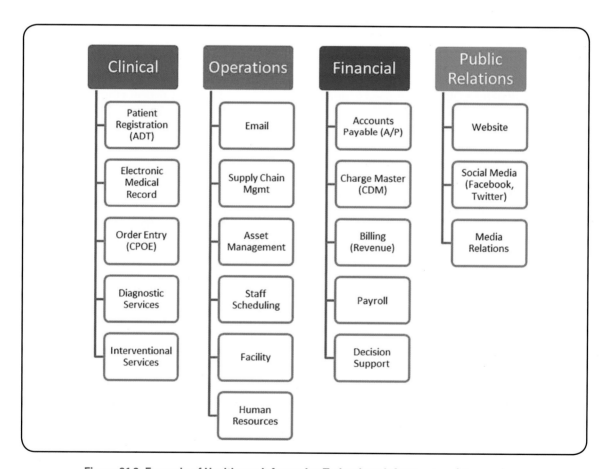

Figure 21.3 Example of Healthcare Information Technology Infrastructure (diagram)

- Centralized patient order entry (CPOE) systems are data portals used by physicians and other authorized caregivers to order tests, medications, supplies and equipment for patient use. The CPOE system also provide alerts when there are potentially conflicting orders created for a patient, such as allergies or medication incompatibility. This is important to CS because automated requests for patient care items are generated by a CPOE system.

- Diagnostic and therapeutic services systems are used to manage the scheduling, procedures performed, and results reported for their respective departments, such as radiology, ultrasound, vascular lab, ekg, respiratory and pulmonary functions lab, physical and occupational therapy, etc.

- Interventional services systems are used to manage scheduling, procedures performed and results reported for their respective departments, such as the OR, Labor & Delivery and cardiac catheterization lab. These systems are important to CS because information is received (schedules, pick lists, etc.) about the daily needs of CS's critical customers.

Operational systems are essential in managing the various functions within the organization that are not directly related to patient care.

- Email systems are a crucial platform for managing communication within any organization. Email has reduced the need for voice mail and pagers.

- Supply chain management or materiels management information systems (MMIS) are used for managing the purchasing, receipt and inventory control functions within an organization. The supply chain system is essential to CS for many reasons, including inventory control, and ordering instruments and/or supplies.

- Asset management (tracking) systems are used to manage the use, processing and location of medical equipment (See **Figure 21.4**) and/or surgical instrumentation throughout an organization. These systems serve as tools for efficiently monitoring and controlling the utilization of surgical instruments and/or patient care equipment.

Figure 21.4 Barcode scanning systems are an example of computerized methods used to track assets, such as equipment.

- Staff scheduling systems can be used to monitor compliance with the organization's time clock policies, provide a mechanism to create work schedules and analyze workforce needs and trends.

- Facility systems are used to manage the physical environment of the organization. Examples of commonly-found facility systems are heating ventilation and air conditioning (HVAC) for monitoring and managing temperature and humidity; fire control for managing fire alarms, sprinklers and magnetically-controlled doors; public address for audible announcements; and access control for managing identification badge access to secure areas within the facility. These are important to CS for managing the safety and quality of areas where items are processed and stored.

- Human resources systems are used not only for the process of recruiting and retaining staff, but also to manage employee benefits and monitor compliance with regulatory requirements for staff competency.

Financial systems are essential in managing the financial activities of the organization. These include the following:

- Accounts payable (AP) systems — Used to manage payment to vendors providing products or services to the organization.

- Charge description master (CDM) systems — Used to manage a listing of services and items that are chargeable to patients. The CDM system is designed to communicate (interface) with other software systems to support government-mandated standard billing requirements.

- Billing or patient accounting (revenue) systems — Used to manage the issuing of bills to patients/insurance payors, and assist with collections of amounts due.

- Payroll systems — Used to track hours, calculate wages, taxes and deductions, and print and deliver checks.

- Decision support systems — Used to analyze operational and financial performance, and provide key metrics to senior leadership. Decision support includes information related to the volume of procedures and services provided, as well as the operational costs and revenue received. This is an essential tool used by leadership to evaluate the financial impact of services and programs offered by the organization.

Public relations systems are essential in managing the public perception of the organization.

- The hospital's website is a significant portal for patients, employees and physicians to obtain information about the services and programs offered: employment or volunteer opportunities; the facility's core mission and values; and other details, such as phone directories, maps and directions.

- Social media portals, such as Facebook and Twitter, are becoming increasingly important to hospitals as they are frequently used by patients to express their opinion about their experience with an organization (or learn about the opinions and viewpoints shared by others).

- Media relations resources include information that resides on other websites not directly controlled by the organization, such as news articles on services provided.

Selection of Department Systems

Many factors must be considered when selecting an information system to support activities used by a specific department or facility. Key issues and requirements must first be evaluated and defined. Before selecting a system, the following questions should be asked and answered:

- Why is the system needed?

- What does the system need to do?

- Is the system capable of doing what is needed?

- Is the system compatible with existing systems?

Issues related to the appropriate range of budget costs and the projected volume of transactions that the system will process are also important. Other concerns may include the types of hardware and operating systems available, and the functional needs of the department (including the number of users). Also, if financial or patient-related information is involved, the system must be able to access the data, in compliance with industry standards and regulatory requirements.

After a system is selected, hardware and software must be installed. Vendor application software can be purchased outright or acquired through a software-based software-as-a-service (SaaS) model. Application software installation typically requires initial implementation support costs and payment of annual maintenance fees if purchased outright. If software and implementation costs are bundled, their costs may be prorated over time through monthly, quarterly or annual payment schedules. Significant costs are generally involved, and this purchase is typically treated as a capital expenditure, even when a subscription-based solution is chosen.

TRACKING SYSTEMS FOR CENTRAL SERVICE

The processes and needs of the CS department have changed over the years. Advances in sterilization and instrument technologies, and durable medical equipment and supply inventory are ongoing, and costs for instrumentation purchase, repair and replacement have led to a greater need for improved asset tracking and management.

Overview

Tracking systems available for use in CS can forecast needs and identify processing costs for trays and single instruments. These tracking systems can also help maximize equipment and inventory utilization to provide pertinent information as future budgets are developed.

Many healthcare environments still use procedures that, while popular for many years, should now be re-evaluated. CS personnel must also move out of their comfort zones as they improve processes to maintain patient care equipment for nursing units, and track supplies, instrument sets and trays used throughout the facility.

Manual methods using handwritten tags, logbooks, wall-mounted bulletin boards, etc., to track equipment are now being replaced with computerized alternatives. Many facilities acquire a **turnkey system** with limited features or support that generate less-than-ideal information. A better strategy involves using a reputable product that provides updates to ensure that the facility receives necessary support and upgrades.

> **Turnkey system** A computer system supplied to a customer in such a complete form that it can be put to immediate use.

Tracking Methods

There are several types of tracking systems and methods available. Examples include use of barcodes to scan an item's last known location, and radio frequency identification (RFID) tags used for real-time tracking of patient care equipment.

System ease of use cost and compatibility with other software systems in use are among the factors affecting purchasing decisions. Additionally, to ensure reliability, the tracking method must be compatible with the processing practices and technologies used by the facility. For example, RFID tags that can be sterilized reliably are a relatively new advancement and can be costly. Barcode based tracking is generally used for tracking sterile surgical trays and instruments, while RFID-based tracking, on the other hand, is generally reserved for tracking patient care equipment, as the devices are not subjected to a sterilization process, and a cost-efficient, reliable tag can be used.

A tracking system may typically be either a traditional installed software application with a database managed by facility information technology (IT) personnel or a web-based application with a database managed (hosted) by the software vendor and accessed through the internet. The latter, commonly referred to as **cloud computing**, may offer several advantages, including cost benefits and ease of installation.

> **Cloud computing** The practice of storing regularly-used data on multiple servers that can be accessed through the Internet.

Integration (interfacing) capabilities are of importance when communicating critical information to and from the tracking system. OR scheduling system interfaces are typically desirable to both CS and the OR because they facilitate information about instruments, supplies and equipment needs, based on the surgery schedule in real-time or near real-time forecasting).

Tracking Systems Meet Specific Needs

A tracking system must meet the specific needs of the facility that uses it. For example, in a multi-hospital health network, there may be certain modules or special features in the system utilized by personnel at one site, but are not implemented or used at other sites. This is generally due to differences in the complexity of processing or logistics between sites or departments. For example, a processing area supporting a small ambulatory surgery department may not have a need for the tracking features that a CS department supporting a large inpatient OR would find beneficial. Conversely, the ambulatory surgery area might have a need for features related to flexible endoscope processing, which may not be as meaningful to a large CS department.

In short, a well-developed tracking system has built-in flexibility and scalability that can allow CS departments to tailor the configuration to meet specific needs and also allow for logical reconfiguration, or changes, as needed.

Computerized Systems in Use

Computerized methods facilitate more effective data tracking for rapid report generating, and are much more comprehensive in scope and efficiency than manual systems. Data integrity is consistently more reliable than with a manual system. Computerized standards are accepted by the **Healthcare Information Management Systems Society (HIMSS)** and are used by applicable facility departments to securely store backup data.

> **Healthcare Information Management Systems Society (HIMSS)** A global, cause-based, nonprofit organization focused on better health through information technology.

More about Tracking Systems

The continual need to update information is critical for the success of any tracking system, regardless of whether its primary use is for instrument processing, case cart pick lists, preference cards, inventory control or other purposes. (See **Figure 21.5**)

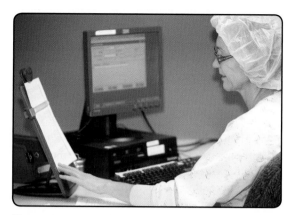

Figure 21.5   A CS technician updates information on preference cards.

Surgical instrument sets or single peel-packed items can be tracked (located) at the packaged and sterilized product level using one dimensional (1D) barcode labels. Small RFID tags, which can be used reliably within the sterilization process, can provide real-time location data when they are affixed to instruments or trays. It is likely that RFID technology will coexist with barcodes because use of a barcode promotes line-of-sight inspection by the user when scanning an item. This is an essential step in ensuring the sterile integrity of packaged products.

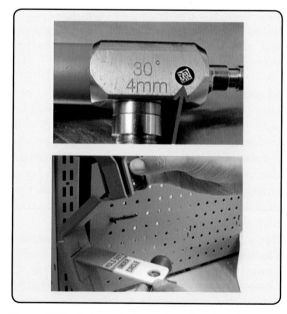

Figure 21.6   Dot matrix barcodes allow individual instrument scanning and tracking.

Individual instruments can be tracked (located) within a set/tray using two-dimensional (2D) data-matrix barcodes. These are marked directly on the instrument using a laser etching/engraving process or through the placement of a dot-type label. (See **Figure 21.6**) Individual instrument tracking ensures specific instruments are kept with a specific set. It can also locate specific high-cost, complex devices, such as powered, endoscopic or robotic instruments for required preventative maintenance inspection. In facilities where the risk of exposure to emerging pathogens, such as Creuztfeldt-Jakob Disease (CJD), is high, individual instrument tracking is crucial for demonstrating the processing or dispensing actions taken in the investigation of a suspected or confirmed exposure.

System documentation and scanning can be done with many different types of devices. These include wireless mobile handheld devices, (See **Figure 21.7**) wired directly to the computer terminal, fixed radio receivers that read RFID transponder signals throughout the facility, and manual entry of information into the computer.

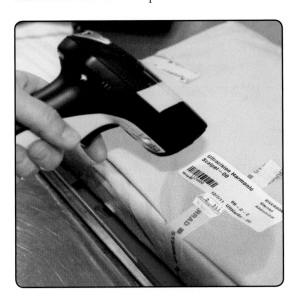

Figure 21.7 – A handheld scanner is used to capture instrument information before an item is sterilized.

Decisions about system utilization should consider the specific environment to which the item(s) will be exposed. For example, the cleaning and sterilization processes for instruments and sets must be evaluated in detail during any implementation planning process to minimize the risk of any adverse impacts on the tracking system. For example, chemical agents designed to be compatible for use with instruments (based on the materials used in their manufacture) may negatively impact laser etchings, fade barcode labels, and make them unreadable to the scanner after repeated use. Heat generated during steam sterilization may damage RFID tags and may impair their functionality. Water, chemicals and drying temperatures used to clean case carts and other equipment may cause the adhesives used to affix the RFID tags to dissolve. When this occurs, they can fall off or become damaged from water leakage. As these risks are recognized, manufacturers generally respond by making improvements to components or processes to ensure reliability.

FEATURES OF INSTRUMENT AND EQUIPMENT TRACKING SYSTEMS

Instrument and equipment tracking systems can provide many different features to assist CS professionals in the facility's OR, finance, nursing and administrative departments. All tracking systems include some basic operating features; however, more advanced systems include additional features to enhance their usefulness.

Basic Systems

Basic instrument and equipment tracking systems typically can track (account for):

- Complete instrument sets and trays.

- Specific equipment items.

- Last known location of a specific instrument set, tray or equipment.

- Cost and value of specific equipment and instruments, and the total cost of an instrument set/tray.

- Number of complete processing and use cycles through which instruments and instrument sets have moved.

- Usage of specific equipment.

- Preventive maintenance schedules and repairs made to specific equipment and instrument sets/trays.

Basic instrument and equipment tracking systems also provide other information, including:

- Complete tray lists for accurate tray assembly (See **Figure 21.8**) and equipment set up, such as:

  › Name of CS technician who assembled and inspected the set or equipment.

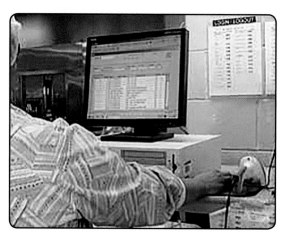

Figure 21.8

  › Date set or equipment was processed.

  › Sterilization and cleaning modality (process).

  › Catalog number and manufacturer name to identify instruments and associated equipment/supplies.

  › Quantity (individual and total) of instruments included within the set or tray.

  › Identification of instruments missing from set. *Note: These can be identified on the list and can then be affixed to the outside of the set for identification and tracking.*

- Productivity reporting information:

  › Sets and instruments processed and completed during a specific work shift.

  › Sets and instruments completed by specific employees. *Note: This information is helpful for educational and training purposes.*

  › Equipment processed and distributed.

Quality assurance data for specific facility-based information, such as:

- Sterilization load quarantines or recalls.

- Biological monitoring standards and regulations.

- Educational and inservice documentation.

Financial data for documenting/managing:

- Instrument replacement and repair.

- Equipment replacement and repair.

- Preventive maintenance notification.

- Preventive maintenance records.

- Utilization of instrument sets, trays and equipment.

- Productivity data and staffing requirements for peak operational workflow.

Integrating/interfacing with clinical systems allows facilities to associate (link) instrument trays, sets and equipment to each patient's medical record. Today's tracking systems can also interface with sterilization and washer/decontamination equipment.

Advanced Systems

Instrument and equipment tracking systems may also include some advanced features that are beneficial in certain healthcare facility applications:

- RFID enables real-time location of an instrument or equipment item as it moves through the facility and the processing cycle. The real-time location of a complete instrument set or tray can also be assessed.

- Set-level tracking features to allow staff members to know the last scanned location of an instrument set/tray.

- Individual instrument level tracking features to allow staff to track a single instrument within a set or tray, and identify the set into which a specific instrument was placed.

Note: This information represents a generalized list of features that software developers typically provide in their instrument and equipment tracking systems. A complete review of a facility's specific needs is required to select the most appropriate tracking system.

CONCLUSION

Central Service professionals must responsibly manage the equipment, instruments and supplies entrusted to them by their healthcare facility. An instrument and equipment tracking system facilitates this goal by capturing pertinent data, logging and documenting processes, practices and CS-related functions, and more.

As computer technology and information systems continue to evolve, additional capabilities will become available to help facilities better address operational activities and facilitate high-quality patient care. Even so, computers are only one part of a total information system. While computers and tracking systems provide numerous benefits, CS professionals are the key to providing efficient and effective services to help their department support the facility's core mission, which is providing safe, high-quality patient care and customer service.

RESOURCE

Glandon GH, Slovensky DJ, Smaltz GL. *Austin & Boxerman's Information Systems for Healthcare Management, 7th Ed.* 2008.

CENTRAL SERVICE TERMS

Turnkey system

Cloud computing

Healthcare Information Management Systems Society (HIMSS)

Chapter 22

Safety and Risk Management for Central Service

Learning Objectives

As a result of successfully completing this chapter, readers will be able to:

1. Explain the importance of safety and risk management in the Central Service department

2. Review three common workplace hazards: Fire, hazardous substances and bloodborne pathogens

3. Explain the importance of ergonomics and health awareness for Central Service technicians

4. Discuss common safety hazards applicable to Central Service functions and work areas, and explain how employee injuries can be prevented

5. Describe special safety precautions for handling ethylene oxide

6. Discuss the basics of internal and external disaster plans for a healthcare facility

7. Review procedures to report employee accidents and injuries

8. Explain the importance of education and reporting in a Central Source safety and risk management system

INTRODUCTION

It has been said that "safety is no accident," and that statement couldn't be more true, especially for healthcare professionals who are responsible for keeping patients, employees and visitors free from injury.

Safety requires ongoing education, safeguards, proper planning and the combined implementation of safety systems to reduce risks, prevent injury and save lives. The Central Service (CS) decontamination area is a perfect example of how safety systems and due diligence is essential for ensuring safety. This area operates in the presence of pathogenic microorganisms and presents a real risk to those who enter. Engineering controls, such as managed air pressure, physical separation from clean areas, and personal protective equipment (PPE) are provided to minimize risk. Employees are educated in biohazard safety and must follow specific regulations, such as those established by the Occupational Safety and Health Administration (OSHA), to reduce the risk of injury. (See **Figure 22.1**) This chapter will identify common risks found in the CS work areas and discuss ways to minimize the risk of injury.

RISK MANAGEMENT

Risk management is a method used to assess the risks of a specific activity and develop programs to reduce that risk. It also involves injury prevention and claims management (the settlement, defense and prevention of lawsuits).

Risk management originated in the insurance industry as the result of the increased number of medical malpractice lawsuits. These lawsuits cost healthcare facilities billions of dollars over the past several years. Healthcare facilities must effectively manage injury prevention for patients and employees as part of a risk management program. Various authorities, including The

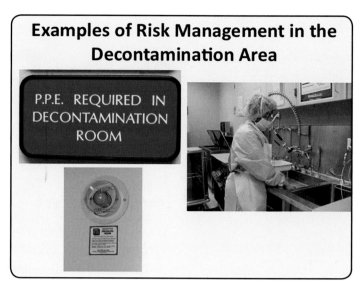

Examples of Risk Management in the Decontamination Area

P.P.E. REQUIRED IN DECONTAMINATION ROOM

Figure 22.1

Joint Commission (TJC), require that healthcare facilities develop and implement procedures to ensure that they meet minimum safety standards.

Risk management programs are designed to prevent accidents and/or injuries, and ensure accurate reporting and follow up to help prevent similar incidents. After a situation is examined and hazards or unsafe practices have been discovered, risk management personnel ensure that corrective actions are taken to improve systems, behaviors and/or physical conditions to help prevent employee and patient accidents and injuries.

By following the protocols outlined in this textbook, as well as the manufacturer's Instructions for Use (IFU), standards and regulations, and CS technicians support patient safety.

> **Risk management** The methods used to assess the risks of a specific activity and develop a program to reduce losses from exposure to those risks.

COMMON WORKPLACE SAFETY HAZARDS

All jobs involve some risks. The key to working safely in any work environment is to understand those risks and take appropriate steps to minimize them. CS technicians must understand potential hazards and pay close attention in work areas within and sometimes outside of their department. The belief that "an accident or injury will never happen to me" creates a false sense of security that results in many injuries each year. Following safety protocols and incorporating them into all work practices is necessary for preventing injuries and accidents.

Central Service Occupational Hazards

In CS, there are three different types of occupational hazards: physical, biological and chemical hazards. (See **Figure 22.2**) Some of those occupational hazards can be present in all areas of the department. For example, physical hazards, such as heavy or awkward lifting, can occur in any work area. Other hazards may be confined to a specific work area. For example, biohazard contamination will most likely occur in the decontamination area.

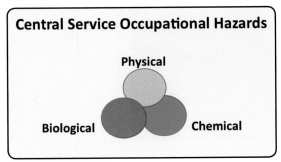

Figure 22.2

Physical safety hazards may be caused by the environment and the tasks performed within that environment. Due to the nature of the tasks performed, there are many potential physical hazards in the CS department. Physical hazards may include: wet floors, cluttered walkways, heavy carts and sharp instruments. Fire is also a physical safety concern.

Biological safety hazards (infectious waste and bloodborne pathogens) can potentially be found in any area of the department. Obviously, the decontamination area is the main area of concern for biological hazards.

Chemical safety hazards may be found throughout the work area. For example, solutions used in the decontamination area, sterilants used in the sterilization area and some patient care products may pose chemical hazards within the department.

The following sections examine general safety hazards and then outline specific safety hazards by work area. The risk of injury from all of these hazards can be minimized by following safety protocols.

GENERAL PHYSICAL HAZARDS

Ergonomic Concerns

General physical hazards include those related to **ergonomics**, slips, falls, electrical, safety and sharps. Ergonomics is the process of changing work or working conditions to reduce physical stress. CS technicians are exposed to many ergonomic stress factors, such as repetitive motion, lifting and pushing.

Ergonomic stressors that employees may encounter include:

- Force - Heavy lifting or manipulating equipment or instrument sets.

- Repetition – Using the same motion, or series of motions, continually or frequently.

- Awkward positions – Assuming positions that place stress on the body, such as reaching or twisting while lifting.

- Vibration – Rapid oscillation of the body or a body part.

- Contact stress – Continuous pressure between the body and a sharp edge.

Exposure to these stressors can cause numerous problems, including ligament sprains, joint and tendon inflammation, pinched nerves, herniated spinal discs and other injuries.

Problems, such as carpal tunnel syndrome from typing at a computer station, may develop gradually, over time, or from a single event, such as from improperly lifting a heavy object. In either case, the injuries may cause pain, loss of work and disability.

The number and severity of ergonomic injuries can be reduced if the work environment and work practices are effectively adjusted. To be effective, management commitment and employee participation are required. This forms the foundation for ergonomic improvements because a sustained effort, allocation of resources, and frequent follow up is needed. Staff member buy in of equipment and work procedure changes is of special importance.

Training can help employees to:

- Recognize the signs and symptoms of injuries, so they can respond to them.

- Report potential problems.

- Recognize jobs/tasks that have ergonomic stressors.

Ergonomics Process of changing work or working conditions to reduce employee stress.

Conducting a work site analysis can help identify conditions and aspects of work activities that increase injury risks to employees. It will also help ensure that corrective actions taken will address the problems creating the hazard. *Note: **Figures 22.3** and **22.4** show overhead lift systems, transport carts and adjustable height work tables that can be used to reduce the risk of back injuries.*

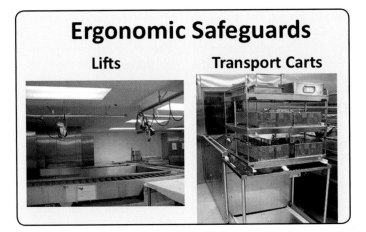

Figure 22.3

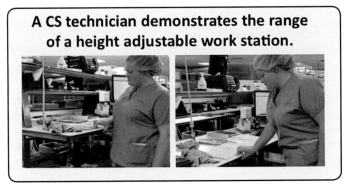

Figure 22.4

Simple changes, such as stretching before work, shifting position, learning and practicing good body mechanics and breaking up repetitive activities can help employees reduce the risks of ergonomic injuries. **Figure 22.5** shows a technician practicing good body mechanics while lifting a tray.

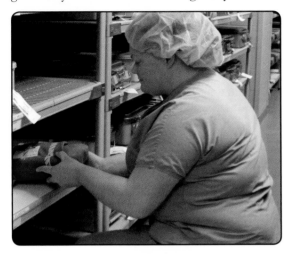

Figure 22.5

Proper lifting and pushing movements can also prevent injuries. When loading and unloading carts from dumbwaiters or elevators, or receiving a cart into the department, it is essential to check the weight on the cart before attempting to move it. **Figure 22.6** provides an example of a heavy cart that must be handled carefully. Ensuring that the wheels are straight, and that they will roll over door spaces or uneven edges is also important, as is unloading some items to lighten the cart if it is too heavy to move easily.

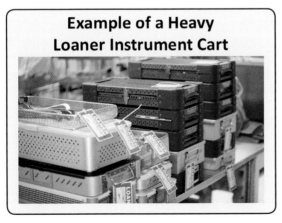

Figure 22.6

Slip and Fall Concerns

Slips and falls are always a concern in the CS department. Mobile equipment and ever-present wet floors increase fall risks. To reduce these risks, mobile equipment should be parked away from common traffic areas. Areas that often have wet floors, such as in the decontamination area, around the cart wash exits, and washer unload areas, must be kept as dry as possible, and spills should be wiped immediately. Non-slip footwear should be worn and attention should be given to slippery floors. Signage, such as the wet floor sign pictured in **Figure 22.7**, alerts people to the potential hazard.

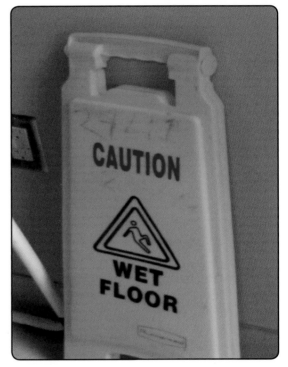

Figure 22.7

Electrical Safety Concerns

Burns and shocks from electric equipment can result if safe handling precautions are not observed.

Carefully check all electrical cords to ensure they are intact, with no breaks in the insulation. Electrical cords on mobile equipment run a greater risk of being kinked or run over by rolling carts, which can make the equipment unsafe. All plugs on electrical equipment must be three-pronged and grounded, and all electrical outlets must accommodate these plugs. Inspecting electrical cords for breaks and plugs for bent prongs is a responsibility of CS technicians. (See **Figure 22.8**) Identifying and reporting a potential hazard during cleaning or delivery can prevent injuries to patients and staff.

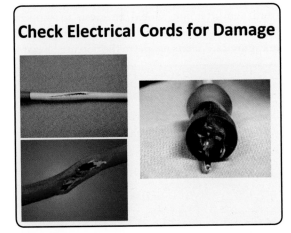

Figure 22.8

Use Caution with Electrical Equipment

All electrical equipment can pose a hazard if it is used in an unsafe manner. For example, radios placed near water sources, such as sinks and ultrasonic cleaners, can lead to staff injury in that work area. Keep the work area safe from electrical hazards.

Sharps Concerns

Cuts and puncture injuries from sharps can happen in any area of the CS department. Sharp instruments can break the skin's surface and produce puncture wounds, lacerations and abrasions. If the injury occurs in the decontamination area, these injuries can result in exposure to disease.

Some general precautions to prevent sharps injuries include:

- Handling all sharps with care.

- Not grasping several objects at the same time.

- Ensuring that sharp ends point away from any part of one's body during transport.

- Placing all disposable sharps, such as needles and blades, in the appropriate sharps container. (See **Figure 22.9**)

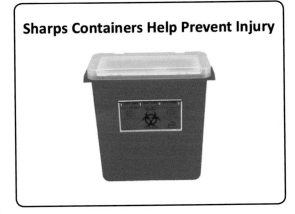

Figure 22.9

General Chemical Hazards

Although most chemicals used in CS are found in the decontamination area, chemical hazards may be found in other areas of the department, as well.

Splashing chemicals is a common cause of eye injuries, so the use of eye protection is required. Eye wash stations are also required in areas where chemical injuries are a concern. (See **Figure 22.10**)

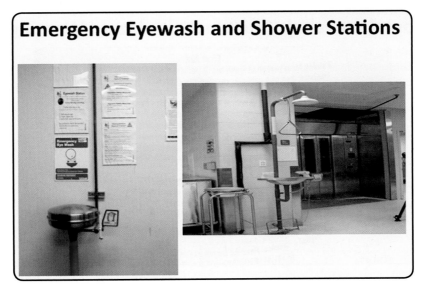

Emergency Eyewash and Shower Stations

Figure 22.10

Hazardous Substance Concerns

Each state categorizes certain chemicals and substances as hazardous. Each CS department should have an easily accessible, understandable, and current list of all hazardous substances with which employees could come in contact. Most facilities today have a comprehensive computerized hazardous chemical list.

If employees are required to perform known hazardous tasks, it is important that they understand the safety procedures developed for that task. Prior to performing such tasks, employees must be given information about the hazards to which they may be exposed. This information should include identification of specific hazards, use of PPE, recommended safety measures and emergency response procedures. Employers should take measures to minimize hazards to employees. These could include increased area ventilation, respirators, presence of other employees to assist, and the rehearsal of emergency procedures.

CS managers must develop a hazardous materials management program to best ensure the health and safety of employees, as required by state and federal regulations and TJC. Information about hazardous chemicals and substances must be available to all employees.

OSHA's "Employee Right to Know" regulations mandate that a comprehensive hazard communication program be in place to help ensure that employees know about hazards around them. Components of an effective departmental hazardous substance management program include container labeling requirements; use of safety data sheets (SDS); employee information and training, procedures to manage and handle hazardous substances; employee monitoring; and **hazardous waste** management.

> **Hazardous waste** Substances that cannot be disposed of in the facility's normal trash system.

Container Labeling

All containers that contain hazardous substances must be clearly labeled to specify contents and appropriate hazard warnings, and must indicate the name and address of the manufacturer. All **secondary containers** must be labeled with an extra

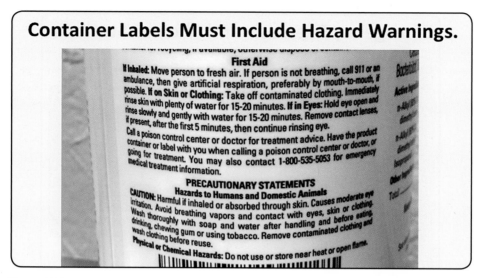

Container Labels Must Include Hazard Warnings.

Figure 22.11

copy of the original manufacturer's label, or with a generic label that identifies hazard warnings and directions.

> **Secondary container** A generic container that is filled from a primary container or filled with a diluted solution. Secondary containers must be clearly labeled with content.

Safety Data Sheets

An SDS (formerly called material safety data sheet - MSDS) contains important information about product materials and properties that employees must know to work safely with any given product. SDS are developed and provided by the manufacturer of the product, and they are specific for each product. SDS contain at least the following information:

- Product identification – Product name, manufacturer's name, address and telephone number, product item number (manufacturer's identification) and synonym names.

- List of hazardous ingredients.

- Physical data – Vapor pressure, evaporation rate, solubility in water, freezing and boiling points, specific gravity, acidity (pH), vapor density, appearance and odor.

- Fire and explosion information – Flash point, flammable units, extinguishing media, special firefighting procedures; and unusual fire and explosion hazards.

- Reactivity data – Stability, incompatibility, hazardous decomposition products and conditions contributing to hazardous **polymerization**.

- Health hazard data – Effects of overexposure.

- Storage recommendations – Incompatible materials and storage temperatures.

- Emergency and first-aid procedures. (See **Figure 22.11**)

- Spill or leak procedures, spill management and waste disposal methods.

- Protection information and control measures.

- Special precautions.

> **Polymerization** A molecular reaction that creates an uncontrolled release of energy.

The employer is responsible to ensure that SDS are readily available to employees who may work with, or be in the vicinity of, hazardous materials. (See **Figure 22.12**) In turn, employees are responsible for becoming familiar with the SDS information and consistently following the instructions given for the products they handle and use.

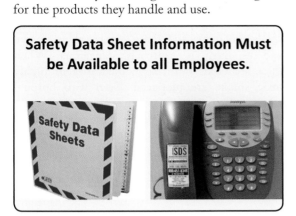

Figure 22.12

Employee Monitoring

To prevent potential health hazards to workers, OSHA has established permissible exposure limits (PELs) for many chemicals used in sterilant and disinfectant formulations. These include ethylene oxide (EtO), hydrogen peroxide (H_2O_2), ozone (O_3) and others.

Glutaraldehyde is a chemical commonly used in CS as a high-level disinfectant. The National Institute for Occupational Safety and Health (NIOSH) recommends that exposure to glutaraldehyde be under 0.2 parts per million (ppm) time weighted average over an eight-hour work shift. The American Conference of Governmental Industrial Hygienists (ACGIH) recommends a ceiling value of 0.05 ppm, which should not be exceeded at any time.

Healthcare facilities are required by OSHA to:

- Provide adequate ventilation systems.

- Establish safe work operating procedures.

- Provide PPE.

- Implement other methods to ensure that occupational exposure limits are not exceeded in the workplace.

Mechanical monitoring systems can aid in the detection of chemicals present in the work area. These systems can detect the presence of chemicals at levels far below the level an employee would be able to detect by smell. (See **Figure 22.13**)

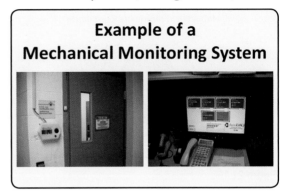

Figure 22.13

Personal monitors that measure individual exposure to chemical vapors by measuring the presence of specific chemicals in the employee's breathing zone are also available. (See **Figure 22.14**)

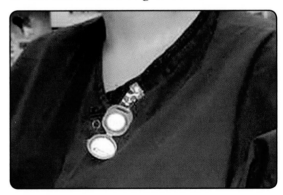

Figure 22.14

Fire Hazards

Fire requires three elements to be present at the same time; these elements make up the "Fire Triangle."

- A **combustible** or flammable substance.

- A source of oxygen.

- A source of ignition.

To prevent fires, at least one of the elements in the triangle must be eliminated. (See **Figure 22.15**)

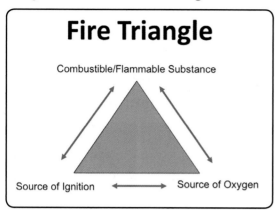

Fire Triangle

Combustible/Flammable Substance

Source of Ignition

Source of Oxygen

Figure 22.15

Fire and Explosions

A fire occurs when the temperature of a flammable or combustible substance is raised high enough for the individual carbon and hydrogen atoms to combine with oxygen, and the resulting energy is released. If the material is a solid, it will burn only at its surface. In contrast, if the material is a volatile liquid, such as alcohol, which readily vaporizes, or a gas, such as EtO, the flame front passes quickly through the substance. The result is an explosion accompanied by the instantaneous generation of large quantities of heated gases. Their rapid expansion creates a very loud pressure wave that can cause great damage.

Combustible loading is the weight of combustible materials per square foot of area where the materials are located.

> **Combustible** A substance that, if ignited, will react with oxygen and burn.
>
> **Combustible loading** The weight of combustible materials per square foot of area in which those materials are located.

Disposable materials, including gowns, caps, masks, shoe covers, tubing, syringes, and their packaging, contribute to heavy combustible loads in hospitals. This problem occurs principally in central storage areas such as CS, Operating Room (OR), delivery suites, nursing units and trash handling facilities.

The presence of large volumes of combustible materials and flammable substances poses unique risks. The large combustible loading created by single-use items and their wrappings in storage and as trash is especially dangerous. When these materials burn, large quantities of highly toxic smoke are produced. Even with hospital compartmentalization features that limit the spread of smoke and fire, a high-risk situation occurs; therefore, healthcare fire safety programs must include:

- Minimization of the combustible load.

- Fire response plans.

- Early detection.

- Containment of the fire and combustible products.

- Extinguishment.

- Evacuation plans.

Minimize Combustible Loads

It is important to minimize the volume of combustible substances because a prime rule of fire protection is: "Don't give fire a place to start."

Strategies to minimize combustible loads include:

- Ensure that single-use items are safely stored by keeping them in areas with the proper temperature and humidity.

- Minimize the volume of combustible substances, even when adequate storage facilities are available. Consider purchase systems in which the supplier retains possession of, but not the title to, items until actually needed.

- Minimize trash build up. Each facility must have an adequate trash handling program that includes covered trash containers of noncombustible construction and adequate volume at each site of trash generation.

Fire Response Plan

Every healthcare facility requires a comprehensive fire response plan and each staff member in every department must know his/her specific role in these plans. The fire safety emphasis should begin at the time of new employee orientation and should continue with ongoing training.

Every healthcare facility is required to have and maintain sprinkler systems, smoke detectors, fire extinguishers and audible alarms to warn and protect staff and patients. (See **Figure 22.16**)

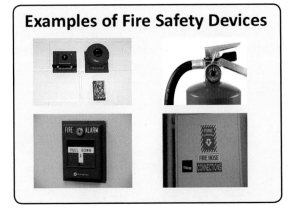

Examples of Fire Safety Devices

Figure 22.16

Each CS technician must participate in their facility's fire training and become aware of the fire safety items within their work area. Carefully following the facility's fire plan is important for both staff and patient safety. When a fire emergency occurs, everyone must understand their role and act quickly.

Workplace Violence

According to OSHA, approximately two million people are the victims of **workplace violence** each year. All employees should pay attention to possible warning signs, and they should:

- Immediately report any direct threats of violence or retaliation to management.

- Note behavior, statements or attitudes that are unusual, threatening or disconcerting.

Employees should be aware of their facility's specific policies on workplace violence and attend education programs designed to provide information on prevention and response.

> **Workplace violence** Any act or threat of physical violence, harassment, intimidation or other threatening disruptive behavior that occurs at the work site.

AREA-SPECIFIC SAFETY CONCERNS

There are safety concerns that are common in specific work areas within the CS department. **Figure 22.17** shows a sign notifying personnel about the need for PPE in the decontamination area.

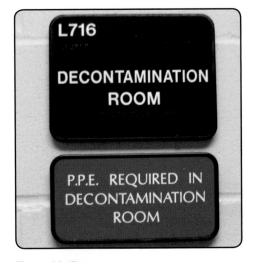

L716

DECONTAMINATION ROOM

P.P.E. REQUIRED IN DECONTAMINATION ROOM

Figure 22.17

Soiled Receiving and Decontamination Areas

Safety tips when working in soiled receiving and decontamination areas include:

- Never reach into a basin or container holding contaminated objects, unless the objects in the basin are clearly visible. Use a sponge forceps to grasp the object or pour out any solution that prohibits visual examination, and then remove objects from basins or containers one at a time. Never use foaming detergents when handling contaminated instruments in the decontamination sink, as the foam can prevent visualization of sharp objects. (See **Figure 22.18**)

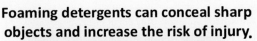

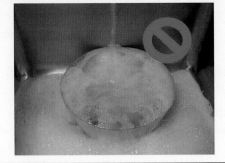

Figure 22.18

- Never reach into trash containers or sharps containers.

- Use extreme caution when disarming scalpel blades. Do not attempt to do so without training. Never disarm by hand. Always use a needle holder or tool specifically designed to remove blades. (See **Figure 22.19**)

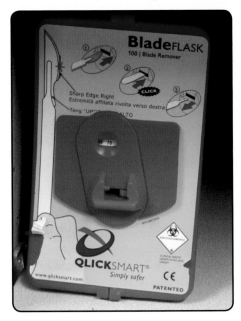

Figure 22.19

- When processing reusable sharps, separate them from other instruments and position them in a manner that protects anyone who may handle them.

- Follow the manufacturer's recommendations for safe use of chemicals. Always wear recommended PPE to protect all skin surfaces and mucous membranes from chemical burns.

- Follow the manufacturer's recommendations for safe operation of cleaning and testing equipment.

- Use caution when walking, and inspect the floor for slippery surfaces. Utilize mats and non-skid footwear. (See **Figure 22.20**)

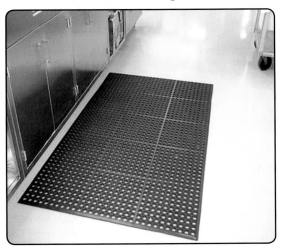

Figure 22.20

- When cleaning instruments in a sink, always scrub below the surface of the water to avoid the formation of **aerosols**. (See **Figure 22.21**)

Aerosol A suspension of ultramicroscopic solid or liquid particles in air or gas; a spray.

- Sinks and other working surfaces should be at levels to afford easy access, and to reduce back and arm strain.

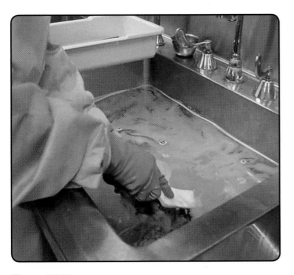

Figure 22.21

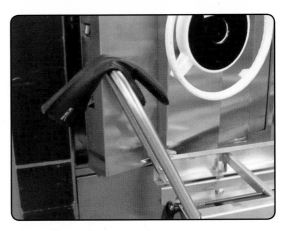

Figure 22.23

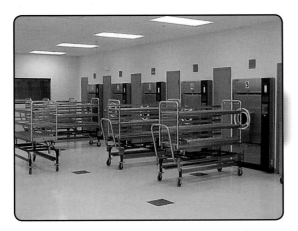

Figure 22.22

Preparation and Sterilization Areas

Safety tips when working in preparation and sterilization areas include:

- Move sterilizer carts to low/no traffic or other designated areas, so co-workers will be less likely to come in contact with hot carts. (See **Figure 22.22**)

- Use thermal insulated gloves when handling steam sterilizer carts, washer baskets and other objects subjected to high temperatures. (See **Figure 22.23**)

- Keep sterilizer doors closed when not loading or unloading the chamber to protect co-workers from coming in contact with the hot inner door. (See **Figure 22.24**)

- Use caution when using heat sealers. Keep away from heated components. Be sure to follow the manufacturer's instructions.

- Be cautious when using a cutting edge to prepare paper/plastic packs.

- Be cautious when testing instruments for sharpness.

- When lifting instrument sets, use the larger muscles in legs and arms. Hold the item as close to the body as possible without actually touching the body.

- Follow procedures for using and disposing of biological indicators.

- Ensure that proper signs and labels are posted to warn of hot surfaces or other hazards.

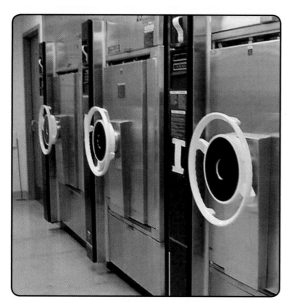

Figure 22.24

Sterilizer Safety

Steam sterilizers
- Use caution to avoid burns when working with steam sterilizers.

Hydrogen Peroxide Sterilizer Safety
- Use caution when handling H_2O_2 containers; damaged containers may release sterilant into the work area.

Ethylene Oxide Sterilizer Safety
EtO has been strongly regulated by the federal government for many years. In 1984, OSHA established a 1 ppm (in air) PEL, and a 0.5 ppm **action level** (AL) for EtO. *Note: AL is the concentration level of airborne EtO in or at breathing level.* The PEL and AL limits are expressed as an eight-hour time weighted average (TWA). They represent the total allowable worker exposure during an eight-hour period and express it as an average exposure during the period.

> **Action level (AL)** Level of exposure to a harmful substance or other hazard at which an employer must take required precautions to protect the workers. It is normally one-half the permissible exposure limit (PEL).

In 1988, OSHA amended its rule on occupational exposure to EtO by adding a 5 ppm **short-term excursion limit (STEL)** over a 15-minute period. The STEL is typically related to tasks, such as transferring or handling of non-aerated goods and performing sterilizer maintenance.

> **Short-term excursion limit (STEL)** The maximum concentration of a chemical to which workers may be exposed continuously for up to 15 minutes without danger to health or work efficiency and safety.

Common Terms:

OSHA – EtO – PEL – TWA – AL – STEL

The Occupational Safety and Health Administration (OSHA) has established several limits on occupational exposure to ethylene oxide (EtO). A permissible exposure limit (PEL) is the average concentration of a chemical in the air to which a worker can be legally exposed over a particular period of time (usually eight hours). The PEL for EtO is 1 part per million (ppm) as an eight-hour time weighted average (TWA). An action level (AL) is the concentration level of airborne EtO in or at breathing level. A short-term excursion limit (STEL) is the maximum concentration of an airborne chemical to which a worker may be exposed over a 15-minute period. OSHA has adopted a STEL of 5 ppm for EtO.

Sterilizer manufacturers now include many safety features on EtO sterilizers. These include negative-pressure air flow to help prevent any exposures if the unit malfunctions during the cycle, and automatic mechanisms keep the sterilizer locked down until the aeration cycle is completed.

Safety precautions when working with EtO equipment include:

- EtO sterilization should be performed in a separate area from other department work areas.

- Healthcare facilities using EtO must have an operational, dedicated ventilation system to remove fumes exhausted during the cycle. This exhaust system should be checked regularly to ensure that any fumes in the employees' breathing zone are captured. It is also necessary to have an audible and visual alarm that will sound in case of any malfunction.

- EtO canisters should be stored in an approved containment locker. Check local regulations for the maximum amount of canisters allowed in the area. (See **Figure 22.25**)

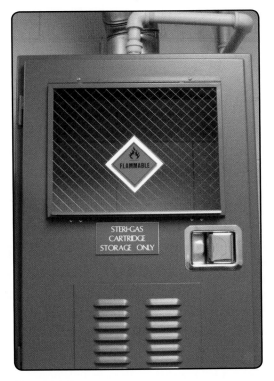

Figure 22.25

- Compliance with all federal, state and local air quality and worker safety regulations relating to employee safety, discharge, air monitoring and recordkeeping.

- The exposure of any person to EtO must be reported immediately to the CS manager, employee health nurse, Emergency Department or employee health service.

Supply Receiving, Breakout and Storage Areas

To ensure a safe and efficient supply receiving area, adequate storage space and traffic access must be available. Supply storage and shelving units must be secure and steady. Shelves should be arranged to facilitate maximum space efficiency and allow employees easy access to supplies. Heavy materials and items used most frequently should be placed on middle shelves to enable them to be easily and safely accessed by employees. Lighter, infrequently-used items should be placed on higher shelves.

Employees should use appropriate equipment (e.g., steps, stands and ladders) to safely reach upper shelves. Climbing on shelves is not acceptable. Procedures for the safe operation of dollies, hand trucks or carts to handle bulk materials must be available, and employees must be trained to consistently comply with them. (See **Figure 22.26**)

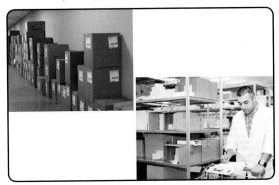

Figure 22.26

Closed trash containers should be available to properly dispose of unwanted materials. Containers for the appropriate storage of hazardous or flammable materials must be readily available to avoid exposure to hazardous substances. Employees working in this area must also follow proper procedures when disposing of and removing hazardous materials. SDS must be available for reference where these substances are used.

Safety tips for supply receiving, breakout and storage include:

- Use caution when removing items from storage units or shelves. Allow time to perform the tasks and ensure adequate space is available to maneuver the items being received.

- When using a box-cutting tool, always cut away from the body or to the side. Retract the blade into the handle, or cover the blade with a sheath when the device is not in use. Scalpels should not be used.

- Avoid twisting and jerking movements when picking up or removing objects from tight spaces.

- Inspect work areas for objects left in pathways or equipment with parts that protrude into a traffic path. Aisles and doorways must be kept clear at all times.

- Perform appropriate stretching exercises prior to work to avoid injuries to the back and other areas affected by lifting, pushing and pulling.

- Use transport carts, when possible, to minimize lifting and carrying.

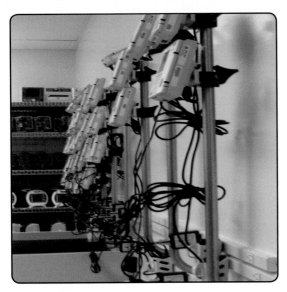

Figure 22.27

Equipment Storage Areas and Equipment Transportation

Areas where supplies and equipment are stored awaiting requests from patient care areas can also be dangerous. These areas can have substantial activity and often have limited space to move about freely. Many types of patient care equipment require electrical charging, so multiple electrical outlets must be available. (See **Figure 22.27**) All portable electrical equipment, including items used in CS and patient care areas, must comply with applicable electrical codes.

Adequate storage space should be provided, and shelving should be of adequate capacity and strength. Rugged, easily controlled carts should be provided for transferring items.

Transporting supplies and equipment through the facility can pose several safety concerns. CS technicians must be aware of their surroundings and take extra care to help ensure they keep themselves and those around them safe as they perform their duties. Food service and patient transportation devices, such as gurneys and wheelchairs, may be in use in patient care areas. There may be hallways, corners and elevators that present hazards if proper techniques are not used by employees transporting patients and other items.

Safety tips include:

- Avoid excessive speed. Be prepared to stop quickly if a person steps into the hallway from a doorway. Always yield to patients.

- Use caution when approaching doorways, hallways, elevators and high-traffic areas.

- Do not use a transport vehicle to push or prop open automatic doors.

- Carts and mobile equipment should not be parked in hallways where it may block traffic or door access. Always keep hallways clear for the free flow of traffic. (See **Figure 22.28**)

- When transporting carts or equipment, make certain that the path in front and on each side of the transport equipment is visible.

- Inspect floors for uneven surfaces or defective tiles or edges to ensure that equipment being transported will not be thrown off balance.

- Use caution when approaching corners or intersections of hallways; use safety mirrors whenever available.

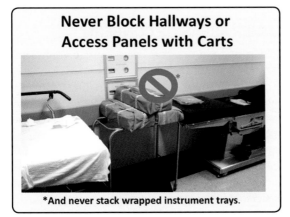

Never Block Hallways or Access Panels with Carts

*And never stack wrapped instrument trays.

Figure 22.28

- Use caution when pushing objects up or down hallway inclines. Push from behind when going up an incline (object goes first) and pull from in front of an object being transported down an incline (person goes first).

- Do not ride or step on wheeled supply carts or other vehicles.

- Consider using powered carts for moving heavy or awkward loads, if available. (See **Figure 22.29**)

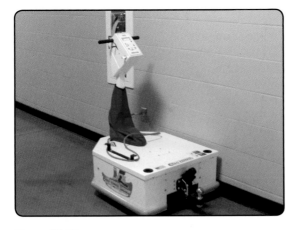

Figure 22.29

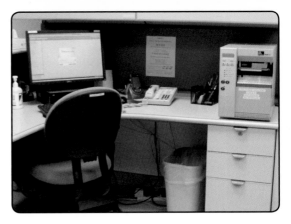

Figure 22.30

Clerical and Other Workstations

Poor workstation design can create issues for CS personnel. Repetitive activities, such as bending over sinks, sitting at a computer desk and standing while assembling instrument sets, should be evaluated in efforts to reduce unnecessary stress and strain. **Figure 22.30** shows a CS clerical workstation.

Safety tips in clerical or other workstations include:

- Assembly work should be performed at levels that will least fatigue and strain employees.

- Floors in work areas where employees must stand should have fatigue mats to relieve leg strain.

- Appropriate chairs should be used at computer, clerical and instrument workstations to properly support employees' backs.

- Items used frequently to perform routine tasks should be stored within easy reach to avoid strain to the upper body from repetitive movements to retrieve these items.

- Caution should be exercised when using filing cabinets. When multiple drawers are open at the same time, the cabinet can tip over. Also, avoid leaving bottom drawers open when not in use because people can trip or fall if they open into a walkway. (See **Figure 22.31**)

Opened File Cabinet

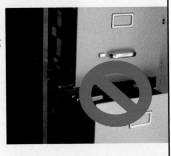

Open one drawer at a time. Opening two drawers may cause the cabinet to tip.

Figure 22.31

Surgical Service Areas

CS technicians may have responsibilities that include services in surgery or other areas where procedures are performed. They should become familiar with possible hazards in all areas they visit, and observe applicable safety policies and signage. These spaces have many of the same hazards found in CS areas. Additionally, they may have hazards applicable to the use of lasers, X-ray equipment, and chemicals utilized during surgical procedures. Caution is required when entering areas when this equipment is in use. Specific safety precautions provided by the manufacturers should be reviewed and followed by employees.

OTHER AREAS OF CONCERN

Central Service Equipment

Equipment that is not functioning correctly may cause injury. TJC and some state and local regulatory agencies require a preventive maintenance (PM) program to ensure optimal operation and function of equipment used for sterile processing activities. This equipment includes sterilizers, washer-disinfectors, heat sealers, and other processing equipment that should be routinely inspected and serviced by certified, experienced service personnel. Inspection records should be maintained with copies available in the CS department. These records should be verified

Handling Compressed Gas Cylinders

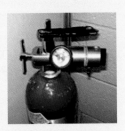

Central Service technicians are often involved in the handling, transport and storage of medical gas cylinders dispensed for direct patient care and treatment or for use as equipment components. These cylinders may contain oxygen, nitrous oxide, helium, nitrogen or other gasses. Specific safety protocols should be used for each specific gas, and should be in compliance with the product's handling instructions in the applicable SDS. Medical gas cylinder safety precautions include:

- No gas cylinder should be dispensed for use without a label.

- Gas cylinders should be secured at all times to prevent tipping. Place them in a secured holder for this purpose, or securely strap or chain them in an upright position.

- Cylinders should be handled carefully during transport. They should never be rolled, dragged or dropped.

- A cover cap should be used to protect the cylinder's valve during transport.

- Cylinder regulators are gas-specific and not necessarily interchangeable, so an appropriate regulator for the cylinder's contents is required.

- Threads on cylinder valves, regulators and other fittings should be inspected for damage before connection.

- All cylinders should be clearly labeled as "full," "in use" or "empty."

- Empty cylinders should not be stored with full ones.

- Gas cylinder regulators are equipped with either a hand wheel or stem valve. Stem valves require a key that should remain with the regulator at all times.

by the department manager to ensure that the equipment used by CS employees is safe for use.

CS personnel should report equipment in need of PM or repair.

CS technicians should also be familiar with any emergency procedures that may be needed when using equipment. For example, CS technicians should be familiar with emergency shut-off procedures for any equipment in their work area. (See **Figure 22.32**)

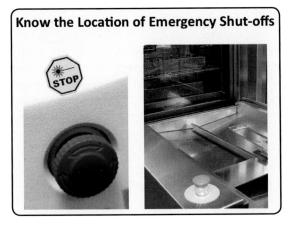

Know the Location of Emergency Shut-offs

Figure 22.32

DISASTER PREPAREDNESS

Disaster preparedness is an important component of the CS safety system. Each facility has developed a comprehensive response plan for internal and external disasters. An **internal disaster** is any situation with the potential to cause harm or injury to the healthcare facility employees or where the loss of utilities may drastically impact departmental operations. Examples of internal disasters include a hazardous chemical spill or leak, loss of power or failure of a utility, such as water, electricity or steam.

An **external disaster** is a situation in which activities outside the facility impact departmental or facility operations. Examples that may necessitate activation of the external disaster plan include earthquakes, floods, hurricanes or other events that result in large numbers of seriously injured patients being sent to the facility. When an external disaster occurs, the entire facility is placed on alert and personnel from each department are expected to perform tasks, based on the situations present.

> **Disaster (internal)** Situation with the potential to cause harm or injury to Central Service or other employees, patients/visitors, or where the loss of utilities may drastically impact departmental operations.
>
> **Disaster (external)** A situation in which activities external to the facility affects departmental or facility operations.

Disaster Plans

CS department disaster plans, like those of other departments, should be consistent with and support, the facility's plans. Most hospitals use an Incident Command System (ICS), a standardized approach to the command, control and coordination of emergency response. CS managers must ensure the CS disaster response activities and expectations are included in the overall ICS plan.

Elements of a CS disaster plan typically include:

- An emergency call list outlining the lines of authority, and the key individuals to be notified in specific types of disasters. *Note: These may differ for each type of disaster.*

- Protocols for inventory replenishment and delivery of emergency supplies. Usually, supply distribution department personnel are responsible for the maintenance of supplies and, in times of disaster, will deliver to an area for emergency patient care.

- Posted evacuation plans and practice drills for employees to ensure that they know alternative ways to leave the department if their safety is at risk.

CS technicians should actively participate in all disaster training and drills. It is important to know responsibilities during a disaster situation and be prepared to perform the assigned duties.

Biological Disasters

Many healthcare facilities have added biological incidents to their disaster plans. As with other types of disasters, CS technicians should know their role. Close communication with the Infection Prevention department is critical in this type of disaster.

CS departments should utilize appropriate resources, such as the Centers for Disease Control and Prevention (CDC; www.cdc.gov) for up-to-date information regarding emerging biological threats. Other resources, such as the World Health Organization (WHO; www.who.org) can also provide guidance. In all instances, coordination between Infection Prevention and all areas impacted by the disaster is very important.

EMPLOYEE ACCIDENTS AND INJURIES

Even significant efforts to emphasize safety and accident prevention cannot eliminate all employee accidents, and CS technicians can still be injured on the job. If an injury occurs, it must be documented and reported to the appropriate administrative personnel, in compliance with OSHA regulations for healthcare facilities. An investigation is needed to provide information about the cause, the situation, and/or the behaviors that were involved to identify contributing factors, hazards or unsafe practices. Then, corrective actions must be implemented to revise the systems or physical conditions, and/or to address the behavior which caused the injury in an effort to prevent future injuries or accidents.

Regardless of how insignificant an injury may seem, the appropriate manager should be informed immediately. Details regarding time, place, tasks performed and a description of exactly what happened must be recorded on the appropriate form. It should then be submitted to the facility's safety officer, personnel department, employee health, or other entity, according to the facility's protocol.

A process should also be in place for CS technicians to report unsafe situations before an accident or injury happens. If an unsafe situation is identified, it should be reported immediately, so the risk of injury can be minimized.

PATIENT ACCIDENTS AND INJURIES

CS professionals have responsibilities to help prevent patient injuries, accidents and infections. They do so as they perform the important tasks of decontaminating, inspecting, testing, assembling, packaging, sterilizing, aseptic handling of sterile items, and delivering items according to established procedures. When their job is done correctly, risk to the patient is greatly reduced.

When a patient incident occurs, it must be promptly investigated and documented. Any practices or physical conditions within the facility that can cause a patient injury must also be investigated and reported. All healthcare workers must report unsafe practices or hazards promptly to minimize accidents and prevent their recurrence.

EMPLOYEE INFORMATION AND TRAINING

No safety and risk management system can be successful without employee involvement. Each employee must understand their role and responsibilities in maintaining a safe environment. This requires education for all staff at all levels of experience.

All new CS employees should attend a health and safety orientation provided by the facility to become familiar with hazards and safety practices throughout the facility. They should also attend a department-specific orientation that focuses on, at least, the following:

- An overview of the requirements contained in the hazard communication regulations, including employees' rights under the regulations.

- Notification of employees about any operations in their work area where hazardous substances are present.

- Location and availability of written hazard communication program information.

- Physical and health effects of any hazardous substances they may encounter.

- Methods and observation techniques used to determine the presence or release of hazardous substances in the work area.

- Strategies to lessen or prevent exposure to these hazardous substances through safe control and work practices, and use of PPE.

- Steps the department has taken to lessen or prevent exposure to these substances.

- Instructions on how to read labels and review SDS to obtain appropriate hazard information.

- Emergency spill procedures.

- Disaster and fire plans, and the role of the CS department in their development and implementation.

EMPLOYEE PREPAREDNESS

An important factor in safety and risk management is employee awareness and preparedness. Every employee should approach each shift and each task with two questions in mind: "What can I do to ensure my safety and the safety of those in the facility?" and "What do I need to know to respond if I am faced with an emergency?" Some strategies to help ensure emergency preparedness include:

- Be familiar with safety policies. Ask questions if specific information is not understood.

- Be familiar with the chemicals used. Know how to handle them safely and what to do in the event of an emergency.

- Know how to work safely around equipment. Understand the hazards and know where emergency shut-off buttons are located.

- Be familiar with evacuation routes, the location of fire extinguishers and fire alarm boxes.

- Leave each area safe. Wipe up spills, prevent trip hazards and do not cross contaminate.

- Maintain a safe environment at all times. Pay attention to detail. Report anything that threatens the safety and well-being of those in the facility.

The success of any safety system is dependent upon the individuals who work within that system. Creating and maintaining a culture of safety reduces the risk for everyone.

CONCLUSION

Central Service technicians play an important role in every healthcare facility's safety program. It is important to know the expectations and be able to perform efficiently and calmly during any type of situation that may arise. For the safety of patients, visitors, other employees and departmental staff, training and safety drills must be taken seriously, as should the adoption of safe work habits that help ensure preparedness for any unplanned emergency.

RESOURCES

Association for the Advancement of Medical Instrumentation. ANSI/AAMI ST79, *Comprehensive guide to steam sterilization and sterility assurance in health care facilities.* 2013.

Occupational Safety and Health Administration *Ergonomics for the Prevention of Musculoskeletal Disorders: Guidelines for Nursing Homes.* 2003.

Occupational Safety and Health Administration *OSHA Fact Sheet Workplace Violence.* www.osha.gov/OshDoc/data_General_Facts/factsheet-workplace-violence.pdf. 2002.

Federal Register 56:64004. December 6, 1991.

CENTRAL SERVICE TERMS

Risk management

Ergonomics

Hazardous waste

Secondary container

Polymerization

Combustible

Combustible loading

Workplace violence

Aerosol

Action level (AL)

Short-term excursion limit (STEL)

Disaster (internal)

Disaster (external)

Chapter 23

Success through Communication

Learning Objectives

As a result of successfully completing this chapter, readers will be able to:

1. Explain why Central Service technicians must use effective communication and human relations skills

2. Define the term "professionalism," list traits of professional Central Service technicians and describe their fundamental beliefs and behaviors

3. Describe behaviors that can impact success on the job

4. Use basic tactics of effective communication in the workplace

5. Practice procedures to enhance and maintain effective working relationships

6. Discuss tactics to improve teamwork

7. Define the term "diversity" and explain why it is important

8. Practice basic customer service skills and utilize tactics to appropriately handle customer complaints

9. Review common workplace communication issues

INTRODUCTION

The responsibilities of Central Service (CS) technicians relate directly to the health and well-being of patients. CS technicians must have the knowledge and skills to address the sophisticated concepts addressed in this technical manual; however, they must also interact with other people in their department—and in other departments within the facility—as well as vendors, suppliers and others. To do so requires the consistent use of communication and human resources skills. A CS department where all employees demonstrate professionalism and utilize effective communication skills is an ideal setting that can be accomplished if each CS technician adopts the behaviors and practices outlined in this chapter.

NEED FOR EFFECTIVE COMMUNICATION AND HUMAN RELATIONS SKILLS

CS technicians, like all other healthcare professionals, must have effective interpersonal skills. Effective communication is one dimension of interpersonal skills because it allows a person to understand someone else's needs and interests. Human relations skills are also important because they enable people to use the information gained from communication to interact effectively with others.

Communication is the process of transmitting information from one person to another by use of words and non-verbal expressions, such as body language. The concept of **human relations** involves the development and maintenance of effective interpersonal (between people) relationships that enhance teamwork and help ensure a positive work environment.

Many communication and human relations principles are applicable on the job and most can be used off the job, as well. While people are unique in many respects, they also share many commonalities, which may include specific needs, wants and desires — all of which help form a framework for human relations.

The use of appropriate communication and human relations skills is important whenever people interact. Human interaction is critical in the CS department. The world of healthcare is very labor intensive: machines do not replace the need for human judgment and skills as CS technicians undertake their job responsibilities. CS technicians must work with their peers, and department supervisors and managers. They also must represent their department as they interact formally and informally with staff members in other departments throughout the facility. CS technicians may also come in contact with patients, their families and visitors to the facility, including those conducting business with department managers. (See **Figure 23.1**) Regardless of the situation, effective communication and solid human relations skills are a must.

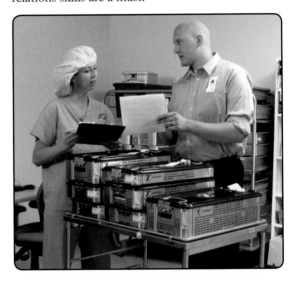

Figure 23.1

These days, when healthcare organizations face public scrutiny, the need for effective communication and the application of appropriate human relation skills continues even when not on the job. What one says (and does not say) and what one does (and does not do) reflects on the individual. All healthcare employees, including CS technicians, reflect not only on themselves, but also on their employer in their off-work words and actions.

COMMON COMMUNICATION BARRIERS

How often do communication problems occur, and what causes them? Interestingly, communication problems happen all too frequently. Even when everyone speaks the same language, common communication errors can lead to errors, frustration and strained relationships. For example:

- Questions that can be interpreted differently, such as, "Can you come to work early?" (What time is "early"?)

- Requests that are vague. Imagine a new technician getting a call to "Send up the old instrument that Dr. Smith used to use." (Which instrument?)

- Answers that do not provide adequate or detailed information. Surgery asks how long until a tray is ready and the response is, "It's in the sterilizer." (For how long? Is the cycle ending or just beginning?)

- The use of **jargon** impedes good communication. "Check the biological on the loaners and get them to eight. The TF has moved to first." (Is this jargon one that a new employee would understand?)

While use of basic communication principles discussed in this chapter will not resolve all communication problems, it will help address many of them.

Communication The process of transmitting information and understanding from one person to another by use of words and non-verbal expressions, such as body language.

Human relations The development and maintenance of effective interpersonal (between people) relationships that enhance teamwork.

Jargon Specialized words or phrases known only by people working in a position.

Some people can easily understand details of inspecting and assembling complex surgical instruments, and can apply specialized skills to operate sophisticated sterilization equipment, but they may have difficulty interacting with others. Proper use of communication and human relations skills is important for the success of all CS technicians in all healthcare facilities. Fortunately, these principles can be learned and are easy to apply on the job. The ability to do so is a characteristic of professional CS technicians.

Professional Central Service Technicians:

- Have a positive attitude and take pride in themselves, and the important work they do.

- Possess the knowledge and skills required to be proficient.

- Demonstrate respect for policies and procedures.

- Are alert to the need for ongoing improvement.

- Contribute 100% (give it their all) to help their team meet its goals.

- Are genuinely interested in helping others.

- Know, attain (and even exceed) their facility's quality and quantity standards.

- Are competent communicators.

- Practice appropriate human relations skills.

- Respect their supervisors and peers.

- Are creative.

- Follow high ethical and moral standards.

- Are self confident.

- Are courteous to their co-workers and all others with whom they have contact.

- Admit mistakes and learn from them.

- Follow appropriate personal hygiene and dress standards.

CENTRAL SERVICE TECHNICIANS ARE PROFESSIONALS

A professional is a person working in an occupation that requires extensive knowledge and skills to be successful. A profession involves membership limited to those with education and experience in a specialized body of knowledge. Membership is usually controlled by licensing, registration and/or certification. This definition certainly applies to CS professionals.

More About Professionalism

Professionals are proud of themselves and the work they do. They tackle their job effectively and efficiently and try to improve their profession in the process. A professional "goes the extra mile," is part of the team, tries to put forth the best possible effort to meet the facility's and department's goals and is truly interested in what is best for their fellow employees and the patient.

Professional CS technicians know what their manager expects of them and strive to consistently meet those expectations. They are effective communicators and are courteous and concerned about the problems encountered by other staff members.

Job success is affected by how well employees get along with their supervisor. Ideally, both parties will demonstrate mutual respect and understanding. Still, friction can sometimes occur. When this happens, it becomes even more important to develop, maintain and improve the relationship. CS technicians should recognize that the boss may not be their friend or "buddy." A professional relationship will address job tasks and human relations concerns.

Those who obtain promotions and pay raises, and most quickly attain career goals often enjoy the respect of their peers and supervisors. This respect is most likely experienced when an employee cooperates, is dependable and ambitious, and is willing to work hard to become successful.

What Should Central Service Technicians Expect from their Employer?

All staff members should expect:

- A job description that outlines expectations of their position.
- Safe working conditions.
- Training to meet job standards and then additional training to maintain performance and, possibly, advance to more responsible positions.
- An environment that values and fosters teamwork.
- An explanation of all applicable policies, rules and regulations.
- A fair evaluation of their work.

Employees who believe that one or more of these considerations are not being provided should discuss the situation with their supervisor. Professionals want to help the team become the best it can be. By working toward solutions, a professional CS technician helps improve the department.

Moral, Legal and Ethical Considerations

CS technicians must follow a professional code of behavior that includes moral, legal and ethical aspects of responsibility.

Moral behavior relates to basic principles about what is right and wrong. Patients who enter the hospital entrust their lives to the staff. CS technicians must honor this trust. They must carry out their duties in compliance with each detail and procedural step. They accept responsibility to follow work schedules, maintain good attendance, and follow established policies and procedures in the best interest of patient care. Professional CS technicians utilize resources wisely. They also do not question or ridicule a patient's religious beliefs or personal possessions. They care for and protect the patient's property, including valuables, clothing, religious and sentimental items.

CS professionals also respect the beliefs and rights of their co-workers. They do not promote gossip or conduct that negatively impacts their department's best interests. They recognize their responsibility to preserve personal values and beliefs, and they do not engage in activities that violate personal moral or religious beliefs.

Legal behavior is determined by the authority of laws, and one must never overstep the limitations of these responsibilities. Laws protect staff, as well as patients. Staff are expected to perform job duties in the way they have been taught. They do not perform duties that have been designated for or assigned to a licensed or registered professional. They pay attention to details, follow each step of written procedures and instructions, and maintain thorough records and documentation.

Ethical behavior relates to what is right and wrong, relative to the standards of conduct for a profession.

Ethical conduct is required of CS technicians at all times; however, the difference between what is "right" and "wrong" can be viewed from different perspectives. Consider the following:

- A CS technician knows that another staff member regularly "beats the system" by arriving late and leaving early. A friend takes care of the time clock; both this employee and the friend spend a lot of time in unproductive work while "on the clock." That technician may assume, "It's none of my business"; however, this situation not only affects the facility, but can also result in suspension or even termination of employment. CS technicians must not have an "it's none of my business" attitude; they must remember they are professionals and conduct themselves accordingly.

How does one decide if a proposed action is ethical? Answering the the following questions may be helpful:

- Is the proposed action legal?

- Does the proposed action hurt anyone (or could it)?

- Is the proposed action fair?

- Am I being honest as I undertake the proposed action?

- Can I live with myself if I do what I am considering?

- What if everyone did it?

- What are the consequences of my actions?

- Would I want my actions to become public knowledge?

Each day, CS technicians are faced with situations that require them to make moral, legal and ethical decisions. Understanding what is right (and the ramifications of what is wrong) can make those decisions easier.

BASICS OF COMMUNICATION

Some employees cannot effectively express their thoughts to co-workers. Others are distracted when someone speaks to them. The first concern relates to speaking and the second involves listening. These are examples of obstacles that create communication breakdowns and interfere with the successful exchange of information from one person to another.

CS technicians play an important role in their facility's communication process. They provide **feedback**, including ideas and suggestions to their supervisors who, in turn, communicate information up and down the chain of command. Each person's role in this communication process is vital to its success. (See **Figure 23.2**)

Feedback A step in communication process that occurs when the listener asks a question, repeats information or otherwise helps the speaker to know if the message has been correctly received. Feedback is also defined as a method to respectfully share ideas and information on a specific issue.

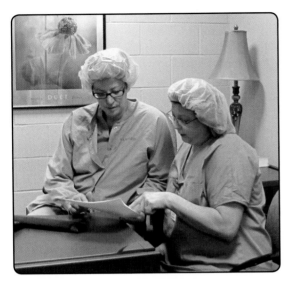

Figure 23.2

Some employees think effective communication is easy (after all, people have been communicating their entire lives). In reality, the process is not difficult, but it does require use of basic principles. Improving communication can be as simple as developing some basic speaking and listening skills.

Basic Speaking Skills

What follows are some principles that should be used when speaking with others:

- Identify the main points in the message; organize what will be said and ensure that, while speaking, each main point is addressed.

- Speak enthusiastically. Be committed to the purpose of the message and show interest and enthusiasm when speaking.

- Be able to support the information provided. If points are well documented, the listener can concentrate on what is said rather than questioning whether your statements are accurate.

- Stay focused. Do not ramble, digress or discuss points that are not critical to your message.

- Concentrate on the listener, rather than on yourself. Remember that the main objective of speaking is to communicate – not to make a good impression.

- Think about the listener's background and speak in a way that will help ensure that the message is accurately received. Use feedback methods, such as asking open-ended questions (e.g., "Why do you think this is a problem?" rather than "Is this a problem?").

- Use language that the listener will understand.

- Be professional. Use appropriate language, tone and volume.

Basic Listening Skills

A good portion of each day is spent speaking and listening. Practice can help enhance good communication skills and the results will benefit oneself, co-workers and others.

Some CS technicians spend more time speaking than listening. Basic techniques to improve listening include:

- Concentrating on the central idea the speaker is trying to convey.

- Focusing on what the speaker is saying and not becoming distracted. Don't let an uncomfortable physical environment cause distraction. There may be few places within a busy CS department where the environment is ideal for effective communication, but it is important to try and make the best of it.

- Not being influenced by emotions. Avoid an immediate evaluation of the message and try to think about its content objectively.

- Staying engaged, even when the message seems familiar or unimportant, or when the speaker's opinion differs from one's own.

- Considering the speaker's perceptions as the message is heard. Understand the speaker's basic ideas before objectively criticizing them.

- Avoiding just listening for specific facts. There may be additional information that is an important part of the message.

- Being aware of the speaker's nonverbal communication. Sometimes the speaker's body language can convey additional information.

- Not tuning out when listening to complicated information. Use feedback such as, "I really don't understand what you are saying," or "Can you please say that in another way" to tell the speaker that the message was not effectively conveyed.

- Concentrating on the message and its content, not on its delivery. Problems with the speaker's voice, speed of speech, and/or pronunciation can cause difficulties, but it is important to attempt to learn the real meaning of the message.

- Allowing the speaker to finish and then reacting fairly to the message that was stated. Don't formulate a response to the message while listening to the speaker.

- Taking notes, when appropriate, if the information is detailed or specific, and/or if it will be helpful in the future.

Types of Communication

Communication flows through formal and informal channels within the CS department.

Examples of formal communication include:

- Instructions, advice and **coaching** by managers and supervisors. (See **Figure 23.3**)

- Facility and departmental policies and procedures that help regulate behavior and work practices.

- Discussions in departmental and other meetings.

- Individual and group training presentations.

- Facility and departmental bulletins, memos, newsletters and related communication tools.

- Performance evaluations.

- Employee work schedules.

- Conversations related to delegated project assignments.

- Monitoring of ongoing work activities

Coaching Positive reinforcement used to encourage Central Service technicians to follow proper work behaviors, and negative reinforcement to discourage inappropriate work behaviors.

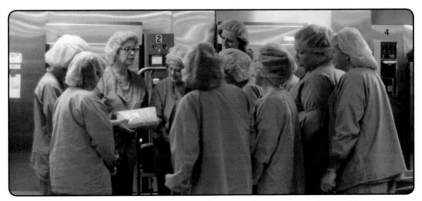

Figure 23.3

Informal methods of communication within CS departments include casual conversations between employees before, during and after work. Much of this communication is beneficial because it can improve working relationships of staff members. Unfortunately, informal communication can also be damaging. Consider, for example, rumors: information circulated without knowledge of its source or with concern about whether it is true.

Rumors and "grapevine gossip" can negatively impact the team and the collective department. False information can cause anxiety and frustration, and increase an already stressful work environment. In some cases, information may be true, but should not be shared with the team. For example, if a co-worker learns of a fellow co-worker's personal problems, that information should not be shared unless the affected co-worker chooses to share it.

Gossip and rumors erode personal relationships and trust. They can waste time and move the CS team's attention away from its real purpose.

Telephone, Email and Technology Etiquette

The manner in which CS technicians answer and speak on the telephone reflects on their department, their facility and themselves. The need to be professional, courteous and helpful is obvious. Each facility has policies and procedures to address professional expectations for telephone and email etiquette. It is important to be aware of your facility's requirements and carefully follow them. (See **Figure 23.4**)

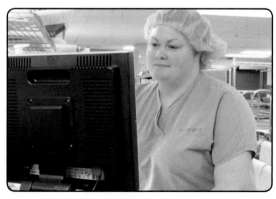

Figure 23.4

Whose Technology Is It?

Healthcare facilities and the Central Service departments within them have invested significant financial resources in communications technology. It is increasingly difficult for many people to imagine how they could manage their professional and personal lives without seemingly constant access to the wide variety of computers, copiers, printers, fax machines, telephones and other electronic communication equipment available. With its convenience, however, comes the opportunity for misuse when facility equipment is used for personal purposes (e.g., shopping on the internet, sending personal emails, and photocopying private or personal materials). Problems include time away from the job, increased facility expenses, and the blurring of the distinction between acceptable and unacceptable behaviors.

These concerns and other related issues are often addressed in facility policies and identified in employee handbooks and other documents. Professional CS technicians know about these policies, understand their importance and consistently comply with them.

Another concern created by advancing technology is the common availability of smart phones and other technologies that enable employees to text, speak, email and take photographs from almost anywhere. In addition to concerns regarding non-productive time, Health Insurance Portability and Accountability Act (HIPAA) and confidentiality concerns can also become an issue if information captured in personal photos and videos is shared outside the facility.

To ensure compliance, review regulations and facility policies, and ask questions, as needed.

Music in the Workplace

Many CS departments allow music to be played in the workplace. Music can promote a more comfortable atmosphere and may make the working experience more enjoyable. What follows are some guidelines for ensuring that music is enjoyed without creating distractions and jeopardizing the professionalism of the department:

Type of music. The type of music listened to at work reflects on the CS department and the healthcare facility. Do not listen to music that would be deemed unprofessional by the facility or its staff. When in doubt, don't play it.

Lyrics. Lyrics should not be offensive to anyone in the department.

Volume. Music should be played on low volume. Background music should allow staff to carry on a normal conversation without having to raise their voice, even when near the speakers. Music should not be heard in other areas of the department, public hallways, department offices, etc. If the telephone rings or a person needs to make a call, the music volume should not have to be turned down; it should barely be detected by the person on the other end of the call.

Productivity. Time spent selecting, arranging and changing music must be kept to a minimum. Meeting the needs of patients and other customers is always the top priority.

Headsets or earphones should not be used because they can reduce the technician's ability to hear the telephone, machine cycle alarms, questions from co-workers, and other important sounds that are a part of the job.

Infection Prevention and Technology

Phones and other personal technologies carried into the department from outside sources may pose an infection prevention concern. Handling those items with clean hands may recontaminate hands. Check with your department for specific policies regarding personal communication technologies.

HUMAN RELATIONS

CS technicians may have the knowledge and skills required to do their job properly, but they cannot be successful unless they know how to get along with their supervisors, peers and customers.

Professional CS employees possess the following human relations skills:

- They recognize each of their fellow employees as individuals and, when possible, incorporate this understanding into how they interact with other staff members.

- They contribute effectively to their team because this benefits the department, facility, profession and the patient.

- They develop a genuine spirit of cooperation and teamwork amongst themselves, their peers and those at higher organizational levels.

It is relatively easy to talk about human relations skills' positive impact on the organization; however, it is much more difficult for CS technicians to consistently apply these skills. The workplace requires staff members to interact with many employees of different backgrounds, interests, challenges and job responsibilities. Such factors make it increasingly difficult to practice effective human relations.

There are numerous ways that CS technicians effectively apply their human relations skills on the job. For example, they:

- Take responsibility for maintaining positive working relationships with supervisors, peers and others in the healthcare facility.

- Act in a professional manner.

- Serve as a contributing member of the department and healthcare team.

- Accept the responsibility to continually learn and, when applicable, help their peers do so, as well.

- Promote cooperation among their peers. This is done by helping others, sharing knowledge and experience, and trying to understand the perspectives of others.

- Accept full responsibility for their own actions (or inaction) and do not try to pass the blame onto another person, shift or department.

Now that we have defined "human relations" and established ways for CS technicians improve communication and relationships with their supervisors, peers and customers, it is necessary to also understand the outcomes of these interactions.

Behaviors That Can Impede Success

Being successful in the workplace involves much more than having the technical skills to perform a job. The following are common behaviors that can impede success:

- Refusing to follow directions, orders, policies and procedures.

- Being unwilling to adapt to change.

- Talking too much and/or conducting personal business while at work.

- Demonstrating inconsistent and unreliable work behaviors.

- Engaging in gossip and other behaviors that reduce group productivity.

- Failing to get along with others.

- Being dishonest and lacking integrity on the job.

- Failing to complete assignments in a timely manner.

- Making or contributing to excessive errors.

- Regularly missing work or being tardy.

- Abusing substances.

CENTRAL SERVICE TECHNICIANS AND TEAMWORK

Individuals must work as part of a team because the work they do relates directly to that being done by others. Consider, for example, that the main goal of every CS technician, like all other staff members employed by the facility, is to help the patients. Teamwork is essential for ensuring that the patients are best served.

What one employee does (or does not do) affects the work of others, and also impacts the success (or failure) of the CS department. For example, staff in the decontamination area may work intently to clean turnaround instruments as quickly and safely as possible, and the assembly technicians may assemble and package them as quickly as is feasible; however, if the instruments are not put in the sterilizer as soon as possible, a delay will occur that could impact the surgical staff and jeopardize patient care.

Teamwork is beneficial to the facility in other ways, as well. For example, it can:

- Improve productivity through increased staff cooperation.

- Increase employee job satisfaction.

- Improve the work environment by creating a common purpose for staff members.

- Decrease job-related stress.

Factors Impacting Teamwork

Developing a culture where teamwork is valued and practiced requires the dedication and equal efforts of each team member.

Several factors must be present for teamwork to occur:

- **Attitude** – A proper attitude is the most important factor driving effective teamwork. Attitudes of CS technicians about their job, peers and patients impact their actions. An employee's attitude is often influenced by co-workers. If everyone on the team gets along, likes their jobs and the facility and wants to provide good service, each staff member will probably have a good attitude. By contrast, if a co-worker has a negative attitude about the job, supervisor or the facility, and does not care about the quality of work, teamwork will suffer.

Attitude Emotions that cause a person to react to people and/or situations in a predetermined way.

Characteristics of Successful Work Groups

Successful work groups generally share the following characteristics:

1. Common goals that are defined and accepted by group members.

2. Group members that cooperate as a team.

3. Group members that have the resources necessary to attain goals.

4. Group members that help one another.

5. A comfortable work atmosphere.

6. Group members that participate in discussions about matters affecting the group.

7. Group members that are creative and contribute ideas without fear of ridicule.

8. Healthy disagreements between group members that do not cause hard feelings.

9. General group consensus – not just a simple majority – about decisions affecting the entire group.

10. Group members who do not subjectively criticize each other's ideas or positions.

11. Group members who feel free to express their feelings.

12. Assignments that are made and accepted when action must be taken.

13. Avoidance of power struggles between group members.

14. A group leader who does not always dominate. Instead, "what must be done" is the primary concern of group members, as opposed to being concerned with who is in control.

15. Group members who know how the group operates.

The following characteristics are vital for an effective team:

- Cooperation – To provide good service, one must be willing to assist and work with other employees.

- Promptness – When an employee is late to work or does not show up, the remaining members of the team must work harder. As a result, work quality and morale can suffer.

- Trust – An effective member of a team trusts co-workers and supervisors. Co-workers and supervisors also trust each team member.

Types of Groups

CS technicians belong to both formal groups and informal groups. Teamwork concerns are important for both types.

A healthcare facility is comprised of a formal group of employees who, at the highest organizational level, have the same boss: the Hospital Administrator and Board of Directors. As staffing plans are developed, smaller work groups are established. The CS department is an example of a formal group. Work in the CS department may be divided into other formal groups, including those relating to specific work areas and shifts.

Each formal work group has a formal leader responsible for coordinating, directing and controlling the group.

A task group is another example of a formal group. Members work together to perform essential non-routine activities. For example, a committee might address a specific concern, and a work team may develop a job breakdown for training purposes. After the work of a task group is completed, the group is typically dissolved.

Informal groups develop for several reasons, including: common interests of members; a desire to be "close" to others in a similar situation; economic reasons; and a desire to satisfy specific, but common, personal needs. Examples of informal groups may include employees who take lunch or other breaks together, work the same shift, participate in after-work activities, and carpool.

Informal work groups are not necessarily good or bad. Each has the ability to assist, harm or have no impact on the facility's efforts to attain goals. Informal groups frequently develop an informal communication system, called the "grapevine." This system can spread rumors (a negative outcome) or provide helpful information.

Teamwork and Decision-Making

In some healthcare facilities, CS technicians can participate in the decision-making process in their department by participating in cross-functional teams. A cross-functional team is a group of employees from different departments within the healthcare facility that works together to resolve operating problems. Consider, for example, a problem that involves instruments that are unavailable when needed in the Operating Room (OR). A traditional problem-solving approach in which OR personnel address the problem may determine that the majority of concerns relate to those in the CS department. While these observations may be correct, there may be other potential causes of the problem that relate to OR personnel. Therefore, a cross-functional team comprised of OR, CS and staff from other departments may yield creative alternatives that would not be considered when a group with a more narrow focus addressed the issue.

Relating Experience to Job Success

Experience should, but does not always, impact job success. The benefit that experience brings to the work situation is not equal to time spent on the job. In the fast-paced world of CS, ongoing professional development and continuing education is critical for one to make a full contribution. Unfortunately, experience can encourage some to develop an attitude of entitlement.

By contrast, experience can be invaluable because it provides insight about what has and has not been successful in the past. This type of input is important when experienced staff members are encouraged to participate in the decision-making process, or when individuals serve on cross-functional teams.

Experience can improve the knowledge and skills that help CS technicians to be successful.

Special Teamwork Concerns

CS technicians may experience anxiety and tension when they begin their employment and join their new team. Most new employees want to know that their decision to work at the facility was a good one and, therefore, new job experiences — both positive and negative — are very meaningful. An evolutionary process, beginning with uncertainty will, hopefully, evolve into mutual respect and trust. Then, new staff members will begin to communicate candidly with other members of the team.

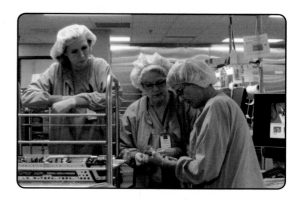

Figure 23.5

Experienced CS technicians should consider how they felt when they first were hired into the department. This can help provide empathy for their newly-hired peers who may share the same concerns, and wish to have the same questions addressed. Facility and departmental orientation programs should provide significant basic information to assist new employees; however, this does not replace the friendly "helping hand" that experienced CS technicians can provide.

CENTRAL SERVICE AND DIVERSITY

Diversity has received a great deal of attention in modern organizations. To some, it means providing equal opportunities to those of certain characteristics, such as age, gender, mental/physical abilities, sexual orientation, race, or ethnic heritage. To others, the concept implies responses to legal concerns, such as equal employment opportunities. Diversity should be defined in the broadest possible way so all employees are included and everyone's diversity is valued.

> **Diversity** The broad range of human characteristics and dimensions that impact the employees' values, opportunities and perceptions of themselves and others at work.

There are numerous other dimensions of diversity that also shape values, expectations and experiences. These include education, family status, organizational role and level, religion, first language, income, geographical location and more. Every person is unique, and brings special qualities to the job.

Developing a work environment where all co-workers are respected provides the following advantages:

- A welcoming and rewarding work environment improves job satisfaction.

- When people are valued, employee turnover and absenteeism are minimized, and associated costs are reduced.

- A culture of understanding, respect and cooperation encourages teamwork.

- Diverse backgrounds create more creative alternatives as decisions are made and as problems are resolved.

CUSTOMER SERVICE SKILLS FOR CENTRAL SERVICE TECHNICIANS

Basics of Customer Service

Customer service refers to the relationship between the CS team and its customers. These customers include anyone who utilizes CS's services, including doctors, nurses, clinicians, patients and vendors. One brief positive or negative encounter with a customer can leave a lasting impression about the entire department. This impression can then be passed on to other customers.

Providing a service is not always easy. Some CS customers are the direct patient caregivers who, themselves, have customers (the patients). CS professionals must be committed to providing excellent support services, so their counterparts throughout the facility can also provide excellent service and care to the patient.

Providing exemplary service requires the consistent delivery of safe, high-quality products and services. Each employee must strive to do their part to support the facility's and department's goals. **Figure 23.6** provides an example of a CS technician problem solving with a customer.

Each functional area and work shift in CS depends on others. The quality of each step in the processing cycle is affected by previous and subsequent steps. If decontamination and cleaning procedures are not done effectively or in a timely manner, the sterilization process may be ineffective, and/or products may not be available when needed. CS technicians must function as a team to achieve quality customer service.

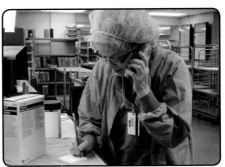

Figure 23.6

Self discipline is very important, especially in difficult situations and encounters. CS team members must stay focused on real issues, maintain composure and not allow emotions or personalities to influence performance. When it is necessary to say "no" to a customer request, explain the reasons and offer alternatives. If an error occurs, it is important to be honest and work toward a resolution. Credibility and trust are essential, and customer trust must always be preserved.

Providing more personalized service is also beneficial. CS professionals should get to know their customers and, when possible, use their names when communicating needs and addressing special requests.

Cheerful, courteous and friendly behavior is also effective for promoting effective customer service. The provision of good service requires CS technicians to constantly assess the quality of their services, follow up on commitments and solicit feedback. Quality service is a reflection of professionalism and it requires maturity, self-esteem, competence, confidence and a positive attitude.

Emergencies and crisis situations are a reality in the healthcare environment; however, even during stressful times, a calm, professional attitude must prevail.

Cooperation with Operating Room Personnel

No two departments in a typical healthcare facility work more closely than the OR and CS. The outcome of every patient procedure depends on effective communication and cooperation between personnel in these two fast-paced, ever-changing departments.

Much of the relationship between OR and CS staff is dependant upon mutual trust, communication and cooperation. To earn and maintain trust, each department must work hand in hand with the other and communicate effectively and often.

Communication is Critical

Differences in communication systems used by different departments can create challenges.

Slang terms, jargon and nicknames used to describe medical instruments and supplies, for example, may not be familiar to all staff working in different departments. Also, instrument and supply needs change (often several times a day) and if information doesn't travel smoothly, frustrations can increase and relationships may become strained.

Communication between OR and CS staff should be ongoing and not just happen when an incident has occurred or after an issue has been identified. Also, simple actions, such as showing appreciation for the efforts and assistance of personnel in the other department, can help establish a stronger bond between both groups.

Handling Customer Complaints

Customer complaints can arise, even when the best procedures and protocols are in place (and even when staff diligently adhere to them). When facilities endorse the concept of empowerment, CS technicians can more easily resolve customer complaints by implementing a practice of **service recovery**.

> **Service recovery** The sequence of steps used to address customer complaints and problems in a manner that yields a win-win situation for the customer and the department.

SETTING PRIORITIES

There may be times when CS technicians face multiple tasks. How should priorities be established in these instances? The most important things should be done first; these might be identified by asking questions, such as:

- What is the immediate need?

- What can I do to help my team?

- What task would I want done if I were the supervisor?

- What is the best use of my time right now?

It is not uncommon for priorities to change during a shift. For example, the addition of a trauma case will necessitate reprioritization of work tasks. CS technicians must be adaptable to changing needs and always put the patient first. **Figure 23.7** provides an example of instrument priorities being communicated through a communication board.

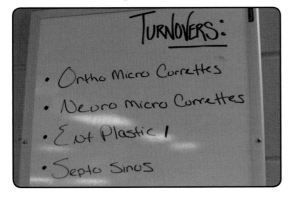

Figure 23.7

AVOIDING WORKGROUP COMPARISONS

Sometimes, CS departments fall into "shift wars" where some (or all) employees assigned to a specific shift begin to believe that the work they do is more important than that of other work groups. For example, a day shift may wonder what the night shift does with their time.

In reality, not all shifts have exactly the same duties and priorities do change throughout each 24-hour period. It is unrealistic to assume that all shifts work in exactly the same way and under exactly the same circumstances.

These types of comparisons can lead to misunderstandings between shifts and individual employees, which can lead to communication breakdown and negatively impact the ability to work as an effective team.

This service recovery example involves an OR nurse who is alleging that an improper instrument tray has been delivered.

Service Recovery Tactic	Service Recovery Tactic in Action
1. Acknowledge the customer.	"Hello, Farrah."
2. Carefully listen to the customer's problem.	The nurse explains that the proper instrument tray must be delivered immediately.
3. Remain calm and give your undivided attention.	The CS technician who is speaking with the OR nurse gives her complete attention and is not distracted by anything else in the area.
4. Ask questions.	"Farrah, I'm sorry about the mix up. What instrument tray do you need?"
5. Empathize with the customer.	"It must be frustrating when this problem occurs. I know this is a very serious problem that must be addressed immediately."
6. Apologize for the problem and accept responsibility to resolve it.	"I'm very sorry, Farrah. I'll be right there with the instruments you need."
7. Do not justify or place blame.	The CS technician does not tell the nurse that the set delivered earlier was the set that was on the order. He/she does, however, relay the information to the CS manager who can initiate discussions to help ensure that problems with instrument tray descriptions do not continue.
8. Provide time frame and remedial action.	"I can return within five minutes with the instruments you need."
9. Monitor problem resolution progress.	The CS technician cannot be distracted as he/she returns to the department and returns with the correct instrumentation.
10. Follow-up with the customer.	The CS technician (or his/her manager who has been notified) later contacts the OR nurse to confirm that the problem has been resolved.
11. Learn from the experience.	The customer complaint has identified a problem. Since it has been brought to the attention of the CS manager, corrective action can be taken to reduce the possibility that improper instrument sets are delivered in the future.

Figure 23.8

COMMITTING TO PATIENT CARE DURING DISASTERS

No one can predict when disasters will occur; however, each healthcare facility, and each CS department, should anticipate the most likely crises that may arise. From there, plans that incorporate the most appropriate responses to such crises can be developed.

All CS technicians should be prepared to provide service during emergencies. To do so, they should:

- Study their department/facility's disaster plans, and ask questions, if necessary.

- Take disaster drills seriously.

- Keep the CS department informed of current contact information, so an accurate call-back roster will be available if it is needed.

- Make personal plans that will allow support of patient care. For example, have a back-up arrangement for child care and family communications if you must remain at the hospital for an extended time.

- Remember to remain calm and positive during a disaster. The stress level will be high, and making a conscious effort not to add to the stressful environment will benefit everyone.

- Focus on the job and what is needed to meet the patient needs.

- Do not share patient information with anyone outside the hospital.

CONCLUSION

Central Service technicians have challenging, critically important and ever-evolving responsibilities. Managing these duties effectively, consistently and efficiently requires good communication and human relation skills and an understanding that a well-operating department can only be had in the presence of a well-functioning team.

RESOURCE

International Association of Healthcare Central Service Materiel Management. Central Service Leadership Manual. Chapters 5-8. 2010.

CENTRAL SERVICE TERMS

Communication

Human relations

Jargon

Feedback

Coaching

Attitude

Diversity

Service recovery

Chapter 24

Personal and Professional Development for Central Service

Learning Objectives

As a result of successfully completing this chapter, readers will be able to:

1. Explain the meaning of personal development and how it can impact a career in the Central Service department

2. List possible Central Service career paths

3. Review strategies for professional goal setting

4. Discuss strategies to enhance professional skills and expertise

5. Discuss resumé development

6. Review the interview process

7. Discuss promotions

INTRODUCTION

Learning is a lifelong endeavor, and change is inevitable. Never have these statements been truer than when applied to the field of Central Service (CS). CS professionals must be prepared to encounter growth regularly, and sometimes profoundly, in their positions. Whether CS professionals wish to stay in their department or seek advancement or promotion, **personal** and **professional development** will enable them to be proactive and more easily prepare for change. This chapter will highlight some of the resources and strategies available to help CS professionals grow and advance in their career.

PERSONAL DEVELOPMENT: WHAT IS IT AND WHY IS IT IMPORTANT?

In some ways, personal development is the first step toward professional development. Personal development may be defined as any activity that identifies and develops talent and personal potential, and improves employability and enhances quality of life. Personal development can help individuals develop personally rewarding goals.

Personal development is usually an individual endeavor – something a person does on their own time; however, more employers are recognizing the importance of investing in personal development. Employers may offer educational programs as part of employee benefit programs to help staff learn more about time management, stress management, teamwork, healthy lifestyles, competency development and career development. Ultimately, these programs are a win-win for both employees and the healthcare facility because personal development can create a workplace that is happier, healthier and more fulfilling. This environment can lead to greater productivity and quality in a department, which helps the healthcare facility meet its strategic goals.

Strategies for Personal Development

How does personal development work? There are four steps:

Step 1: Identify your goal. What do you want to achieve?

Step 2: Identify the requirements for your goal. What will you need to achieve the goal?

Step 3: Identify your strengths and areas that need improvement. What can you build on? What do you need to improve?

Step 4: Create an action plan with a time line for meeting that goal. How do you plan to move forward?

Personal development Activities that identify and develop talent and personal potential, improve your employability and enhance quality of life.

Professional development Commitment to continuous learning and improvement; taking responsibility for your own development.

Personal development should be a lifelong process, and it is more of a journey than a destination. Choose smaller goals that are attainable and build onto those successes. For example, if a long-term goal is a college degree, set the first goal as successfully completing one college class. Upon successful completion of that goal, the individual can set their next goal for the next class.

PROFESSIONAL DEVELOPMENT: WHAT IS IT AND WHY IS IT IMPORTANT?

Professional development specifically refers to the skills and knowledge attained for both personal and career advancement. It provides the information and experience needed to progress in a career, stay competitive with other job seekers and, ultimately, become more employable.

Common Learning Opportunities

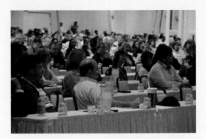

Conferences and Workshops

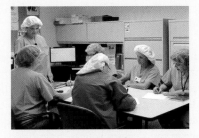

Facility-provided Education

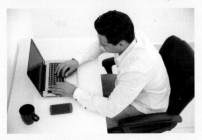

Independent Study

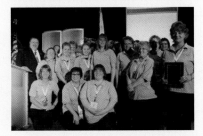

CS Professional Groups

Figure 24.1

Two Types of Professional Development

Professional development can be divided into two categories:

Professional development to keep current in an existing job. Growth is inevitable in the field of CS, and some professional development is mandatory. For example, changes in procedures, policies, instrumentation, products, and sterilization technologies, as well as changes in regulations and standards, must be adapted by every employee. Job growth in an effort to stay current is required of all CS professionals.

Professional development to advance in one's career. Some CS professionals have goals to advance their careers through position advancement and promotion. They participate in activities to improve their professional competency, enhance their existing skills and develop new ones. They move out of their comfort zone to take on new responsibilities and learn new things.

The job market, technology, regulations and practices are always evolving, and an employer may not provide staff with all the skills needed to keep up or move forward in the profession. Whether a person prefers to remain in a current position or dreams of advancement, it is essential to consider the benefits of taking ownership of one's career by continually improving knowledge and skills.

Learning opportunities through conferences, continuing education, and on-the-job training help CS technicians keep up with trends and changes in the CS field. (See **Figure 24.1**) This allows technicians to anticipate change more easily, and helps them recognize professional opportunities.

If a CS technician is a leader or would like to become one, then professional development will provide the knowledge and confidence to influence and lead others by example.

Taking part in activities to improve professional competency will give CS technicians the skills they need to become more effective in their position. This will demonstrate a continuing commitment to the profession, improve employability with current and future employers, and lead to a more fulfilling and rewarding career.

A CS technician may be familiar with sterilization standards as a requirement of the job. If they are able to step out of their comfort zone and teach those standards to new employees, this will increase their understanding of the standards. Teaching an inservice or short course can sharpen your technical skills and help develop training and public speaking skills. (See **Figure 24.2**)

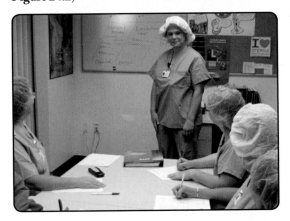

Figure 24.2

CENTRAL SERVICE CAREER PATHS

While most CS professionals choose to remain employed in a CS department and become experts at their assigned duties, some seek different career paths. Common career opportunities for CS professionals include lead technician positions in the CS department, CS management positions, OR core technicians, OR liaisons, CS department educator, faculty positions in local community and technical colleges, consultant, and vendor positions, such as sales representatives and on-site product/service facilitators. (See **Figure 24.3**)

Each career path has specific requirements. It is advisable to research the needed requirements, and develop personal and professional goals to move forward on a specific career path.

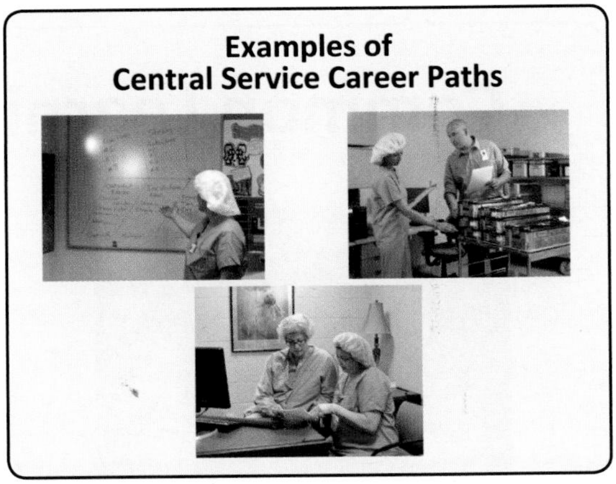

Examples of Central Service Career Paths

Figure 24.3

PLANNING CAREER GOALS

Those professionals looking to make their career more personally meaningful and rewarding, should establish goals and periodically review them. This will identify activities and steps that will help meet those objectives.

As with personal development, professional development requires working toward identifying areas in a present position in need of improvement, and then moving forward with set goals. In many ways, the steps to take for professional development are similar to those one would take for personal development, with a specific emphasis on developing one's position and career advancement.

Strategies for Planning Career Goals

Step 1: Determine the goal for improving professional employability or skills.

Step 2: Identify the requirements for the goal. What will be needed to achieve it?

Step 3: Identify personal strengths and areas that need improvement.

Step 4: Create an action plan with a timeline for meeting that goal.

SOME ADVICE ABOUT CAREER GOALS

Just as personal development is a lifelong process, professional development is a career-long process. Sometimes, employees get discouraged because they set lofty goals that do not materialize immediately. Most goals are achievable, but there may be many smaller goals to accomplish along the way. For example, if the goal is to be the CS department director, that requires achieving some educational goals and will most likely first require attaining some other leadership positions, such as lead technician or supervisor. When identifying what is necessary to achieve the final goal, be sure to identify individual steps that may be needed to prepare for that goal.

Those steps may include:

- Certification.

- Attending educational conferences.

- Becoming active in professional groups.

- Engage in on-the-job training in leadership, job and task-related skills.

THE IMPORTANCE OF RESOURCES

One of the most important factors in attaining goals is finding the right resources to help provide direction and support. There are many resources that can aid in professional development.

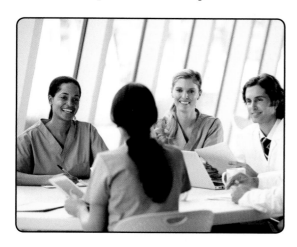

Figure 24.4

Educational resources include publications, printed resources, courses, conferences, online information and other types of information designed to enhance knowledge about a specific process or topic.

A Note about Online Resources

When using online resources, make sure the information and source is valid and current.

Developing professional resources within the field of CS can provide a network with which to share information on issues pertinent to the department. CS peers may have already faced similar situations and may be able to share insights and information.

Do not underestimate the importance of developing a network outside of one's current specialty. OR professionals, infection preventionists, safety officers and Biomedical engineers are a few of the healthcare specialists that can help CS professionals increase their knowledge about specific aspects of the field — and healthcare, in general.

There are several ways to build a network of resources. Becoming active in a local professional group is a great place to start. If there is no group in the area, contact local CS departments and explore the possibility of starting one. The first step can be as simple as gathering some interested individuals at a local business establishment.

PROFESSIONAL DEVELOPMENT ACTIVITIES

There are also ways to enhance existing skills and develop new ones to increase professional knowledge, develop professional behaviors and attain more expertise. **Figure 24.5** explores some ideas for professional development activities.

DEVELOPING A RESUMÉ

A resumé is a compilation of skills, education and accomplishments. It provides a prospective employer with information to help them determine if an employee has the necessary knowledge and skills to be successful in a specific job.

Professional Development Skills Building

Desired Skill	Skill Building Activities
Public speaking • Teaching • Presentations • Speaking in larger groups	• Start with smaller presentations, such as reports and small in-services. Work up to larger presentations for larger groups. • Join a speaking development group. • Take a public speaking class.
Technical expertise	• Pursue additional knowledge through courses, certifications, job shadowing, self study. • Participate in committees through your facility or local and national professional organization. • Take steps to keep up with changes in regulations, standards and technologies.
Writing skills	• Practice writing and ask someone to review what you have written for accuracy, clarity, grammar, spelling and punctuation. • Take a writing class.
Team building skills	• Start by examining your relationships and role with your current team. What can you improve? • Move outside your comfort zone and work with different teams for short projects. • Read articles on team building.

Figure 24.5

One concept of professional development is building a resumé through the advancement of skills. For example, if one aspires to become a CS staff educator, gaining experience presenting inservices, training new employees or developing educational tools for the department can strengthen those skills.

Sometimes, obtaining a new position, either externally or through a promotion within the current healthcare facility, can be decided by a very small margin. For example, if an individual's resumé includes past experience in staff education, that may offer an advantage in the selection process for an educator position.

Many templates exist to assist with resumé writing. Regardless of the chosen format, be certain to follow these simple rules:

• Be truthful.

• Research the duties of the job being sought and use personal experiences to help convince the employer that you are the best candidate for the job.

• Organize information in a logical fashion.

• Keep information clear and concise.

• Check for typographical errors.

UNDERSTANDING THE INTERVIEW PROCESS

CS technicians are involved in interviews as part of their initial selection process, and they participate in performance evaluations that typically include an interview-like component. While much of the interview process is controlled by the manager or another person conducting the interview, the interviewee (CS technician) can benefit from the use of basic speaking and listening techniques (as discussed in Chapter 23) during these sessions. This is especially important because contemporary interviewing methods emphasize a participative approach in which the person conducting the interview interacts with rather than "lectures to" the interviewee.

There are two types of questions that interviewers may ask:

- Open-ended questions that permit the interviewee to respond in an unstructured manner. Examples may include:

  › "What do you think the role of a CS technician should be?"

  › "Give an example of a time when you communicated successfully with another person, even when that individual may not have agreed with your point of view."

- Closed-ended questions call for a brief response. Examples may include:

  › "Do you like your job?"

  › "Do you understand the correct way to do this task?"

Many interviews include both types of questions. One important step in preparing for any interview is to anticipate the types of questions likely to be asked, and then plan a response for them. A good response will answer the question and provide supporting details. This is an opportunity to display knowledge and an understanding for the profession, not to provide "textbook answers." Along with well-thought-out responses, an interviewee should also prepare some questions for the interviewer. This demonstrates an interest for the position and also allows the interviewee to participate in the interview process.

Steps in an Interview

There are four basic steps in any type of interview:

Step 1: It must be planned. Be sure you know the exact purpose of the interview and the "mechanics" of it (time, location and estimated duration).

Step 2: The opening conversation is helpful. Hopefully, there will be an initial discussion of mutual topics of interest to move the discussion away from ongoing work considerations to the specific topic. Professional CS technicians should have the confidence, pride, expertise and positive attitude to reduce tension and allow them to be confident during the interview.

Step 3: Questions will be asked. This is where the interviewee's anticipation of potential questions and ability to effectively speak and listen will be most useful. It is also where application of the speaking and listening tactics outlined previously will be most helpful.

Step 4: The interview discussion can be reviewed. Hopefully, the interviewer will provide a summary. The CS technician should provide reactions to this review, so both parties can agree on what was decided and which, if any, follow-up activities should be undertaken.

Interviews are important. Dress professionally, be punctual and take the interview seriously. Even if you are interviewing for a position at your current place of employment, be sure to follow general interview protocols. Doing so will demonstrate readiness for a change and added responsibilities.

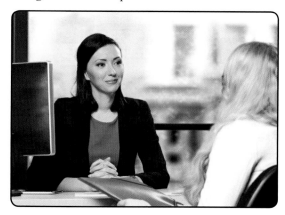

Figure 24.6

PROMOTIONS

Many CS technicians who perform their jobs well have opportunities for promotion to positions with additional responsibilities and higher compensation. Those who accept these positions will likely find many differences in tasks, especially if they assume supervisory duties. Challenges arise when a staff member who has been a peer to other employees becomes their supervisor. Relationships change and they must reflect the new supervisor/**subordinate** dynamic.

> **Subordinate** An employee who is supervised by someone in a higher organizational position.

All management positions must consider the broader needs of the department and the healthcare facility before the specific needs of individual staff members. This can be difficult when they have personal (friendship) relationships with some of those whom they supervise.

CS technicians considering promotions should also recognize that some tasks will be different. One with the knowledge and skills to perform cleaning, decontamination and related tasks may not be as comfortable performing supervisory activities, such as planning, coordinating, directing, controlling and evaluating.

Long-term planning leading to promotion decisions should be an integral part of professional development considerations of interested CS technicians.

PERSONAL AND PROFESSIONAL DEVELOPMENT TIMELINES

Some personal and professional development goals are easier to attain than others. Promotions usually don't happen overnight, but neither does preparing for them. Personal and professional development timelines should be realistic and achievable. Goals for each require planning, commitment and an understanding that things don't always go as planned. When setbacks occur, and they sometimes do, it is essential to regroup and continue moving toward established goals.

CONCLUSION

The field of Central Service is dynamic and ever-evolving, and it requires professional and dynamic individuals to help lead the way in education, systems development, and departmental management. Through personal and professional development, CS technicians can not only enhance the skills necessary to improve upon their current positions, but they can also create new opportunities for career fulfillment and growth.

RESOURCES

Safani B. *Happy about My Resume. 50 Tips for Building a Better Document and Securing a Brighter Future.* 2008.

McDaniel A. *The Young Professional's Guide to the Working World: Savvy Strategies to Get in, Get ahead, and Rise to the Top.* 2013.

International Association of Healthcare Central Service Materiel Management. *Central Service Leadership Manual.* 2010.

CENTRAL SERVICE TERMS

Personal development

Professional development

Subordinate

Glossary

A

AAMI Abbreviation for Association for the Advancement of Medical Instrumentation.

ABC analysis Inventory management strategy that indicates storeroom controls should first address the relatively few items with the greatest value (A items), and should lastly consider the many items with the lowest value (C items).

abdomen Part of the body between the chest and the pelvis.

abduction Movement away from the midline; turning outward.

abort Failed or incomplete machine cycle caused by a malfunction.

abrasive Any of a wide variety of natural or manufactured gritty substances used to grind,wear down, rub away, smooth or scour.

abscess Area of tissue breakdown; a localized space in the body containing pus and liquefied tissue.

absolute pressure (steam sterilizer) Gauge pressure (machine produced) + atmospheric pressure (14.7 pounds per square inch at sea level).

absorbent towel All-cotton towel having a plain weave with only the warp yarns tightly twisted.

acceptance sampling Inspection of a sample from a larger lot to decide whether the lot should be accepted.

ACGIH Abbreviation for American Conference of Governmental Industrial Hygienists.

acid Compound with a pH of less than 7.0 and with a sour, sharp or biting taste; a compound with a water solution that contains positive hydrogen ions (example: HCl).

acid detergent Organic, acid-based cleaning agent; best used for removing mineral deposits.

acid-fast bacteria Bacteria that do not de-colorize when acid is added to the stained smear.

acidity Measurement of the amount of acid present.

acidosis Condition that results from a decrease in the pH of body fluids.

acid scrubber Type of ethylene oxide emission control device.

acquired immune deficiency syndrome (AIDS) Viral disease that attacks the immune system.

acquired immunity Immunity acquired by a person after birth.

action level Level of exposure to a harmful substance or other hazard at which an employer must take required precautions to protect the workers. It is normally one half of the permissible exposure limit.

activated (activation) Process by which a solution is combined with an activating chemical before use. Glutaraldehydes must be activated before initial use.

acute Short in time; relatively severe in degree.

acute disease A disease or disorder that lasts a short time, comes on rapidly and is accompanied by distinct symptoms.

adhesion Holding together of two surfaces or parts; a band of connective tissue between parts that are normally separate; the molecular attraction between contacting bodies.

adipose Referring to fatty tissue.

adrenal Endocrine gland located above the kidney; suprarenal gland.

aerate To expose gas-sterilized items to warm, circulating air.

aeration A process in which sterilized packages are subjected to moving air to facilitate removal of toxic residuals after exposure to a sterilizing agent, such as ethylene oxide.

aerator (ethylene oxide) Machine designed to speed up removal of ethylene oxide residuals from sterilized items by subjecting them to warm, circulating air.

aerobe Microorganism that requires the presence of air or oxygen for growth.

aerobic (bacteria) Capable of growing in the presence of free oxygen; requiring oxygen.

aerosol Suspension of ultramicroscopic solid or liquid particles in air or gas; a spray.

affinity Attraction.

agar Extract of red seaweed used as a solidifying agent in culture media.

AIDS Abbreviation for acquired immune deficiency syndrome; the advanced symptomatic and often fatal disease in the progression of an HIV infection.

airborne Suspended or carried in a gas or air stream.

air count Method of estimating the number of bacteria or microbes in a specific quantity of air.

albumin Protein in blood plasma and other body fluids that helps to maintain the osmotic pressure of the blood.

alimentary canal Pathway that food takes through the body's digestive system.

alkalies Chemicals that release an excess of hydroxyl ions (OH) in a solution to yield a pH of more than 7.

alkaline In solution; having a pH greater than 7.

alkalosis Condition that results from an increase in the pH of body fluids.

alkylation A chemical reaction where hydrogen is replaced with an alkyl group, this causes the cell to be unable to normally metabolize or reproduce, or both.

allergen Substance that causes hypersensitivity; substance that induces allergy.

allergic Caused by allergy.

allergy Tendency to react unfavorably to a certain substance that is normally harmless to most people; hypersensitivity.

alveolus (pl. alveoli) One of millions of tiny air sacs in the lungs through which gases are exchanged between the outside air and the blood; tooth socket.

ambient condition Environmental conditions such as pressure, temperature and humidity, which are normal for a specific location.

ameba (pl. amebas) Protozoon that moves by extruding finger-like elements (pseudopods); also spelled amoeba (pl. amoebae).

amebiasis Infection with pathogenic amebas; acute amebiasis is called amebic dysentery.

amino acid Building block of protein; organic chemical compounds containing an amino group and a carboxyl group; forms the chief structure of proteins.

amitosis Direct cell division.

amniocentesis Removal of fluid and cells from the amniotic sac for prenatal diagnostic tests.

amniotic sac Fluid-filled sac that surrounds and cushions the developing fetus.

amoeboid movement Crawling movement of cells that occurs as the cell successively becomes longer and then retracts.

anaerobe Microorganism that grows only or best in the absence of oxygen.

anaerobic (bacteria) Capable of growing in the absence of free oxygen; not requiring oxygen.

analgesic Relieving pain; a pain-relieving agent that does not cause loss of consciousness.

anaphylaxis State of hypersensitivity to a protein resulting from a previous introduction of the protein into the body; may result in death without treatment.

anastomosis Surgical or pathological formation of a passage between two normally distinct structures, such as tubular organs.

anatomy The study of the structure and relationships between body parts.

anemia Reduction in the amount of red cells or hemoglobin in the blood resulting in inadequate delivery of oxygen to the tissues.

anesthesia Loss of sensation (particularly of pain).

aneurysm Bulging sac in the wall of a vessel.

angina Severe choking pain; disease or condition producing such pain.

angina pectoris Suffocating pain in the chest usually caused by lack of oxygen supply to the heart.

angstrom A unit used to measure the length of light waves.

animate Having life.

anion Negatively-charged particle (ion).

anionic Compounds with a negative electrical charge on the large organic portion of the molecule which are relatively hydrophobic and lipophilic; used as synthetic detergents.

anorexia Loss of appetite.

anoxia Lack of oxygen.

ANSI Abbreviation for American National Standards Institute.

antagonist Muscle with an action opposite that of a given movement; substance that opposes the action of another substance.

anterior Toward the front or belly surface; ventral.

anthrax Infectious disease of cattle and sheep caused by a spore-forming bacterium (Bacillusanthracis) which may be transmitted to man through handling of infected products.

antibacterial serum Antiserum that destroys or prevents the growth of bacteria.

antibiotic Substance produced by one microorganism that will kill or inhibit another microorganism.

antibody Protein produced in the body which reacts against a specific foreign molecule (antigen).

antigen Substance which causes the body to produce antibodies.

antiseptic Solution that inhibits the growth of bacteria; usually used topically and only on animate (living) objects.

antiserum Serum containing antibodies given to provide passive immunity.

antitoxin Immune serum that neutralizes the action of a toxin.

anus Lower opening of the alimentary canal.

anvil One of the three middle ear bones; attaches to the hammer and stirrup.

AORN Abbreviation for Association of peri-Operative Registered Nurses.

aorta Largest blood vessel in the body.

APIC Abbreviation for Association for Professionals in Infection Control and Epidemiology.

aqueous humor Watery-like fluid between the cornea and the eye lens.

aqueous solution Liquid in which a chemical substance is dissolved in water.

areriole Vessel between a small artery and a capillary.

arrhythmia Abnormal rhythm of the heartbeat.

arteries Vessels that carry blood away from the heart.

arteriosclerosis Hardening of the arteries.

arthritis Inflammation of the joints.

asepsis Absence of microorganisms that cause disease.

asepsis (medical) clean technique Procedures performed to reduce the number of microorganisms to minimize their spread.

asepsis (surgical) surgical technique Procedures to eliminate the presence of all microorganisms and/ or to prevent the introduction of microorganisms to an area.

aseptic Free from pathogenic organisms; a means of preventing infection.

aseptic technique Activity or procedure that prevents infection or breaks the chain of infection.

ASHCSP Abbreviation for American Society of Healthcare Central Service Personnel.

asphyxia Condition caused by lack of oxygen in inspired air.

aspirate To draw by suction. Examples: when fluid is removed with a syringe and material is drawn into the lungs during inspiration.

assembly area A clean area of the Central Service department where inspection, assembly and packaging functions are performed. The assembly area is sometimes called the Preparation and Packaging (prep and pack) area.

asset Something of value owned by an organization or person.

Glossary

asset (current) Asset that is expected to be used within one year.

Asymptomatic Shows no signs or symptoms of disease or infection.

atherosclerosis Hardening of the arteries caused by deposits of yellowish, fat-like material on blood vessel linings.

atom Fundamental unit of a chemical element.

atria The two upper chambers of the heart.

atrium One of the two upper chambers of the heart.

atrophy Wasting or decreasing in size of a part.

attenuated Weakened attitude; a person's emotions or willingness that cause him/her to react in a predetermined way to people or situations.

attitude Emotions that cause a person to react to people and/or situations in a predetermined way.

austenitic (stainless steel) This material is also known as 300 stainless steel. It is nonmagnetic, cannot be heat hardened and is more corrosion-resistant than martensitic stainless steel.

autoclave Equipment that uses steam under pressure to sterilize, usually at temperatures of 250° or 270°F (121°C or 132°C).

automated supply replenishment system Replenishment system in which items removed from inventory are automatically identified and tracked. When a reorder point is reached, item information is generated on a supply pick list in the central storeroom or at a contracted vendor. Items are then issued and transferred to the appropriate user area.

automatic endoscope reprocessor (AER) Automated equipment designed to clean, disinfect and rinse flexible endoscopes.

autonomic nervous system Part of the nervous system that controls smooth muscle, cardiac muscle and glands; motor portion of the visceral or involuntary nervous system.

autopsy Examination of the internal organs of a dead body.

axilla Hollow beneath the arm where it joins the body; armpit.

B

bacillus (pl., bacilli) Rod-shaped bacteria; a genus of the family *Bacillaceae.*

bacillus atrophaeus Resistant microorganism used to challenge ethylene oxide sterilizers.

bacillus stearothermophilus See *geobacillus stearothermophilus.*

bacillus subtilis See bacillus atrophaeus.

bacteremia Condition in which bacteria are in the bloodstream.

bacteria (sing. bacterium) Single-celled, plant-like microbes that reproduce by splitting; some cause diseases; also called "germs."

bacterial count Method of estimating the number of bacteria in a sample unit.

bactericidal Relating to the destruction of bacteria.

bactericide Substance that kills bacteria.

bacteriology Science of the study of bacteria.

bacteriophage Virus that parasitizes and multiplies exclusively in bacteria.

bacteriostasis Condition in which bacterial growth is inhibited, but the organisms are not killed.

bacteriostat Substance that inhibits the growth of bacteria.

bacteriostatic Inhibition of bacterial growth without their destruction.

balance sheet Financial summary of what a healthcare facility owns (assets), owes (liabilities) and is worth (equity) at a specific point in time. Example: the last day of every month.

bar code Numerous machine-readable rectangular bars and spaces arranged in a specific way to represent letters, numbers and other symbols.

barrier cloth Fabrics made of blends or cotton/polyester.

barrier packaging Minimum package that prevents ingress of microorganisms and allows aseptic presentation of the product at the point of use.

barrier properties Ability of a material to resist the penetration of liquids and/or microorganisms.

basal ganglia Gray masses in the lower part of the forebrain that assist with muscle coordination.

base Compound with a pH above 7.0, a compound whose water solution yields negative hydroxyl ions (e.g., NaOH), and combines with an acid to form a salt and water; turns red litmus paper blue.

basophil Granular white blood cell that shows large, dark blue cytoplasmic granules when stained with basic stain.

BCG (Bacillus of Calmette-Guerin) Vaccine against tuberculosis made from a bovine strain of tubercle bacilli attenuated through long culturing.

benign Tumor that does not spread, is not recurrent or becoming worse; not malignant.

best practice - A method or technique that has consistently shown results superior to those achieved with other means.

bevel Angle at which the point of a needle is ground.

bile Substance produced in the liver that emulsifies fats.

binary fission Typical method of bacterial reproduction in which a cell divides into two equal parts.

bioburden The number of microorganisms on a contaminated object; also called bioload or microbial load.

biocide A substance or microorganism that kills or controls the growth of living organisms. Examples: antibiotics and disinfectants.

biodegradable Readily decomposed by bacteria or enzymatic actions.

biofilm A collection of microorganisms that attach to surfaces and each other and form a colony. The colony produces a protective gel that is very difficult to penetrate with detergents and disinfectants.

biohazard signage notices posted in easily-seen locations that alert persons in the area about the presence of harmful bacteria, viruses or other dangerous biohazardous agents or organisms.

biohazardous waste Wastes containing infectious agents that present a risk or potential risk to human health either directly through infections or indirectly through the environment.

biological Relating to biology.

biological indicator (BI) Sterilization process monitoring device consisting of a standardized, viable population of microorganisms (usually bacterial spores) known to be resistant to the mode of sterilization being monitored.

biological transfer of infection Mode of transfer of infection from host to host by an animal or insect in which the disease-causing agent goes through a development cycle.

biology Science which studies living things, both animals and plants.

Biomedical/Clinical Engineering department The hospital department responsible for performing safety inspections and function tests on medical equipment; frequently abbreviated "Biomed Department." Also known as Healthcare Technology Management department.

biopsy Removal of tissue or other material from the living body for examination, usually under the microscope.

blood Connective tissue fluid that transports many substances throughout the circulatory system.

borosilicate Alkaline-free silicate glass having at least 5% boric oxide and used especially in heat-resistant glassware; a very hard glass (Pyrex).

botulism Food poisoning caused by the toxin of an anaerobic, spore-forming bacterium, (clostridium botulinum) in contaminated canned or smoked foods.

Bowie-Dick test Test run daily to validate the vacuum function of the sterilizer. The test should be run in an empty load and at the same time each day.

box locks Point where the two jaws or blades of an instrument connect and pivot.

bradycardia Heart rate of less than 60 beats per minute.

brain Main control unit of the central nervous system.

brain stem Controls many automatic body functions such as heartbeat and breathing.

breakout The process of removing commercially-sterilized items from their outer shipper containers in an area adjacent to the storage area to prevent contamination that is present on the containers from being introduced into the storage area.

broad spectrum Term indicating that an antibiotic is effective against a large array of microorganisms.

bronchi The main passageway for air to travel from the trachea to the lungs.

bronchiole One of the small bronchial subdivisions that branch throughout the lungs.

brownian motion Dancing motion of finely divided particles in suspension.

buffer Substance that prevents sharp changes in the pH of a solution.

bursa Small, fluid-filled sac in an area subject to stress around bones and joints.

C

calibration Comparison of a measurement system or device of unknown accuracy to a national standard of known accuracy to detect, correlate, report or adjust any variation from the required performance limits of the unverified measurement system or device.

cancer Uncontrolled growth of a tumor that spreads to other tissue; a malignant neoplasm.

cannulas Surgical instruments with a hollow barrel (or lumen) through their center; often inserted for drainage.

capillaries Vessels that connect veins and arteries.

capillary action Attraction or repulsion force caused by the surface tension of liquids in hair-like tubes.

capital equipment Item of major importance; usually defined by a set dollar amount and which is depreciated over the useful life of the equipment rather than being expensed at purchase.

capital (equipment) Assets that are relatively expensive such as sterilizers or washers that require significant advance planning for their purchase.

capsule Gelatinous, colorless envelope or slime layer surrounding the cell wall of certain microorganisms; a membrane or sack containing a body part.

carbohydrate Simple sugar or compound made from simple sugars linked together.

carbon dioxide Gaseous waste product of cellular metabolism; CO_2.

carcinogen Cancer-causing substance.

carcinoma Malignant growth of epithelial cells; a form of cancer.

cardiopulmonary resuscitation Method to restore heartbeat and breathing by mouth-to-mouth resuscitation and closed chest cardiac massage; also called "CPR."

carditis Inflammation of the heart; myocarditis.

career ladder Plan projecting progressively more responsible professional positions that serves as a foundation for a professional development program.

caries Tooth decay.

carpals Wrist bones.

carrier A person or organism infected with an infectious disease agent, but displays no symptoms. Although unaffected by the disease themselves, carriers can transmit it to others.

cartilage Type of flexible connective tissue.

case cart A cart prepared for an individual procedure. Case carts usually contain all instruments, supplies and utensils needed for a specific procedure.

case cart pull sheet (pick list) A list of specific supplies, utensils and instruments for a specific procedure. Central Service technicians use these lists to assemble the items needed for individual procedures.

case cart system An inventory control system for products/equipment typically used in an Operating Room that involves use of an enclosed or covered cart generally prepared for one surgical case, and not used for general supply replenishment.

CAT scan See computed tomography.

catalyst Substance that influences the speed of a chemical reaction without being consumed.

catalytic converter Type of ethylene oxide emission control device.

cataract Opacity of the eye lens or lens capsule.

catheter Slender, flexible tube of rubber, plastic or metal used for draining a body cavity or injecting fluids through a body passage.

cation Positively charged particle (ion).

cation resin tank Tank into which untreated hard water flows, and in which sodium ions are exchanged for calcium and magnesium ions to produce soft water.

cationic Compounds containing a positive electrical charge on the large organic hydrophobic molecule which exhibit germicidal properties.

causative agent (chain of infection) Microorganism that causes an infectious disease.

caustic Corrosive and burning; agent, particularly an alkali, that will destroy living tissue.

cautery Burner; a means of destroying tissue by electricity, heat or corrosive chemicals. Thermocautery consists of a red hot or white hot object, usually a wire or pointed metallic instrument, heated in a flame or with electricity.

cavitation Process used by an ultrasonic cleaner in which low-pressure bubbles in a cleaning solution burst inward to dislodge soil from instruments.

CDC Abbreviation for Centers for Disease Control and Prevention (part of the Department of Health and Human Services) whose primary function is to investigate outbreaks of and control various diseases.

cecum Small pouch at the beginning of the large intestine.

ceiling limit The maximum safe airborne concentration of a potentially toxic substance.

cell Basic unit of life; the smallest structural unit of living organisms capable of performing all basic life functions.

cell membrane Outer covering of a cell; regulates what enters and leaves the cell.

cellulitis Diffuse inflammation of connective tissues.

centigrade Thermometer temperature scale with 100° between the melting point of ice at 0° and the boiling point of water at 100°.

central nervous system (CNS) Part of the nervous system that includes the brain and spinal cord.

centrifuge Device used to spin test tubes; used in the laboratory.

cerebellum Second largest part of the brain. It controls muscle coordination, body balance and posture.

cerebrospinal fluid (CSF) Fluid that circulates in and around the brain and spinal cord.

cerebrovascular accident (CVA) Condition involving bleeding from the brain or obstruction of blood flow to brain tissue, usually resulting from hypertension or atherosclerosis; also called stroke.

cerebrum Largest part of the brain. It that controls mental activities and movement.

certification Association and industry recognition given to individuals with educational and/or work experience requirements who successfully complete an examination process that demonstrates their knowledge of subject-matter to be mastered for success in the position.

cervix Lower end (neck) of the uterus.

chlorofluorocarbon (CHC) Inert (inflammable) gas often mixed with a flammable gas to create an inflammable solution; has been used with ethylene oxide to create an inert gas.

chain of infection A way of gathering the information needed to interrupt or prevent an infection. Each of the links in the chain must be favorable to the organism for the infection to continue. Breaking any link in the chain can disrupt the infection. Which link is most effective to target will depend on the organism.

challenge test pack Used in qualification, installation and ongoing quality assurance testing of hospital sterilizers.

chamber Enclosed area that holds products to be sterilized.

chelating agents Chemicals that hold hard water minerals in solution and prevent soaps or detergents from reacting with the minerals.

chemical indicators (CIs) Devices used to monitor the presence or attainment of one or more of the parameters required for a satisfactory sterilization process.

chemical sterilization Process using a chemical agent to render a product free of viable microorganisms.

chemotherapy Treatment of disease without injury to patient with chemicals having a specific effect on microorganisms.

chickenpox Varicella; a rather mild, highly contagious virus disease characterized by fever and the appearance of vesicles.

chisels Wedge-shaped instruments used to cut or shape bone.

CHL Abbreviation for Certification in Healthcare Leadership, a certification offered by the International Association of Healthcare Central Service Materiel Management.

CHMMC Abbreviation for Certification in Healthcare Materiel Management Concepts (International Association of Healthcare Central Service Materiel Management).

chloride Compound commonly found in water created when chlorine is combined with another element or radical. Examples: salt and hydrochloric acid.

chlorophyll Molecule in plants that absorbs sunlight and converts it to energy in a process called photosynthesis.

cholesterol Organic, fat-like compound found in animal fat, bile blood, myelin, liver and other parts of the body.

chromium Blue-white metallic element found naturally only in combination and used in alloys and electroplating.

chromogenic Producing a pigment.

chromosomes Rod-shaped structures responsible for inherited characteristics passed from parent to child.

chronic Referring to a disease (illness) that is not severe, but is continuous, recurring, protracted and prolonged.

cilia (sing. cilium) Hair-like elements that spring from certain cells and, by their action, create currents in liquids; if the cells are fixed, the liquid is made to flow; if the cells are unicellular organisms suspended in the liquid, the cells move.

circumduction Circular movement at a joint.

cirrhosis Chronic disease (usually of the liver) in which active cells are replaced by inactive scar tissue.

CIS Abbreviation for Certified Instrument Specialist, a certification offered by the International Association of Healthcare Central Service Materiel Management.

CJD Abbreviation for Creutzfeld-Jakob Disease; a debilitating, fatal brain disease; see prions.

class 5 (chemical integrators) Integrating indicators designed to react to all critical parameters over a specified range of sterilization cycles.

cleaning Removal of all visible and non-visible soil, and any other foreign material from medical devices being processed.

clostridium Genus of cylindrical-shaped bacteria that are anaerobic, gram positive and spore forming.

cloud computing The practice of storing regularly used computer data on multiple servers that can be accessed through the Internet.

coaching Positive reinforcement used to encourage Central Service technicians to follow proper work behaviors, and negative reinforcement to discourage inappropriate work behaviors.

coagulase Enzyme that causes coagulation or clotting of blood serum.

coagulation Clotting (as in blood).

coccus Round-shaped (spherical) bacterium.

coccyx Tailbone.

cochlea Coiled portion of the inner ear that contains the organs of hearing.

cold boil Cavitation that is not dependent upon heat for its bubbling action.

coliform bacteria Group of intestinal microorganisms of which Escherichia coli is a member.

collagen Flexible white protein that gives strength and resilience to connective tissue, including bone and cartilage.

colon Main portion of the large intestine.

colonization Occurs when microorganisms live on or in a host organism, but do not invade tissues or cause damage.

colony Visible growth of microorganisms seen in culture medium; usually obtained from a single organism.

colony count Determination of the number of visible clumps of bacteria derived from the multiplication of specific microorganisms on or in a culture medium.

combining vowel Letter, usually an "o," that is sometimes used to ease the pronunciation of a medical word.

combustible Substance that, if ignited, will react with oxygen and burn.

combustible Loading weight of combustible materials per square foot of area in which the materials are located.

combustion Chemical process accompanied by the rapid production of heat and light.

commissioning (installation qualification) Obtaining and documenting evidence that equipment has been provided and installed in accordance with its specifications, and that it functions within predetermined limits when operated in accordance with operational instructions.

communicable Disease whose causative agent is easily transmitted from person to person by direct or indirect contact.

communication Process of transmitting information and understanding from one person to another by use of words and nonverbal expressions including body language.

complication Secondary illness imposed upon a person with a primary illness.

compound Substance composed of two or more chemical elements.

computed tomography Imaging method in which multiple x-ray views taken from different angles are analyzed by computer to show a cross section of an area; used to detect tumors and other abnormalities; abbreviated "CT" or "CAT" (computed axial tomography).

conditioning Treatment of products within the sterilization cycle but before sterilant admission to attain a predetermined temperature and relative humidity; may be carried out at atmospheric pressure or under vacuum.

conduction Heat transfer method in which heat is absorbed by an item's exterior surface and passed inward to the next layer.

conduction heating Process in which heat is transmitted in a solid substance from molecule to molecule by molecular impact or agitation.

conductivity (of water) A measurement of the ability of water to carry an electrical current.

congenital Present at birth.

conjunctiva Membrane that lines the eyelid, and covers the anterior part of the sclera.

conjunctivitis Inflammation of the conjunctiva of the eye.

consumable (inventory) Assets such as wrapping supplies, processing chemicals and other items that are consumed (used up) as healthcare services are provided to patients.

contagious Highly communicable; easily transmitted.

contaminate To render unfit for use through introduction of a substance which is harmful or injurious.

contamination State of being soiled or infected by contact with infectious organisms or other material.

continuous quality improvement (CQI) Scientific approach which applies statistical methods to improve work processes.

contraception Prevention of fertilization of an ovum or implantation of a fertilized ovum; birth control.

convalescence Period during which recovery takes place following illness.

convection Process of heat transfer by the circulation of currents from one area to another.

convection heating Transfer of heat in a fluid or gas from one place to another by the motion of the fluid or gas.

copious Present in a large amount (such as large volume of rinsing water).

cornea Clear portion of sclera that covers the front of the eye.

coronary Referring to the heart or to the arteries supplying blood to the heart.

corrosion Act of wearing away gradually by a chemical reaction.

corrosive Having the power to corrode or wear away.

cortex Outer layer of an organ, such as the brain, kidney or adrenal gland.

counterstain Second stain of a contrasting kind applied to a smear for the purpose of making the microorganisms treated with a primary stain more distinct.

CPR Abbreviation for cardiopulmonary resuscitation.

CPU Abbreviation for central processing unit.

craze Spider web cracking of plastics under chemical stress.

CRCST Abbreviation for Certified Registered Central Service Technician, a certification offered by the International Association of Healthcare Central Service Materiel Management.

crisis Change in a disease which indicates whether the result will be recovery or death.

critical devices Refers to the Spaulding medical device classification system. Instruments or objects introduced directly into the bloodstream or other normally sterile body areas.

critical parameters Parameters that are essential to the sterilization process and that require monitoring.

cross contamination Migration of contaminants from one person, object or work location to another.

cross-functional team Group of employees from different departments within the healthcare facility that work together to resolve operating problems.

cross infection Infection acquired from an animate or inanimate contaminated environment, usually accidentally.

culture Growth of microorganisms on a nutrient medium; to grow microorganisms on such medium.

culture medium Substance or preparation used for the growth and cultivation of microorganisms.

customer (internal) Physicians, nurses and other professional personnel served by Central Service personnel.

cutaneous Referring to the skin.

cyanosis Bluish color of the skin and mucous membranes resulting from insufficient oxygen in the blood.

cycle buying Purchasing method in which an order is placed at a scheduled interval.

cycle (gravitation-displacement type; steam sterilization) Sterilization cycle in which incoming steam displaces residual air through a port or drain in or near the bottom of the sterilizer chamber.

cycle (sterilization) Defined sequence of operational steps designed to achieve sterilization; carried out in a sealed chamber.

cycle time Total elapsed time of a sterilization cycle from when the sterilizer door is closed and the cycle is activated until the cycle is completed and the door is opened.

cystitis Inflammation of the urinary bladder.

cytology Study of cells.

cytoplasm Clear, jelly-like substance of a cell between the cell membrane and nucleus.

D

D-value Amount of time required to kill 90% of the microorganisms present.

debridement Surgical removal of dead or unhealthy tissue.

decontamination To make safe by removing or reducing contamination by infectious organisms or other harmful substances; the reduction of contamination to an acceptable level.

decontamination area Location within a health care facility designated for collection, retention and cleaning of soiled and/or contaminated items.

defecation Act of eliminating undigested waste from the digestive tract.

defect Variance from expected standards.

deflocculate To reduce or break up into very fine particles.

degeneration Breaking down (as from age, injury or disease).

degerm To remove bacteria and other microbes by mechanical cleaning and applying antiseptics or disinfectants.

dehydration Excessive loss of body fluid.

deionization Process by which ions with an electrical charge are removed from water.

deionize To remove ions from (as water by ion exchange); demineralize.

deionized (DI) water Water that has had all minerals removed by using an ion exchange process.

denatured alcohol Alcohol that has been rendered unfit for use as a beverage by the addition of substances which impart an unpleasant odor and taste. Examples: wood alcohol and benzene.

density Degree of compactness; closely set or thickness.

deoxyribonucleic acid (DNA) One of two nucleic acids; essential for biological inheritance.

dermatitis Inflammation of the skin.

dermis True skin; deeper part of the skin.

detergent Cleaning agent composed of a "surface wetting agent" that reduces surface tension; a "builder" which is the principle cleaning agent, and a "sequestering" or "chelating agent" to suspend the soil; detergents may also have additional additives, such as blood solvents or rust inhibitors; any chemical that causes oil or grease to dissolve in water and cleans the item on which it is used. Unlike soap, detergent does not contain fats and lye.

detergent/germicide Combination of a cleaning agent and a disinfectant.

detergent/sanitizer Combination of chemicals that possesses antibacterial and cleaning properties.

dextrose Glucose; simple sugar

diabetes mellitus Disease in which glucose is not oxidized in body tissues for energy because of insufficient insulin.

diagnosis Identification of an illness.

dialysis Method to separate molecules in solution based on differences in their rates of diffusion through a semi-permeable membrane; method for removing nitrogen waste products from the body by hemodialysis or peritoneal dialysis.

diaphragm Dome-shaped muscle under the lungs that flattens during inhalation; a separating membrane or structure.

diarrhea Loose and frequent bowel movements.

differential staining Staining techniques to distinguish between different bacteria.

diffusion Movement of molecules from a region of higher concentration to a region of lower concentration.

digestion Process of breaking down food into absorbable particles.

dilation Widening of a part (e.g., pupil of the eye, blood vessel or uterine cervix).

diphtheria Acute, infectious disease of the mucous membranes of the upper respiratory tract; characterized by patches of *pseudomembrane* and caused by *Corynebacterium diphtheriae.*

diplococci Pairs of cocci.

direct contact Spread of disease from person to person.

disaster (external) Situation in which activities external to the facility affect departmental or facility operations.

disaster (internal) Situation with the potential to cause harm or injury to Central Service or other employees, or where the loss of utilities may drastically impact departmental operations.

disease State of illness characterized by marked symptoms caused by an infectious agent producing a definite pathological pattern.

disinfectant Chemical that kills most pathogenic organisms, but not all spores.

disinfectant/detergent Chemical compound that contains both detergent and disinfectant. Usually, the action of both is compromised because of the combination.

disinfection Destruction of nearly all pathogenic microorganisms on an inanimate (non-living) surface.

disinfestation Destruction of insects, rodents or other animals that transmit infections to other animals, humans or their surroundings.

displacement Ionic change in which one element exchanges with another element by oxidation or reduction; a chemical change in which one element, molecule or radical is removed by another.

dissection The process of cutting apart or separating tissue.

dissociation Physical breaking apart of a molecule.

distal The end of an item that is farthest away from the point of origin; the end of the instrument farthest away from the operator; the distal end of the femur is closest to the knee.

distill To vaporize by heat, and condense and collect the volatilized product.

distillation Changes from liquid to vapor to liquid; a process for removing impurities from liquids.

distilled water Water that has been heated to boiling point, vaporized, cooled and condensed into liquid form. Distillation removes impurities and like gases and organic material, it also removes some bacteria.

distribution Movement of supplies (primarily consumable supplies from storeroom to clinical units and reprocessed supplies from Central Service to the Operating Room) throughout the facility.

diversity The broad range of human characteristics and dimensions that impact employees' values, opportunities and perceptions of themselves and others at work.

DNA See deoxyribonucleic acid.

doctor's (physician's) preference card Document that identifies a physician's needs (requests and preferences) for a specific medical procedure. Preference cards usually contain information regarding the instruments, equipment, supplies and utensils used by a specific physician. They may also include reminders for the staff of the physician's preferences regarding patient draping, instruments and supplies.

dominant Referring to a gene that is always expressed if present.

dorsal Toward the back; posterior.

down time rate (equipment) Number of down days/number of devices (x) 365.

droplet infection Infection transmitted by small drops (particles) of sputum or nasal discharges expelled into the air while talking, coughing or sneezing.

duct Tube or vessel.

duodenum First portion of the small intestine.

dust cover Protective plastic bag used to maintain the sterility of an item by protecting it from the environment; also known as a sterility maintenance cover.

dye Coloring material used for staining or coloring bacteria for microscopic examination.

dyspnea Difficult or labored breathing.

E

ebonize Exposure of an instrument to a chemical dip that blackens the metal.

ECG Short for electrocardiogram; a picture of the electrical activity of the heart used to determine if heart disease is present.

economic order quantity (EOQ) Specific mathematical formula used to determine the most appropriate order quantity based upon usage and other variables.

ectoplasm Outer clear zone of the cytoplasm of a one-celled organism.

edema Presence of abnormally large amounts of fluid in intercellular tissue spaces of the body.

EDI Abbreviation for electronic data interchange. Orders, invoices and other transactions are transferred electronically between the customer and the vendor to create a paperless and more efficient system.

EEG Abbreviation for electroencephalogram; a picture of the electrical activity of the brain.

effusion Escape of fluid into a space or part; the fluid itself.

ejaculation Expulsion of semen through the urethra.

ejaculatory duct Duct formed by the joining of the seminal vesicle with the vas deferens, through which semen moves during ejaculation.

electrocardiograph (ECG or EKG) Instrument to study the electric activity of the heart; record made is an electrocardiogram.

electroencephalograph (EEG) Instrument used to study electric activity of the brain; record made is an electroencephalogram.

electrolyte Compound that forms ions in solution; substance that conducts an electric current in solution.

electron Negatively-charged particle that moves around the nucleus (central core) of an atom.

electroplating To plate with an adherent continuous coating by electrodeposition.

electrostatic Pertaining to the attractions and repulsions of electrical charges.

element One substance from which all matter is made; a substance that cannot be decomposed into a simpler substance.

embolus Blood clot or other obstruction in the circulation system; the condition is an embolism.

embryo Developing offspring during the first two months of pregnancy.

emesis Vomiting.

emphysema Pulmonary disease characterized by dilation and alveoli destruction.

empowerment Granting authority (power) to employees to make decisions within their areas of responsibility.

empyema Accumulation of pus in a body cavity, especially the chest.

emulsification Dispersion of two mutually immiscible (unable to be mixed) liquids.

emulsifier Any ingredient used to bind together substances that normally do not combine, such as oil and water.

emulsify To break down large volumes of fats, oils and greases into small globules, which are held in suspension.

encephalitis Inflammation of the brain.

encephalomyelitis Inflammation of the brain and spinal cord.

endemic disease One that occurs more or less continuously throughout a community.

endocarditis Inflammation of the endocardium (lining membrane) of the heart, including heart valves.

endocardium Membrane that lines the heart chambers and covers the valves.

endocrine Gland that secretes directly into the bloodstream.

endogenous Originating within the organism.

endometrium Lining of the uterus.

endoscope An instrument used to examine the interior of a hollow organ or body cavity.

endothelium Epithelium that lines the heart, blood vessels and lymphatic vessels.

engineering controls Controls (e.g., sharps disposal containers and self-sheathing needles) that isolate or remove bloodborne pathogen hazards from the workplace.

enteric Pertaining to the intestines.

enteric bacteria Bacteria living in or isolated from the intestinal tract.

entrained Trapped in the stream. Example: water can be trapped in the stream of steam.

environment Space that surrounds or encompasses a person or object.

enzymatic solution Solution containing special enzymes that dissolves proteinaceous materials.

enzyme Substance that initiates chemical changes, such as fermentation, without participating in them; a catalyst, usually protein, produced by a living cell with a specific action and optimum activity at a definite pH value.

EPA Abbreviation for Environmental Protection Agency.

epicardium Membrane that forms the outermost layer of the heart wall and is continuous with the lining of the pericardium; visceral pericardium.

epidemic Occurrence of a disease among many people in a given region at the same time.

epidemiology Study of the occurrence and distribution of disease; usually refers to epidemics.

epidermis Outermost layer of the skin.

epididymis Tube that carries sperm cells from the testes to the vas deferens.

epiglottis Leaf-shaped cartilage that covers the larynx during swallowing

equipment (capital) Relatively expensive assets, such as sterilizers or washers, that require significant advance planning for their purchase.

equipment utilization rate Days used/Number of devices (x) 365.

ergonomics Process of changing work or working conditions to reduce employee stress.

erythema Redness of the skin.

erythrocyte Red blood cell (corpuscle).

esophagus Tube that carries food from the throat to the stomach.

estrogen Group of female sex hormones that promotes development of the uterine lining and maintains secondary sex characteristics.

ethylene oxide (EtO or EO) Chemical (gas) used in low-temperature sterilization; performs as a very effective general purpose sterilant for heat- or moisture-sensitive items.

etiology Study of the cause of a disease or the theory of its origin.

eustachian tube Tube that connects the middle ear cavity to the throat; auditory tube.

exacerbation Increase in the severity of a disease.

exchange cart system Inventory system in which desired inventory items are placed on a cart assigned a specific location. A second duplicate cart is maintained in another location and the two carts are exchanged on a scheduled to ensure that sufficient supplies are available at all times.

excretion To eliminate or give off waste products (e.g., feces, perspiration, urine).

exfoliate To come off in strips or sheets; particularly the stripping of the skin after certain exanthematous diseases.

exotoxin Soluble poisonous substance excreted by a living microorganism; can be obtained in bacteria-free filtrates without death or disintegration of the microorganism.

expiration date Date calculated by adding a specific period of time to the date of manufacture or sterilization of a medical device or component that defines its estimated useful life.

expiration statement Statement indicating that the contents of a package are sterile indefinitely, unless the integrity of the package is compromised.

exposure time Time in which the sterilizer's chamber is maintained within the specified range for temperature, sterilant concentration, pressure and humidity.

external solutions Solutions normally used for irrigating, topical application and surgical use given orally or by inhalation.

extracellular Outside the cell.

extraction Use of physical force (usually centrifugal or strike/impact) to remove excess water from a wash load prior to drying.

extraneous Outside the organism; not belonging to it.

extrinsic Coming or operating from outside.

exudate Accumulation of a fluid in a cavity or matter that penetrates through the vessel walls into adjoining tissue.

F

facultative Having the power to do something, but not ordinarily doing it; capable of adapting to different conditions. Example: a facultative anaerobe can live in the presence of oxygen, but does not ordinarily do so.

fahrenheit Thermometer scale in which the space between the freezing point and the boiling point of water is 180°; 32° is the freezing point and 212° is the boiling point. To convert from Fahrenheit to Centigrade scales: 5/9 (°F - 32) = °C.

failure mode and effect analysis (FMEA) Process to predict the adverse outcomes of various human and machine failures to prevent future adverse outcomes.

fallopian tubes Slender tubes that convey the ova (eggs) from the ovaries to the uterus.

families (chemicals) Groups of chemicals that have similar characteristics.

fascia Band or sheet of fibrous connective tissue.

FCS Abbreviation for Fellowship in Central Service, a designation offered by the International Association of Healthcare Central Service Materiel Management.

FDA Abbreviation for U.S. Food and Drug Administration.

febrile Characterized by or pertaining to fever.

feces Waste material discharged from the large intestine; excrement; stool.

feedback Step in communication that occurs when the listener asks a question, repeats information or otherwise helps the speaker know if the message has been correctly received; also defined as a method to respectfully share ideas and information on a specific issue.

femur Upper leg bone.

fenestrated Having openings.

fermentation Decomposition of complex organic molecules under the influence of ferments or enzymes; usually associated with living microorganisms.

fertilization Union of an ovum and a spermatozoon.

fetus Developing offspring from the third month of pregnancy until birth.

fever Abnormally high body temperature.

fibrin Blood protein that forms a blood clot.

fibula Smaller bone of the lower leg.

filter Device secured to a rigid sterilization container's lid and/or bottom that allows passage of air and sterilants, but provides a microbial barrier.

filter retention system Mechanism on a rigid sterilization container that secures disposable filters in place.

filtrate Liquid that has passed through a filter.

fimbriae Finger-like projections extending from the fallopian tubes that draw ova (eggs) into the fallopian tube.

first in, first out (FIFO) Stock rotation system in which the oldest product (that which has been in storage the longest) is used first.

fissure Deep groove.

flagella Long, hair-like structures extending from the cell wall of a microorganism that help an organism to move (especially in liquids).

flammable Combustible substance that ignites very easily, burns intensely or has a rapid rate of flame spread.

flash sterilization Process by which unwrapped instruments were sterilized for immediate use when an emergency situation arises; process of sterilizing an item that is not packaged. This term is no longer used in the healthcare industry (it has been replaced with the term "immediate use steam sterilization").

flash sterilizer Sterilizer that uses higher temperatures for shorter exposure times for emergency sterilization of dropped instruments.

flatus Gas in the digestive tract.

Glossary

flexion Bending motion that decreases the angle between bones at a joint.

fluid invasion Damage to powered surgical instruments when water or solution enters the instrument's internal components.

focal infection Localized site of more or less chronic infection from which bacteria or their byproducts are spread to other parts of the body.

fomite Inanimate object that can transmit bacteria.

foot candle Amount of light equivalent to that produced by one standard candle at a distance of one foot.

forceps Instruments used for grasping, holding firmly or exerting traction upon objects.

forging To form by heating and hammering.

formaldehyde Class of disinfectants most often used to disinfect hemodialysis equipment; also used as a preservative and fumigant. Should be used with caution because of its potential carcinogenic effect and irritating fumes.

fractional sterilization Sterilization performed at separate intervals, usually for 15-minute periods over three to four days, so spores will develop into bacteria that can then be destroyed.

fumigation Disinfection by exposure to a lethal gas/fumigant.

fumes Emanating from a gas or vapor (such as from a disinfectant).

fungicide Substance that kills fungi.

fungus (pl. fungi) Type of plant-like microorganism; unicellular and multi-cellular vegetable organisms that feed on organic matter (e.g., molds, mushrooms and toadstools).

G

gamma globulin Protein component of blood plasma that contains antibodies.

ganglion Collection of nerve cell bodies located outside the central nervous system.

gangrene Death of tissue due to loss of blood supply; accompanied by bacterial invasion and putrefaction.

gas State of matter in which molecules are practically unrestricted by cohesive forces. A gas has neither shape or volume, nor is it liquid nor solid.

gas cylinder safety relief device Device installed in a gas cylinder or container to prevent rupture of a cylinder by overpressures resulting from certain conditions of exposure; device may be a frangible (breakable) disc, fusible plug or relief valve.

gasket Pliable strip on sterilization containers that seals the lid and the container to prevent entry of microorganisms.

gas pressure regulator Device that may be connected to the cylinder valve outlet to regulate the gas pressure delivered to a system.

gastroenteritis Inflammation of the stomach and intestines with symptoms similar to enteritis and dysentery; often caused by enteric group of bacteria (e.g., *Salmonella paratypih* and *Salmonella schottmuller*).

gastrointestinal (GI) Pertaining to the stomach and intestine or the digestive tract, as a whole.

gauge pressure (steam sterilizer) The pressure inside the sterilizer chamber above atmospheric pressure (14.7 psi at sea level).

gene Biological unit of heredity, self-reproducing and located in a definite position (locus) on a specific chromosome.

generalized infection One involving the whole body.

genetic Pertaining to genes or heredity.

genus Group of one or more related species.

geobacillus stearothermophilus Highly resistant, but relative harmless nonpathogenic microorganism used to challenge steam and dry heat sterilizers.

germ Microorganism that causes disease.

germicidal Related to destroying germs.

germicide Agent that kills germs.

glucagon A hormone that can increase the blood sugar level.

glaucoma Disorder involving increased fluid pressure within the eye.

glucose Simple sugar; main energy source for the cells; dextrose.

gonad Sex gland; ovary or testis.

gonorrhea Contagious venereal disease of the genital mucous membranes; caused by *Neisseria gonorrhoeae*.

gram Basic unit of weight in the metric system.

gram-negative Losing the purple stain or decolorized by alcohol in Gram's method of staining; a primary identification characteristic of certain microorganisms

gram-positive Retaining the purple stain or resisting decolorization by alcohol in Gram's method of staining.

gram stain Differential stain used to classify bacteria as gram positive or gram negative, depending upon whether they retain or lose the primary stain (crystal violet) when subjected to a decolorizing agent.

gravity Pull toward the center of the earth.

greenhouse gases Any of the gases that absorb solar radiation and are responsible for the greenhouse effect, including carbon dioxide, methane, ozone and fluorocarbons.

gross soil Tissue, body fat, blood and other body substances

H

HAI – See "healthcare-acquired infection."

halogen Any of the four very active non-metallic chemical elements: chlorine, iodine, bromine and fluorine.

hammer One of the three middle ear bones; attaches to the tympanic membrane.

hand bacterial count Method of estimating the number of bacteria present on one's hand.

hand hygiene Act of washing one's hands with soap and water or using an alcohol-based hand rub.

hardness Amount of dissolved minerals in water, which alters the effectiveness of many disinfectants, detergents and soaps.

hazardous waste Substances that cannot be disposed of in the facility's normal trash system.

HCFC Abbreviation for hydrochlorofluorocarbon gas; when mixed with other gases, it yields an inflammable gas.

health care products Medical devices, medicinal products (pharmaceuticals and biologics) and invitro diagnostics.

Health Insurance Portability And Accountability Act (HIPAA) The HIPAA privacy rule provides federal protections for individually identifiable health information held by covered entities and their business associates, and gives patients an array of rights with respect to that information.

healthcare-associated infection (HAI) - An infection that is not present when a patient is admitted to a hospital or healthcare facility. If the infection develops in a patient on or after day three of admission to the hospital or healthcare facility, the infection is referred to as hospital-acquired or healthcare-associated.

Healthcare Information Management Systems Society (HIMSS) Global, cause-based, not-for-profit organization focused on better health through information technology.

heart Muscular organ that pumps blood throughout the body.

heat sink Heat-absorbent material; a mass that readily absorbs heat.

heat-up time Time required for entire load to reach a pre-selected sterilizing temperature after

the chamber has reached that temperature.

hematocrit (Hct) Volume percentage of red blood cells in whole blood; packed cell volume.

hematoma Swelling filled with blood.

hematuria Blood in the urine.

hemodialysis Removal of impurities from the blood by passage through a semi-permeable membrane.

hemoglobin Iron-containing protein in red blood cells that transports oxygen; abbreviated "Hb."

Glossary

hemolysis The destruction of red blood cells, which leads to the release of hemoglobin from within the red blood cells into the blood plasma.

hemolytic Destruction of red blood cells with the liberation of hemoglobin.

hemorrhage Loss of blood.

hemostasis Stoppage of bleeding.

hemostatic forceps Surgical instrument used to control flow of blood.

heparin Substance that prevents blood clotting; anticoagulant.

hepatitis Inflammation of the liver; usually caused by the hepatitis virus.

heredity Transmission of characteristics from parent to offspring by genes.

hernia Protrusion of an organ or tissue through the wall of the cavity in which it is normally enclosed.

herpes simplex Mild, acute, eruptive, vesicular virus disease of the skin and mucous membrane.

herpes zoster Shingles; an acute virus disease characterized by a vesicular dermatitis, which follows a nerve trunk.

high efficiency particulate air filter (HEPA) Special filters with minimum efficiency of 99.97%.

high-level disinfection The destruction of all vegetative microorganisms, mycobacterium, small or non-lipid viruses, medium or lipid viruses, fungal spores and some bacterial spores.

HIPAA See Health Insurance Portability and Accountability Act

histology Study of tissues.

HIV Abbreviation for human immunodeficiency virus; an HIV infection is a chronic viral infection characterized by progressive destruction of the T-cell, which impairs the body's immune system; disease severity is relates to the degree of immune suppression.

HMO Abbreviation for health maintenance organization.

homeostasis State of balance within the body; maintenance of body conditions within set limits.

hormones Chemical messengers that travel through the blood and act on target organs.

host Animal, plant or human that supports the growth of microorganisms.

huck towel All-cotton surgical towel with a honeycomb-effect weave.

human immunodeficiency virus Virus that causes AIDS.

human relations The development and maintenance of effective interpersonal (between people) relationships that enhance teamwork.

humerus Upper arm bone.

hydration Act of combining with water.

hydrocarbon Chemically identifiable compound of carbon and hydrogen.

hydrogen ion concentration Degree of concentration of hydrogen ions in a solution used to indicate the reaction of that solution; expressed as pH (the logarithm of the reciprocal of the hydrogen ion concentration).

hydrologic cycle Continual movement of water from the atmosphere to the earth and back to the atmosphere.

hydrolysis Splitting of large molecules by the addition of water (as in digestion).

hydrophilic Refers to a substance that absorbs or adsorbs water.

hydrophobic Refers to a substance that does not absorb or adsorb water.

hyperglycemia Abnormal increase in the amount of glucose in the blood.

hypertension High blood pressure.

hypertonic Solution with a higher osmotic pressure than that of a reference solution.

hypoglycemia Abnormal decrease in the amount of glucose in the blood.

hypotension Low blood pressure.

hypothermia Abnormally low body temperature.

hypotonic Solution that is of less than isotonic concentration.

hypoxia Reduced oxygen supply to the tissues.

I

IAHCSMM Abbreviation for International Association of Healthcare Central Service Materiel Management.

icteric Yellow pigmentation of the tissues, membranes and secretions caused by the deposit of bile pigment; usually a sign of liver or gall bladder disease.

idiopathic Of unknown cause.

idiosyncrasy Individual and peculiar susceptibility or sensitivity to a drug, protein or other matter.

ileum Last portion of the small intestine.

Immediate use steam sterilization (IUSS) Process designed for the cleaning, steam sterilization and delivery of patient care items for immediate use. Previously known as flash sterilization.

immune Exempt from a given infection.

immunity Power of an individual to resist or overcome the effects of a particular disease or other harmful agent.

immunization Process of conferring immunity on an individual.

impact marker Tool which engraves with a forceful impact that indents and "breaks" the polished metal surface, leaving an inscribed marking.

impingement Spray-force action of pressurized water against instruments being processed to physically remove bioburden.

implosion Bursting inward; the opposite of an explosion; occurs when cavitation in an energized solution collapse.

inactivation To stop or destroy activity.

inanimate Not endowed with life or spirit; not alive.

incipient Just beginning.

incompatible Not capable of being mixed without undergoing destructive chemical changes or antagonism.

Incubate To maintain under optimum environmental conditions favorable for growth.

incubation period Period between when infection occurs and appearance of first symptoms.

incubator Apparatus for maintaining a constant and suitable temperature for the growth and cultivation of microorganisms.

indefinite Shelf life of hospital-sterilized items without a definite expiration date; based on premise that shelf life is event related, not time related. User must assure the integrity of the packaging is intact, clean and properly identified.

indicator (quality) Measurable variable that relates to the outcome of patient care or employee safety.

indirect contact Transfer of infection by means including inanimate objects, contaminated fingers, water and food.

infarct Area of tissue damaged from lack of blood supply caused by blockage of a vessel.

infection Invasion of body tissue by microorganisms that multiply and produce a reaction.

infection control Control of active infectious disease; requires (a) working knowledge of the usefulness and applications of physical and chemical agents that suppress or kill microorganisms and (b) familiarity with the sources of potentially dangerous microorganisms, routes by which they spread, and their portals of entry into the body.

infectious Having the ability to transmit disease.

inferior Below or lower.

infestation Lodgment, development and reproduction of arthropods on a body or clothing.

inflammation Reaction of the tissues to an injury; a protective mechanism to an irritant on tissues.

inhibition Act of checking or restraining.

inoculate To implant or introduce causative agents of disease into an animal or plant or microbes onto culture media.

inoculated carrier Carrier on which a defined number of test organisms has been deposited.

inorganic Composed of matter other than plant or animal; minerals.

Glossary

installation qualification (IQ) Obtaining and documenting evidence that equipment has been provided and installed in accordance with its specifications.

instructions for use (IFU) See manufacturer's instructions for use.

instrument Utensil or implement.

instrument washer sterilizer (IWS) Combination units that wash and sterilize instruments to ensure the safety of processing personnel.

issue Act of withdrawing supplies from storage for transfer to areas for use.

insulin Hormone that reduces the level of sugar in the blood.

integrated delivery network (IDN) System of healthcare providers and organizations that provides (or arranges to provide) a coordinated range of services to a specific population.

integrating indicator Chemical indicator (CI) designed to react to all critical parameters over a specified range of sterilization cycles, and whose performance has been correlated to the performance of the relevant biological indicator (BI) under the labeled conditions of use.

intercellular Between cells.

interfaced An area or system through which one machine is connected to another machine in order to share information. Example: Two computers may be interfaced or a computer and a sterilizer may be interfaced.

Intermediate-level disinfection The destruction of viruses, mycobacteria, fungi and vegetative bacteria, but not bacterial spores.

intermittent (fractional) sterilization Destruction of microorganisms by moist heat for given periods of time on several successive days to allow spores during the rest periods to germinate into vegetative forms (which are most easily destroyed).

interstitial Between; pertaining to spaces or structures in an organ between active tissues.

intracellular Within a cell or cells.

intravenous Within or into the veins.

in-use testing Evaluation of infection control chemicals, aseptic techniques and sanitary and sterilization procedures under actual working conditions.

inventory Reusable equipment and consumable items used to provide healthcare services for patients.

inventory (consumable) Assets, such as wrapping supplies, processing chemicals and other items, that are consumed as healthcare services are provided to patients.

inventory (official) Consumable products found in Central Service and other storerooms, warehouses and satellite storage areas. Official inventory is included as an asset on a healthcare facility's balance sheet.

inventory (reusable) Relatively inexpensive assets, such as medical devices and sterilization containers, that can be reused as healthcare services are provided to patients.

inventory service level Percentage of items filled (available) when an order is placed.

inventory stock out rate Percentage of items that cannot be filled (are not available) when an order is placed.

inventory turnover rate Number of times per year (or other time period) that inventory is purchased, consumed and replaced.

inventory (unofficial) Consumable products found in user areas, such as surgical locations and labs. Unofficial inventory has usually been expensed to user units and is stored in various locations on the units.

in vitro Referring to a process or reaction carried out in a culture test tube or petri dish.

in vivo In the living body.

iodophor Disinfectant that is a combination of iodine and a solubilizing agent (or a carrier), which slowly liberates or releases free iodine when diluted with water.

ion Electronically-charged particle formed by the loss or gain of one or more electrons.

ionize To dissociate into ions or to become electrically charged.

iris Circular colored region of the eye around the pupil.

ischemia Lack of blood supply to an area.

islets Groups of cells in the pancreas that produce hormones; islets of Langerhans.

ISO 9000 International standards used by participating organizations to help ensure that quality services and products are consistently delivered.

isolate To place by itself; to separate from others.

isotonic Solution having the same osmotic pressure as that of another solution taken as a standard reference.

isotope Form of an element with the same atomic number as another, but with a different atomic weight.

IUSS – See immediate use steam sterilization.

J

jargon Specialized words or phrases often known only by individuals working in the same job or position.

jaundice Excess of bile pigments in blood, skin and mucous membranes, with a resulting yellow appearance of the individual.

jaw Two or more opposable parts that open and close for holding or crushing something between them.

jejunum Second portion of the small intestine.

JIT Abbreviation for "just in time," a method of inventory distribution where a vendor holds inventory for an organization and on a regular basis delivers items that go directly to supply carts.

job description A human resources tool that identifies the major tasks performed by individuals in specific positions.

joint Any place where two bones meet.

julian date - The Julian day or Julian day number (JDN) is the number of days that have elapsed since January 1 of a specific year.

K

kidneys Organs that remove excess water and waste substances from the blood in a process that yields urine.

killing power Ability of a chemical to kill bacteria under laboratory conditions and during in-use testing.

L

labeling Legend, work or mark attached to, included in, belonging to or accompanying any medical device.

lacrimal Referring to tears or the tear glands.

lactation Secretion of milk.

lactic acid Organic acid that accumulates in muscle cells functioning without oxygen.

laminar airflow Filtered air moving along separate parallel flow planes to surgical suites, nurseries, bacteriology work areas and pharmacies; prevents collection of bacterial contamination or hazardous chemical fumes in work areas.

large intestine (colon) Digestive organ that dehydrates digestive residues (feces).

larynx Voice box.

laser Device that produces a very intense beam of light.

latching mechanism Mechanical device that secures a rigid sterilization container's lid to the container's bottom.

latent heat Additional heat required to change the state of a substance from solid to liquid at its melting point, or from liquid to gas at its boiling point after the temperature of the substance has reached either of those points.

lateral Farther from the midline; toward the side.

latex Common form of rubber used in the manufacture of hospital and medical supplies.

latex sensitivity Sensitivity (allergic reaction) of some people to latex caused by exposure to latex that is improperly processed; symptoms range from skin rash, primarily on the hands, to an anaphylactic reaction.

leak test (endoscope) Endoscope processing procedure that ensures the device's flexible covering and internal channels are watertight.

lean A quality process that focuses on eliminating waste in the production of products.

LED Abbreviation for light emitting diode, a semiconductor diode that emits light when voltage is applied.

lens Biconvex structure of the eye that changes in thickness to accommodate near and far vision; crystalline lens.

lesion Wound or local injury; a specific change or morphological alteration by disease or injury.

lethal Pertaining to death.

leukemia Malignant blood disease characterized by abnormal development of white blood cells.

leukocyte White blood cell.

ligament Band of connective tissue that connects a bone to another bone.

lipids Group of fats or fatty substances characterized by insolubility in water.

lipid virus A virus whose core is surrounded by a coat of lipoprotein. Viruses included in this structural category are generally easily inactivated by many types of disinfectants, including low-level disinfectants.

liquid-proof Material that prevents the penetration of liquids and microorganisms.

liquid-resistant Material that inhibits the penetration of liquids.

liter Basic unit of volume in the metric system.

liver Organ that filters the blood to remove amino acids and neutralize some harmful toxins.

load configuration All attributes defining the presentation of products to sterilization process including (a) orientation of products within the primary package (b) quantity and orientation of primary packages(s) within secondary and tertiary packages (c) quantity, orientation and placement of tertiary packages on sterilizer pallets or within carriers and (d) quantity and placement of the pallets (or carriers) within the vessel or area.

load control number Label information on sterilization packages, trays or containers that identifies the sterilizer, cycle run and date of sterilization.

loaner instrumentation Instruments or sets borrowed from a vendor for emergency or scheduled surgical procedures that will be returned following use.

local exhaust hood System that captures contaminated air and conducts it into an exhaust duct; also called a venting hood.

local infection One confined to a restricted area.

logarithm Exponent indicating the power to which a fixed number (the base) must be raised to produce a given number.

lot (load) control number Numbers and/or letters by which a specific group of products can be traced to a particular manufacturing or sterilization operation.

low-level disinfection The destruction of vegetative forms of bacteria, some fungi, and lipid viruses, but not bacterial spores.

lumen Interior path through a needle, tube or surgical instrument.

lungs Main organs of the respiratory system whose function is transporting oxygen into the blood and removing carbon dioxide from the blood.

lux A unit of illumination equal to one lumen per square meter.

lymph Fluid in the lymphatic system.

lymphatic system Series of tiny vessels throughout the body that carry lymph fluid to protect the body against disease.

lymphocyte White blood cell involved in antibody production.

M

macromolecules Large molecules (proteins, carbohydrates, lipids and nucleic acids) within a microorganism.

macroscopic Visible to the naked eye.

magnet status Award given by the American Nurses Credentialing Center to hospitals that satisfy factors measuring the strength and quality of nursing care.

magnetic resonance imaging (MRI) Method for studying tissue based on nuclear movement following exposure to radio waves in a powerful magnetic field.

maintenance insurance Equipment outsourcing alternative in which a hospital retains control of its equipment, but contracts with an insurance organization to manage and insure the costs involved in maintaining it.

malaise Indisposition, discomfort or feeling of ill health.

malignant Describing a tumor that spreads or a disorder that worsens and can lead to death.

malnutrition State resulting from lack of food, lack of an essential component of the diet, or faulty use of food in the diet.

mandible Lower jaw bone.

manufacturer's instructions for use (IFU) Information developed by a device manufacturer that provides detailed instructions on how to properly use and process the device.

Mantoux test Tuberculin skin test.

manufacturer Maker or producer of items or equipment.

martensic This metal is also known as 400 series stainless steel; it is magnetic and may be heat-hardened.

materiel management department Healthcare department responsible for researching, ordering, receiving and managing inventory (consumable supplies).

mastectomy Removal of the breast; mammectomy.

mastication Act of chewing.

measles Rubeola; acute, infectious virus disease characterized by fever, catarrh, coryza, Koplik spots on buccal mucous membrane, and a papular rash.

medial Nearer the midline of the body.

mediastinum Region between the lungs and the organs and the vessels it contains.

Medicaid Federal and state assistance program paying covered medical expenses for low-income individuals. It is run by state and local governments within federal guidelines.

medical device Any instrument, apparatus, appliance, material or other article used alone or in combination, including software necessary for its proper application intended by the manufacturer; to be used for human beings for a) diagnosis, prevention, monitoring, treatment or alleviation of disease (b) diagnosis, monitoring, treatment, alleviation of or compensation for an injury or handicap (c) investigation, replacement or modification of the anatomy or of a physiological process, or (d) control of conception.

Medicare Federal medical insurance program that primarily serves those over 65 years of age, regardless of income, people under 65 with certain disabilities and people of all ages with end stage renal disease.

MedWatch Safety information and adverse event reporting system from the U.S. Food and Drug Administration that serves healthcare professionals and the public by reporting serious problems suspected to be associated with the drugs and medical devices they prescribe, dispense or use.

meiosis Process of cell division that halves the chromosome number in the formation of the reproductive cells.

membrane Thin sheet of tissue.

memory Inherent ability of a substance to return to its original shape and contours.

meningitis Inflammation of the meninges.

menopause Time at which menstruation ceases.

menses Monthly flow of blood from the female reproductive tract.

mesentery Membranous peritoneal ligament that attaches the small intestine to the dorsal abdominal wall.

mesophiles Bacteria that grow best at moderate temperatures: 68°F to 113°F (20°C to 45°C).

metabolic rate Rate at which energy is released from nutrients in the cells.

metabolism Total chemical changes by which the nutritional and functional activities of an organism are maintained.

metacarpals Hand bones.

metallurgy Science and technology of metals.

metastasis Spread of tumor cells.

metatarsals Bones of the foot.

meter Basic unit of length in the metric system.

methicillin-resistant Staphylococcus aureus (MRSA) Staphylococcus aureus bacteria that have developed a resistance to methicillin, the drug of choice; usually occurs with patients who have had antibiotic therapy for a long time.

microaerophilic Microorganisms which require free oxygen for their growth, but in an amount less than that of the oxygen in the atmosphere.

microbes Organisms of microscopic or submicroscopic size generally, including viruses,

rickettsiae, bacteria, algae, yeasts and molds.

microbiology The study of microorganisms. The scientific study of the nature, life and action of microorganisms.

micron Unit of measurement; 1/1000 of a millimeter or 1/25,000 of an inch or one millionth of a meter. *Note: meter equals 39.37 inches.*

microorganisms Forms of life which are too small to see with the naked eye. Bacteria, viruses and fungi are types of microorganisms; also called "germs" and "microbes."

midbrain Upper portion of the brain stem.

mil Unit of length or thickness equal to .001 of an inch.

mineral Inorganic substance; diet element needed in small amounts for health.

min/max (minimum/maximum) System in which orders are placed to reach a predetermined maximum when a predetermined minimum level is reached.

minimally invasive procedure A surgical procedure done in a manner that causes little or no trauma or injury to the patient; often performed through a cannula using lasers, endoscopes or laparoscopes. Compared with other procedures, minimally invasive procedures involve less bleeding, anesthesia and pain, and minimal scarring.

minimum effective concentration (MEC) Percentage concentration of the active ingredient in a disinfectant or chemical sterilant that is the minimum concentration at which the chemical meets all label claims for activity against specific microorganisms.

mitosis Cell division that produces two daughter cells exactly like the parent cell.

mitral valve Valve between the left atrium and left ventricle of the heart; bicuspid valve.

mixed culture Growth of two or more microorganisms in the same medium.

mixed infection Simultaneous process of two or more microorganisms causing an infection.

mixture Blend of two or more substances.

mode of transmission (chain of infection) Method of transfer of an infectious agent from the reservoir to a susceptible host.

molds See fungus.

molecular attraction Adhesive forces exerted between the surface molecules of two bodies in contact.

molecule Smallest quantity of matter that can exist in a free state and retain all of its properties.

monel A trademark used for an alloy of nickel, copper, iron and manganese.

monitor To systematically check or test to control the concentration of a specific ingredient or the execution of a process; may include qualitative and/or quantitative measurements.

monitor To watch, observe, listen to or check (something) for a special purpose over a period of time.

mouth Opening through which air, food and beverages enter the body; beginning of the alimentary canal.

MRC Abbreviation for minimum recommended concentration; minimum concentration at which the manufacturer tested the product and validated its performance.

MRI See magnetic resonance imaging.

MRSA See methicillin-resistant staphyloccus aureus.

mucosa Lining membrane that produces mucus; mucous membrane.

mucous Thick, protective fluid secreted by mucous membranes and glands.

mucous membrane Mucus-secreting membrane that lines all body cavities that open externally, including mouth, nose and intestines.

multi-parameter indicator An indicator designed for two or more critical parameters that indicates exposure to a sterilization cycle at stated values of the parameters.

murmur Abnormal heart sound.

muslin Broad term describing a wide variety of plain-weave cotton or cotton/polyester fabrics with approximately 140 threads per square inch.

mutation Change or alteration in the gradual evolution of a microorganism.

mycology Study of molds, yeasts and fungi.

myocardium Middle layer of the heart wall; heart muscle.

N

nasopharynx Portion of the pharynx above the palate.

natural immunity Immunity with which a person or animal is born.

necropsy Postmortem examination or autopsy.

necrosis Death of a mass of tissue while part of the living body.

needle holders Surgical instruments to drive suture needles to close or rejoin a wound or surgical site; also known as needle drivers.

negative air pressure Situation that occurs when air flows into a room or area because the pressure in the area is less than that of surrounding areas.

neoplasm Abnormal growth of cells; tumor.

nephron Microscopic functional unit of the kidney.

nerve Nerve fibers outside the central nervous system.

neuritis Inflammation of a nerve.

neuron Nerve cell.

neutral Neither acid nor base.

neutralizer Substance added to a medium, which stops the action of a antimicrobial agent.

NFPA Abbreviation for National Fire Protection Association.

node Small mass of tissue, such as a lymph node; space between cells in the myelin sheath.

nomenclature System of names used to identify parts of a mechanism or device.

noncritical devices Refers to the Spaulding medical device classification system; devices that come in contact with intact skin.

noncritical zone Area of a gown or drape where direct contact with blood, body fluids and other potentially infectious materials is unlikely to occur.

nonionic Atoms with no electrical charges; compounds containing a non-dissociated hydrophilic group, which forms a bond with water.

nonlipid virus A virus whose nucleic acid core is not surrounded by a lipid envelope. These viruses are generally more resistant to inactivation by disinfectants.

nonpathogenic Not capable of producing disease.

nonpyrogenic Free from fever-causing substances.

nonstock items Items that are not carried in the central storeroom or in Central Service storage area; purchased from an outside vendor, as they are needed, and delivered to the requesting department.

nontoxic Not poisonous; not capable of producing injury or disease.

nonwoven Fabric made by bonding (as opposed to weaving) fibers together

normal flora Normal bacterial population of a given area.

nose Organ of smell; also filters the air we breath.

nosocomial Hospital-acquired infection (HAI); pertaining to a hospital; applied to a disease caused in the course of being treated in a hospital.

noxious Physically harmful or destructive to living beings.

nucleotide Building block of deoxyribonucleic acid (DNA) and ribonucleic acid (RNA).

nucleus Functional center of a cell that governs activity and heredity.

O

occluded Closure of an opening.

ohm Unit of measurement that expresses the amount of resistance to the flow of an electric current.

olfactory Pertaining to the sense of smell.

oncology Study of tumors.

operational supplies Supplies that are needed for the operation of the CS department. Examples: detergents, sterilization wrap, sterilization testing products, etc.

ophthalmic Pertaining to the eye.

opportunists Microbes that produce infection

only under especially favorable conditions.

optimum temperature Applied to bacterial growth, the temperature at which bacteria grow best.

order point (order quantity system) Method of reordering a predetermined quantity of products when a predetermined on-hand level is reached.

organ Part of the body containing two or more tissues that function together for a specific purpose.

organic Describing compounds containing oxygen, carbon and hydrogen; characteristic of, pertaining to or derived from living organisms.

organic material Compounds containing oxygen, carbon and hydrogen; derived from living organisms. Organic matter in the form of serum, blood, pus, or fecal or lubricant material can interfere with the antimicrobial activity of disinfectants and sterilants.

organism Living thing, plant or animal; may be unicellular or multicellular.

origin Source; beginning; end of a muscle attached to a nonmoving part.

OSHA Abbreviation for Occupational Safety and Health Administration; concerned with safe work environment and employee safety.

osmosis Net movement of solvent molecules across a selectively permeable membrane from areas of higher to lower concentrations.

osmotic pressure Tendency of a solution to draw water into it; directly related to the concentration of the solution.

ossification Process by which cartilage is replaced by bone.

osteoblast Bone-forming cell.

osteomyelitis Inflammation of bone marrow.

osteoporosis Abnormal loss of bone tissue with tendency to fracture.

osteotomes Chisel-like instruments used to cut or shave bone.

otitis media Inflammation of the middle ear.

outsourcing (equipment) Transfer of control of a hospital's equipment management system to an external entity.

ovaries Female reproductive glands.

ovulation Release of a mature ovum from a follicle in the ovary.

ovum Female sex cell.

oxidation The process by which several low-temperature sterilization processes, including hydrogen peroxide gas plasma, vaporized hydrogen peroxide and ozone, destroy microorganisms. Oxidation involves the act or process of oxidizing: addition of oxygen to a compound with a loss of electrons.

oxidative chemistries Class of compounds containing an additional atom of oxygen bound to oxygen that uses oxidation to interrupt cell function.

oxidize To change by increasing the proportion of the electronegative part or change (an element or ion) from a lower to higher positive valence.

oxidizing agent Material that removes electrons from another substance.

oxygen Gas needed to completely break down nutrients for energy within the cell.

ozone A reactive and unstable oxygen molecule.

P

packaging Application or use of appropriate closures, wrappings, cushioning, containers, and complete identification up to, but not including, the shipping container and associated packing.

pandemic Very widespread epidemic (even of worldwide extent).

papers (kraft-type) Medical grade paper packaging material used for numerous sterilization applications.

paracentesis Puncture through the wall of a cavity (usually to remove fluid or promote drainage).

parametric release Declaring product to be sterile on the basis of physical and/or chemical process data, rather than on the basis of sample testing or biological indicator results.

parasite Plant or animal that lives upon or within another living organism (host) from which it obtains nourishment and at whose expense it grows without giving anything in return.

par cart Distribution method in which a supply cart remains in a given location is inventoried and replenished on a regular basis.

parenteral Something that is put inside the body, but not by swallowing, for example, an injection given into the muscle.

parenteral solutions Solutions administered to patients intravenously.

parietal Pertaining to the wall of a space or cavity.

par level (inventory) Desired amount of inventory which should be on hand.

particle Piece of matter with observable length, width and thickness; usually measured in microns.

particulate matter General term applied to matter of miniature size with observable length, width and thickness (contrasted to nonparticulate matter without definite dimension).

parturition Childbirth; labor.

patient care equipment Portable (mobile) equipment used to assist in the care and treatment of patients. Examples: suction units and heat therapy units.

passivation Chemical process applied during instrument manufacture that provides a corrosion-resistant finish by forming a thin, transparent oxide film.

passive carrier Carrier who harbors the causative agent of a disease without having had the disease.

passive immunity Immunity produced without the body of the person or animal that becomes immune participating in its production. Example: production of immunity to diphtheria by injection of diphtheria antitoxin.

pasteurization Process of heating a fluid to a moderate temperature for a definite period of time to destroy undesirable bacteria without changing its chemical composition.

patella Kneecap.

pathogen Capable of causing disease; disease-producing microorganism

patient care equipment Portable (mobile) equipment that is used to assist in the care and treatment of patients. Examples: suction units, temperature management units, infusion therapy devices, etc.

patient care supplies Supplies that will be dispensed for patient treatment and care. Examples: catheters, implants, bandages, etc.

pathogenic Capable of producing disease.

pathology Study of disease.

Glossary

pawl Pivoted tongue or sliding bolt on one part of an instrument adapted to fall into notches or interdental space on another part to permit motion in only one direction.

PEL Abbreviation for permissible exposure limit.

pelvis Basin-like structure; lower portion of the abdomen; large bone of the hip.

penicillin Antibiotic produced by the mold, *Penicillium notatum*.

penis Male organ of urination and intercourse.

peracetic acid (PA) Liquid oxidizing agent that is an effective biocide at low temperatures; used in a sterilization system that processes immersible diagnostic and surgical instruments (primarily flexible and rigid scopes); items must be used immediately after sterilization because they are wet and cannot be stored.

performance qualification (PQ) Obtaining and documenting evidence that equipment, as installed and operated in accordance with operational procedures, consistently performs according to predetermined factors and meets specifications.

perineum Pelvic floor; external region between the anus and genital organs.

periodic automatic replenishment (PAR) Also known as PAR-Level or PAR System; an inventory replenishment system in which the desired amount of products that should be on hand is established, and inventory replenishment returns the quantity of products to this level.

periosteum Membrane of connective tissue that closely invests all bones except at the articular surface.

peripheral Located away from a center or central structure.

peripheral nervous system All nerves and nerve tissue outside the central nervous system.

peristalsis Wavelike movements in the wall of an organ or duct that propel its contents forward.

peritoneum Serous membrane that lines the abdominal cavity, and forms the outer layer of abdominal organs; forms supporting ligaments for some organs.

peritonitis Inflammation of the peritoneum.

permissible exposure limit (PEL) The maximum amount or concentration of a chemical that a worker may be exposed to under OSHA regulations.

perpetual inventory system System that tracks all incoming and issued supplies to determine, on an ongoing basis, the quantity of supplies in storage.

personal development Activities that identify and develop talent and personal potential; improves employability and enhances quality of life.

personal protective equipment (PPE) A part of standard precautions for all healthcare workers that prevents skin and mucous membrane exposure when in contact with blood and body fluid of any patient. PPE includes fluid-resistant protective clothing, disposable gloves, eye protection and face masks and shoe covers.

pertussis Whooping cough.

petri dish Shallow, covered cylindrical glass or plastic dish used to culture bacteria and in which bacterial colonies may be observed without removing the cover.

pH Measure of alkalinity or acidity on a scale of 0 to14; pH of 7 is neutral (neither acid or alkaline); pH below 7 is acid; pH above 7 is alkaline.

phagocyte Cell capable of ingesting bacteria or other foreign particles.

phagotization Process by which some cells can ingest bacteria or other foreign particles.

phalanges Bones that comprise the fingers and toes.

pharynx Throat.

phenol Carbolic acid (phenyl alcohol); a colorless crystalline compound (C_6H_5OH) with strong disinfectant properties.

phenol coefficient Method of designating the disinfecting properties of a chemical by comparing its activity to that of phenol.

phlebitis Inflammation of a vein.

physiology The study of the functions of body parts and the body as a whole.

PI Abbreviation for performance improvement; a process to continually improve patient care that identifies performance functions and associated costs that affect patient outcomes, and the perception of patients and families about the quality and value of services provided.

pick and pack Inventory control system for forms and office supplies. Items are shipped/charged to the customer as ordered in minimal quantities, and the customer is financially responsible for the vendor's agreed-upon inventory.

pick list A list of specific instruments and supplies needed for a surgical case or a medical procedure.

placenta Structure that nourishes and maintains the developing individual during pregnancy.

plague Acute, often fatal epidemic disease caused by *Pasteurella pestis* and transmitted to man by fleas from rats and other rodents.

plasma The largest component of the blood. Plasma transports nutrients throughout the body and helps remove waste from the body.

plasmolysis Shrinkage of a cell or its contents due to withdrawal of water by osmosis.

plasmoptysis Escape of protoplasm from a cell due to rupture of the cell wall.

platelets Blood cells that function to help blood to clot.

pleura Serous membrane that lines the chest cavity and covers the lungs.

pneumonia Inflammatory consolidation or solidification of lung tissue due to presence of an exudate blotting out the air-containing spaces; see exudate.

pneumothorax Accumulation of air in the pleural space.

Point-of-use processing That which occurs when a medical device is processed immediately before use and/or close to the patient care area.

poliomyelitis Virus disease in which there is inflammation of the gray substance of the spinal cord; commonly called infantile paralysis.

pollution State of rendering unclean or impure by adding harmful substances.

pounds per square inch gauge (psig) Measure of ambient air pressure; the pressure that a gas would exert on the walls of a one cubic-foot container.

polycarbonate Type of plastic.

polyethylene Thermoplastic polymer capable of being produced in thin sheets; exhibits good moisture-vapor barrier qualities, but has a high sloughing tendency.

polymerization A molecular reaction that creates an uncontrolled release of energy

polymerize Process of joining many simple molecules into long chains of more complex molecules whose molecular weight is a multiple of the original and whose physical properties are different.

polyp Protruding growth (often grapelike) from a mucous membrane.

polypropylene Type of plastic.

polystyrene Type of plastic.

polyurethane Type of plastic.

polyvinyl chloride (PVC) Type of plastic.

porous Possessing or full of pores (minute openings).

portability Not fixed; can be transported.

portal of entry (chain of infection) Path used by an infectious agent to enter a susceptible host.

portal of exit (chain of infection) Path by which an infectious agent leaves the reservoir.

positive air pressure Situation in which air flows out of a room or area because the pressure in the area is greater than that of surrounding areas.

posterior Toward the back; dorsal.

ppm Abbreviation for parts per million.

preconditioning Treatment of product prior to the sterilization cycle in a room or chamber to attain specified limits for temperature and relative humidity; see conditioning.

preconditioning area Chamber or room in which preconditioning occurs.

prefix (word element) Word element that comes before the root word element.

preservative Substance that prevents biologic decomposition of materials when added to them.

preventive maintenance (equipment) Service provided to equipment to maintain it in proper operating condition by providing planned inspection and by detecting and correcting failures before they occur; often abbreviated "PM."

primary infection First of two or more infections.

Prion An infectious protein particle that, unlike a virus, contains no nucleic acid, does not trigger an immune response and is not destroyed by extreme heat or cold.

procedure area – An area within the healthcare facility that conducts invasive and minimally invasive procedures requiring instruments, supplies and equipment.

process challenge device (PCD) Object that simulates a predetermined set of conditions when used to test sterilizing agent(s).

process equivalency Documented evaluation that the same sterilization process can be delivered by two or more pieces of sterilization equipment.

process improvement Activity to identify and resolve work task-related problems that yield poor quality; the strategy of finding solutions to eliminate the root causes of process performance problems.

process indicators Devices used with individual units (e.g., packs or containers) to demonstrate that the unit has been exposed to the sterilization process, and to distinguish between processed and unprocessed units.

processes (work) Series of work activities which produce a product or service.

processing area Area in which decontaminated, clean instruments and other medical and surgical supplies are inspected, assembled into sets and trays and wrapped, packaged or placed into container systems for sterilization; commonly called the "preparation and packaging area" if part of Central Service, and "pack room" if textile packs are assembled there.

processing group Collection of products or product families that can be sterilized in the same ethylene oxide sterilization process. All products within the group have been determined to present an equal or lesser challenge to the sterilization process.

product adoption Process of formally including a candidate product into an existing validated sterilization process.

product family Collection of products determined to be similar or equivalent for validation purposes.

professional development Commitment to continuous learning and improvement, taking responsibility for one's own development.

progesterone Hormone produced by the corpus luteum and placenta; maintains the lining of the uterus for pregnancy.

prognosis Prediction of the probable outcome of a disease, based on the patient's condition.

prophylactic Agent used to prevent infection or disease.

prophylaxis Prevention of disease.

prostate gland Organ that produces a fluid element in semen that stimulates the movement of sperm.

prosthesis Artificial replacement of a body part such as an arm or leg.

protein Complex combinations of amino acids containing hydrogen, nitrogen, carbon, oxygen and, usually, sulfur and sometimes other elements; essential constituents of all living cells.

prothrombin Clotting factor; converted to thrombin during blood clotting.

proton Positively-charged particle in the nucleus of an atom.

protoplasm Thick, mucous-like substance that is colorless and translucent and forms the biochemical basis of life found within the cell nucleus.

protozoan One-celled animal-like microorganism of the subkingdom, protozoa.

proximal The end of an item that is closest to the point of origin; the end of the instrument closest to the operator; the proximal end of the femur is closest to the hip.

prudent Marked by wisdom or judiciousness; wise.

pseudopodia "False feet;" temporary protrusions of ectoplasm to provide locomotion.

psia Abbreviation for pounds per square inch absolute.

psychrophiles (bacteria) Cold-loving bacteria whose optimum temperature for growth is 59°F to 68°F (15°C to 20°C) or below.

pulse Wave of increased pressure in blood vessels produced by contraction of the heart.

pupil Opening in the center of the eye through which light enters.

pure culture Specific bacterial growth of only one species of microorganism.

purulent Containing pus.

pus Semifluid, creamy product of inflammation consisting of blood cells (mainly white), bacteria, dead tissue cells and serum.

pyogenic Pus producing.

pyrex Type of hard glass made from borosilicate, which is alkaline free.

pyrexia Fever.

pyrogen A substance typically produced by a bacterium that produces fever when introduced/released into the blood .

pyrogenic Fever producing; byproducts of bacterial growth or metabolism.

Q

quadrant One part of four; to be divided into four equal parts.

qualified personnel Prepared by training and experience to perform a specified task.

quality Consistent delivery of products and services according to established standards. Quality "integrates" the concerns for the customers (including patients and user department personnel) with those of the department and facility.

quality assurance Comprehensive and measured efforts to provide total quality; a technical, statistical sampling method that measures production quality.

quality control Technical, statistical sampling method that measures production quality.

quarantine Isolation of infected people and contacts who have been exposed to communicable diseases for the time equal to the longest incubation period of the disease to which they have been exposed.

quaternary compound Group of disinfectants having derivatives of benzalkonium chloride as the active ingredient.

quiescent Not active.

R

radiation heat Transmission of heat from one object to another without heating the space in between; process of emitting radiant energy in the form of waves or particles.

radical Group of atoms that behaves as a single atom in a chemical reaction.

radio frequency identification (RFID) Term used to describe a system in which the identity (serial number) of an item is wirelessly transmitted with radio waves.

radius One of the two bones in the forearm.

random numbers (table) Compilation of numbers generated in an unpredictable, haphazardous sequence used to create a random sample.

ratchet (or rachet) Part of a surgical instrument that "locks" the handles in place.

rationale Underlying reason; basis.

recessive Gene that is not expressed if a dominant gene for the same trait is present.

rectum Last several inches of the large intestine.

red blood cells Blood cells that carry oxygen throughout the body.

reflex Involuntary response to a stimulus.

refraction Bending of light rays as they pass from one medium to another of a different density.

regulation Rules issued by administrative agencies that have the force of law.

relative humidity (RH) Amount of water vapor in the atmosphere; expressed as a percentage of the total amount of vapor the atmosphere could hold without condensation.

remission Diminution or abatement of disease symptoms.

reorder point (ROP) Inventory level available when an order is placed to replenish inventory.

repair (equipment) Procedures used to return equipment to proper operating condition after it becomes inoperative.

requisition system Method of inventory distribution in which items needed are requested (requisitioned) and removed from a central storage location for transport to the user department.

reservoir Carrier of an infectious microorganism; generally refers to a human carrier.

reservoir of agent (chain of infection) Place where an infectious agent (microorganisms) can survive.

resident bacteria Bacteria normally occurring at a given anatomical site.

residual (EtO) Amount of ethylene oxide that remains inside materials after they are sterilized.

residual property Capacity of an antiseptic or disinfectant to kill microorganisms over a long period of time after initial application.

resistance Ability of an individual to ward off infection.

resorption Loss of substance (such as bone).

respiration Exchange of oxygen and carbon dioxide between outside air and body cells.

retina Innermost layer of the eye; contains light-sensitive cells (rods and cones).

retractors Surgical instruments primarily used to move tissues and organs to keep the surgical site exposed throughout surgery.

retroperitoneal Behind the peritoneum (kidneys, pancreas and abdominal aorta).

reusable (inventory) Assets that are relatively inexpensive, such as medical devices and sterilization containers, that can be reused as healthcare services are provided to patients.

reusable medical device Devices intended for repeated use on different patients, with appropriate decontamination and other processing between uses.

reusable surgical textile Drape, gown, towel or sterilization wrapper intended to be used during surgery or to assist in preparing for surgery; made from a fabric (usually woven or knitted), fabric/film laminate, or non-woven material intended to be used more than once, with appropriate reprocessing between uses.

reverse osmosis (RO) A water purification process by which a solvent, such as water, is removed of impurities after being forced through a semipermeable membrane.

rhinitis Inflammation of the mucous membrane of the nose.

rib spreaders Retractor used to expose the chest.

rigid container system Instrument containers that hold medical devices during sterilization and also protect devices from contamination during storage and transport

ribonucleic acid (RNA) One of two types of nucleic acids; found in nucleus and cytoplasm and involved in protein synthesis.

risk management The methods used to assess the risks of a specific activity and to develop a program to reduce risk.

rod Straight, slim mass of substance related to microorganisms. Example: rod-shaped bacteria.

roentgenogram Film produced with of x-rays.

rongeurs Surgical instruments to cut or bite away at bone and tissue.

root cause analysis (RCA) Process that "looks backwards" at an event to help prevent its future occurrence.

root (word element) Tells the primary meaning of a word; also called base word element.

rubeola Measles.

S

sacrum Lower portion of vertebral column.

safety data sheet (SDS) – A written statement providing detailed information about a chemical or toxic substance including potential hazards and appropriate handling methods. An SDS is provided by the product manufacturer to the product buyer, and it must be posted and/or made available in a place that is easily accessible to those that will use the product.

safety stock Minimum amount of inventory that must be on hand.

saline Containing or pertaining to salt; an isotonic aqueous solution of sodium chloride for temporarily maintaining living cells.

saliva Secretion of salivary glands; moistens food and contains an enzyme that digests starch.

sanitary Relating to health; characterized by or readily kept in cleanness.

sanitize To reduce the microbial flora in materials or on articles, such as eating utensils, to levels judged safe by public health standards.

saponification Action of detergent alkalies on an item's fat or soil contents to form soaps.

sarcoma Malignant tumor of connective tissue; a form of cancer.

saturated steam Steam that contains the maximum amount of water vapor.

scapula Shoulder blade.

schizomycetes Plant class to which all bacteria belong.

scissors Surgical instruments used to cut, incise and/or dissect tissue.

scissors Surgical instruments used to cut, incise and/or dissect tissue.

sclera Outermost layer of the eye; "white" of the eye.

scrotum Sac in which testes are suspended.

SDS Abbreviation for safety data sheet

seals (tamper-evident) Sealing method for sterile packaging that allows users to determine if packaging has been opened (contaminated) and helps them identify packages unsafe for patient use.

sebaceous Secreting or pertaining to sebum.

sebum Oily secretion of sebaceous gland that lubricates the skin.

Secondary container A generic container that is filled from a primary container or filled with a diluted solution; secondary containers must be clearly labeled with content.

secondary infection Superimposed infection occurring in a host who is already suffering from an earlier infection.

selective action Ability to inhibit or kill one group of microbes and not another.

semen Mixture of sperm cells and secretions from several male reproductive glands.

semi-critical devices Refers to the Spaulding medical device classification system; devices that come in contact with nonintact skin or mucous membranes.

seminal vesicle Gland that produces semen.

sensitivity State of being susceptible.

sensitization Process of sensitizing or making susceptible.

sentinel event An unexpected occurrence involving death, serious physical or psychological injury, or the risk thereof.

sepsis Condition, usually with fever, that results from the presence of microorganisms or their poisons in the bloodstream or other tissues.

septic Relating to the presence of pathogens or their toxins.

Septicemia Presence of pathogenic microorganisms or their toxins in the bloodstream; blood poisoning.

septum Dividing wall (e.g., between heart chambers or sides of the nose).

sequestering agents Chemicals that remove or inactivate hard water minerals.

Glossary

sequestration Removal or inactivation of water hardness elements by formation of a soluble complex or chelate.

serology Science that deals with serum.

serrations Parallel grooves in the jaws of surgical instruments.

serum Clear fluid exuded when blood coagulates.

service Activity that helps one or more people or groups of people.

service recovery The sequence of steps used to address customer complaints and problems in a manner that yields a win-win situation for the customer and the department.

sex-linked Gene carried on a sex (usually X) chromosome.

shank The straight, narrow part of a tool that connects the part that does the work with the handle.

sharps Cutting instruments, including knives, scalpels, blades, needles and scissors of all types. Other examples include chisels and osteotomes, some curettes, dissectors and elevators, Rongeurs and cutting forceps, punches, saws and trocars.

shelf life Period of time during which product sterility is assumed to be maintained.

shelf life (disinfectants) Length of time a disinfectant can be properly stored after which it must be discarded.

shock Pertaining to circulation: inadequate output of blood by the heart.

short-term exposure limit (STEL) The maximum concentration of a chemical to which workers may be exposed continuously for up to 15 minutes without danger to health or work efficiency and safety.

sigmoid colon Last portion of large intestine.

sign Manifestation of a disease noted by an observer.

silicate Mineral commonly in water derived from silica in quartz and other components.

simple stain Staining technique using only one dye.

single-parameter indicator Designed for one critical parameter that indicates exposure to a sterilization cycle at a stated value of the chosen parameter.

six sigma Quality process that focuses on developing and delivering near-perfect products and services.

skin Organ containing sweat glands that, through perspiration, produces and eliminates sweat.

sloughing To cast off one's skin; to separate dead tissue from living tissue.

small intestine Digestive organ where the greatest amount of digestion and nutrient absorption into body cells occurs.

smear Thin layer of material spread on a glass slide for microscopic examination.

SMS (spunbond-meltblown-spunbond) Non-woven packaging material that is the most popular flat wrap.

soap Compound of one or more fatty acids, or their equivalent, with an alkaline substance.

softening (sequestering) Process of removing selected substances from hard water.

soft glass Glass made from alkaline materials that cannot be subjected to high temperatures without causing chemical reactions and possible shredding of the glass.

soluble Able to be dissolved.

solution Mixture with components evenly distributed.

solvent Liquid capable of dissolving another substance.

Spaulding classification system A system developed by Dr. E.H. Spaulding that divides medical devices into categories based on the risk of infection involved with their use.

species One kind of organism; the subdivision of a genus.

sperm Male sex cell.

spermatozoon Male reproductive cell; gamete.

sphincter Muscular ring that regulates the size of an opening.

sphygmomanometer Device used to measure blood pressure.

spirillum Spiral-shaped bacterium of the genus spirillum; chief pathogens causing rat bite fever and Asiatic cholera.

spirochete Slender, corkscrew-like or spiral-shaped bacteria found on man, animals and plants, and in soil and water; moves in a waving and twisting motion; some cause disease.

spleen Lymphoid organ in the upper left region of the abdomen.

sporadic disease Disease that occurs in neither an endemic nor epidemic.

spore Microorganisms capable of forming a thick wall around themselves to enable survival in adverse conditions; a resistant form of bacterium.

spore strip Paper strip impregnated with a known population of microorganisms and that meets the definition of biological indicator.

sporicide Agent that destroys spores.

stain Substance used to color cells or tissues to differentiate them for microscopic examination and study; see gram stain.

stainless steel An alloy of steel with chromium and sometimes another element, such as nickel or molybdenum, that is highly resistant to rusting and ordinary corrosion.

standard Uniform method of defining basic parameters for processes, products, services and measurements.

standards (AAMI) Voluntary guidelines representing a consensus of AAMI members intended for use by healthcare facilities and manufacturers to help ensure the safety of medical instrumentation for patient use.

standards (regulatory) Comparison benchmarks mandated by a governing agency. Noncompliance with regulatory standards may lead to citations and legal penalties.

standards (voluntary) Guidelines or recommendations for best practices to provide better patient care; developed by industry, non-profit organizations, trade associations and others.

standardization Being made uniform.

standard precautions Method of using appropriate barriers to reduce the risk of transmission of bloodborne and other pathogens from both recognized and unrecognized sources. It is the basic level of infection control to prevent transmission of infectious organisms from contact with blood and all other body fluids to non-intact skin and mucous membranes. This standard applies to all patients, regardless of diagnosis or presumed infectious status.

staphylococci Gram-positive bacteria that grow in grape-like clusters.

stasis Stoppage in the normal flow of fluids, such as blood, lymph, urine or contents of the digestive tract.

stat. Abbreviation for the Latin "statim," meaning immediately or at once.

statute Written and enforceable law enacted by a governing body.

steam Water vapor at 212°F (100°C) or above.

steam purity Degree to which steam is free of dissolved and suspended particles, water treatment chemicals and other contaminants.

steam quality Weight of dry steam present in a mixture of dry saturated steam and entrained water.

STEL Abbreviation for short term exposure limit.

stenosis Narrowing of a duct or canal.

stereotype Preconceived belief or opinion about a group of people applied to every person in that group.

sterilant/sterilization Physical or chemical entity, or combination of entities, that has sufficient microbicidal activity to achieve sterility under defined conditions.

sterile Completely devoid of all living microorganisms.

Glossary

sterile field Immediate environment around trauma site or surgical incision; includes all materials in contact with the wound, gowns worn by the surgical team (front panel from chest to the level of the operative field and sleeve from the cuff to two inches above the elbow), patient drapes (area adjacent to the wound) and table covers (top surface).

sterile storage area Area of healthcare facility designed to store clean and sterile supplies and protect them from contamination.

sterility assurance level (SAL) Probability of a viable microorganism being present on a product unit after sterilization.

sterility (event-related) Items are considered sterile unless the integrity of the packaging is compromised (damaged) or suspected of being compromised (damaged), regardless of the sterilization date; sometimes referred to as ERS (event-related sterility).

sterility (time-related) A package is considered sterile until a specific expiration date is reached.

sterilization Process by which all forms of microbial life, including bacteria, viruses, spores and fungi, are completely destroyed.

sterilization area Location of steam sterilizers, including the space for loading, queuing carts, cool down and unloading carts.

sterilization process monitor Physical/chemical device used to monitor one or more parameters to detect failures due to packaging, loading and/or sterilizer functioning. These devices cannot guarantee, assure or prove sterilization; they measure physical conditions.

sterilization wrap Device intended to enclose another medical device to be sterilized by a healthcare provider, and maintain sterility of the enclosed device until used.

sterilizer Equipment to sterilize medical devices, equipment and supplies by direct exposure to sterilizing agent.

sterilizer (ethylene oxide) Sterilization equipment that utilizes ethylene oxide under defined conditions of gas concentration, temperature and percent relative humidity.

sterilizer (steam) Sterilization equipment that uses saturated steam under pressure as the sterilant.

sterilizer (steam, dynamic-air-removal type) Steam sterilizer in which air is removed from the chamber and the load by means of pressure and vacuum excursions, or by means of steam flushes and pressure pulses.

sternum Breast bone.

stethoscope Instrument that conveys sounds from the patient's body to the examiner's ears.

stilet (or stylet) Small, sharp, pointed instrument used to probe, stabilize needles or catheters for insertion, and remove obstructions from lumens of needles and tubes.

stockless inventory Distribution method in which supplies are stored by an outside vendor and delivered to the hospital on a regular basis in case lot quantities. Advantage: minimum inventory is held and paid for by the facility.

stock outs (inventory) Condition that occurs when reusable or consumable inventory items required to provide healthcare services to patients are not available.

stomach Pouch that serves as a reservoir for food that has been consumed.

strain Specific specimen or "culture" of a given species.

streptococci Bacteria which divide to form chains; members of the genus streptococcus which are Gram-positive, chain-forming bacteria.

strikethrough Penetration of liquid or microorganism through a fabric.

subcutaneous Under the skin.

subordinate Employee who is supervised by someone in a higher organizational position.

suction devices Surgical instruments used to extract blood and other fluids from a surgical site.

surfactant A substance that lowers the surface tension of the water and increases the solubility of organic compounds.

suffix (word element) Word element that comes after the root word element.

Super-heated steam Occurs when dry steam becomes too hot compared to saturated steam; dry steam rises to a temperature higher than the boiling point of saturated steam. This commonly occurs when dehydrated linen is processed in a steam sterilizer. Due to the lack of moisture, dry steam is not an effective sterilant and will often char or burn items in the sterilizer.

superior Above; in a higher position.

surface tension Contractile surface force of a liquid that makes it tend to assume a spherical form (example:, to form a meniscus); also exists at the junction of two liquids.

surgical drape Device made of natural or synthetic materials and used as a protective patient covering. Its purpose is to isolate a site of surgical incision from microbial and other contamination.

surgical gown Devices worn by Operating Room personnel during surgical procedures to protect the patient and Operating Room staff from transfer of microorganisms, body fluids and particulate matter.

surgical site infection An infection that occurs after surgery in the part of the body where the surgery took place.

surgical towel Absorbent product, typically made of cotton, intended to be used in a patient care procedure.

susceptible host (chain of infection) Person or animal that lacks the ability to resist infection by an infectious agent.

suspension Mixture that will separate unless shaken.

sustainability Processes designed to reduce harm to the environment or deplete natural resources, thereby supporting long-term ecological balance.

suture Joint in which bone surfaces are closely united (e.g., skull); stitch used in surgery to bring parts together.

symbiosis Living together or close association of two dissimilar organisms with mutual benefit.

symptom Subjective disturbance due to disease.

synapse Junction between two neurons or between a neuron and an effecter.

syndrome Group of symptoms characteristic of a disorder.

synergism Action of an inactive material that improves or increases the action of an active material; case in which the sum of the actions of two or more active materials mixed together is greater than the sum of their individual actions.

synovial Pertaining to a thick, lubricating fluid found in joints, bursae and tendon sheaths; pertaining to freely movable (diarthrotic) joint.

synthetic Produced by chemical synthesis rather than of natural origin.

system Group of organs that work together to carry out a specific activity.

systole Contraction phase of cardiac cycle.

T

tabletop sterilizer Compact steam sterilizer with a chamber volume of not more than two cubic feet that generates its own steam with distilled or deionized water added by the user.

tachycardia Heart rate greater than 100 beats per minute.

tamper-evident seals Sealing methods for sterile packaging that allow users to determine if the packaging has been opened. Tamper-evident seals allow users to determine if packages have been opened (contaminated) and help users identify packages that are not safe for patient use.

tap water Treated water that is acceptable for drinking.

tarsals Ankle bones.

t cell Lymphocyte active in immunity that matures in the thymus gland; destroys foreign cells directly; T lymphocyte.

technical information report (TIR) Reports developed by experts in the field that contain valuable information needed by the healthcare industry. TIRs do not undergo the formal approval system that standards are and may be recised or withdrawn at any time because they address a rapidly evolving field or technology.

Glossary

technical quality control indicators Process control measures utilized to assure that planned technical conditions within sterilizers and aerators are met.

tendinitis Inflammation of a tendon.

tendon Cord of fibrous tissue that attaches a muscle to a bone.

terminal disinfection Disinfection of a room after it has been vacated by a patient.

terminal infection Infection with streptococci or other pathogenic bacteria that occurs during the course of a chronic disease and causes death.

terminal sterilization The process by which surgical instruments and medical devices are sterilized in their final containers, allowing them to be stored until needed.

testes Male reproductive gland that forms and secretes sperm and several fluid elements in semen.

testosterone Male sex hormone produced in the testes; promotes the development of sperm cells and maintains secondary sex characteristics.

tetanus Constant contraction of a muscle; infectious disease caused by a bacterium (*Clostridium tetani*); lockjaw.

tetany Muscle spasms due to abnormal calcium metabolism as in parathyroid deficiency.

therapy Treatment of disease.

thermal disinfection Use of heat to reduce the amount of microorganisms (excluding spores) on a medical device.

thermal equilibrium Condition in which all parts of a system have reached the same temperature; in a steam autoclave or hot-air oven, when the temperature throughout the entire load is the same.

thermocouple Device composed of two lengths of wire, each of which is made of a different homogenous metal; used to measure temperature changes by connecting a potentiometer or pyrometer into the thermocouple circuit.

thermolabile Easily altered or decomposed by heat.

thermophiles (bacteria) Bacteria which grow best at a temperature of 122°F to 158°F (50°C to 70°C).

thermostable Not easily affected by moderate heat.

thermostatic Controlled by temperature.

thorax Chest; thoracic.

threshold limit value (TLV) Refers to airborne concentrations of substances and represents conditions under which it is believed that nearly all workers may be repeatedly exposed day after day without adverse health effects.

Thrombocyte Blood platelet; participates in clotting.

thrombus blood clot within a vessel.

thumb forceps Tweezer-like instrument with smooth tip; used to grasp objects.

thyroid Endocrine gland in the neck. tibia Large bone in lower leg.

Time-weighted average (TWA) The amount of a substance employees can be exposed to over an eight-hour day

tincture Liquid in which a chemical is dissolved in alcohol.

tissue Group of similar cells that performs a specialized function.

tissue culture Cultivation of tissue cells in vitro.

tissue forceps Tweezer-like instrument with teeth to grasp tissue.

titer Concentration of infective microbes in a medium; amount of one substance to correspond with given amount of another substance.

titration Volumetric determination against standard solutions of known strength.

TLV-C The concentration that should not be exceeded during any part of the working exposure. If instantaneous monitoring is not feasible, the TLV-C can be assessed by sampling over a 15-minute period, except for substances that may cause immediate irritation when exposures are brief.

TLV-TWA The time-weighted average concentration for a normal eight-hour workday and a 40-hour work week, to which nearly all workers may be repeatedly exposed, day after day, without adverse effect.

TLV-STEL A 15-minute TWA exposure that should not be exceeded at any time during a workday, even if the eight-hour TWA is within the TLV-TWA Exposure above the TLV-TWA, up to the STEL, should not exceed 15 minutes and should not occur more than four times per day. There should be at least 60 minutes between successive exposures in this range.

tolerance Ability to withstand or endure without ill effects.

tonsil Mass of lymphoid tissue in the pharynx region.

total acquisition costs All costs incurred by a facility to purchase a specific supply or equipment item from the point of authorization through its disposal.

total quality improvement (TQI) Concept of measuring the current output of a process or procedure and then modifying it to increase the output, efficiency and/or effectiveness.

total quality management (TQM) Quality management approach based on participation of all members aimed at long-term success through customer satisfaction and benefits to all members of the organization and society.

toxemia General intoxication caused by absorption of bacterial products, usually toxins, formed at a local source of infection.

toxic Poisonous.

toxic anterior segment syndrome (TASS) An acute postoperative inflammatory reaction in which a noninfectious substance enters the anterior segment and induces toxic damage to the intraocular tissues.

toxin Poisonous substance produced by and during the growth of certain pathogenic bacteria.

toxoid Detoxified toxin that produces specific antibodies; neutralized specific toxins used to immunize against bacteria that produce specific toxins.

TQM A for total quality management.

trachea Windpipe.

tracheostomy Surgical opening into the trachea to introduce a tube through which the patient may breathe.

trait Characteristic.

transducer Device that converts energy from one form to another; ultrasonic transducer changes high-frequency electrical energy into high-frequency sound waves.

transmission Transfer of anything (such as a disease).

transplant Portion of a bacterial culture which has been transferred from an old pure culture to a fresh new medium.

triage System designed to sort out or classify emergency room patients according to severity of injury or disease.

tricuspid valve Valve between the right atrium and right ventricle of the heart.

tuberculin Filterable substance produced in the growth of mycobacterium tuberculosis in culture media; when injected intracutaneously in people exposed to the tuberculosis bacillus or its products, a reaction is produced in 24 to 48 hours that consists of infiltration and hyperemia.

tuberculocidal Having the ability to kill tubercle bacilli.

tuberculosis Highly variable and communicable disease of man and some animals caused by the tubercle bacillus (Mycobacterium tuberculosis) and characterized by the formation of tubercles in the lungs or elsewhere.

turbidity Occurs when water contains sediments or solids that, when stirred, make the water appear cloudy.

turnkey A computer system supplied to a customer in such a complete form that it can be put to immediate use.

turnover/turnaround Term used to describe instruments or equipment that must receive priority reprocessing in order to be made available for another procedure.

tympanic membrane Membrane between the external and middle ear that transmits sound waves to the bones of the middle ear; eardrum.

Glossary

U

ubiquitous Present everywhere or in many places.

ulcer Area of the skin or mucous membrane in which the tissues are gradually destroyed.

ulna One of the two bones in the forearm.

ultrasonics Physical science of acoustic waves that oscillate in approximate range of 18 to 80 KHz.

ultraviolet radiation (UV) Invisible component of sun's radiation; used infrequently to degerm air and inanimate objects.

umbilical cord Structure that connects the fetus with the placenta; contains vessels that carry blood between the fetus and placenta.

umbilicus Small scar on the abdomen that marks the former attachment of the umbilical cord to the fetus; navel.

unicellular Composed of a single cell.

universal precautions See standard precautions.

unsanitary Deficient in sanitation; unclean to such a degree as to be injurious to health.

UPC Abbreviation for universal product code.

ureters Tube-like structures extending from the kidneys to the urinary bladder that move urine between these organs.

urethra Tube that discharges urine.

urinary bladder Reservoir for urine.

urine Liquid waste excreted by kidneys.

use life (disinfectants) Length of time (or number of times) a disinfectant can be used after which the efficacy of a disinfectant is diminished.

utensil Instrument or container for domestic use; in hospitals, an item used for basic patient care, such as a bed pan or wash basin.

uterus Female organ within which the fetus develops during pregnancy.

uvula Soft, fleshy, V-shaped mass that hangs from the soft palate.

V

vaccination Introduction of vaccine into the body.

vaccine Substance used to produce active immunity; usually a suspension of attenuated or killed pathogens given by inoculation to prevent a specific disease.

vagina Muscular canal in a female that extends from an external opening to the neck of the uterus.

validation Procedures used by equipment manufacturers to obtain, record and interpret test results required to establish that a process consistently produces a sterile product.

value analysis Study of the relationship of design, function and cost of a product, material or service.

valve Structure that prevents fluid from flowing backward (as in the heart, veins and lymphatic vessels).

vancomycin-resistant enterococcus (VRE) Enterococcus bacteria that are no longer sensitive to vancomycin; transmission can occur either by direct contract or indirectly by hands.

vapor Substance in the gaseous state that is usually a liquid or solid.

variance Difference between the amount of a supply that should be available (from records), and the amount that is available (from physical count) when a perpetual inventory system is used.

varicella Chickenpox.

varicose Pertaining to an unnatural swelling; Example: varicose vein.

variola Smallpox.

vas deferens Duct that transfers sperm from the epididymus to the seminal vesicle.

vasoconstriction Decrease in the diameter of a blood vessel.

vasodillation Increase in the diameter of a blood vessel.

VD Abbreviation for venereal disease.

vector Carrier of pathogenic microorganisms from one host to another (Examples: flies, fleas, mosquitoes).

vegetative bacteria Non spore-forming bacteria or spore-forming bacteria in a nonsporulating state.

vegetative stage State of active growth of microorganisms (as opposed to resting or spore stages.)

veins Vessels that carry blood back to the heart.

vena cava One of two large veins that carry blood into the right atrium of the heart.

venereal disease (VD) Disease transmitted through sexual activity.

venous Relating to vein or veins.

ventilation Movement of air into and out of the lungs.

ventral Toward the front or belly surface; anterior.

ventricles The two lower chambers of the heart.

venule Very small vein that collects blood from the capillaries.

verification Procedures used by healthcare facilities to confirm that the validation undertaken by the equipment manufacturer is applicable to the specific setting.

vertebra One of the bones of the spinal column.

vesicle Small sac or blister filled with fluid.

viable Living; having the ability to multiply.

virology Study of virus and viral diseases.

virucide Agent that destroys or inactivates viruses.

virulence Capacity of microorganisms to produce disease; power of an organism to overcome defenses of the host.

virus One of a group of minute infectious agents that grow only in living tissues or cells

viscera Organs in the ventral body cavities (especially the abdominal organs).

vital Characteristic of life; necessary for life; pertaining to life.

vitreous humor Fluid-filled compartment that gives shape to the eye.

VRE Abbreviation for vancomycin resistant enterococcus. When enterococcus bacteria are no longer sensitive to vancomycin, treatment is a challenge. Transmission occurs by direct contract or indirectly by hands.

W

warranty Guarantee or an assurance from a seller to the buyer that the goods or property is or shall be as represented.

washers Automated equipment used to clean, decontaminate or disinfect (low, intermediate, or low level) and dry medical devices.

wet pack Package or containers with moisture after the sterilization process is completed.

wetting agent Substance that reduces the surface tension of a liquid and allows the liquid to penetrate or spread more easily across the surface of a solid.

wetting power Reduction of the water surface tension, which allows the water to run or spread evenly over the surface.

white blood cells Blood cells that circulate in the blood and help defend the body against infection or foreign invaders.

wicking material Approved absorbent material that allows for air removal and steam penetration, and facilitates drying.

word elements Parts of a word.

workplace violence Any act or threat of physical violence, harassment, intimidation, or other threatening disruptive behavior that occurs at the work site.

work practice controls Controls that reduce the likelihood of exposure by altering the manner in which a task is performed. Example: prohibiting recapping needles with a two-handed technique.

work-related musculoskeletal disorder (WMSD) Injury to or disorder of the musculoskeletal system where exposure to workplace risk factors may have contributed to the disorder's development or aggravated a pre-existing condition.

Glossary

X

x-ray Radiation of extremely short wave length that can penetrate opaque substances and affects photographic plates and fluorescent screens.

Y

yeasts Any of several unicellular fungi of the genus, Saccharomyces, which reproduce by budding.

Z

Index